Introduction to
Clinical Neurology

Introduction to Clinical Neurology

Sixth Edition

Douglas J. Gelb, MD, PhD
Department of Neurology
University of Michigan Medical School
Ann Arbor, Michigan

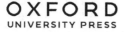

OXFORD
UNIVERSITY PRESS

OXFORD
UNIVERSITY PRESS

Oxford University Press is a department of the University of Oxford. It furthers
the University's objective of excellence in research, scholarship, and education
by publishing worldwide. Oxford is a registered trade mark of Oxford University
Press in the UK and certain other countries.

Published in the United States of America by Oxford University Press
198 Madison Avenue, New York, NY 10016, United States of America.

Library of Congress Cataloging-in-Publication Data
Names: Gelb, Douglas James, 1957– author.
Title: Introduction to clinical neurology / Douglas J. Gelb.
Description: 6. | New York, NY : Oxford University Press, [2024] |
Includes bibliographical references and index.
Identifiers: LCCN 2023054203 (print) | LCCN 2023054204 (ebook) |
ISBN 9780197772904 (paperback) | ISBN 9780197772928 (epub) |
ISBN 9780197772935
Subjects: MESH: Nervous System Diseases
Classification: LCC RC346 (print) | LCC RC346 (ebook) |
NLM WL 140 | DDC 616.8—dc23/eng/20240105
LC record available at https://lccn.loc.gov/2023054203
LC ebook record available at https://lccn.loc.gov/2023054204

DOI: 10.1093/med/9780197772904.001.0001

Printed by Marquis Book Printing, Canada

In memory of my father, the best teacher I've ever known.

Contents

Contributors *xix*
Preface to the Sixth Edition *xxi*
Preface to the First Edition *xxiii*

PART I: The Basic Approach

1. Where's the Lesion? (How We Localize) 3
   I. Sample Localization Problems 3
  II. The Game 5
 III. The Rules 7
 IV. The Play: The Long Version 8
  V. The Play: The Abbreviated Version 15
 VI. More Examples 39
VII. Rules for Speed Play 39

2. The Neurologic Examination (What We Localize) 45
   I. More Localization Problems 45
  II. General Comments on the Neurologic Examination 46
 III. How to Do the Neurologic Examination 50
     A. Mental Status Examination 50
     B. Cranial Nerve Examination 53
     C. Motor Examination 56
     D. Reflex Examination 59
     E. Sensory Examination 60

    IV. Additional Comments on Terminology and
        Examination Technique *62*
        A. Mental Status Examination *62*
        B. Cranial Nerve Examination *67*
        C. Motor Examination *68*
        D. Reflex Examination *71*
        E. Sensory Examination *72*
    V. Interpretation of the Neurologic Examination *73*
        A. Mental Status Examination *73*
        B. Cranial Nerve Examination *75*
        C. Motor Examination *84*
        D. Reflex Examination *88*
        E. Sensory Examination *88*
    VI. Modifications of the Neurologic Examination *90*
        A. Screening Neurologic Examination *90*
        B. Video Examination *92*
        C. Examination of Patients with Altered Level of
           Consciousness *94*
        D. Inconsistent or Anomalous Examination
           Findings *99*
    VII. Supplementary Table for Reference *100*
    VIII. Discussion of Localization Problems *105*
**3. Diagnostic Reasoning: What's the Lesion? (Why
We Localize)** *107*
James W. Albers and Douglas J. Gelb
    I. Case Histories *107*
    II. Beyond Localization *109*
        A. Localization *111*
        B. Temporal Profile *111*
        C. Epidemiology *112*
    III. Etiology *112*
        A. Degenerative Diseases *112*
        B. Neoplastic Diseases *112*

C. Vascular Diseases *113*

D. Inflammatory Diseases *113*

E. Toxic and Metabolic Diseases *113*

F. Traumatic Diseases *114*

G. Congenital and Developmental Diseases *114*

IV. Discussion of Case Histories *116*

PART II: Common Diseases

4. Stroke *123*

I. Case Histories *123*

II. Approach to Stroke *124*

III. Background Information *125*

A. Definitions *125*

B. Classification of Strokes by Etiology *125*

C. Pathophysiology *127*

IV. Diagnosis *128*

A. Clinical Features *128*

B. Imaging *133*

V. Management of Acute Stroke *134*

A. Restoration of Blood Flow in Ischemic Stroke *134*

B. Limitation of Deficits *136*

C. Rehabilitation *138*

VI. Secondary Prevention of Ischemic Stroke *139*

A. Lipid Management *141*

B. Antiplatelet Medication *142*

C. Blood Pressure *142*

D. Other Risk Factors *143*

E. Cardioembolic Disease *144*

F. Cervical Carotid Stenosis *146*

G. Ischemic Stroke Mechanisms Other Than Cardioembolism and Cervical Carotid Stenosis *148*

H. Determining the Underlying Mechanism of Stroke *149*

VII. Secondary Prevention of Cerebral Hemorrhage *151*

VIII. Primary Prevention *152*

    A. Hypertension *152*

    B. Smoking *153*

    C. Diabetes *153*

    D. Dyslipidemia *153*

    E. Mechanical Heart Valves *154*

    F. Atrial Fibrillation *154*

    G. Cervical Carotid Stenosis *155*

    H. Sickle Cell Disease *156*

    I. Other Factors *156*

IX. Supplementary Tables for Reference *157*

X. Discussion of Case Histories *160*

5. Seizures *165*

    I. Case Histories *165*

    II. Approach to Seizures *166*

    III. Background Information *167*

        A. Definitions *167*

        B. Clinical Characteristics of Seizures *168*

        C. Seizures vs. Epilepsy *171*

        D. Epilepsy Classification *172*

        E. Electroencephalography *172*

        F. Pathophysiology of Seizures and Epilepsy *174*

    IV. Diagnosis *175*

        A. Characterizing the Presenting Spell *175*

        B. Identifying Prior Spells *176*

        C. Recognizing Spells That Are Not Seizures *176*

    V. Determining the Cause of Seizures *179*

        A. Provoked Seizures *179*

        B. Epilepsy *180*

        C. The Diagnostic Evaluation *181*

    VI. Management of Seizures and Epilepsy *182*

        A. People with Seizures But No Proven Epilepsy *182*

B. People with Epilepsy 182

C. Patient Education (for People with Isolated Seizures or Epilepsy) 187

D. Restrictions (for People with Isolated Seizures or Epilepsy) 189

VII. Special Clinical Problems 189

    A. Status Epilepticus 189

    B. Seizures and Pregnancy 190

    C. Refractory Seizures 192

VIII. Supplementary Tables for Reference 192

IX. Discussion of Case Histories 198

6. Neuromuscular Disorders 201

Mark B. Bromberg and Douglas J. Gelb

    I. Case Histories 201

    II. Approach to Neuromuscular Diseases 203

    III. Background Information 204

        A. Functional Divisions of the Peripheral Nervous System and Associated Symptoms 204

        B. Proximal-to-Distal Organization of the Peripheral Nervous System 205

        C. Electrodiagnostic and Other Laboratory Studies 208

    IV. Specific Neuromuscular Diseases 209

        A. Motor Neuron Diseases 209

        B. Nerve Root Disorders (Radiculopathies) 214

        C. Plexus Disorders (Plexopathies) 215

        D. Peripheral Nerve Disorders (Neuropathies) 215

        E. Neuromuscular Junction Disorders 222

        F. Muscle Disorders (Myopathies) 226

    V. Symptomatic Treatment 229

        A. Emergency Measures 229

        B. Non-Urgent Measures: Motor Symptoms 230

        C. Non-Urgent Measures: Sensory Symptoms 230

VI. Supplementary Tables for Reference 231

VII. Discussion of Case Histories 234

7. Dementing Illnesses 237
Linda M. Selwa and Douglas J. Gelb

I. Case Histories 237

II. Approach to Dementing Illnesses 240
   A. Is It Abnormal? 240
   B. Are There Any Potentially Reversible Components? 242
   C. Which Primary Degenerative Dementing Illness Is Most Likely? 245

III. Primary Dementing Illnesses 248
   A. Alzheimer Disease (AD) 248
   B. Dementia with Lewy Bodies (DLB) 257
   C. Frontotemporal Dementia (FTD) 258
   D. Vascular Cognitive Impairment 260
   E. Limbic-Predominant Age-Related TDP-43 Encephalopathy (LATE) 262
   F. Creutzfeldt-Jakob Disease (CJD) 262
   G. Other Neurologic Diseases That Produce Dementia 265

IV. Supplementary Tables for Reference 266

V. Discussion of Case Histories 268

8. Movement Disorders 271
Linda M. Selwa and Douglas J. Gelb

I. Case Histories 271

II. Approach to Movement Disorders 272

III. Background Information 272
   A. Anatomic Definitions 272
   B. Clinical Definitions 273
   C. Classification of Movement Disorders 274

IV. Specific Movement Disorders 276
   A. Essential Tremor 276
   B. Parkinson Disease (PD) 277

    C. Other Parkinsonian Syndromes *283*

    D. Hereditary Ataxias *287*

    E. Huntington Disease *290*

    F. Tardive Dyskinesia *292*

    G. Dystonias *292*

    H. Wilson Disease *294*

    I. Tourette Syndrome *296*

  V. Supplementary Tables for Reference *297*

  VI. Discussion of Case Histories *302*

9. Sleep Disorders *305*

  I. Case Histories *305*

  II. Approach to Sleep Disorders *306*

  III. Background Information *307*

    A. Definitions *307*

    B. Sleep Physiology *307*

    C. Diagnostic Tests *310*

    D. Classification of Sleep Disorders *311*

  IV. Trouble Staying Awake *311*

    A. Insufficient Sleep *312*

    B. Sleep Apnea *312*

    C. Narcolepsy *314*

    D. Other Causes of Hypersomnolence *316*

  V. Trouble Sleeping *316*

    A. Sleep-Onset Delay *316*

    B. Early Morning Awakening *318*

    C. Sleep Fragmentation *319*

    D. Sleep State Misperception *319*

  VI. Abnormal Behavior During Sleep *319*

    A. Nonrapid Eye Movement (NREM) Sleep Parasomnias *320*

    B. Rapid Eye Movement (REM) Sleep Parasomnias *323*

  VII. Discussion of Case Histories *324*

10. Multifocal Central Nervous System Disorders *327*

    I. Case Histories *327*

    II. Approach to Multifocal Disorders *329*

    III. Focal Diseases with Multifocal Propagation *329*

        A. Neurologic Manifestations of Systemic Cancer *329*

        B. Central Nervous System Infections *333*

    IV. Inherently Multifocal Diseases *349*

        A. Multiple Sclerosis (MS) and Related Disorders *349*

        B. Rheumatologic Diseases *357*

        C. Sarcoidosis *360*

        D. Coagulation Disorders *361*

        E. Functional Disorders *362*

    V. Supplementary Tables for Reference *364*

    VI. Discussion of Case Histories *370*

PART III: Common Symptoms

11. Acute Mental Status Changes *377*

    I. Case Histories *377*

    II. Background Information *378*

        A. Definitions *378*

        B. Focal Mental Status Changes vs. Altered Level of Consciousness *379*

        C. Physiology of Normal and Altered Consciousness *380*

    III. Approach to Acute Changes in Level of Consciousness *381*

        A. ABCs: Airway, Breathing, Circulation *381*

        B. Oxygen, Glucose, Naloxone *382*

        C. Pupils, Doll's Eyes, Motor Asymmetry *383*

        D. Other Electrolytes, Renal, Hepatic, Temperature Abnormalities *386*

        E. Everything Else *386*

IV. Special Circumstances *388*
    A. Head Trauma *388*
    B. Increased Intracranial Pressure *391*
    C. Brain Death *392*
V. Discussion of Case Histories *393*

12. Headache *395*
    I. Case Histories *395*
    II. Approach to Headache *396*
    III. Background Information *396*
        A. Primary vs. Secondary Headaches *396*
        B. Pathophysiology of Migraine *396*
    IV. Headache Emergencies: Subarachnoid Hemorrhage and Bacterial Meningitis *398*
    V. Other Secondary Headaches *402*
        A. Viral Meningitis or Encephalitis *402*
        B. Fungal or Tuberculous Meningitis *403*
        C. Mass Lesions *404*
        D. Giant Cell (Temporal) Arteritis *404*
        E. Idiopathic Intracranial Hypertension (IIH) *405*
        F. Spontaneous Intracranial Hypotension *406*
        G. Cerebral Venous Thrombosis *407*
        H. Arterial Dissection *407*
        I. Reversible Cerebral Vasoconstriction Syndrome (RCVS) *407*
        J. Systemic Conditions *408*
        K. Secondary Headache Syndromes with Diagnostic Ambiguity *408*
    VI. Primary Headaches *410*
        A. Migraine and Tension Headaches *410*
        B. Trigeminal Neuralgia *414*
        C. Glossopharyngeal Neuralgia *415*
        D. Cluster Headaches *416*

E. Other Trigeminal Autonomic Cephalalgias
(TACs) *417*

F. Primary Stabbing Headache *418*

G. Persistent Idiopathic Facial Pain *418*

VII. Supplementary Tables for Reference *419*

VIII. Discussion of Case Histories *423*

13. Visual Symptoms *425*

I. Case Histories *425*

II. Background Information *426*

A. Definitions *426*

B. Overview of the Visual System *426*

III. Approach to Visual Symptoms *426*

IV. Monocular Vision Loss *427*

A. Acute or Subacute Monocular Vision Loss in
Young People *427*

B. Acute, Subacute, or Chronic Monocular Vision
Loss in Older People *428*

V. Transient Vision Loss (Monocular or Binocular) *429*

VI. Persistent Binocular Vision Loss *430*

VII. Diplopia *430*

A. Localization *430*

B. Differential Diagnosis and Management *432*

VIII. Discussion of Case Histories *433*

14. Dizziness and Disequilibrium *435*

I. Case Histories *435*

II. Approach to Dizziness *437*

III. Localization *437*

IV. Differential Diagnosis *438*

A. Central Vertigo *439*

B. Peripheral Vertigo *439*

V. Disequilibrium *445*

VI. Discussion of Case Histories *446*

15. **Back Pain and Neck Pain** *449*

    I. Case Histories *449*

    II. Approach to Back or Neck Pain *450*

        A. Emergency Situations *450*

        B. Non-Urgent Indications for Surgery *451*

    III. Specific Conditions Causing Back or Neck Pain *451*

        A. Musculoskeletal Pain *451*

        B. Disc Herniation *452*

        C. Spinal Stenosis *454*

    IV. Discussion of Case Histories *454*

16. **Incontinence** *457*

    I. Case Histories *457*

    II. Background Information *458*

    III. Approach to Incontinence *458*

        A. Non-neurologic Causes of Incontinence *459*

        B. Central vs. Peripheral Nervous System Causes of Incontinence *460*

    IV. Supplementary Table for Reference *462*

    V. Discussion of Case Histories *462*

PART IV: Bookends

17. **Pediatric Neurology** *467*

    I. Case Histories *467*

    II. Developmental Considerations *469*

    III. Hypotonic Infants *470*

    IV. Developmental Delay and Developmental Regression *472*

    V. Paroxysmal Symptoms *475*

        A. Migraine *475*

        B. Seizures *476*

        C. Breath-Holding Spells *476*

        D. Benign Paroxysmal Vertigo *477*

VI. Gait Disturbance *477*

   A. Spasticity *478*

   B. Weakness *478*

   C. Ataxia *478*

VII. Functional Disorders *479*

VIII. Discussion of Case Histories *479*

18. Geriatric Neurology *485*

   I. Case Histories *485*

   II. Geriatric Issues *487*

   III. Effects of Aging on the Neurologic Examination *487*

      A. Mental Status *489*

      B. Cranial Nerves *489*

      C. Motor System *489*

      D. Reflexes *490*

      E. Sensation *490*

   IV. Common Neurologic Symptoms in the Elderly *490*

      A. Dizziness *490*

      B. Gait Disturbance *491*

      C. Incontinence *491*

      D. Dementia *492*

      E. Pain *492*

   V. Discussion of Case Histories *492*

19. Practice Cases *495*

   I. Case Histories *495*

   II. Answers *498*

Index *505*

Contributors

James W. Albers, MD, PhD
Professor Emeritus
Department of Neurology
University of Michigan Medical School
Ann Arbor, MI, USA

Mark B. Bromberg, MD, PhD
Professor
Department of Neurology
University of Utah School of Medicine
Salt Lake City, UT, USA

Linda M. Selwa, MD
Professor
Department of Neurology
University of Michigan Medical School
Ann Arbor, MI, USA

Preface to the Sixth Edition

In the preface to the 1995 first edition of this book I wrote about chess-playing computers and advances in imaging technology; today's news brings stories of full-body MRI fads and the threats and opportunities presented by artificial intelligence. It seems that the characters may change, but the plot doesn't. There are plenty of new or maturing characters in this edition. Mechanical thrombectomy, perfusion imaging, antiseizure medications, genetic therapy (especially for spinal muscular atrophy), classification of inflammatory myopathies and neuropathies, genetic testing, amyloid-targeted treatment for Alzheimer disease, disease-modifying treatment for multiple sclerosis and neuromyelitis optica spectrum disorder, and migraine medications have all evolved dramatically since the most recent (2016) edition of this book. "Functional disorders," a topic I've purposely avoided discussing in previous editions, has received so much attention that I felt compelled to include it in this edition. And, of course, a new virus took its place on the world stage. The treatment options for some conditions and the diagnostic considerations for others have multiplied so profusely that it would be unrealistic to expect non-neurologists to have more than a glancing familiarity with them. For that reason, in this edition I've removed many details from the body of the text and placed them in supplementary tables near the ends of chapters. As with previous editions, I've tried to focus on general concepts relevant to the neurologic conditions most clinicians are likely to encounter.

As a general neurologist working in an academic neurology department, I'm surrounded by people who know more than I do about the disorders covered in this book. I haven't asked them to write about those diseases because I've wanted to preserve the perspective of what a non-specialist might want to know. To avoid glaring errors, however, I've asked a few of them to skim what I wrote and set me straight where necessary. Thank you to Sami Barmada, Devin Brown, Kelvin Chou, Praveen Dayalu,

Rachel Gottlieb-Smith, Judy Heidebrink, Steve Leber, and Mollie McDermott for their thoughtful comments. The errors that remain are my fault. I'd also like to acknowledge my debt to Marty Samuels, who encouraged me to publish this book many years ago and supported me at many stages of my career. He was the exemplar of the clinician-teacher and his recent death is a great loss to all involved in neurologic education. My final thanks, as always, go to Karen, Elizabeth, and Molly, for everything.

D.J.G.

Preface to the First Edition

Is neurology obsolete? Two current trends prompt this question. First, dramatic biologic and technologic advances have resulted in increasingly accurate diagnostic tests. It is hard to believe that CT scans have only been widely available since the 1970s; MRI scans, PET scans, and SPECT scans are even more recent, and they are constantly being refined. While chess-playing computers have not quite reached world champion status yet, neurodiagnostic imaging studies have long since achieved a degree of sensitivity that neurologists cannot hope to match. There is more than a little truth to the joke that "one MRI scan is worth a roomful of neurologists." Moreover, advances in molecular genetics and immunochemistry now permit more accurate diagnosis of many conditions than could have been imagined 25 years ago. Some conditions can even be diagnosed before any clinical manifestations are evident. With tests this good, what is the point of learning the traditional approach to neurologic diagnosis, in which lesion localization is deduced from patients' symptoms and signs?

The second major trend challenging the current status of neurology is health care reform. As of this writing, the first great national legislative debate concerning health care reform has ended, not with a bang but a whimper. Yet the problem itself has not disappeared. The already unacceptable costs of health care will continue to escalate if the current system remains unchanged. While the various reform plans that have been proposed differ in many fundamental respects, there appears to be a consensus that there should be more primary care physicians and fewer specialists. Indeed, several forces are already pushing the medical profession in that direction even in the absence of a comprehensive national legislative plan. As a concrete example, it is anticipated that the number of residency training positions in neurology will drop, perhaps to only half of the current level. With so much nationwide emphasis on primary care, what is the point of studying neurology?

Ironically, these two trends together provide a compelling reason to study neurology. In coming years, there will be increasing pressures on primary care physicians to avoid referring patients to specialists (and there will be fewer specialists in the first place). One response of primary care physicians might be to order more diagnostic tests. Unfortunately, the only thing more impressive than the sensitivity of the new tests is their price tag. Just at the time when diagnostic tests are reaching unprecedented levels of accuracy, the funds to pay for the tests are disappearing. Rather than replacing neurologists with MRI scans and genetic testing, primary care physicians will have to become neurologists (to some degree) themselves.

In short, the role currently played by neurologists may well be obsolete, but neurology itself is not. All physicians, regardless of specialty, must become familiar with the general principles of neurologic diagnosis and management. That is the rationale for this book.

The purpose of this book is to present a systematic approach to the neurologic problems likely to be encountered in general medical practice. The focus throughout the book is on practical issues of patient management. This is a departure from the traditional view of neurologic diseases as fascinating but untreatable. Neurologists are often caricatured as pedants who will pontificate interminably on the precise localization of a lesion, produce an obscure diagnosis with an unpronounceable eponym, and smugly declare the case closed. In years past, this stereotype was not wholly inaccurate. Even when therapeutic options existed, there were few controlled studies of efficacy, so it was easy to take a nihilistic approach to therapy. "First do no harm" could often be legitimately interpreted to mean "Do nothing." This was obviously a frustrating position for physicians, and even more so for patients, but at least it kept things simple. All this has changed. Controlled trials of both new and traditional therapies are being conducted with increasing frequency. In the two years since the original versions of some of the current chapters were first prepared, sumatriptan has been approved for treatment of headache, beta interferon for use in multiple sclerosis, ticlopidine for stroke, and tacrine for Alzheimer's disease. Felbamate has appeared and (practically) disappeared. Gabapentin and lamotrigine have been approved for use in epilepsy. The long-term results of a large cooperative study of optic neuritis have challenged traditional practices involving the use of steroids for that condition and for multiple sclerosis. Preliminary reports have appeared concerning the value of endarterectomy for asymptomatic carotid stenosis, a new preparation of beta interferon for MS, and Copolymer I for MS.

PREFACE TO THE FIRST EDITION | xxv

These are exciting developments, but many of the studies raise as many questions as they answer. They certainly change the way physicians have traditionally approached many neurologic diseases. This book reflects that change. Esoteric diagnostic distinctions with little practical relevance are avoided. Distinctions that affect treatment are emphasized. In most chapters, the available treatment options and general approach to management are presented first, to clarify which diagnostic distinctions are important and why.

For many physicians and medical students, the most difficult aspect of neurology is deciding where to start. It is relatively straightforward to manage a patient who has had a stroke; it is often harder to determine whether the patient had a stroke in the first place. When does hand weakness indicate carpal tunnel syndrome, and when is it a manifestation of multiple sclerosis? When does back pain signify metastatic cancer or a herniated disk? These general issues are addressed in the three chapters of Part I. In Part II, common neurologic disease categories are discussed. Part III concerns common symptoms and issues that cross disease categories. Features that distinguish neurologic problems in the pediatric and geriatric populations are discussed in Part IV.

This book is not meant to be comprehensive. Certain topics are omitted, notably specialized management issues that primary care physicians will probably not need to address and other conditions for which treatment is a matter of standard medical care. For example, most patients with primary brain cancer will probably be referred to specialists even in an age of health care reform, so the different types of brain cancer and their treatment are not addressed in this book. Diabetes, chronic alcohol abuse, vitamin B12 deficiency, and other metabolic disturbances can affect many parts of the nervous system. These conditions are mentioned in the relevant sections of this book, but there is no chapter devoted specifically to metabolic problems and their management because these topics are covered in standard medical textbooks. Even for the topics that are included in the book, much detail has been omitted. Again, detailed discussions are available in standard reference books. Use of those books requires some sophistication about neurology, however. A physician trying to figure out why a patient's hand is weak may be overwhelmed by a one-or two-thousand page textbook. Even when the patient's diagnosis is known, the standard references often fail to distinguish the forest from the trees, making it difficult to glean the main principles governing patient management. Those principles are the focus of this book.

Each chapter in this book begins with a set of clinical vignettes and associated questions. These are intended to help the reader focus on practical clinical questions while reading the chapter. Readers should try to answer the questions before reading the rest of the chapter. After finishing the chapter (but before reading the discussion of the clinical vignettes) readers should return to the questions and revise their answers as necessary. Readers can then compare their answers with those given in the discussion at the end of the chapter.

The vignettes are also intended to convey the message that neurology is fun. Many students who used the original version of this book reported that they enjoyed working through the vignettes, and they even suggested that more be included. This response is gratifying. Still, the best "clinical vignettes" come from patients themselves, not from books. Ideally, readers of this book will be inspired to seek out patients with neurologic problems, and will approach them not only with confidence, but with enthusiasm.

I

The Basic Approach

Chapter 1

Where's the Lesion?
(How We Localize)

I. Sample Localization Problems[1]

Example 1. A patient is found to have neurologic deficits that include the following:

1. weakness of abduction of the little finger on the right hand, and
2. reduced pinprick sensation on the palmar surface of the little finger of the right hand.

Where's the lesion?

Example 2. A patient is found to have neurologic deficits that include the following:

1. reduced pinprick sensation on the left forehead, and
2. reduced pinprick sensation on the palmar surface of the little finger of the right hand.

Where's the lesion?

Example 3. A patient is found to have neurologic deficits that include the following:

1. reduced joint position sense in the left foot, and
2. reduced pinprick sensation on the palmar surface of the little finger of the right hand.

Where's the lesion?

---

[1] An on-line tutorial you can use to work through these and similar problems is available at http://neurologic.med.umich.edu

Example 4. A patient is found to have neurologic deficits that include the following:

1. reduced joint position sense in the left foot,
2. reduced pinprick sensation on the palmar surface of the little finger of the right hand,
3. weakness of left ankle dorsiflexion, and
4. hyperreflexia at the left knee.

Where's the lesion?

Example 5. A patient is found to have neurologic deficits that include the following:

1. reduced joint position sense in the left foot,
2. reduced joint position sense in the right foot,
3. reduced joint position sense in the left hand, and
4. reduced joint position sense in the right hand.

Where's the lesion?

Example 6. A patient is found to have neurologic deficits that include the following:

1. reduced joint position sense in the left foot,
2. reduced pinprick sensation on the palmar surface of the little finger of the right hand, and
3. reduced visual acuity in the left eye.

Where's the lesion?

Example 7. The findings on a patient's neurologic examination include the following:

1. reduced joint position and pinprick sensation in the left foot,
2. reduced joint position and pinprick sensation in the right foot,
3. reduced joint position and pinprick sensation in the left hand,
4. reduced joint position and pinprick sensation in the right hand, and
5. normal strength and sensation proximally in all four limbs.

Where's the lesion?

II. The Game

In medicine, as in most endeavors, the first step in addressing a problem is figuring out where it is. For patients with dyspnea, the diagnostic considerations will be different depending on whether the underlying problem is in the lungs or the heart. If it's in the lungs, the diagnosis and management will depend on whether the problem is in the alveoli or the airways. If the problem is in the alveoli, is it a diffuse process affecting all lobes of both lungs, or is it confined to one region in a single lobe of one lung? Similarly, if the underlying problem is in the heart, is it in a valve or in the myocardium—and if a valve, which one? For patients with gastrointestinal bleeding, endoscopy is commonly necessary, but the likely location of the bleeding within the gastrointestinal tract will determine whether the scope is introduced from above or below. For patients with limb pain, the diagnostic and therapeutic plan will depend on whether the pain is in the joints or the soft tissues. For patients with abdominal pain—well, you get the idea.

If localization is so fundamental in all branches of medicine, why are neurologists the only ones who seem to be obsessed by it, always asking: "Where's the lesion?" The answer is that most organ systems have a narrow range of functions and they can be examined directly, so localization is straightforward and almost intuitive. In contrast, the nervous system has many different functions, each one mediated by anatomic structures that overlap or abut structures responsible for other functions, and most of those anatomic structures are inaccessible to direct examination. The nervous system can't be inspected, auscultated, percussed, or palpated. It is, in effect, a black box—we can observe what goes in (sensory input) and what comes out (a person's movements, language output, and behaviors), but not what happens inside the box. Fortunately, we know enough about the structure and function of the nervous system that by observing the "output" that results from a known sensory "input," we can typically deduce the site of nervous system dysfunction.

As an analogy, suppose you are trying to find a broken track in an urban subway system, but the only information available to you is a map of the subway lines and continuous satellite video footage (see Figure 1.1).

Having monitored the video footage every day, you recognize certain people who routinely enter a particular station at the same time each day and always exit the system at some other station. Reviewing today's video, you see that some of those people have maintained their routine, which means that the tracks connecting their entry and exit stations are intact. Other people have revised their routine, indicating a disruption

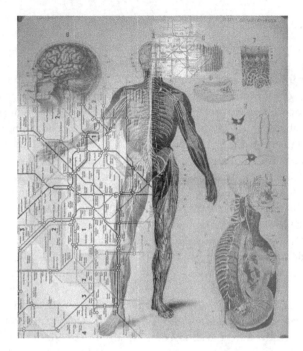

Fig. 1.1 Superposition of the human nervous system and a subway system.

somewhere on the track between their usual entry and exit stations. By analyzing which people had to alter their routines and which did not, and referring to your map of the subway system, you should be able to pinpoint the damage.

Over the years, astute clinicians, anatomists, and physiologists have provided us with a detailed "subway map" of the nervous system. We also have plenty of "previous days' video footage"—patients can tell us how they functioned at baseline, and we know what to expect when we perform a neurologic examination on a healthy individual. By comparing a patient's current symptoms to their baseline and comparing their current exam findings to the expectations for a healthy person (or to the patient's own baseline, if they have been examined previously), we can determine which functions of the nervous system remain intact and which are disrupted. From this, we can deduce which pathways (which "subway lines") are blocked, and we can identify the site (or sites) of disease based on where those pathways intersect. Neurologic localization is essentially an exercise in logic—a game, but hardly a frivolous one. Once you learn to play the game, you can approach patients with neurologic symptoms and signs in a systematic manner rather than relying on pattern recognition (an overwhelming prospect given how many diseases affect the nervous system) or even worse, a shotgun approach, testing for every possible disease.

The rules of the game are presented in Part III of this chapter. For practicing neurologists, the reasoning involved in localization is so instinctive that explicit rules are unnecessary, but most would agree that localization ultimately depends on the kind of logical, stepwise approach summarized in these rules.

III. The Rules

1. Each symptom or abnormal physical finding can be thought of as a line segment connecting the central nervous system to the periphery (a muscle or sensory receptor). (In terms of the subway analogy in Part II, *each symptom or physical finding corresponds to a subway line.*)
2. If all these line segments intersect at a single point, that point is the site of the lesion (i.e., *a station that is on every one of the damaged subway lines.*)
3. There may be two or more points where all the line segments intersect, and hence, two or more potential lesion sites. If so, each potential site must be evaluated further by determining whether the patient has the other symptoms or signs that would be expected with a lesion in that location. (*For every station common to all the damaged subway lines, check to see whether any additional subway lines travel through that station, then look to see if trains are running normally along those lines.*)
4. There may be no points that fall on all the line segments. If so, the goal is to explain all the patient's symptoms and physical findings on the basis of just two lesions (i.e., to find two points such that every line segment passes through one or the other point; or, in our analogy, to find *two stations that together account for all the damaged subway lines*).
5. If even two lesion sites are not sufficient to explain all the symptoms and findings, the process is likely to be either multifocal or diffuse. The goal then becomes one of detecting a unifying property that applies to all the lesion sites. For example, they may all be located at the neuromuscular junction, or they may all be in the white matter of the central nervous system (*all the stations that are above ground, say, or all the stations that are in suburbs*).

When stated in this way, the rules appear abstract and somewhat obscure, but in practice they are straightforward. This is demonstrated in the following three parts of this chapter by considering specific examples. It might seem that detailed knowledge of neuroanatomy would be required. Certainly, more precise neuroanatomic knowledge permits more refined localization, but for most purposes, rough neuroanatomic approximations are adequate. To show this, several examples of careful neuroanatomic analysis are presented in Part IV, and simpler analyses of the same clinical scenarios are presented in Part V. Part VI provides a link (https://neurolo gic.med.umich.edu/) to a computer tutorial that can be used to practice the analytic approach and learn the pathways explained in Parts IV and V. In Part VII, the kind of reasoning applied in Parts IV and V is used to derive some general principles that can expedite localization.

IV. The Play: The Long Version

Note: If the following discussion seems too complicated, you might want to proceed directly to the explanations in Part V and the additional prac- tice problems available in the computer tutorial of Part VI. In fact, you could skip even further ahead and focus on the simple rules presented in Part VII, which can be used to localize the majority of neurologic lesions. At some point, however, you should return to Part IV to understand the detailed reasoning process that underlies the more simplified approaches.

Example 1. A patient is found to have neurologic deficits that include the following:

1. weakness of abduction of the little finger on the right hand, and
2. reduced pinprick sensation on the palmar surface of the little finger of the right hand.

Where's the lesion?

Item 1 in Example 1 could be caused by a lesion anywhere in the line segment shown in Figure 1.2. The pathway begins in the precentral gyrus of the left cerebral cortex (i.e., the motor strip). The representation of the hand in this strip is midway between the leg representation medially and the face representation laterally. From this point of origin, the segment descends in order through the corona radiata, the internal capsule, the cerebral peduncle—also called the crus cerebri (in the midbrain), and the base of the pons (basis pontis), until it reaches the pyramid in the medulla.

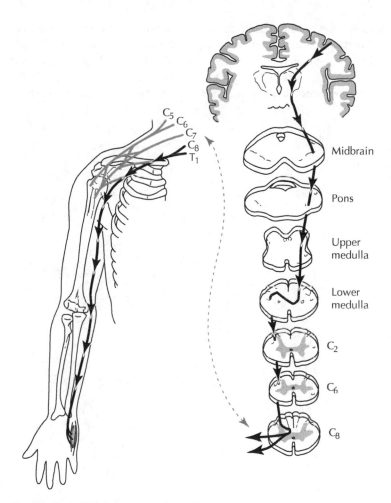

Midbrain

Pons

Upper medulla

Lower medulla

C_2

C_6

C_8

C_5 C_6 C_7 C_8 T_1

Fig. 1.2 The solid black arrows show the pathway corresponding to weakness of abduction of the little finger on the right hand.

At this point, the pathway crosses to the right side, and proceeds downward in the lateral white matter of the spinal cord. At the C8 and T1 levels of the spinal cord, the pathway enters the anterior aspect of the gray matter (where the cortical neuron synapses on a motor neuron whose cell body is in the anterior horn), then exits the spinal cord via the right C8 and T1 roots, proceeds through the lower trunk and then the medial cord of the brachial plexus, exits in the ulnar nerve, passes through the neuromuscular junction, and terminates in the abductor digiti minimi muscle.

The line segment corresponding to item 2 is shown in Figure 1.3. It starts in sensory receptors in the little finger of the right hand, continues in the ulnar nerve, proceeds proximally through the medial cord and lower trunk

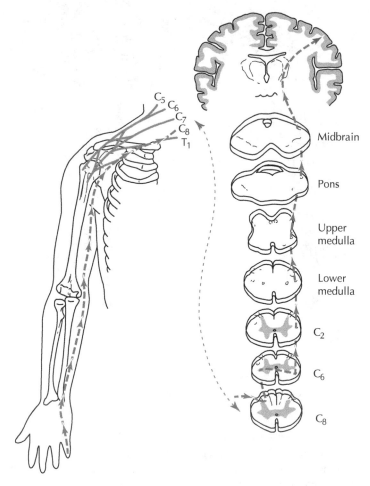

Fig. 1.3 The dashed gray arrows depict the pathway corresponding to reduced pinprick sensation on the palmar surface of the little finger on the right hand.

of the brachial plexus, and enters the spinal cord via the right C8 nerve root. It ascends one or two segments in the spinal cord, synapses in the dorsal horn, and then crosses to the left spinothalamic tract, ascending in this tract through the medulla, pons, and midbrain. After synapsing in the ventral posterolateral nucleus of the thalamus, the pathway continues through the internal capsule and corona radiata, terminating in the parietal cortex (just posterior to the region of the motor strip where the line segment for item 1 originates).

Figure 1.4 illustrates both of these line segments together. One obvious point of intersection is in the frontoparietal cortex, where one segment lies directly behind the other. In addition, there is a whole set of possible intersection sites falling between the ulnar nerve distally and the C8/T1 nerve roots proximally. To decide which of these potential localization sites is the true focus of pathology, the next step is to consider what other signs and symptoms might be expected from a lesion at each site. For example, a lesion in the C8/T1 nerve roots or the lower trunk of the brachial plexus would be likely to affect fibers destined for the median nerve, affecting muscles innervated by that nerve, whereas these muscles would clearly be spared by a lesion in the ulnar nerve itself. In contrast, a cortical lesion affecting the arm could extend far enough laterally or medially to affect the cortical representation of the right face or leg, whereas a nerve, plexus, or root lesion would not affect anything outside the right upper extremity. Abnormalities of vision or language function would also imply a cortical localization and would be inconsistent with a lesion in the peripheral nervous system.

Example 2. A patient is found to have neurologic deficits that include the following:

1. reduced pinprick sensation on the left forehead, and
2. reduced pinprick sensation on the palmar surface of the little finger of the right hand.

Where's the lesion?

The line segment corresponding to item 2 in Example 2 was already discussed in the previous example (see Figure 1.3). The pathway for item 1 is shown in Figure 1.5. It starts in sensory receptors in the left forehead and continues in the first division (the ophthalmic division) of the trigeminal nerve (cranial nerve V). This nerve travels through the superior orbital fissure and enters the lateral wall of the cavernous sinus. It then emerges

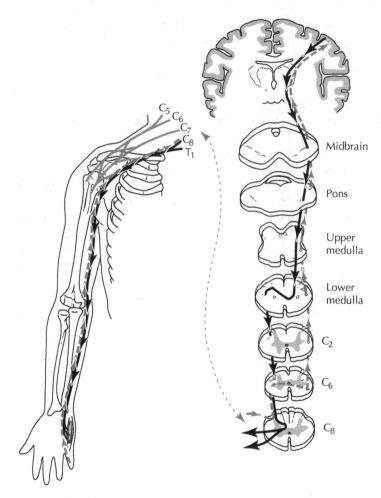

Fig. 1.4 Diagram illustrating both the pathway corresponding to weak abduction of the right little finger (black, descending arrows) and reduced pinprick sensation (gray dashed ascending arrows) in that finger (i.e., the pathways of both Figure 1.2 and Figure 1.3). The regions common to both pathways are in the left frontoparietal cortex and in the peripheral nervous system (from the right C8/T1 nerve roots to the right ulnar nerve).

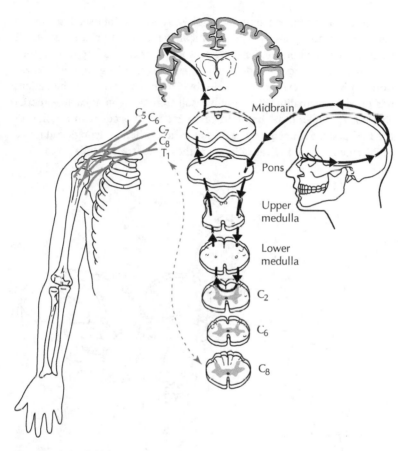

Fig. 1.5 The solid black arrows show the pathway corresponding to reduced pinprick sensation on the left forehead.

to join the other two divisions of the trigeminal nerve in the trigeminal (gasserian) ganglion. From here, the pathway enters the pons, descends in the left spinal tract of the trigeminal nucleus, and synapses in the nucleus of that tract at about the C2 spinal level. At this point, the pathway crosses to the right side of the spinal cord and ascends in the ventral trigemino-thalamic tract to synapse in the ventral posteromedial nucleus of the right thalamus. The final section of the line segment runs from the ventral posteromedial nucleus through the internal capsule and corona radiata to terminate in the lateral aspect of the postcentral gyrus of the parietal lobe.

Figure 1.6 combines Figures 1.3 and 1.5. Potential intersection sites lie between the mid-pons and the high spinal cord (C2) on the left. At all other points, the line segments are nowhere near each other. In fact, they are generally on opposite sides of the nervous system! Again, the localization can be made even more precise by determining whether the patient has other abnormalities that might result from a lesion at each potential site. For example, facial nerve involvement could occur with a lesion in the mid-pons, but not at any of the lower sites, whereas hypoglossal nerve involvement would indicate a lesion at the level of the medulla.

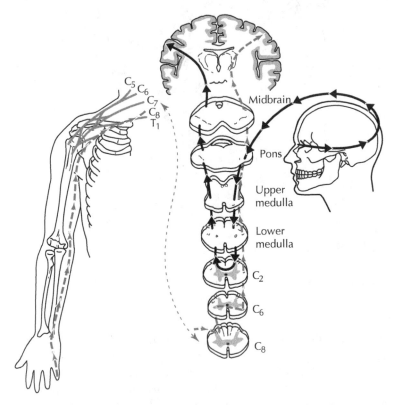

Fig. 1.6 Diagram illustrating both the pathway corresponding to (gray dashed arrows) reduced pinprick sensation in the right little finger and (black arrows) reduced pinprick sensation on the left forehead (i.e., the pathways of both Figure 1.3 and Figure 1.5). The regions common to both pathways lie between the mid-pons and the C2 level of the spinal cord on the left.

Although Figures 1.2 through 1.6 may seem excessively detailed, they are still simplified approximations of the underlying anatomy. For example, Figure 1.2 reflects a tacit assumption that the lateral corticospinal tract is the principal descending pathway affecting limb muscles. The ventral corticospinal tract and other descending motor pathways (such as the vestibulospinal, tectospinal, rubrospinal, reticulospinal, and ceruleus-spinal projections) are not included in the figure. The importance of these other descending pathways can be appreciated by recognizing that a selective lesion of the corticospinal tract (e.g., in the medullary pyramid, one of the few locations where it is physically isolated from other descending tracts) results in minimal long-term weakness. Even so, the pathway presented in Figure 1.2 proves to be very useful in clinical localization. Presumably, the contributions of all the descending tracts sum up in such a way that the net effect is something similar to the pathway shown in the figure. As another example, the entire spinal tract of the trigeminal nucleus appears to descend to the level of C2 in Figure 1.5. In reality, some axons in that tract synapse on second-order neurons almost as soon as they enter the brainstem, and other axons descend varying distances in the pons or medulla before synapsing; only a few descend all the way to C2. Nonetheless, for the purpose of localizing all possible lesion sites, the pathway can be treated as if all the axons descend to C2. These are just two examples of how approximations and simplifications that we know are inaccurate can nonetheless lead to conclusions that are clinically useful. In fact, we can ignore the cross-sectional anatomy and many other anatomic details and still localize most lesions reliably. Part V illustrates this.

V. The Play: The Abbreviated Version

The best way to identify all plausible lesion localization sites (and only those sites) is to follow the approach outlined in Part IV. In many cases, however, much coarser analysis of the symptoms and signs will give nearly the same results. In particular, the lesion can often be localized with surprising precision simply by considering where the relevant nervous system pathways cross the midline.

Example 1 Revisited. Figure 1.7 shows a schematic diagram of the pathway portrayed in Figure 1.2, corresponding to weakness of the right abductor digiti minimi muscle. Much of the detail has been eliminated. In fact, the same diagram would apply to any muscle in the right upper extremity.

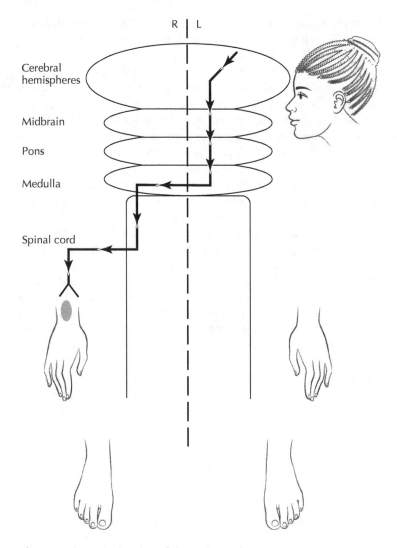

R | L

Cerebral
hemispheres

Midbrain

Pons

Medulla

Spinal cord

Fig. 1.7 Schematic drawing of the pathway shown in Figure 1.2, representing weakness of right little finger abduction. The same diagram would be used to represent weakness in any muscle of the right upper extremity.

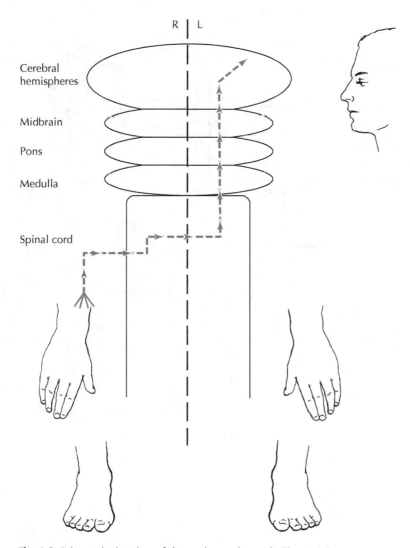

Fig. 1.8 Schematic drawing of the pathway shown in Figure 1.3, representing reduced pinprick sensation in the right upper extremity.

Figure 1.8 shows a schematic diagram for the reduced pain sensation in the right hand represented in Figure 1.3. Figure 1.9 combines Figures 1.7 and 1.8. It is clear even from this simplified diagram that within the spinal cord the two pathways are on opposite sides, so the lesion could not possibly be

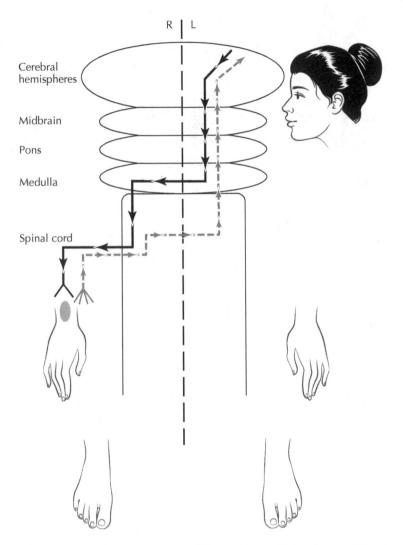

R | L

Cerebral
hemispheres

Midbrain

Pons

Medulla

Spinal cord

Fig. 1.9 Schematic representation of Figure 1.4, combining Figures 1.7 and 1.8. The only regions common to both pathways are at the level of the mid-medulla or above on the left, or in the peripheral nervous system on the right.

located there. Instead, it must either be in the periphery (i.e., at the level of nerve roots, plexus, or peripheral nerves) or rostral to the level at which the motor pathway crosses in the medulla. Although the more detailed analysis presented in Part IV results in a more refined final localization (ruling out all of the rostral structures except the cortex), this additional refinement may not be that important in practice. The entire region from the medulla to the cortex is visualized on magnetic resonance imaging (MRI) of the brain, so as long as the lesion can be localized to somewhere within this region the appropriate diagnostic study will be performed. In contrast, elimination of the cervical spinal cord from consideration does have a significant practical result, because it makes an MRI scan of the cervical spine unnecessary.

Example 2 Revisited. Figure 1.10 presents a schematic diagram for the pathway shown in Figure 1.5, representing left forehead numbness. Again, Figure 1.8 represents a schematic diagram for right hand numbness. Both pathways are shown together in Figure 1.11. It is clear from the diagram that the only potential intersection points lie in the region extending from the left mid-pons down to the left side of the spinal cord at the C2 level. This is exactly the same localization deduced earlier from the more detailed analysis.

Because the level at which a pathway crosses the midline is the most important feature for localizing central nervous system lesions, many different symptoms can be portrayed by the same schematic diagram. For example, Figure 1.7 represents weakness in any muscle of the right upper extremity, and an analogous figure can be drawn for weakness in any other limb. Figure 1.8 portrays a deficit in pain or temperature sensation anywhere in the right upper extremity, and analogous figures apply to pain/temperature deficits in other limbs. Figure 1.10 portrays the pathway for impaired pain and temperature sensation anywhere in the face.

A deficit in proprioception or vibration sense is represented by Figure 1.12 (or something analogous in another limb). The pathway for facial weakness is represented in Figure 1.13, and analogous figures can be drawn for the motor components of other cranial nerves. These pathways are complicated because there is bilateral cortical input to many of these cranial nerve nuclei, making interpretation difficult at times (see Chapter 2, Part V, Section B). Analogously, the auditory and vestibular pathways project bilaterally once they enter the central nervous system, making peripheral lesions much more straightforward to localize than central lesions. For example, unilateral hearing loss implies a lesion in the ipsilateral eighth nerve, cochlea, or inner ear. Dysfunction of the auditory pathway above the medulla results in bilateral hearing loss.

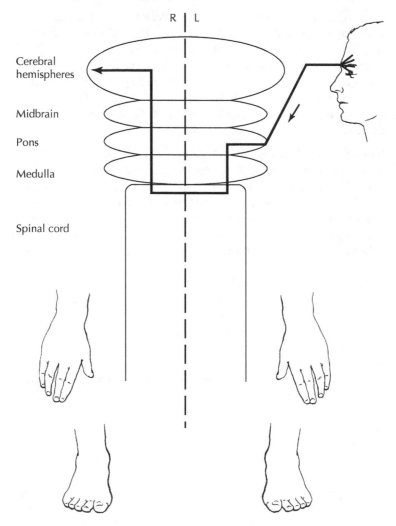

Fig. 1.10 Schematic drawing of the pathway shown in Figure 1.5, representing left facial numbness.

The distinction between the central and peripheral portions of a pathway can be very powerful. When considered schematically, the peripheral portion of a pathway (connecting a muscle or sensory receptor organ to the spinal cord or brainstem) is perpendicular to the "long axis" of the nervous

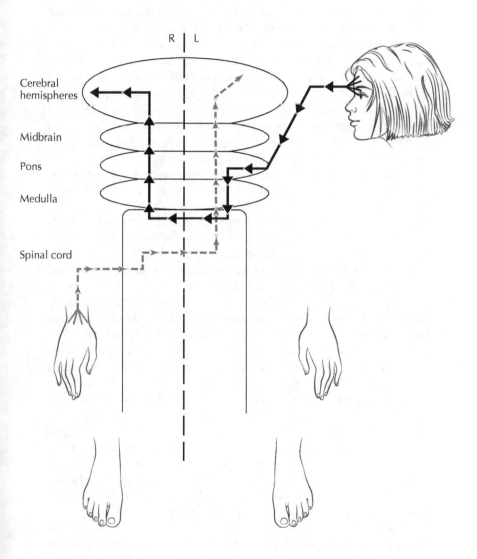

Fig. 1.11 Schematic representation of Figure 1.6, combining Figures 1.8 and 1.10. The only regions common to both pathways lie between the mid-pons and the C2 level of the spinal cord on the left.

system (the neuraxis), which runs from the cortex to the base of the spinal cord. A lesion that can be localized to the peripheral limb of one pathway (pathway X in Figure 1.14) and the central limb of another (pathway Y) is thus "caught in the cross-hairs," permitting very precise localization (the subway equivalent would be involvement of both a north–south line and an east–west line).

For example, someone who has a lesion compressing the spinal cord typically has hypoactive deep tendon reflexes at the level of the lesion and hyperactive reflexes below that level. *Hypoactive reflexes indicate dysfunction in the peripheral portion of the reflex pathway, the reflex arc.* The reflex arc begins in a sensory receptor located inside a muscle, travels along sensory nerve fibers to the spinal cord, then synapses with a motor neuron in the anterior horn at the same level, and proceeds out along motor nerve fibers to the original muscle. The afferent limb of the reflex arc is identical to the initial, peripheral portion of the pathway for vibration/position sensation (see Figure 1.12). The efferent limb of the reflex arc is identical to the final, peripheral portion of the motor pathway (see Figures 1.2 and 1.7)—this is called the lower motor neuron (LMN) portion of the motor pathway. In normal individuals, the deep tendon reflexes are continually suppressed by descending motor tracts. These tracts constitute the central, or upper motor neuron (UMN), portion of the motor pathway. *When there is a lesion in this central pathway, the peripheral reflex arc is no longer suppressed, and a hyperactive reflex results.* Several different descending tracts are involved, but the central limb of the pathway shown in Figure 1.7 approximates the net effect (as already discussed with regard to weakness). Both the peripheral (LMN) and the central (UMN) portions of the pathway for the right biceps reflex are represented schematically in Figure 1.15. A compressive lesion at the C5 level of the spinal cord interrupts the peripheral portion of the biceps reflex pathway and at the same time interrupts the central portion of the pathways mediating the triceps and lower extremity reflexes. Other examination findings useful in distinguishing UMN from LMN lesions are discussed in Chapter 2.

Visual information is transmitted from the eyes to the brain by another pathway that is perpendicular to the neuraxis (Figure 1.16). Detailed understanding of this pathway can lead to elegant and precise localization, but at the most basic level it suffices to know that the optic nerves from each eye converge at the optic chiasm. Anterior to the chiasm, a structural lesion will affect vision from only one eye, whereas a lesion at the chiasm or posterior to it will produce visual problems in both eyes. Moreover, when the fibers meet at the chiasm, they sort themselves so that all the fibers on one side of the brain correspond to visual input from the opposite side of

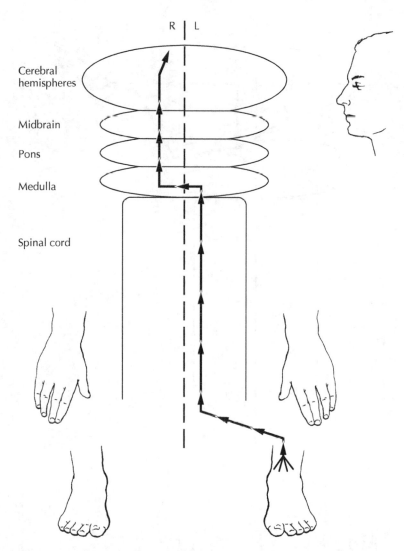

Fig. 1.12 Schematic drawing of the pathway corresponding to reduced position or vibration sense in the left lower extremity.

the visual world. To be specific, stimuli in the right half of the visual world are focused by the lens system of each eye onto the left side of the retina. This is the temporal half of the left retina and the nasal half of the right retina. The ganglion cells in the left half of each retina send information

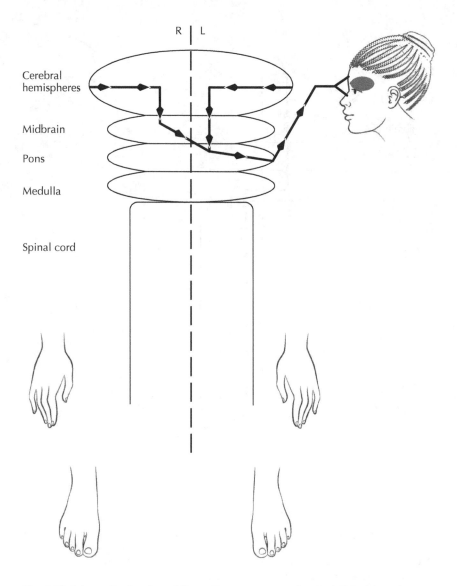

Fig. 1.13 Schematic drawing of the pathway corresponding to left facial weakness.

to the left occipital cortex. Thus, the left occipital cortex processes visual input from the right half of the visual world. To accomplish this, the fibers from the nasal half of the right retina must cross the midline. Analogously, the fibers from the nasal half of the left retina cross the midline to send

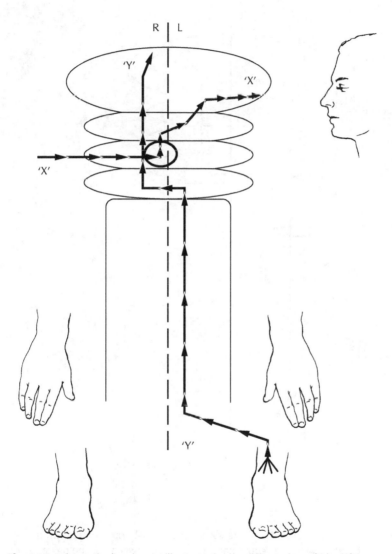

Fig. 1.14 Schematic drawing to illustrate the localizing value of identifying dysfunction in the peripheral portion of one pathway ('X') and the central portion of another pathway ('Y'), thereby localizing the lesion "in the cross-hairs" (small circle).

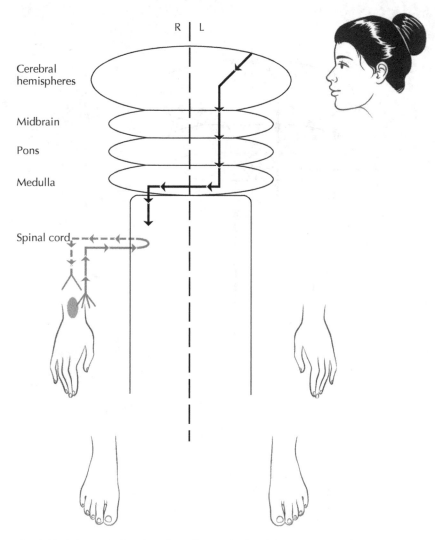

Fig. 1.15 Schematic drawing of a reflex arc in the right upper extremity (gray arrows), together with the central pathway (black arrows) providing descending inhibitory input to the reflex arc. Within the reflex arc, the solid arrows depict the afferent limb, and the dashed arrows depict the efferent limb.

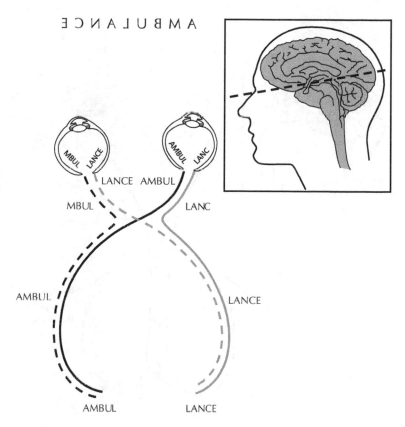

Fig. 1.16 Schematic drawing representing the visual pathways.

information to the right visual cortex. This crossing occurs in the optic chiasm. A single large lesion at the chiasm can damage all the crossing and uncrossing fibers, resulting in total blindness. A smaller, centrally placed lesion may damage only the crossing fibers. Since these fibers originate in the nasal retina of each eye, the result is impaired vision in the temporal field of each eye (a bitemporal hemianopia).

The pupillary light reflex is mediated by another pathway that is perpendicular to the neuraxis (Figure 1.17). The pathway runs from the eye through the optic chiasm, just as in Figure 1.16, but soon after leaving the chiasm some fibers diverge from the rest of the visual fibers to synapse in the dorsal midbrain on parasympathetic nerve fibers that travel with

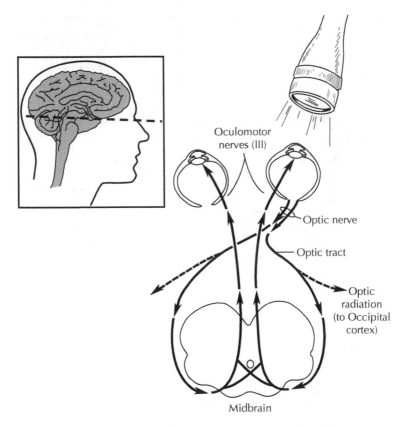

Fig. 1.17 Schematic drawing of the pathway mediating bilateral pupillary constriction in response to light in one eye.

the oculomotor nerve (cranial nerve III) and terminate in the pupillary constrictor muscles. Note that even with input to just one eye, the bilateral projections in the optic chiasm and again in the midbrain result in bilateral output—that is, both pupils constrict. The net output is actually a function of the input to both eyes. In most natural circumstances, the overall illumination is the same in both eyes, so the input to each eye is the same. When the input to each eye is different (e.g., when an examiner holds a bright flashlight up to one eye, or when one optic nerve is defective), the midbrain essentially averages the illumination from the two eyes to produce a single net output signal that is the same for the two pupils.

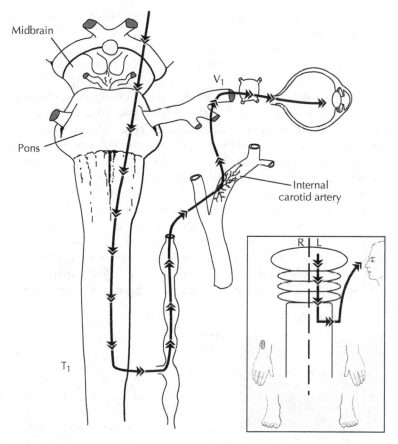

Fig. 1.18 Schematic drawing illustrating the pathway for sympathetic innervation of the left pupil.

Pupillary size is determined not only by the parasympathetic pathway but also by the sympathetic pathway, represented in Figure 1.18. This pathway begins in the hypothalamus, descends through the brainstem to the spinal cord at about the T1 level, then exits the spinal cord to enter the sympathetic chain and synapse in the superior cervical ganglion. From here, the pathway follows first the internal carotid artery and then the ophthalmic division of the trigeminal nerve (cranial nerve V), ultimately terminating in the pupil. Unlike most other pathways, the sympathetic pathway controlling the pupil remains on one side of the nervous system throughout its course. This is often extremely helpful in pinning down the site of a lesion.

Several neurologic deficits with localizing value do not readily lend themselves to a formulation in terms of line segments. For example, coordinated movements involve the interplay of motor cortex, basal ganglia, cerebellum, and brainstem nuclei. The interconnections between these structures result in "double-crossing" and "triple-crossing" pathways. It is often simplest to localize a lesion on the basis of other clinical features, and then check to see that the resulting localization is consistent with the patient's coordination problem, rather than starting by trying to reason through all the potential sites that could cause the coordination abnormality.

Cognitive processing is another example of neural circuitry that is so complicated that it does not lend itself to simple diagrams based on isolated line segments. For example, the neurophysiologic mechanisms involved in linguistic processing involve intricate connections between many different brain regions. Despite this complexity, clinicians often refer to the model of language processing depicted in Figure 1.19A and 1.19B. According to this model, Wernicke's area in the posterior temporal cortex is involved in

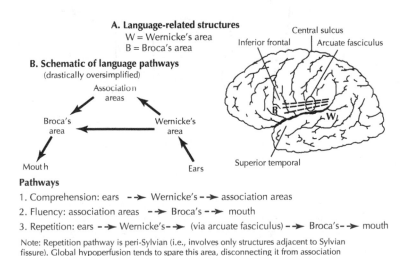

A. Language-related structures
W = Wernicke's area
B = Broca's area

Central sulcus
Inferior frontal | Arcuate fasciculus

B. Schematic of language pathways
(drastically oversimplified)

Association areas

Broca's area ← Wernicke's area

Mouth   Ears   Superior temporal

Pathways

1. Comprehension: ears - ➤ Wernicke's - ➤ association areas
2. Fluency: association areas - ➤ Broca's - ➤ mouth
3. Repetition: ears - ➤ Wernicke's- ➤ (via arcuate fasciculus) - ➤ Broca's- ➤ mouth

Note: Repetition pathway is peri-Sylvian (i.e., involves only structures adjacent to Sylvian fissure). Global hypoperfusion tends to spare this area, disconnecting it from association areas and producing transcortical aphasias (see Panel C).

Fig. 1.19 Schematic diagrams representing language processing in the brain.

Panel D reproduced, with permission, from Chang EF, Raygor KP, Berger MS. Contemporary model of language organization: an overview for neurosurgeons. J Neurosurg 2015;122:250–261.

C. Traditional aphasia classification scheme
(again, oversimplified)

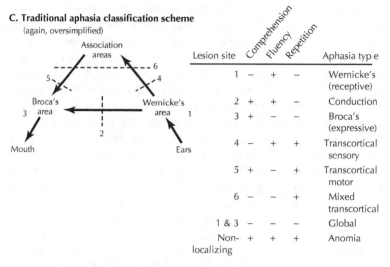

Lesion site	Comprehension	Fluency	Repetition	Aphasia type
1	–	+	–	Wernicke's (receptive)
2	+	+	–	Conduction
3	+	–	–	Broca's (expressive)
4	–	+	+	Transcortical sensory
5	+	–	+	Transcortical motor
6	–	–	+	Mixed transcortical
1 & 3	–	–	–	Global
Non-localizing	+	+	+	Anomia

D. Dual stream model

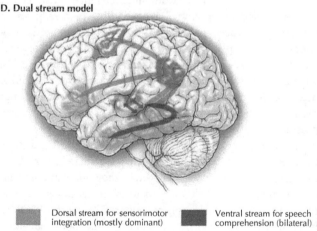

	Dorsal stream for sensorimotor integration (mostly dominant)		Ventral stream for speech comprehension (bilateral)

Fig. 1.19 Continued

recognizing the linguistic structures incorporated in a string of sounds. Areas of "higher" association cortex process these linguistic structures to extract meaning. Broca's area in the inferior lateral frontal lobe (just anterior to the region of the motor strip representing the face) translates linguistic structures into the motor programs necessary for producing speech. Thus, the comprehension of spoken language is represented in Figure 1.19B by pathway 1 from the ear to auditory cortex to Wernicke's area and thence to association areas. The ability to produce fluent, meaningful speech output is represented by pathway 2 traveling from cortical association areas to Broca's area to regions of the motor cortex and brainstem involved in movements of the lips, tongue, pharynx, larynx, and diaphragm. The ability to repeat a string of words is represented by pathway 3 from the ear to auditory cortex to Wernicke's area, and from there through the arcuate fasciculus to Broca's area to the motor strip and thence to the cranial nerves innervating the appropriate muscles of the face, tongue, pharynx, larynx, and diaphragm. This model was derived primarily from clinical observations of patients who had suffered strokes or other focal lesions, and many of these observations were made long before the invention of computed tomography (CT) scans and MRI scans. The model is an oversimplification and incorrect in many respects. It fails to explain many clinical observations. For example, many patients with lesions in the arcuate fasciculus are able to repeat normally, and most patients with the clinical syndrome of conduction aphasia have cortical lesions that spare the arcuate fasciculus. Evidence from functional imaging studies, other imaging modalities, and electrophysiologic recording (generally performed during neurosurgical procedures) suggests that the brain networks underlying word comprehension are different from those mediating sentence comprehension, and different networks process different semantic categories (such as verbs and nouns, or even different categories of nouns, such as animals and tools). Moreover, it is now recognized that the anterior pole of the temporal lobe and numerous subcortical structures and fiber bundles are critical to language processing. Recent models of language organization propose two streams of information processing, each involving both cortical and subcortical structures (Figure 1.19D). The ventral stream, centered in the temporal lobe of each hemisphere, is involved in speech recognition and the representation of lexical concepts. The dorsal stream, which includes structures and fiber bundles in the dominant hemisphere's posterior temporoparietal region, parietal lobe, and frontal lobe, is involved in mapping phonologic information onto motor programs involved in speech production.

As a way to conceptualize these streams, I find it helpful to consider two things I do simultaneously when I'm having trouble thinking of a person's name. First, I silently cycle through the letters of the alphabet in my mind. Somehow, even though I can't recall the name, I often have a powerful feeling that it must begin with a certain letter, or at least I can narrow it down to a few letters. Sometimes, I also have a strong sense of what the name rhymes with. At the same time, I try to think of things I know about the person, how I have interacted with them, and other people I associate with them. As

I keep concentrating on the likely letters and rhymes while thinking about associated names and facts, I have the impression that I'm getting closer and closer until suddenly the name pops into my head. Presumably, reciting the letters activates the dorsal (phonologic) stream, whereas thinking about the associations activates the ventral (semantic) stream, and the points of intersection that are reinforced and amplified by this simultaneous activation correspond to the neural circuits relevant to the name I was trying to recall.

The "dual-stream" models of language processing are more accurate than the traditional model shown in Figure 1.19A, 1.19B, and 1.19C, but they are more complicated and less intuitive. Despite being simplistic and unrealistic, the traditional dimensions of fluency, comprehension, and repetition still provide a convenient way to categorize language problems, and the traditional model provides a convenient way to think about those dimensions and draw some general conclusions about lesion localization (primarily whether the lesion is likely to be located anteriorly or posteriorly).

Example 3. A patient is found to have neurologic deficits that include the following:

1. reduced joint position sense in the left foot, and
2. reduced pinprick sensation on the palmar surface of the little finger of the right hand.

Where's the lesion?

The line segment corresponding to item 2 in Example 3 has already been discussed (see Figure 1.8). The line segment corresponding to item 1 is shown in Figure 1.12. Both line segments are shown together in Figure 1.20. The two line segments are on opposite sides of the nervous system except for a short segment running from the lower medulla on the left to about the C6/7 level of the spinal cord on the left. This region is the only potential localization site.

Example 4. A patient is found to have neurologic deficits that include the following:

1. reduced joint position sense in the left foot,
2. reduced pinprick sensation on the palmar surface of the little finger of the right hand,
3. weakness of left ankle dorsiflexion, and
4. hyperreflexia at the left knee.

Where's the lesion?

The first two items are the same as in Example 3 and imply a lesion localization somewhere between the low medulla and the C6/7 level of the spinal cord on the left (see Figure 1.20). Within this region, the line segments corresponding to the third and fourth items essentially coincide with the line segment for item 1. Thus, the additional deficits help to confirm the region of potential localization, but they don't help to refine it. One way to narrow the region would be to examine the left biceps reflex. This would be represented by a mirror image of the pathway shown in Figure 1.15. A depressed biceps reflex would imply a lesion in the reflex arc at the C5 or C6 level of the spinal cord. In contrast, a hyperactive biceps reflex would imply a lesion above the level of C5.

Example 5. A patient is found to have neurologic deficits that include the following:

1. reduced joint position sense in the left foot,

2. reduced joint position sense in the right foot,

3. reduced joint position sense in the left hand, and

4. reduced joint position sense in the right hand.

Where's the lesion?

Figure 1.12 shows the line segment corresponding to item 1 in **Example 5**. Figure 1.21 includes this line segment together with analogous line segments from each of the other three limbs representing items 2, 3, and 4. At first glance, it appears that there is only one level at which all these segments intersect: in the medulla, where they all cross. At every other level, two of the segments are on one side of the nervous system and two are on the other. On closer scrutiny, however, additional localization sites are evident. Even though the segments lie on both sides of the nervous system, there are two places where they are contiguous across the midline. Thus, whereas a unilateral lesion could not affect all four line segments, a bilateral lesion centered in the midline and extending out to each side could explain the pattern of deficits. The sites where this is possible are in the cervical spinal cord (at the level of C7 and above) and the postcentral gyrus of the cortex. The presence or absence of additional deficits (corresponding to additional line segments) would help to distinguish between these three potential lesion sites (medulla, cervical cord, and cortex).

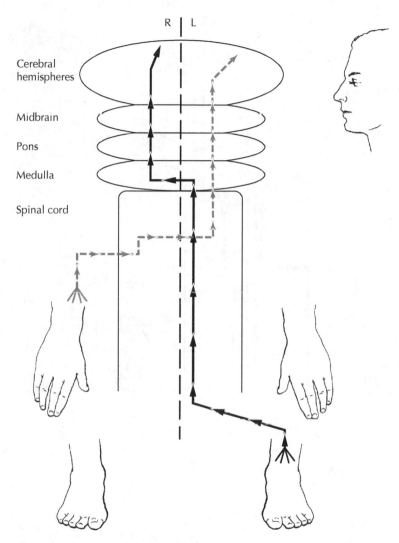

Fig. 1.20 Schematic drawing combining Figures 1.8 and 1.12, corresponding to reduced pinprick sensation in the right upper extremity and reduced joint position sense in the left lower extremity. The only regions common to both pathways lie between the low medulla and the C6/7 level of the spinal cord on the left.

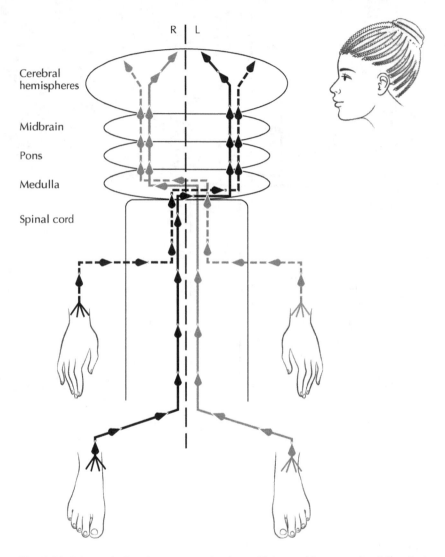

R | L

Cerebral hemispheres

Midbrain

Pons

Medulla

Spinal cord

Fig. 1.21 Schematic drawing representing loss of joint position sense in all four limbs. Potential lesion sites lie in the midline and extend bilaterally, at the levels of the cortex, low medulla, or high cervical spinal cord.

Example 6. A patient is found to have neurologic deficits that include the following:

1. reduced joint position sense in the left foot,

2. reduced pinprick sensation on the palmar surface of the little finger of the right hand, and

3. reduced visual acuity in the left eye.

Where's the lesion?

The first two items are the same as in Examples 3 and 4 and imply a lesion localization somewhere between the low medulla and the C6/7 level of the spinal cord on the left (see Figure 1.20). This region is not even close to the line segment representing the patient's visual loss (see Figure 1.16). This means that no single lesion site could produce all of this patient's findings. By the rules of the game, the next objective is to explain all the deficits on the basis of two lesion sites. This can obviously be achieved by assuming that one lesion is in the previously identified region of the medulla or spinal cord and the other lesion is in the left retina or optic nerve. The next step is to decide whether these two lesions are related or coincidental, using the approach to be presented in Chapter 3.

Example 7. The findings on a patient's neurologic examination include the following:

1. reduced joint position and pinprick sensation in the left foot,

2. reduced joint position and pinprick sensation in the right foot,

3. reduced joint position and pinprick sensation in the left hand,

4. reduced joint position and pinprick sensation in the right hand, and

5. normal strength and sensation proximally in all four limbs.

Where's the lesion?

The deficits in joint position sense in all four limbs were discussed in **Example 5.** They imply a lesion site lying in the midline and extending bilaterally either in the cortex or in the region extending from the low medulla to the C7 level of the spinal cord. Within this latter region, the line segments representing pinprick sensation lie laterally (see Figure 1.3). Unlike the pathways for joint position sense, they are not contiguous across the midline, and only an extremely large lesion could affect them bilaterally. This is shown in Figure 1.22, which represents a cross section

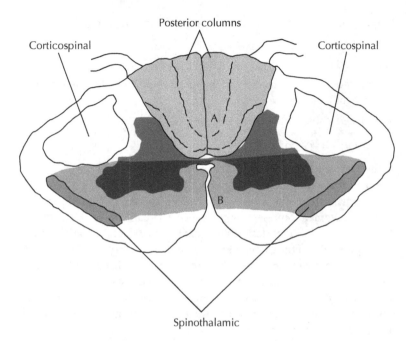

Posterior columns

Corticospinal

Corticospinal

A

B

Spinothalamic

Fig. 1.22 Cross section of the high cervical spinal cord. Region A corresponds to the area that must be affected to produce loss of joint position sense in all four limbs. Region B corresponds to the area that would produce reduced pinprick sensation in all four limbs. Any lesion large enough to affect both region A and region B would also include the lateral corticospinal tracts and the anterior horns, resulting in motor symptoms.

of the spinal cord (the reasoning would be the same for the medulla). Region A is the area corresponding to the loss of position sense in all four limbs and region B is the area corresponding to the loss of pinprick sensation. Because the lateral corticospinal tracts lie between these two regions, a single lesion large enough to encompass both regions A and B would necessarily result in weakness throughout the lower extremities. The preserved proximal strength (item 5) therefore eliminates this potential lesion site.

Similar reasoning eliminates the cortex as a potential localization. The representation of the body surface along the postcentral gyrus is organized in the following order from medial to lateral: distal lower extremity, proximal lower extremity, proximal upper extremity, distal upper extremity, face. The only way a single lesion could produce sensory deficits in both the distal upper extremity and the distal lower extremity would be to involve the proximal portions of the limbs also.

In short, no single lesion site can explain all the findings in this patient. The findings cannot even be explained by positing two lesions. This patient has a multifocal or diffuse condition. By the rules of the game, the next goal is to identify some common characteristic unifying all the lesion sites. In this case, all the findings are sensory deficits restricted to the distal portions of the limbs. This suggests a process affecting peripheral nerves, specifically involving the longest sensory nerves. *Peripheral polyneuropathy* is the term for such a condition (see Chapter 6).

VI. More Examples

The approach presented in Parts III, IV, and V focuses on deductive reasoning rather than memorizing syndromes and patterns of clinical deficits. Nonetheless, it still involves memorizing the location of midline crossing for a core group of pathways. One way to accomplish this memorization and to gain confidence in applying this approach is to practice with multiple examples. A computer tutorial providing such examples is available (https://neurologic.med.umich.edu/).

To use this tutorial, click on the link near the top ("Click Here to Enter the NeuroLogic Modules"). This brings you to the Main Menu page. Click on the "Sorted Cases" box, which brings you to a set of 35 CNS cases and 16 brachial plexus cases; the CNS cases are the ones relevant to this chapter. They can be accessed in any order.

VII. Rules for Speed Play

Even in the limited number of examples presented in Part V, several themes emerge repeatedly. Many of these themes can be summarized as general principles that are often sufficient for localizing a lesion without actually drawing line segments for each symptom and looking for the points of intersection. Most neurologists have internalized these rules. When they encounter a patient like the one described in Example 4, they immediately think of a spinal cord lesion; in fact, this is even a named syndrome (Brown-Séquard syndrome). The patient described in Example 7 is so typical of a patient with polyneuropathy that no neurologist would require diagrams to reach that conclusion.

The following principles summarize many of the "shortcuts" used by neurologists in localizing a lesion. They are useful in many clinical situations, but they are simplifications. If they are applied without thinking, they may result in errors or omissions. Even neurologists sometimes fall into this trap. When a case is confusing, it is always best to analyze it systematically as described in Part V. In fact, with more confusing cases, even the analysis of Part V may be inadequate, and the kind of detailed analysis presented in Part IV may be required.

With those caveats, the following principles may be presented. They are derived from the kind of reasoning already presented in analyzing Examples 1–7; a brief explanation follows each principle.

1. *If someone has deficits of both strength and pain/temperature sensation in a single limb, and no other neurologic abnormalities, the lesion is either in the periphery (nerve/plexus/root) or in the cortex.*

   Explanation: The pathway for pain and temperature sensation crosses the midline soon after entering the spinal cord. The motor pathway crosses in the low medulla. Between these two levels of crossing (i.e., between the low medulla and the spinal cord at the level of the affected limb), the motor pathway is on the opposite side of the nervous system from the sensory pathway. Above the low medulla, the motor pathway is on the same side as the sensory pathway but they are not aligned except in the cortex (see Figures 1.4 and 1.9).

2. *If pain/temperature sensation is reduced in one limb and position/vibration sensation is reduced in a contralateral limb, the lesion is somewhere in the spinal cord (on the same side as the position/vibration deficit).*

   Explanation: The pathway for pain and temperature sensation crosses the midline soon after entering the spinal cord; the pathway for position and vibration sense does not cross until it reaches the low medulla. Between the two sites of crossing (i.e., within the spinal cord), the pathway for pain and temperature in one limb lies on the same side of the nervous system as the pathway for position and vibration sense in the contralateral limbs (see Figure 1.20).

3. *Bilateral sensory and motor deficits throughout the body below a roughly horizontal level on the trunk, with normal function above that level, indicate a spinal cord lesion (at or above that level).*

   Explanation: A large spinal cord lesion will disrupt all ascending fiber tracts from all parts of the body below the lesion, and it will disrupt all descending fiber tracts traveling to those body parts. A smaller spinal cord lesion may spare portions of those fiber tracts. The tracts are arranged in such a way that the spared portions typically contain the fibers corresponding to the uppermost part of the affected region of the body. Hence, a given sensory/motor level can indicate a large spinal cord lesion at that level, or a smaller lesion higher up in the spinal cord.

4. *Increased reflexes in a symptomatic limb suggest a central lesion; reduced reflexes in a symptomatic limb suggest a peripheral lesion.*

   Explanation: The nerve root, plexus, peripheral nerve, and muscle are all included in the reflex arc, which is tonically inhibited by descending pathways from above (see Figure 1.15).

5. *Reduced pain/temperature sensation on one side of the face and the opposite side of the body implies a lesion between the pons and C2 (ipsilateral to the facial numbness). Reduced pain/temperature sensation on one side of the face and the same side of the body implies a lesion in the high brainstem or above.*

   Explanation: The pathway for pain and temperature sensation from the face enters the pons via the trigeminal nerve, descends on the same side to about the C2 level of the spinal cord, crosses, and ascends on the opposite side. The descending pathway (from the pons to C2) is close to the ascending pathway conveying pain and temperature sensation from the contralateral body. After crossing at the C2 level, the tract conveying facial sensation is on the same side as the tract conveying ipsilateral trunk and limb sensation, but the two tracts are not close to each other until reaching the high brainstem (see Figures 1.6 and 1.11).

6. *Facial weakness ipsilateral to body weakness implies a lesion in the high pons or above.*

   Explanation: The facial nerve (supplying the muscles of the face) exits from the pons; no lesion below that level can affect facial strength.

7. *Both a third nerve palsy and Horner syndrome can result in ptosis and pupillary asymmetry, but with a third nerve palsy, the ptosis is on the side of the large pupil; with Horner syndrome, the ptosis is on the side of the small pupil.*

   Explanation: A third nerve palsy often results in dysfunction of parasympathetic fibers traveling with the third nerve, causing a large pupil because of impaired constriction. Horner syndrome is due to damage to the sympathetic system, causing inadequate pupillary dilation and therefore a small pupil. With either lesion, the ptosis is always on the same side as the abnormal pupil (see Chapter 2, Part V, Section B).

8. *Binocular diplopia is always due to a lesion in the brainstem or periphery (nerve/neuromuscular junction/muscle), but not the cortex. A gaze palsy (impaired movement of both eyes in one direction, but both eyes move congruently and remain aligned in all positions of gaze) is due to a lesion in the cortex or brainstem but not in the periphery.*

Explanation: Cortical and brainstem gaze centers control movements of both eyes in parallel; individual eye movements are controlled by brainstem nuclei and mediated by individual cranial nerves. This is discussed further in Chapters 2, 11, and 13.

9. *Visual symptoms restricted to one eye imply a lesion anterior to the chiasm.*

Explanation: From the chiasm back to the occipital cortex, information from the two eyes is combined in the visual system, so that any lesion affecting the visual pathways at the chiasm or behind it will generally affect vision from both eyes. Only prior to the chiasm is visual information from each eye segregated (see Figure 1.16). This point is also discussed in Chapters 2 and 13.

10. *Aphasia or dysphasia (abnormal language processing resulting in difficulty understanding words, recalling words, or organizing words grammatically) implies a lesion in the dominant cerebral hemisphere. Dysarthria (abnormal motor control of speech resulting in disturbances of articulation, rate, rhythm, or voice quality) in the absence of dysphasia suggests a subcortical, brainstem, or cerebellar lesion.*

Explanation: The cognitive processing necessary for language comprehension and production takes place largely in the dominant cerebral hemisphere. The cerebral hemispheres are also involved in the specific motor sequences involved in speech, but there is enough redundancy of function that the unaffected hemisphere can often compensate for a unilateral hemispheric lesion as long as the areas involved in language processing are intact. There is less redundancy at lower levels, so a unilateral subcortical, brainstem, or cerebellar lesion can produce significant dysarthria.

11. *An altered level of consciousness indicates either dysfunction of both cerebral hemispheres or a lesion in the brainstem or the thalamus.*

Explanation: The physiologic basis of "consciousness" is not well understood. Even if it were, it would surely be too complicated to represent in terms of line segments. Suffice it to say that the thalamus and wakefulness-promoting pathways in the brainstem are critical elements, but there is no localized region in the cerebral cortex essential for maintenance of consciousness. A lesion that completely destroys the function of the cerebral cortex on one side will not affect consciousness as long as the brainstem, thalamus, and contralateral cortex are intact. This is discussed further in Chapter 11.

Chapter 2

The Neurologic Examination (What We Localize)

I. More Localization Problems

Example 1. In the dark, a patient's right pupil is 3 mm larger than the left. In bright light, the right pupil is only 1 mm larger than the left.

Questions:

1. Which pupil is abnormal, the right or the left?
2. Which pathway is abnormal, the sympathetic or the parasympathetic?
3. Is this patient likely to have ptosis? If so, on which side?

Example 2. A patient has weakness of the right face, arm, and leg.

Question:

Which is likely to be weaker, the forehead or the lower face?

Example 3. A patient has weakness of hip flexion, knee flexion, and ankle dorsiflexion in the left lower extremity.

Questions:

1. Is this distribution of weakness consistent with a single nerve root lesion?
2. Is this pattern of weakness suggestive of any other lesion localization?

II. General Comments on the Neurologic Examination

A careful history can elicit most of the information necessary to localize a patient's lesion, especially if you follow up open-ended questions with questions that focus on specific nervous system pathways. For example, to investigate temperature sensation, you can ask patients if they have any problems detecting water temperature when washing their hands or stepping into a bathtub. Regarding fine touch discrimination, you can ask patients whether they have problems pulling the correct coin or other objects out of their pockets. Position sense can be explored by asking whether they have problems knowing where their feet are on the accelerator and brake pedals of their cars. Even a history of clonus may sometimes be deduced from patients who experience uncontrollable, rhythmic jerking of the foot when slamming on the brakes. This type of directed questioning may also allow you to differentiate proximal weakness from distal, horizontal diplopia from vertical, monocular vision loss from binocular, aphasia from dysarthria, and so forth.

No matter how accurate and detailed the history, however, the neurologic examination is the most reliable way to identify certain abnormalities, such as subtle weakness, eye movement abnormalities, pupillary defects, sensory deficits, and asymmetric reflexes. Moreover, the information obtained from a history depends on the reliability of the informant. If the informant is a poor observer, has trouble communicating, or for some reason provides misleading information, it is essential to have an independent source of information. The neurologic examination serves this purpose.

The nervous system has many functions, and there are many ways to test each function. The components of a standard neurologic examination are listed in Table 2.1. It would not be practical to perform all possible tests on each patient. Instead, the examination must be tailored to the situation. In patients with no neurologic symptoms, a screening examination is adequate (see Part VI, Section A of this chapter). In patients who do have neurologic symptoms, it is best to try to narrow the list of potential localization sites as much as possible based on the history so you can perform a focused examination aimed at verifying the salient features of the history and refining the localization even further.

One constraint on the neurologic examination is that it requires patient cooperation. Some people are unable or unwilling to cooperate fully with the examination, so findings must be interpreted with caution and checked for internal consistency. A second constraint on the examination, even

Table 2.1 Organization of the Neurologic Examination (* indicates components that are rarely performed)

A. Mental status
  1. Level of alertness
  2. Language
    a. Fluency
    b. Comprehension
    c. Repetition
    d. Naming
    e. Reading
    f. Writing
  3. Memory
    a. Immediate
    b. Short-term
    c. Long-term
      i. Recent (including orientation to place and time)
      ii. Remote
  4. Calculation
  5. Visuospatial function
  6. Abstraction
B. Cranial nerves
  1. Olfaction (CN I)*
  2. Vision (CN II)
    a. Visual fields
    b. Visual acuity
    c. Funduscopic examination
  3. Pupillary light reflex (CNs II, III)
  4. Eye movements (CNs III, IV, VI)
  5. Facial sensation (CN V)
  6. Facial strength
    a. Muscles of mastication (CN V)
    b. Muscles of facial expression (CN VII)
  7. Hearing (CN VIII)
  8. Vestibular function (CN VIII)
  9. Palatal movement (CN X)
  10. Dysarthria (CNs VII, IX, X, XII)
  11. Head rotation (CN XI)
  12. Shoulder elevation (CN XI)
  13. Tongue movements (CN XII)

(continued)

Table 2.1 Continued

C. Motor
  1. Gait
  2. Coordination
  3. Involuntary movements
  4. Pronator drift
  5. Individual muscles
     a. Strength
     b. Bulk
     c. Tone (resistance to passive manipulation)
D. Reflexes
  1. Tendon reflexes
  2. Plantar responses
  3. Superficial reflexes*
  4. "Primitive" reflexes*
E. Sensory
  1. Light touch
  2. Pain/temperature
  3. Joint position sense
  4. Vibration
  5. Double simultaneous stimulation
  6. Graphesthesia*
  7. Stereognosis*

---

when cooperation is not an issue, is the fact that the range of normal findings can be broad. It is frequently difficult to determine whether a given finding is outside the range of normal. For example, one individual may be much stronger than another, but the weaker individual does not necessarily have anything wrong with their nervous system. Weakness that has developed recently is much more indicative of neurologic disease than lifelong weakness. The same is true of hyperreflexia and many other neurologic findings. Unfortunately, it is not always clear whether an examination finding is new or old unless previous examinations have been documented. When no baseline examination is available for comparison, patients can sometimes "serve as their own controls." The two sides of the body should be compared directly at each step of the examination. A finding on the right that is substantially different from the corresponding finding on the left is strong evidence of a neurologic lesion. Even in that circumstance, the lesion could be chronic and irrelevant to the patient's current symptoms. Although the examination supplements the history, it cannot supplant it.

To facilitate side-to-side comparisons and enhance sensitivity to subtle asymmetry, any exam maneuver on one side of the body should be followed directly with the same maneuver on the opposite side before proceeding to a different maneuver. Other than that, the neurologic examination can be performed in any order. Examiners may even change the sequence of the examination from one patient to the next, depending on the patient's symptoms, mobility, and ability to cooperate. Sensory testing and mental status testing are the parts of the examination most likely to make patients uncomfortable, so I typically perform these tests last, but each examiner's style and preferences differ.

The sequence in which the neurologic examination is *presented* is more standardized, primarily to make it easier for a listener or reader to focus and organize the information. If I am particularly interested in a patient's deep tendon reflexes, for example, it helps me to know when the presenter is likely to discuss them. Among other things, it helps me avoid interrupting the presentation to ask about details that the presenter was going to discuss in due course. It doesn't really matter what the sequence of presentation is, as long as it is consistent. Different medical centers have different conventions. A fairly standard sequence is shown in Table 2.1. It can be thought of as "zooming in" on the patient. The component presented first, mental status, could almost be tested by telephone. Little direct observation of the patient is necessary. Gait is tested by observing the patient, but no physical contact is required. The remainder of the motor examination requires some physical contact. The sensory exam is presented last because it requires the closest and most refined physical interactions, such as the small limb movements used when testing joint position sense or the stimuli applied in testing pain sensation. The cranial nerves are inserted as a bridge between mental status and the rest of the examination, and the deep tendon reflexes are positioned between the motor and the sensory exams because the reflex arc includes both sensory and motor components.

The portion of the examination for which presentation in a consistent sequence is most important is the mental status examination. Certain findings on the mental status examination can only be interpreted by knowing a patient's ability to perform other, more fundamental tasks. For example, difficulty with simple calculations may have some localizing significance in a patient who is otherwise cognitively intact, but not in a patient who is unable to answer any questions at all. To give the listener a sense of whether a cognitive deficit is isolated or simply a consequence of some more elemental problem (such as impaired language function or a depressed level of consciousness), it is best to present the level of alertness first, then language function, and then memory. The remainder of the mental status examination can be presented in any order.

III. How to Do the Neurologic Examination

The neurologic examination outlined in Table 2.1 is seldom performed in its entirety, but one must be able to perform each of the components of the neurologic examination when appropriate. This part of the chapter presents instructions for doing so.

A. Mental Status Examination

1. Level of alertness

No special testing is required. While taking the history and examining the patient, observe whether the patient is alert, attentive, sleepy, or unresponsive.

2. Language

a. Fluency

No special testing is required. Throughout the course of the patient interaction, assess whether the patient's phrases and sentences are of normal length, are spoken effortlessly and at a normal rate, and have normal grammatical structure. Note that fluency is independent of content; speech can be completely fluent and still be incomprehensible.

b. Comprehension

Comprehension is often adequately assessed during the routine history and physical but can also be tested explicitly. Give the patient progressively more complex commands, such as one step (e.g., "Touch your nose"), two steps (e.g., "Touch your nose, then stick out your tongue"), and three steps (e.g., "Touch your nose, then stick out your tongue, and then raise your right foot"). Commands that require a body part to cross the midline (e.g., "Touch your right ear with your left thumb") are more complex than those that don't. Increasingly advanced vocabulary ("Point to the entryway." "Point to a source of illumination.") or grammatical constructions can also be used (e.g., "Touch the coin with the pencil." "With the comb, touch the straw.."). Ask the patient progressively more complex questions, either yes/no (e.g., "Does a stone sink in water?" "Do you put on your shirt before your coat?") or otherwise. Again, more complex grammatical constructions such as passive voice or possessive may be useful (e.g., "Is a car's owner a person or an object?" "If a lion was killed by a tiger, which one is still alive?").

c. Repetition

Ask the patient to repeat phrases or sentences of progressively greater length and complexity (e.g., "It is cold outside." or "We all went over there together." or "The lawyer's closing argument convinced the jury." or "Many people admired the airplane pilot's courage and judgment.").

d. Naming

Throughout the interaction, observe whether the patient frequently pauses and struggles to think of words. In addition, test "confrontation naming" by asking the patient to name items as you point to them (e.g., shirt, shoe, phone, collar, lapel, shoelace, heel, receiver). Less common objects are generally harder to name, and parts of an object are harder to name than the entire object. Test "responsive naming" with questions such as "What do you use to dry yourself after a shower?" or "What do you call a person who fixes sinks and toilets?" or "What do you use to pound in a nail?"

e. Reading

Ask the patient to follow a written command. This can be one of the same commands used to test comprehension of spoken language.

f. Writing

Ask the patient to write an original sentence, and to write a sentence from dictation. Look for omitted or added words, or for word substitutions.

3. Memory

a. Immediate memory

Tell the patient "repeat after me," and then recite a string of seven digits. Lengthen or shorten the string until you find the longest string the patient can repeat correctly. This is called the *digit span*. Note: Despite its categorization as "immediate memory," this is really more appropriately considered "attention."

b. Short-term memory

Ask the patient to memorize three unrelated words (e.g., horse, purple, anger), and then distract the patient for 5 minutes (usually by performing other parts of the exam). Then ask the patient to recall the list. If the patient misses an item, give clues (e.g., "One was an animal"), and if this isn't enough, offer a multiple choice (e.g., "It was a cat, a bear, or a horse").

c. Long-term memory

Long-term memory includes both recent and remote memory. Assess recent memory by testing the patient's orientation to time (e.g., day, date, month, season, year), and place (e.g., state, city, building), and by asking questions about events of the past few days or weeks (e.g., "Who are the current candidates for president?" or, assuming an independent source is available for verification, "What did you have for supper last night?"). Remote memory can be tested by asking for the names of the presidents in reverse order as far back as the patient can remember, or by asking about important historical events and dates. The patient can also be asked about details of personal life such as full name, birth date, names and ages of children and grandchildren, and work history, assuming independent verification is available.

4. Calculation

Ask some straightforward computation problems (e.g., 5 + 8 = ?; 6 × 7 = ?; 31 − 18 = ?) and some "word problems" (e.g., "How many nickels are there in $1.35?" "How many quarters in $3.75?").

5. Visuospatial function

Ask the patient to draw a clock, including all the numbers, and to place the hands at 4:10. Ask the patient to draw a cube; for patients who have trouble doing so, draw a cube and ask them to copy it.

6. Abstraction

Ask the patient to explain similarities (e.g., "What do an apple and an orange have in common? . . . a basketball and a grapefruit? . . . a tent and a cabin? . . . a bicycle and an airplane? . . . a sculpture and a symphony?") and differences (e.g., "What's the difference between a radio and a television? . . . a clock and a calendar? . . . a bookstore and a library? . . . a fact and an opinion? . . . character and reputation?").

B. Cranial Nerve Examination

1. Olfaction

Although I do not usually test olfaction, it can be assessed by having the patient occlude one nostril and identify a common scent (e.g., coffee, peppermint, cinnamon) placed under the other nostril.

2. Vision

a. Visual fields

Have the patient cover their left eye. Stand facing the patient from two arm's-lengths away, close your right eye, and stretch your arms forward and to the sides so that your hands are positioned at about 1:30 and 10:30 and just barely visible in your peripheral vision. They should be the same distance from you and the patient. Ask the patient to keep looking directly at your nose and tell you how many fingers you hold up. Quickly flash either one or two fingers on your left hand, right hand, or both. Do this several times; for at least one of the trials, raise fingers on both hands. Next, move your hands down to roughly 4:30 and 7:30 and test again. Then test analogous portions of the visual field of the patient's left eye (closing your left eye and using your right eye as a control).

b. Acuity

Place a handheld visual acuity card 14 inches in front of the patient's right eye, while the left eye is covered. The patient should wear their usual corrective lenses. Ask the patient to read the lowest line on the chart (20/20). If the patient cannot do so, move up a line, and continue doing so until you reach a line where most items are read correctly. Note which line this is, and how many errors the patient makes on this line. Repeat the process for the left eye.

c. Funduscopic examination

Funduscopic examination is described in standard physical examination textbooks.

3. Pupillary light reflex

Reduce the room illumination as much as possible. Shine a penlight on the bridge of the patient's nose, so that you can see both pupils without directing light at either of them. Check that they are the same size. Now move the penlight so that it is directly shining on the right pupil and check to see that both pupils have constricted to the same size. Next, move the penlight back to the bridge of the nose so that both pupils dilate, and then shine the light directly on the left pupil, again checking for equal constriction in the two eyes. Finally, move the penlight rapidly from the left pupil to the right; the pupil size should not change. Swing the light back to the left pupil; again, the pupil size should remain constant. Repeat this "swinging" maneuver several times to be sure there is no consistent tendency for the pupils to be larger when the light is directed at one eye than when it is directed at the other one.

4. Eye movements

Observe the patient's eyelids for *ptosis* (drooping). Have the patient fixate on your finger held about two feet away, in the vertical and horizontal midline. Observe for *nystagmus*—a slow drifting movement of the eyes in one direction, alternating with a quick movement of the eyes in the opposite direction, repeated several times or more.

To evaluate smooth pursuit movements, ask the patient to keep watching your finger without moving their head. Slowly move your finger to the patient's right while observing the smoothness and range of the patient's eye movements. Keep your finger at the far right of the patient's gaze ("3:00") for several seconds while observing again for nystagmus. Move your finger slowly up ("1:00") while making the same observations. Continue making these observations as you move your finger slowly down ("5:00"), back up to the vertical midline ("3:00"), then to the patient's left ("9:00"), up ("11:00"), and down ("7:00"), pausing for a few seconds at the end of each movement to observe for nystagmus. You will have traced an "H."

To evaluate voluntary saccades, hold up your right index finger about 10° to the left of the patient's nose, and hold up your left thumb about 10° to the patient's right. Ask the patient to look at your nose. Then ask the patient to look at your finger. Then ask the patient to look back at your nose. Then ask the patient to look at your thumb. Continue to have the patient move from one target to another in random order several times and observe whether there is a consistent tendency to overshoot or undershoot the target.

5. Facial sensation

Lightly touch the patient's right forehead once, and then repeat on the opposite side. Ask the patient if the two stimuli feel the same. Repeat this procedure on the cheek and on the chin. This is usually adequate testing, unless the patient reports asymmetric facial sensation, in which case you should lightly touch each side of the forehead with a sharp pin and ask the patient if the stimuli feel equally sharp, then repeat the procedure on the cheek and on the chin. Testing of the corneal reflex is not routinely necessary, but it is useful when patients have difficulty following instructions or when the rest of the exam suggests that there may be a problem with facial sensation or strength. It is tested by having the patient look to the far left, then touching the patient's right cornea with a fine wisp of cotton (introduced from the patient's right, outside the field of vision) and observing the reflexive blink that occurs in each eye. The process is then repeated with the left eye.

6. Facial strength

a. Muscles of mastication
Have the patient open the jaw against resistance, and then close the jaw against resistance. Have the patient move the chin from side to side.

b. Muscles of facial expression
Have the patient close their eyes tightly. Observe whether the lashes are buried equally on the two sides and whether you can open either eye manually. Then have the patient look up and wrinkle the forehead; note whether the two sides are equally wrinkled. Have the patient smile and observe whether one side of the face is activated more quickly or more completely than the other.

7. Hearing

For a bedside examination, it usually suffices to perform a quick hearing assessment by holding your fingers a few inches away from the patient's ear and rubbing them together softly. Alternatively, you can hold your hand up as a sound screen and ask the patient to repeat a few numbers that you whisper behind your hand while rhythmically tapping the opposite ear to keep it from contributing. Each ear should be tested separately.

8. Vestibular function

Ask the patient to fixate on your nose as you turn the patient's head to one side as quickly as possible while you observe the patient's eyes to see if they remain fixed on the target. Repeat several times in each direction. This is called the *head impulse test* or the *head thrust maneuver*. It assesses the vestibulo-ocular reflex, which is the mechanism by which the nervous system keeps the eyes pointed in a stable direction even while the head is moving.

9. Palatal movement

Ask the patient to say "aaah" or to yawn; observe whether the two sides of the palate move fully and symmetrically. The palate is most readily visualized if the patient is sitting or standing, rather than supine. There is generally no need to test the gag reflex in a screening neurologic examination. When you have reason to suspect reduced palatal sensation or strength or the patient has difficulty following instructions, the gag reflex can be checked by observing the response when you touch the posterior pharynx on one side with a cotton swab; compare this to the response elicited by touching the other side.

10. Dysarthria

When the patient speaks, listen for articulation errors, abnormalities of voice quality, and irregularities of rate or rhythm.

11. Head rotation

Have the patient turn the head all the way to the left. Place your hand on the left side of the jaw and ask the patient to resist you as you try turning the head back to the right. Palpate the right sternocleidomastoid (SCM) muscle with your other hand at the same time. Repeat this maneuver in the other direction to test the left SCM.

12. Shoulder elevation

Ask the patient to shrug the shoulders while you resist the movement with your hands.

13. Tongue movement

Have the patient protrude the tongue and move it rapidly from side to side. Ask the patient to push the tongue against the left cheek from inside the mouth while you push against it from outside, and then do the same on the right side of the mouth.

C. Motor Examination

1. Gait

Observe the patient's casual gait, preferably with the patient unaware of being observed. Have them walk toward you while walking on the heels, then walk away from you walking on tiptoes. Finally, have the patient walk in tandem, placing one foot directly in front of the other as if walking on a tightrope (i.e., the "drunk-driving test"). Note if the patient is unsteady with any of these maneuvers, or if there is any asymmetry of movement.

Also observe how the arms swing, and look for *festination,* an involuntary tendency for steps to accelerate and become smaller.

2. Coordination

a. Finger tapping
Ask the patient to make a fist with the right hand, then to extend the thumb and index finger and tap the tip of the index finger on the tip of the thumb as quickly as possible. Repeat with the left hand. Observe the speed, accuracy, and regularity of rhythm.

b. Rapid alternating movements
Have the patient alternately pronate and supinate the right hand against a stable surface (such as a table, or the patient's own thigh or left hand) as rapidly as possible; repeat for the left hand. Again, observe speed, accuracy, and rhythm.

c. Finger to nose testing
Ask the patient to use the tip of their right index finger to touch the tip of your index finger, then the tip of their nose (or chin), then your finger again, and so forth. Hold your finger so that it is near the extreme of the patient's reach, and move it to several different positions during the testing. Repeat the test using the patient's left arm. Observe for accuracy, smoothness, and tremor.

Finger chase is a similar test that may be more sensitive. Point your finger toward the patient and ask them to point to your finger with their right index finger, getting as close as possible to your finger without touching it. Then ask the patient to try to keep their finger in the same position relative to your finger as you quickly move your finger to random destinations. Repeat using the patient's left index finger. Observe for undershoot and overshoot (or oscillation between the two).

d. Heel-knee-shin testing
Have the patient lie supine, place the right heel on the left knee, and then move the heel smoothly down the shin to the ankle. Repeat using the left heel on the right shin. Again, observe for accuracy, smoothness, and tremor.

3. Involuntary movements

Observe the patient throughout the history and physical for *tremor, myoclonus* (rapid, shock-like muscle jerks), *chorea* (rapid, sudden, often jerky twitches, similar to myoclonus but more random in location and more likely to blend into one another), *athetosis* (slow, writhing movements of the limbs), *ballismus* (large-amplitude, flinging limb movements), *tics* (abrupt, stereotyped, coordinated movements or vocalizations), *dystonia* (maintenance of an abnormal posture or repetitive twisting movements), or other involuntary motor activity.

4. Pronator drift

Have the patient stretch out the arms so that they are level and fully extended, with the palms facing straight up, and then ask them to close their eyes. Watch for five to ten seconds to see if either arm tends to pronate (so that the palm turns inward) and drift downward.

5. Individual muscles

a. Strength

In the upper extremities, test shoulder abduction, elbow extension, elbow flexion, wrist extension, wrist flexion, finger extension, finger flexion, and finger abduction. In the lower extremities, test hip flexion, hip extension, knee flexion, knee extension, ankle dorsiflexion, and ankle plantar flexion. For each movement, place the limb near the middle of its range, and then ask the patient to resist you as you try to move the limb from that position. For example, in testing shoulder abduction, the patient's arms should be horizontal, forming a letter "T" with the body, and the patient should try to maintain that position while you press down on both arms at a point between the shoulders and the elbows. When possible, place one hand above the joint being examined to stabilize the joint and exert pressure with your other hand just below the joint, to isolate the specific movement you are testing.

b. Bulk

While testing strength, inspect the muscles active in each movement and palpate them for evidence of atrophy. You can usually do this with the hand you have placed above the joint to stabilize it. Fasciculations (random, involuntary muscle twitches) should also be noted.

c. Tone

Ask the patient to relax and let you manipulate their limbs passively. This is harder for most patients than you might imagine, and you may need to try to distract them by engaging them in unrelated conversation, or ask them to let their limbs go limp, "like a wet noodle."

D. Reflex Examination

1. Tendon reflexes (muscle stretch reflexes)

The biceps, triceps, brachioradialis, knee (patellar), and ankle (Achilles) reflexes are the ones commonly tested. The joint under consideration should be at about 90° and fully relaxed. It is often helpful to cradle the joint in your own arm to support it. With your other arm, hold the end of the hammer and let the head of the hammer drop like a pendulum so that it strikes the tendon (specifically, just anterior to the elbow for the biceps reflex, just posterior to the elbow for the triceps reflex, about 10 cm above the wrist on the radial aspect of the forearm for the brachioradialis reflex, just below the patella for the knee reflex, and just behind the ankle for the ankle reflex). You should strive to develop a technique that results in a reproducible level of force from one occasion to the next. When a patient has reflexes that are difficult to elicit, you can amplify them by using reinforcement procedures: Ask the patient to clench their teeth or (when testing lower extremity reflexes) to hook together the flexed fingers of both hands and pull. This is also known as the *Jendrassik maneuver*.

Clonus is a rhythmic series of muscle contractions induced by stretching the tendon. It most commonly occurs at the ankle, where it is typically elicited by suddenly dorsiflexing the patient's foot and maintaining light upward pressure on the sole.

2. Plantar response

Using a blunt, narrow surface (e.g., a tongue blade, key, or handle of a reflex hammer), stroke the sole of the patient's foot on the lateral edge, starting near the heel and proceeding along the lateral edge almost to the base of the little toe, then curve the path medially just proximal to the base of the other toes. This should take the form of a smooth "J" stroke. Always start by applying minimal pressure. This is usually adequate, but if no response occurs, repeat the maneuver with greater pressure.

The normal response is for all the toes to flex (a "flexor plantar response"). When there is damage to the central nervous system motor pathways, a normally suppressed reflex is disinhibited, so an abnormal response is observed: The great toe extends (dorsiflexes) and the other toes fan out. This is called an extensor plantar response; it is also known as a *Babinski sign*.

3. Superficial reflexes

The abdominal reflexes, cremasteric reflexes, and other superficial reflexes are described in standard physical examination textbooks. They are only rarely useful.

4. Primitive reflexes

The grasp, root, snout, and palmomental reflexes are known as primitive reflexes or frontal release signs. These tests do not fit easily into any examination category. They are reflex responses, but their pathways are far more complicated than the monosynaptic arcs of the deep tendon reflexes. I do not test these reflexes. They have very little localizing value; in particular, there is no convincing evidence that they reflect frontal lobe pathology. They are not even reliable indicators of abnormal function, because except for the grasp, each of these reflexes is present in a substantial proportion of normal individuals, especially older individuals.

E. Sensory Examination

1. Light touch sensation

Have the patient close their eyes and tell you whether you are touching their left hand, right hand, or both simultaneously. Repeat this several times, using as a stimulus a single light touch applied sometimes to the medial aspect of the hand and sometimes to the lateral aspect. Note whether the patient consistently fails to detect stimulation in one location. Also note whether the patient consistently "extinguishes" the stimulus on one side of the body when both sides are stimulated simultaneously. Next, touch the patient once lightly on the medial aspect of each hand simultaneously, and ask if they feel the same. Ask the same question for the lateral aspect of each hand. If any abnormalities are detected, extend your region of testing proximally in the limb to map out the precise area of abnormality. Perform analogous testing on the feet.

2. Pain/temperature sensation

Explain to the patient that you will be touching each finger with either the sharp or the dull end of a safety pin, and demonstrate each. Be sure the safety pin is previously unused. Then, with the patient's eyes closed, lightly touch the palmar aspect of the thumb with the sharp point of the pin and ask whether the stimulus is painful. Repeat this for each finger of each hand, usually using the sharp point but including at least one dull stimulus on each hand to be sure the patient is paying attention. Next, touch the patient with the pin once lightly on the medial aspect of each hand, and ask if the two hands feel equally painful. Ask the same question for the lateral aspect of each hand. If any abnormalities are detected, extend your region of testing proximally in the limb to map out the precise area of abnormality. Perform analogous testing on the feet. Discard the pin in a container for contaminated medical "sharps."

It is not usually necessary to test both pain and temperature – either will suffice. You can test temperature in a fashion analogous to pain; a reasonable stimulus is the flat portion of a tuning fork after it has been immersed in cold water and dried.

3. Joint position sense

With the finger and thumb of one hand, stabilize the distal interphalangeal joint of the patient's left thumb by holding it on the medial and lateral aspects. With the finger and thumb of your other hand, hold the medial and lateral aspects of the tip of the thumb and move it slightly up or down. Have the patient close their eyes and identify the direction of movement. Repeat several times. Most normal patients can identify movements of a few degrees or less. Perform analogous testing of the patient's right thumb and both great toes. If abnormalities are detected, proceed to more proximal joints in the same limb until a joint is found where position sense is intact.

The *Romberg* test also helps to assess position sense. Have the patient stand with both feet together, and then note whether they can maintain balance after closing their eyes.

4. Vibration sense

Tap a 128-Hz tuning fork lightly against a solid surface to produce a slight (silent) vibration. With the patient's eyes closed, hold the base of the tuning fork firmly on the distal interphalangeal joint of the patient's left thumb and ask if they can detect the vibration. Let the vibration fade until the patient no longer detects it, then apply the tuning fork to your own thumb to see if you can still feel any vibration. You can even quantify the result by measuring how much time elapses between the point where the patient stops detecting the vibration and when you stop feeling it (although you might need to strike the tuning fork more forcefully to be sure the patient can detect it initially). Repeat this testing on the patient's right thumb and both great toes. For one of the limbs, stop the vibration before applying the tuning fork to the limb to be sure that the patient is paying attention. If not, remind the patient to respond only when they feel a definite vibration, not just pressure. If any abnormalities are detected, apply the tuning fork to progressively more proximal joints until one is found where the vibration is detected normally.

5. Double simultaneous stimulation

The test for double simultaneous stimulation is performed while testing light touch sensation (see *1. Light touch sensation*, above).

6. Graphesthesia

Ask the patient to close their eyes. Draw a number (between 0 and 9) on their index finger using a ballpoint pen (with the tip retracted) or the dull side of a safety pin and ask them to identify the number. Repeat with several other numbers and compare to the other hand. This test is rarely necessary. It is almost never performed on the feet.

7. Stereognosis

Ask the patient to close their eyes and identify a small object (e.g., nickel, dime, quarter, penny, key, paper clip) you place in their right hand. Test the left hand in the same way. This test is rarely necessary, and it is never performed on the feet.

IV. Additional Comments on Terminology and Examination Technique

When reporting examination findings, you must be familiar with some basic definitions and standard conventions. In this part of the chapter, I present some of the more commonly used terms, as well as some hints and comments regarding common sources of confusion. Many of these latter comments reflect my personal observations or opinions, and other neurologists might disagree.

A. Mental Status Examination

1. Terminology

A number of specialized terms often confuse students. Here is a partial glossary.

abulia: loss of initiative, willpower, or drive

acalculia: inability to calculate

agnosia: inability to recognize one or more classes of environmental stimuli, even though the necessary intellectual and perceptual functions are intact

agraphia: inability to write

alexia: inability to read for comprehension

amnesia: inability to retain new information

anomia: inability to name objects or think of words; in practice, often used as a synonym for *dysnomia*

anosognosia: inability to recognize one's own impairment

aphasia: literally, a complete loss of language function, but in practice, used as a synonym for *dysphasia*

aphemia: complete loss of the ability to speak, but retained comprehension and writing ability

apraxia: inability to perform a previously learned set of coordinated movements even though the necessary component skills (including intellect, language function, strength, coordination, and sensation) remain intact

Broca aphasia: acquired language disorder characterized by nonfluent verbal output with omission of relational words (prepositions, conjunctions, articles, and minor modifiers), abnormal *prosody*, impaired repetition, and relatively intact comprehension. See *nonfluent aphasia;* see also Figure 1.19

conduction aphasia: acquired language disorder characterized by prominent impairment of repetition, relatively intact comprehension, and verbal output that is *fluent* but contains *literal paraphasias;* see Figure 1.19

delirium: an acute, transient, fluctuating confusional state characterized by impairment in maintaining and shifting attention, often associated with agitation, disorientation, fear, irritability, illusions, or hallucinations

dementia: an acquired, persistent decline of intellectual function that causes impaired performance of daily activities, without clouding of the sensorium or underlying psychiatric disease

dysnomia: difficulty naming objects or finding the desired words

dysphasia: acquired disorder of language not due to generalized intellectual impairment or psychiatric disturbance

fluent: an adjective used to describe verbal output that is normal to excessive, easily produced, with normal phrase length (five or more words) and normal *prosody*

fluent aphasia: acquired language disorder in which verbal output is *fluent.* See *Wernicke aphasia* and *conduction aphasia*

Gerstmann syndrome: the constellation of (1) *agraphia,* (2) *acalculia,* (3) *right-left confusion,* and (4) *finger agnosia;* classically associated with lesions in the angular gyrus of the dominant hemisphere (but the subject of endless debate)

jargon: verbal output containing so many *literal paraphasias* that the words are unrecognizable

nonfluent: an adjective used to describe verbal output that is sparse, with only one to four words per phrase

nonfluent aphasia: acquired language disorder in which verbal output is *nonfluent.* See *Broca aphasia*

paraphasia: a substitution error in which the word produced is similar in sound or meaning to the intended word. A *literal* or *phonemic* paraphasia is a sound substitution error resulting in production of a word that is phonemically related to the intended word (e.g., "greed" or "greeb" instead of "green"). A *semantic* or *verbal* paraphasia is a word substitution error in which the word produced is semantically related to the intended word (e.g., "blue" instead of "green")

prosody: the rhythm and tempo of speech

prosopagnosia: inability to recognize faces

transcortical aphasia: acquired language disorder in which the ability to repeat is relatively intact; see Figure 1.19

Wernicke aphasia: acquired language disorder characterized by markedly impaired comprehension and repetition, with verbal output that is *fluent* but contaminated by numerous *paraphasias* or, in severe cases, *jargon.* See *fluent aphasia*; see also Figure 1.19

The following terms are discouraged:

expressive aphasia (discouraged term): acquired language disorder in which verbal output is *nonfluent.* See *Broca aphasia* and *nonfluent aphasia*

receptive aphasia (discouraged term): acquired language disorder in which comprehension is impaired. See *fluent aphasia* and *Wernicke aphasia*

2. Patient willingness to participate

Many patients resist formal mental status testing. Some find it threatening. Others are offended by it ("What do you mean, do I know my name?"), and some just don't see the point. In fact, formal mental status testing is often unnecessary, and I generally reserve it for patients whose mental status is suspect, based on information I obtain in the history or the rest of the examination (see Part VI, Section A of this chapter). When I do see the need to do a formal mental status examination, I usually introduce it by saying, "Now I'm going to test your memory. I'm going to ask you to remember some words. Then I'm going to distract you with a bunch of questions, some of which will be easy and some will be hard. Then I'll test you on those words." Most patients can understand the need for testing memory, and they are more willing to accept all the other components of the mental status examination if they are presented as "distractions."

Even so, some patients find the mental status examination so annoying that they won't participate, and some even refuse to proceed with any other portion of the physical examination. For this reason, I usually defer formal mental status testing until I have nearly completed the rest of the examination. By then, I will have observed the patient's ability to express themselves, follow instructions, remember their history, and respond to questions, and this will help me tailor my examination.

3. Tailoring the examination to the patient

For each cognitive domain tested in the mental status examination, the goal is to determine the patient's level of function as precisely as possible: the patient can correctly perform tasks at or below that level of difficulty, but has trouble with more difficult tasks. Try to guess the approximate level of performance you expect from a patient and then ask a screening question that might be a little too tough. If the patient gets the correct answer, you can skip the easier questions. If the patient doesn't get the correct answer, you can gradually reduce the difficulty of your questions until you have reached the patient's level. This approach saves time. Try to stockpile questions of various levels of complexity, so you don't have to think them up on the spot. For example, it is useful to remember sentences of different word lengths for testing repetition. A reasonably tough math problem that I often use as my initial screening question for people who have completed high school is "How much change would you get from a dollar if you bought six items at twelve cents each?"

4. Aphasia terminology

People with aphasia usually have at least some degree of impairment in all three of the fundamental dimensions of language—fluency, comprehension, and repetition—but the relative severity of impairment varies. When describing aphasia, I recommend explicitly describing the pattern of language deficits, focusing especially on the degree to which each of the three dimensions is impaired, rather than trying to find a single term that summarizes the pattern.

Do not confuse speech and language. *Dysarthria* is an impairment of the motor functions necessary for speech production. Dysarthria is not a language disorder, and it is not a component of the mental status examination.

5. Cultural and educational factors

A patient's background will obviously influence performance on mental status testing, and the examiner must try to take this into account. There is no reliable way to do this; it is ultimately a matter of gestalt. Your estimate of the expected level of performance will be influenced by your interactions with the patient during the history and examination and also by their medical and social history, especially their occupational and educational experiences. Some tests are affected more than others by these factors. For example, the ability to copy a sequence of repetitive hand movements is relatively independent of education. In contrast, the interpretation of proverbs is so dependent on an individual's cultural and educational exposure that I consider it practically useless and instead rely on the interpretation of similarities and differences for assessing abstract thought.

6. Standardized screening tests

Don't confuse the mental status examination with the Mini-Mental State Examination (MMSE) or the Montreal Cognitive Assessment (MoCA). These are specific batteries of questions commonly used as quick screening instruments (the MoCA is a little more comprehensive than the MMSE). Their value lies in the fact that they are simple, don't take much time to administer, and yield a numerical value that can be followed over time, but they are no substitute for a thorough mental status examination. Accurate assessment of a patient's level of function in specific cognitive domains requires tailoring the examination to the patient or else referring the patient for comprehensive neuropsychological testing.

7. Reporting findings

It is most informative to report patients' actual responses, rather than interpretations such as "mildly abnormal" or "slightly concrete."

B. Cranial Nerve Examination

1. Olfaction

I almost never test the sense of smell. When patients give a history of olfactory problems, I take them at their word. Formal instruments for testing olfaction are available. They are particularly useful for research purposes, especially with respect to Parkinson disease and other degenerative diseases that are associated with an impaired sense of smell. The olfactory loss associated with COVID-19 infection is discussed in Chapter 10.

2. Visual fields

There are many alternatives to the technique for testing visual fields described in Part III of this chapter. You can ask patients to tell you when they first see a test stimulus as you slowly move it in from the periphery at various orientations. You can place your hands in various spots in the field, wiggle a finger on one or both hands, and ask patients to point to the finger that moved (or say "both"). You can ask patients to tell you when they can detect that a stimulus is red as you move it in from the periphery of the field (the "kinetic red target" method). Each of these techniques has advantages and disadvantages, and some neurologists have very strong opinions about which technique is best. I prefer the method described in Part III or the "Which finger wiggled?" technique because the visual stimulus can be presented very briefly, minimizing the opportunity for the patient to shift fixation (which could result in testing a different region of the visual field than I thought I was testing). Also, I find the other techniques harder to interpret when patients have mental status abnormalities—even counting fingers may be too great a cognitive load in some cases. Regardless of the technique used, each eye must be tested separately. Otherwise, if there is a defect in a portion of the visual field of only one eye, the other eye will be able to compensate and the defect will not be detected. One example of this situation is the bitemporal hemianopia that can occur with a lesion in the optic chiasm (see Chapter 1, Part V)—the defective hemifield of each eye corresponds to the intact hemifield of the other eye, so the patient may be completely unaware of the deficit until each eye is tested separately.

3. Eye movements

Eye movement abnormalities may be masked by convergence if the target is too close to the patient, but if you stand too far away, it may be difficult for you to see subtle abnormalities. I often position my head close to the patient and off to the side while holding the target (my finger or my reflex hammer) as far away from the patient as possible.

4. Corneal and gag reflexes

Because testing the corneal reflex and the gag reflex is uncomfortable for the patient, I only perform these tests when I am trying to answer a specific question. When I check the gag reflex, I always check it bilaterally. About 20% of normal individuals do not have a gag reflex, so the test is most informative when the responses are asymmetric.

5. Weber and Rinne tests

Most physical diagnosis textbooks advocate the Weber and Rinne tests for distinguishing conductive hearing loss from sensorineural deafness. I do not. I find that patients have difficulty understanding what is being asked, and they give inconsistent responses (especially on the Weber test). Even if these tests gave consistently reliable results, they would still not be as sensitive or as informative as an audiogram. I use the examination to determine whether or not there is hearing loss; if there is, I send the patient for an audiogram.

C. Motor Examination

1. Grading muscle strength

The most common convention for grading muscle strength is the 0 to 5 Medical Research Council (MRC) scale:

0 = no contraction

1 = visible muscle twitch but no movement of the joint

2 = weak contraction insufficient to overcome gravity

3 = weak contraction able to overcome gravity but no additional resistance

4 = weak contraction able to overcome some resistance but not full resistance

5 = normal; able to overcome full resistance

The most compelling feature of this scale is its reproducibility. For example, an examiner is unlikely to assign a score of 1 to a muscle that another examiner graded 3 or stronger. A major limitation of the scale is that it is insensitive to subtle differences in strength. In particular, grade 4 covers a wide range, so that in most clinical situations the MRC scale does not allow precise differentiation of the severity of weakness from one muscle to the next. Similarly, it is not a sensitive tool for documenting moderate changes in strength over time. Many clinicians try to compensate for this by using intermediate grades, such as 3+ or 5-, but there is no consensus on how these intermediate grades should be defined so they are less reproducible.

2. Terminology

a. Patterns of weakness

Weakness of a single limb is called *monoparesis*. *Hemiparesis* is weakness of one side of the body; *paraparesis* is weakness of both lower extremities; and *quadriparesis* is weakness of all four limbs. *Monoplegia, hemiplegia, paraplegia*, and *quadriplegia* are analogous terms that refer to complete or nearly complete paralysis of the involved limbs. *Diplegia* is a term that is best avoided because different authors use it differently.

b. Tone (resistance to passive manipulation)

Several forms of increased resistance to passive manipulation are distinguished. *Spasticity* depends on the limb position and on how quickly the limb is moved, classically resulting in a "clasp-knife phenomenon" when the limb is moved rapidly: the limb moves freely for a short distance, but then there is a "catch" such that the examiner must use progressively more force to move the limb until at a certain point there is a sudden release and the limb moves freely again. Spasticity is generally greatest in the flexors of the upper extremity and the extensors of the lower extremity. These are the muscles that are usually least affected when someone has the upper motor neuron (UMN) pattern of weakness discussed in Part V, Section C. This pattern is easy to remember for anyone who has seen patients with long-standing hemiparesis (especially if the patients did not receive physical therapy): these patients hold the hemiparetic arm flexed at the elbow, wrist, and fingers and pressed tightly to the chest, and they walk with the hemiparetic leg stiffly extended and the ankle plantar flexed, forcing them to circumduct the leg. *Rigidity*, in contrast to spasticity, is characterized by abnormally high resistance throughout the movement. *Lead-pipe* rigidity applies to resistance that is uniform throughout the movement. *Cogwheel* rigidity is characterized by rhythmic interruption of the resistance, producing a ratchet-like effect. Rigidity is usually accentuated by distracting the patient. *Paratonia*, or *"gegenhalten,"* is increased resistance that becomes less prominent when the patient is distracted; without such distraction, the patient seems unable to relax the muscle. This is particularly common in patients who are anxious or who have dementia. When paratonia is prominent, other abnormalities of tone are difficult to assess.

c. Coordination

Coordination testing is often referred to as cerebellar testing, but this is a misnomer. Although the cerebellum is very important in the production of coordinated movements and particular abnormal findings on coordination testing may suggest cerebellar disease, other systems also play critical roles. As an obvious example, severe arm weakness will prevent a patient from performing finger-to-nose testing, even though the cerebellum and its pathways may be intact.

3. Modifications of strength testing

a. Selection of muscles to test

The eight upper-extremity movements and six lower-extremity movements tested in the examination described in Part III of this chapter are sufficient for a screening examination. If some of these muscles are weak, or if the patient reports focal weakness, additional testing may be necessary to determine if the weakness is in the distribution of a specific nerve or nerve root.

b. Limb position

The position of the joint during strength testing determines the mechanical advantage of the patient relative to the examiner. For example, it is much easier to overcome patients when they are trying to extend the elbow from a fully flexed position than it is when they are starting from a position of nearly maximal extension. In most cases it is reasonable to test the muscle with the joint at about mid-position, although positions that increase the patient's mechanical advantage may be preferable for particularly strong examiners or frail patients.

Some examiners test corresponding muscles on both sides (e.g., the left and right biceps muscles) simultaneously. I usually do not do this because it prevents me from using one hand to stabilize the joint and palpate the muscle.

An alternative to the strength examination technique presented in Part III in this chapter is to position the patient's limb and then ask the patient to move the limb steadily in a specified direction while the examiner resists the movement. I generally prefer to follow the format presented in Part III because it allows me to give essentially the same instruction ("Don't let me move your limb") for all movements. This is especially helpful when patients are confused, when they have aphasia or dementia, or when we are communicating through an interpreter. It may take them a while to understand the instruction initially, but once they understand the task for one or two muscles they usually comprehend it much more readily for subsequent muscles.

D. Reflex Examination

1. Grading reflexes

The most common convention for grading deep tendon reflexes is simple but imprecise:

0 = absent

1 = reduced (hypoactive)

2 = normal

3 = increased (hyperactive)

4 = clonus

Some examiners use a grade of 5 to designate sustained clonus, reserving 4 for unsustained clonus that eventually fades after 2 to 10 beats. Also, some examiners include a reflex grade of 1/2 to indicate a reflex that can only be obtained using reinforcement.

The obvious limitation of this terminology is that it provides no guidelines for determining when reflexes are reduced, normal, or increased. This is left up to individual judgment, based on the examiner's sense of the range of reflexes present in healthy individuals.

2. Detection and documentation of subtle asymmetry

Comparison between reflexes in one part of the body and another is much more important than the absolute reflex grade. The most important comparison is between corresponding reflexes on the right and left, where even subtle asymmetry may be clinically meaningful. For example, patients with an S1 radiculopathy may have an ankle reflex that would be considered normal, yet it is clearly less brisk than the ankle reflex on the other side. This is another limitation of the reflex grading scale: It does not express subtle distinctions that may be clinically important. For this reason, many examiners augment the scale by using "+" or "−" to designate intermediate grades. These grades have very little reproducibility from one examiner to another (or even from one examination to the next by a single examiner). They are only useful for indicating that asymmetry exists, not for quantifying it in any meaningful way.

When reflexes are brisk, it is difficult to detect slight asymmetry. For the most sensitive comparison, it is best to reduce the stimulus until it is just barely above threshold for eliciting the reflex. In patients with brisk reflexes, I can often set the reflex hammer aside and elicit the reflex by tapping lightly with my fingers. Once I have found the threshold stimulus for a given reflex, I look for two manifestations of asymmetry. First, is the threshold stimulus the same on each side, or do I consistently need to hit harder on one side than the other? Second, if the threshold stimulus is the same on each side, does it elicit the same magnitude of response on each side? Such subtle asymmetry is most readily detected by testing the reflex on one side immediately after testing the corresponding reflex on the other side, rather than testing all reflexes in one limb before testing the contralateral limb.

Another technique I use to heighten sensitivity to subtle reflex asymmetry is to place my thumb on the patient's tendon and strike my thumb rather than striking the tendon directly. This helps me aim more accurately and allows me to feel the tendon contraction. Moreover, it demonstrates to patients that I am willing to "share the pain," thereby gaining their sympathy and cooperation.

3. Relaxing the patient

Relaxation is critical in the reflex examination. Tendon reflexes are difficult to elicit when patients tense the muscles being tested. It is helpful to distract patients by engaging them in conversation while testing their reflexes. I take this opportunity to ask questions that I forgot to ask earlier, or if I have decided that formal mental status testing is necessary, I often do it while testing reflexes.

4. Significance of a Babinski sign

The Babinski sign is not graded. It is an abnormal finding that is either present or not. It is one of the few neurologic examination findings that can be interpreted without comparison to the contralateral response or consideration of patient effort.

E. Sensory Examination

The sensory examination can be the most frustrating part of the neurologic examination. The instructions often must be repeated several times or more before patients understand what they are being asked to do. Even then, some patients overinterpret negligible distinctions while others have difficulty attending to the task and fail to report important abnormalities. This part of the examination is also tiresome and somewhat uncomfortable for patients. For these reasons, the sensory examination is usually one of the last things I test. That way, I have a fairly good sense of whether the patient is likely to overinterpret small differences, and I can adjust accordingly. Furthermore, if a patient gets exasperated and insists on terminating the exam altogether (which sometimes happens), I already have most of the information I need from the other parts of the exam.

V. Interpretation of the Neurologic Examination

The general principles governing lesion localization were discussed in Chapter 1. The following discussion presents some additional principles that are often helpful in deducing lesion localization based on specific examination findings.

A. Mental Status Examination

Cognition is poorly understood. All of the categories used to describe mental status (e.g., calculation, abstraction) are convenient simplifications, but they do not necessarily reflect the way in which the brain actually functions. For example, it is very unlikely that any region or circuit in the brain is devoted specifically or exclusively to mathematical calculation.

This complicates the interpretation of the mental status examination. For example, students often ask whether the subtraction of serial sevens ("Count backwards from 100 by 7") is a test of calculation or of attention. The answer is both, and neither. For patients to subtract serial sevens successfully they must (1) be alert, (2) comprehend language well enough to understand a fairly abstract command, (3) retain the command in memory long enough to process it, (4) possess the necessary calculation skills, (5) verbalize the response, and (6) maintain attention on the task so that the current result can be taken as the basis for generating the next one. It is not possible to assign a one-to-one correlation between a task on the mental status examination and a single cognitive function in the same way that abduction of an eye correlates to the function of a single lateral rectus muscle. When a patient is unable to perform a cognitive task, there are always multiple possible explanations. The examiner must observe the response to a variety of tasks, determine which ones are difficult for the patient, and try to determine the kinds of cognitive processing common to those tasks. Inferences about lesion localization are then possible.

Decreased level of alertness occurs only with dysfunction of both cerebral hemispheres, the thalamus, or the wakefulness-promoting pathways in the brainstem (see Speed Rule 11 in Chapter 1). The usual cause is a generalized metabolic abnormality, such as hypoxia or hyperglycemia. Less commonly, appropriately placed structural lesions (especially expanding ones) may produce the same result. The implications and management options are very different for structural causes and metabolic causes, and a major goal of the examination is to distinguish between these two possibilities (see Chapter 11).

Mental status changes in alert patients can result from either focal or generalized processes. Generalized processes usually affect all cognitive functions about equally, although the initial manifestations may just be inattention or word-finding difficulty. Focal lesions typically affect some cognitive functions more than others, and the pattern of cognitive deficits can have some localizing significance.

Many of the best known examples of selective mental status abnormality involve language function. Figure 1.19 A, B, and C illustrates the traditional model for conceptualizing these disorders. As discussed in Chapter 1, this model is both inaccurate and incomplete, but its principal dimensions— fluency, comprehension, and repetition—still provide a fairly simple way to classify language disorders.

For example, a classic Wernicke aphasia (lesion site #1 in Figure 1.19 C) is characterized by impaired comprehension and repetition with relative sparing of fluency. Any aphasia in which repetition is relatively intact is called *transcortical:* transcortical *sensory* when comprehension is impaired, transcortical *motor* when verbal output is nonfluent, and *mixed* transcortical when both comprehension and fluency are abnormal (lesion sites #4, #5, and #6 in Figure 1.19C).

Other cognitive abnormalities that may be seen in relative isolation include *acalculia, agraphia, alexia,* and *apraxia.* Each of these deficits is associated with focal lesions in the dominant hemisphere. The left hemisphere is dominant for language in almost all right-handed individuals. The left hemisphere is also language-dominant in most left-handed subjects, but the relationship is less predictable.

Neglect of one side of the environment can be seen with a focal lesion in either hemisphere, but it is much more common and tends to be more severe when the lesion is in the nondominant hemisphere (i.e., the hemisphere that is not dominant for language), especially the non-dominant parietal lobe. Nondominant parietal lesions may also produce anosognosia, which is the inability to recognize the existence or severity of one's own impairment.

Unilateral disease of the prefrontal cortex often has surprisingly few clinical consequences, but bilateral prefrontal disease is typically associated with difficulty maintaining and shifting attention. Such patients will demonstrate both impersistence (an inability to stick with a task or topic of conversation) and perseveration (a tendency to continue returning to tasks and topics of conversation even when they are no longer appropriate).

None of these focal findings has any localizing significance unless it occurs out of proportion to other cognitive deficits. Each of them can occur as part of a general dementing illness such as Alzheimer disease. In fact, it is often impossible to assess language function or other "focal" functions when significant dementia is present, or when there is reduction in the level of alertness. People with generalized cognitive impairment perform poorly on all aspects of the mental status examination, and it is usually futile to try to determine if one function is more severely affected than another.

B. Cranial Nerve Examination

1. Visual field defects
Because of the precise spatial organization of the visual pathways throughout their course, visual field defects can be exquisitely localizing at times.

The basic principles of visual field defects and their localizing value are discussed in Chapter 1 (see Figure 1.16) and Chapter 13.

2. Pupillary abnormalities

a. Asymmetric pupils (anisocoria)
The sympathetic and the parasympathetic pathways that determine pupillary size were discussed in Chapter 1 (see Figures 1.17 and 1.18). In most circumstances, the sympathetic and parasympathetic systems are both active simultaneously, and pupillary size is determined by the relative activity in the two systems. This results in potential ambiguity when one pupil is larger than the other (*anisocoria*): the sympathetic pathway (which dilates the pupil) could be damaged on the side of the smaller pupil or the parasympathetic pathway (which constricts the pupil) could be malfunctioning

on the side of the larger pupil. To decide, the pupils should be examined both in bright light and in the dark. If the pupillary asymmetry is greatest in the dark, then the lesion is in the sympathetic system because darkness induces maximal dilation (Figure 2.1A). Conversely, pupillary asymmetry that is greatest in bright light indicates a lesion in the parasympathetic pathway (Figure 2.1B). When the pupillary asymmetry is of equal magnitude in dark and in light, it is generally physiologic (i.e., a normal variant).

Another clue to the lesion site in a patient with anisocoria may be provided by ptosis. Because the parasympathetic fibers travel with the third cranial nerve for much of their course, a parasympathetic lesion often produces other signs of third nerve dysfunction, including eye movement abnormalities or pronounced ptosis (because the levator palpebrae muscle is innervated by the third nerve). Sympathetic lesions also produce ptosis, because they innervate Müller's muscle in the eyelid, but this is a much smaller muscle than the levator palpebrae, so the ptosis is much less dramatic. Thus, ptosis on the side of the larger pupil indicates a parasympathetic (and third nerve) lesion on that side. Mild ptosis on the side of the smaller pupil indicates a sympathetic lesion on that side (Horner syndrome). This is a restatement of Speed Rule 7 in Chapter 1.

b. Afferent pupillary defect

The pupillary reflex has both an afferent and an efferent limb. Anisocoria indicates an efferent defect (i.e., a lesion in the efferent fibers supplying the pupillary sphincter and dilator muscles). In contrast, an afferent defect (i.e., a lesion in the retina or optic nerve) does not produce anisocoria. Instead, an afferent defect produces abnormal findings on the "swinging flashlight test." To understand this test, you must recognize two facts. First, pupillary size is determined by an average of the illumination detected by each eye. For a simple demonstration of this, observe a normal subject's right pupil while covering their left eye: The pupil enlarges, because the average illumination has been effectively halved. Second, the efferent limb of the pupillary reflex is bilateral, so in normal subjects both pupils receive the same "instructions" and they are always the same size. Even if there is an afferent problem, so that one of the eyes registers less light than it should, this input projects bilaterally in the brainstem and affects both pupils equally, so the pupils are still equal in size. The pupils will only be unequal in size when the efferent pathways are not working properly.

Now consider what happens when a patient has an optic nerve lesion. For purposes of illustration, assume the lesion is in the left optic nerve and that it halves the amount of illumination that eye registers. If you shine a

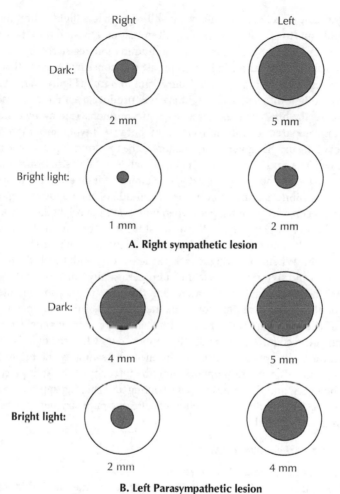

Fig. 2.1 Diagram illustrating the distinction between sympathetic and parasympathetic lesions producing anisocoria. When the left pupil is larger than the right, it could mean a right sympathetic lesion (A) or a left parasympathetic lesion (B). With sympathetic lesions, the pupillary asymmetry is greatest in the dark, whereas with parasympathetic lesions, the asymmetry is greatest in bright light.

bright light directly in the left eye, it will register less illumination than it should, but it will still register more illumination than it did in the ambient room light, so the average of the illumination registered by the two eyes will increase. As a result, both pupils will constrict. Assume that this produces a change in pupil size from 5 mm to 3 mm (Figure 2.2A and B). A bright light directed at the right eye will produce a similar response: In this case, the brain will register an even greater increase in average illumination compared to ambient room light, because it will register the "full" effect of the bright light, not just half of it. The resulting pupillary constriction will be even stronger—producing a change in pupil size from 5 mm to 2.5 mm, for example (Figure 2.2C). It is difficult for an examiner to appreciate this subtle a distinction in the magnitude of the pupillary response. But now consider what happens when you swing the bright light back and forth between the two eyes. When you shine it in the left eye, both pupils are 3 mm. When you swing the light to the right eye, both pupils constrict to 2.5 mm. When you swing it back to the left eye, both pupils dilate back to 3 mm, and so forth. Because the examiner usually can observe the pupil under the bright light more readily than the other pupil, you will note the left pupil dilating each time you shine the light in it. This result might seem paradoxical, as if the pupil were dilating in response to bright light, but not when you recognize that the dilation only occurs when the light is swung from the right eye to the left one. In effect, by swinging the bright light back and forth, you are simply varying the intensity of the light perceived by the brain, and the pupils are constricting and dilating appropriately in response. This finding is termed a left afferent pupillary defect, or a left Marcus Gunn pupil.

3. Eye movement abnormalities

a. Muscle/movement correlations

When you ask a patient to watch your finger as you trace an "H" in the air, every movement tests a pair of muscles, one in each eye. The right eye's lateral rectus muscle and the left eye's medial rectus muscle move the eyes to the patient's right. The left lateral rectus and right medial rectus muscles move the eyes to the patient's left. When an eye is fully abducted, the superior rectus moves it up and the inferior rectus moves it down. When an eye is fully adducted, the inferior oblique muscle moves it up and the superior oblique muscle moves it down. For example, when a patient who is looking to their right moves their eyes upward from "3:00" to "1:00," they activate their right superior rectus muscle and their left inferior oblique muscle.

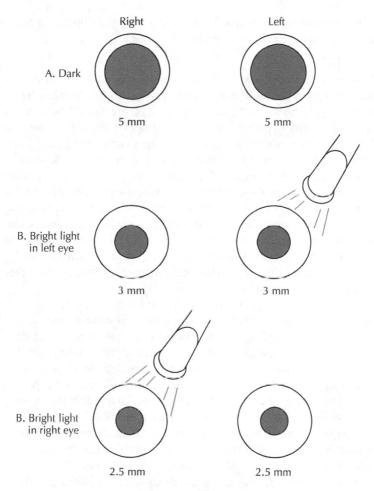

Left afferent pupillary defect

Fig. 2.2 Diagram illustrating a left afferent pupillary defect. The left pupil is the same size as the right under all conditions of illumination (A–C), because the efferent pathways are intact, but both pupils are smaller when light is directed at the right eye (C) than when it is directed at the left eye (B), because light is detected better by the right eye. Alternate swinging of the light between the two eyes therefore produces dilation each time the light is directed to the left eye.

When they then look down to "5:00," they activate their right inferior rectus muscle and their left inferior oblique muscle.

b. Gaze palsy

To keep both eyes focused on the same target even when the head or the target is moving, the two eyes must move conjugately. Conjugate eye movements are governed by cortical and brainstem "gaze centers." The horizontal gaze center in the left cerebral cortex directs gaze to the right. It accomplishes this by sending a message to the brainstem gaze center that directs gaze to the right, which is the right sixth nerve nucleus in the pons. Some of the cells in this nucleus have axons that travel in the right sixth nerve to innervate the lateral rectus muscle of the right eye, turning it to the right (abduction); others have axons that travel in the left *medial longitudinal fasciculus (MLF)*, crossing the midline and traveling up to the left third nerve nucleus and synapsing on cells whose axons travel in the left third nerve to innervate the medial rectus muscle of the left eye, turning it to the right also (adduction). Analogous gaze centers in the right cerebral cortex and left sixth nerve nucleus direct gaze to the left.

When there is malfunction of a cortical or brainstem gaze center or the pathway connecting them, the result is a *gaze palsy*: the eyes are aligned and they move conjugately, but they have limited movement in one direction. Because gaze palsies don't cause ocular misalignment, they don't cause double vision. When the lesion is in the sixth nerve nucleus (the brainstem gaze center), the neurons there cannot be activated either voluntarily or via the vestibulo-ocular reflex (discussed in Part VI, Section C of this chapter). This is called a *nuclear* gaze palsy. When the lesion is in a cortical gaze center, only voluntary gaze is impaired; the vestibular connections with the brainstem gaze center remain intact, so the vestibulo-ocular reflex is preserved. This is called a *supranuclear* gaze palsy.

Someone with a lesion in the left cerebral cortex affecting both the gaze center and the motor pathway will have difficulty directing gaze to the right, so they will have a "left gaze preference," and they will also have right arm and leg weakness. Someone with a lesion in the right sixth nerve nucleus will also have difficulty directing gaze to the right (a left gaze preference), but if they have weakness of the arm or leg it will be on the left side of the body because the descending motor pathway doesn't cross until it reaches the low medulla. This leads to another speed rule: *If someone has a gaze preference for the direction away from their weak limbs, the lesion is in the cerebral cortex; if someone has a gaze preference toward their weak limbs, the lesion is in the pons.*

c. Internuclear ophthalmoplegia

Dysfunction of cranial nerve III, IV, or VI (or of the nuclei of cranial nerve III or IV) results in ocular misalignment, so when both eyes are open the patient sees two images (dysfunction of the nucleus of cranial nerve VI causes a gaze palsy, not double vision, as discussed in the previous two paragraphs). Specific patterns of these eye movement abnormalities and their localizing significance are discussed in Chapter 13. Isolated impairment of adduction in a single eye merits special recognition. This could conceivably result from damage to a single medial rectus muscle, a lesion in one tiny branch of one third nerve, or a focal neuromuscular junction problem, but it is much more commonly due to a lesion in the MLF on the side of the eye that isn't adducting normally. An MLF lesion is termed an *internuclear ophthalmoplegia*, or *INO*, because it is located between the nucleus of cranial nerve VI on one side and the nucleus of cranial nerve III on the other side. When someone with a left-sided INO tries to look to their right, their left cortical gaze center and right brainstem gaze center activate normally and the message gets transmitted appropriately to the right lateral rectus muscle, but the message intended for the left medial rectus muscle is disrupted. The adduction difficulty is accompanied by nystagmus in the right eye as it abducts; in fact, in subtle cases, this may be the most prominent finding. A left-sided INO only causes problems when the patient is attempting to move both eyes to the right; the left third nerve and medial rectus muscle continue to function normally in situations that do not require conjugate eye movements (e.g., convergence on a near object). Analogously, someone with a right-sided INO has problems when trying to look to their left.

4. Facial weakness

The cell bodies of upper motor neurons (UMNs) are in the motor cortex and their axon terminals are in the brainstem or spinal cord, so they reside entirely in the central nervous system. UMNs synapse on lower motor neurons (LMNs). LMN cell bodies are in the brainstem or spinal cord, but their axons run primarily in the peripheral nervous system. As a result, differentiation of UMN and LMN findings can be very helpful in determining the level of the nervous system that is malfunctioning.

For the neurons controlling the muscles of facial expression, the LMN cell bodies are located in the facial nerve nucleus in the pons and the axons travel in the facial nerve. The pattern of facial weakness can help differentiate between UMN and LMN lesions. When one entire side of the face is weak, the lesion is usually in the LMN. With a lesion affecting UMNs (such as a stroke affecting the motor cortex on one side), the forehead muscles are often spared. The traditional explanation for this (though the evidence is sparse) is that the portion of the facial nerve nucleus containing the cell bodies of LMNs that innervate the forehead muscles typically gets input from the motor strips of both cerebral hemispheres, so it can still be activated by the cortex contralateral to the lesion. In contrast, the portion of the facial nerve nucleus that controls the lower face receives its input predominantly from the contralateral cortex so the ipsilateral cortex can't serve as a "backup."

5. Hearing loss and vertigo

As explained in Chapter 1, a central lesion affects hearing in both ears almost equally. The only way to produce hearing loss restricted to one ear is with a peripheral lesion. Examination findings that help to distinguish between central and peripheral vertigo (including the head impulse test described in Part III) are discussed in Chapter 14.

6. Dysarthria and dysphagia

Unilateral weakness of muscles of the palate, pharynx, or larynx indicates a lesion at the level of the LMN, neuromuscular junction, or muscle. These muscles are innervated by LMNs whose cell bodies are in the nucleus ambiguus in the medulla and whose axons travel in the glossopharyngeal and vagus nerves (cranial nerves IX and X, respectively). A unilateral cortical lesion does not usually produce focal palatal, pharyngeal, or laryngeal weakness because the nucleus ambiguus receives descending input from both cerebral hemispheres, so its input from the other hemisphere remains intact.

Dysarthria and dysphagia are prominent symptoms of LMN lesions of cranial nerves IX and X. These symptoms tend to be less prominent after unilateral cortical lesions because of the bilateral cortical input to the nucleus ambiguus. Bilateral cortical lesions often produce dramatic speech and swallowing problems, however. This is known as *pseudobulbar palsy* because the interruption of bilateral descending input to the brainstem simulates a lesion in the brainstem itself (a "bulbar" lesion). On close examination, the character of the dysarthria is different in patients with UMN lesions and those with LMN lesions. There is classically a strained, strangled character to the speech of the former, whereas the latter typically sound breathy, hoarse, and hypernasal. In fact, dysarthria can result from any conditions that damage motor control of the structures necessary for speech production, including cerebellar or basal ganglia disorders, and the specific characteristics of the dysarthria can be useful in localization and differential diagnosis.

7. Neck weakness

The accessory nerve (cranial nerve XI) is a prime candidate for the most confusing of all the cranial nerves. The motor nerves innervating the SCM and trapezius muscles originate in the cervical spinal cord (at the C1-2 level for the SCM and the C3-4 level for the trapezius). They then ascend alongside the spinal cord and enter the skull through the foramen magnum, only to exit the skull again (through the jugular foramen) as the accessory nerve. The nerve cells in the spinal cord at C3-4 that control the trapezius muscle receive descending cortical input that originates almost exclusively in the contralateral cerebral hemisphere. The cortical input to the C1-2 neurons that control the SCM muscle comes from both hemispheres, but predominantly the ipsilateral one. An additional confounding feature is that the left SCM rotates the head to the right (and vice versa).

As a result, LMN lesions produce weakness of the ipsilateral SCM and trapezius muscles, resulting in weakness of shoulder elevation on that side and impaired head rotation to the opposite side. UMN lesions produce weakness of the ipsilateral SCM and the contralateral trapezius, resulting in weakness of shoulder elevation on the side opposite the cortical lesion, and impaired head rotation away from the cortical lesion. Consequently, patients with hemiparesis due to a lesion in the brainstem or above have weakness of shoulder elevation on the side of the hemiparesis and weakness of head rotation toward the side of the hemiparesis.

8. Tongue weakness

The hypoglossal nerve (cranial nerve XII) receives descending cortical input from both hemispheres about equally, except that the fibers destined for the genioglossus muscle receive their cortical input only from the contralateral hemisphere. There appears to be variability in this pattern, so unilateral UMN lesions sometimes produce ipsilateral tongue weakness, more often produce contralateral tongue weakness, and most often produce no significant tongue weakness at all. Unilateral LMN lesions produce weakness of the ipsilateral tongue muscles, resulting in difficulty protruding the tongue to the opposite side. Thus, when the patient is asked to protrude the tongue in the midline, it deviates toward the side of the lesion. Atrophy and fasciculations are often prominent with peripheral lesions, as with LMN lesions throughout the body (see the discussion of the motor examination in Section C).

C. Motor Examination

1. UMN vs. LMN lesions affecting the limbs

In the same way that certain patterns on the examination differentiate lesions in the UMN and LMN portions of the cranial nerve pathways, several examination findings help to distinguish UMN from LMN lesions in patients with abnormal motor function in the limbs. As discussed in Chapter 1 (see Speed Rule 4), deep tendon reflexes are typically hyperactive with an UMN lesion and hypoactive with a LMN one. The Babinski sign is a reliable indicator of an UMN lesion. Spasticity (described in Part IV) is also characteristic of an UMN lesion, whereas tone is normal or reduced with a LMN lesion. Atrophy and fasciculations are common with LMN dysfunction and unusual with UMN dysfunction. The pattern of muscle involvement is also helpful. An UMN lesion usually results in weakness that is more pronounced in the flexors of the lower extremities than in the extensors, but in the upper extremities the extensors are weaker than the flexors. Note that the muscles in which strength is relatively preserved (the flexors of the upper extremities and the extensors of the lower extremities) are the same ones in which spasticity is usually most pronounced. This pattern is sometimes referred to as pyramidal weakness, but it does not occur with pure lesions of the pyramidal tracts. Instead, it is the net result of disrupting all the descending motor tracts, so a more appropriate term is *UMN pattern of weakness*. The UMN pattern of weakness also causes supination of the upper extremity to be weaker than pronation; this accounts for the finding of a pronator drift, in which the arm pronates and drifts downward when the patient is asked to hold it extended with palms up (supinated). This is a fairly sensitive indicator of subtle UMN weakness.

To summarize, UMN lesions are characterized by the pattern of weakness (most prominent in the extensors of the upper extremity and the flexors of the lower extremity), spasticity (most pronounced in the opposite muscles), hyperreflexia, and the Babinski sign. LMN lesions are characterized by weakness, hypotonia, hyporeflexia, atrophy, and fasciculations.

2. Patterns of LMN weakness

For *diffuse* diseases of the peripheral nervous system, the pattern of muscle involvement often provides useful localizing information. For example, predominantly distal weakness usually suggests a disease of peripheral nerves, whereas predominantly proximal weakness is typical of muscle disorders and neuromuscular junction diseases (see Chapter 6). For *focal* lesions in the peripheral nervous system, the most reliable approach to localization is to consult a reference book, but in most cases it is sufficient to remember a few simple patterns.

In each extremity, consider three principal joints: the hip, knee, and ankle in the lower extremities, and the elbow, wrist, and knuckle in the upper extremities (it really doesn't matter which knuckle; the pattern applies equally well to interphalangeal joints and metacarpophalangeal joints). At each joint, consider flexion and extension separately. This gives six principal movements in each limb. Most localization problems can be solved by remembering the innervation patterns for these six principal movements (plus shoulder abduction and finger abduction in the upper extremities).

Figure 2.3 shows which nerve roots provide innervation for each of these principal movements. In the upper extremities, the pattern can be remembered by ordering the movements in a kind of spiral that proceeds down the arm: shoulder abduction (A), elbow flexion (B), elbow extension (C), wrist extension (D), wrist flexion (E), finger flexion (F), finger extension (G), and finger abduction (H). The corresponding roots then proceed in order: C5 (A), C5-6 (B), C6-7 (C), C6-7 (D), C7-8 (E), C8 (F), C8 (G), and T1 (H).

In the lower extremities, the pattern is even simpler (Figure 2.4). The movements can be considered in sequence down the front first and then the back: hip flexion (A), knee extension (B), ankle dorsiflexion (C), hip extension (D), knee flexion (E), and ankle plantar flexion (F). The corresponding roots are: L2-3 (A), L3-4 (B), L4-5 (C), L4-5 (D), L5-S1 (E), and S1-2 (F).

The peripheral nerves providing innervation for these same principal movements are listed in Figures 2.3 and 2.4. There is no simple pattern, but fortunately, there aren't many nerves to remember. In the upper extremities, all the extension movements in Figure 2.3 (C, D, and G) are innervated by the radial nerve. The two distal flexion movements (E and F) are supplied by the median nerve, and the proximal one (elbow flexion, B) by the musculocutaneous nerve. The axillary nerve supplies the deltoid muscle, which is the main shoulder abductor (A), and the interosseous muscles (H) are innervated by the ulnar nerve.

In the lower extremities, the sciatic nerve innervates the muscles responsible for knee flexion (E); its peroneal branch supplies ankle dorsiflexion (C), while its tibial branch supplies ankle plantar flexion (F). The femoral nerve innervates knee extensor muscles (B). The innervation of the iliopsoas muscle, which flexes the hip (A), arises very proximally from the L2 and L3 nerve roots; some consider this to be part of the femoral nerve, and others simply call it the "nerve to iliopsoas." The gluteus muscles, responsible for hip extension (D), are innervated by the gluteal nerves.

The nerve root corresponding to each commonly tested deep tendon reflex can also be derived from Figures 2.3 and 2.4. In particular, the biceps

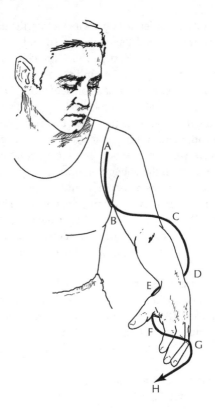

Fig. 2.3 Nerve roots and peripheral nerves corresponding to the principal movements of the upper extremity. The letters labeling the movements form a spiral down the extremity. The nerve roots and peripheral nerves corresponding to each movement are listed in the accompanying table.

Table for Figure 2.3

Movement	Roots	Peripheral Nerve
A. Shoulder abduction	5	Axillary
B. Elbow flexion	5/6	Musculocutaneous
C. Elbow extension	6/7	Radial
D. Wrist extension	6/7	Radial
E. Wrist flexion	7/8	Median
F. Finger flexion	8	Median
G. Finger extension	8	Radial
H. Finger abduction	T1	Ulnar

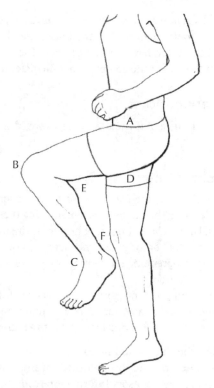

Fig. 2.4 Nerve roots and peripheral nerves corresponding to the principal movements of the lower extremity. The letters labeling the movements proceed in order from proximal to distal down the front of the limb, and then repeat from proximal to distal down the back of the limb. The nerve roots and peripheral nerves corresponding to each movement are listed in the accompanying table.

Table for Figure 2.4

Movement	Roots	Peripheral Nerve
A. Hip flexion	2/3	Femoral ("nerve to iliopsoas")
B. Knee extension	3/4	Femoral
C. Ankle dorsiflexion	4/5	Peroneal
D. Hip extension	4/5	Gluteal
E. Knee flexion	5/1	Sciatic
F. Ankle plantar flexion	1/2	Tibial

and brachioradialis reflexes are mediated by the C5-6 roots, the triceps reflex by the C6-7 roots (mainly C7), the knee reflex by the L3-4 roots (mainly L4), and the ankle reflex by the S1 root. The internal hamstring reflex is less often tested, but the L5 nerve root mediates it.

D. Reflex Examination

The localizing significance of the tendon reflexes was discussed in Section C and in Chapter 1.

E. Sensory Examination

As explained in Chapter 1, the pathways for different sensory modalities cross at different levels in the nervous system, making them very useful for localizing lesions. Unlike the features that help to distinguish UMN lesions from LMN lesions in the motor pathways, there are not really any examination findings that differentiate the central portion of a sensory pathway from the peripheral portion.

For most localization problems, precise knowledge of the sensory fields of specific peripheral nerves and nerve roots is unnecessary. It is usually sufficient to remember the following facts (refer to Figures 2.5 and 2.6):

1. Sensation from the thumb and index finger travels via the C6 nerve root, the C7 root carries sensory information from the middle finger, and the C8 root conveys sensory information from the fourth and fifth fingers.

2. For the remainder of the upper extremity, the root innervation "fans out" from the hand (see Figure 2.5).

3. These innervation patterns cover both the anterior and posterior aspects of the upper extremity.

4. The L 5 dermatome includes the large toe and the lateral lower leg; the S 1 dermatome includes the small toe and sole. Roots L4, L3, and L2 cover the region fanning out medially and proximally from the L5 dermatome. The S2 dermatome extends from the S1 dermatome up the back of the leg (see Figure 2.5).

5. The median nerve carries sensation from all fingers except the fifth finger and half of the fourth, which are served by the ulnar nerve. These nerve territories extend proximally up to the wrist on the palmar aspect of the hand. On the dorsal aspect, the ulnar nerve territory still extends to the wrist, but the median nerve territory fades

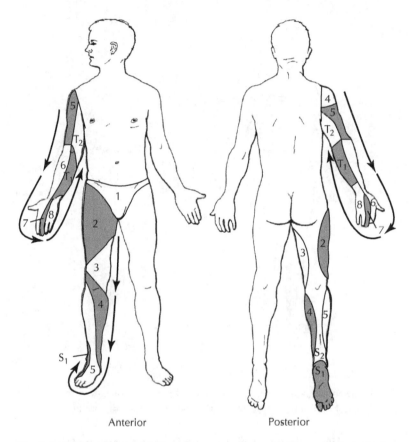

Fig. 2.5 Diagram illustrating the nerve roots corresponding to the principal dermatomes in the upper and lower extremities.

into radial nerve territory at the metacarpal-phalangeal joints (see Figure 2.6).

6. The common peroneal nerve innervates the lateral leg and the dorsum of the foot; the tibial nerve innervates the sole.

For the peripheral nerve innervations of more proximal limb regions, it is best to consult diagrams in reference books.

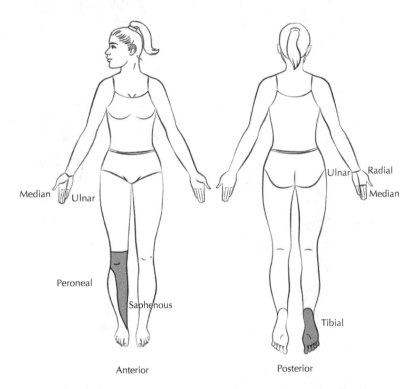

Median   Ulnar
Ulnar
Peroneal
Saphenous
Ulnar   Radial
Median
Tibial

Anterior   Posterior

Fig. 2.6 Diagram illustrating the territories of sensory innervation for the principal peripheral nerves of the distal upper and lower extremities.

VI. Modifications of the Neurologic Examination

A. Screening Neurologic Examination

Medical students should always try to perform complete physical examinations (including complete neurologic examinations) on all patients they evaluate, so they can gain a sense of the range of normal variation and ask questions about the findings they observe. House officers and practicing physicians usually do not have the time to perform complete examinations on all patients, however. They must be able to perform a rapid examination that screens for most common abnormalities. They can then use the results of this screening examination—together with the history—to decide whether certain components of the examination must be conducted in

more detail. For such screening purposes, the following neurologic examination is generally adequate and can be completed in 5 minutes or less. It
may be performed in any order. This examination is offered as a suggestion
for students to use in future practice; it is not adequate for students examining patients during a neurology clerkship.

1. Mental status

Make sure patients can follow at least one complicated command, taking care not to give them any nonverbal cues. Test them for orientation
to person, place, and time. If their responses are appropriate and they
are able to relate a detailed and coherent medical history, no further
mental status testing is necessary (unless they are reporting cognitive
problems).

2. Cranial nerves

Test visual fields in one eye, both pupillary responses to light, eye movements in all directions, facial strength, and hearing to finger rub.

3. Motor system

Test strength in the following muscles bilaterally: deltoids, triceps, wrist
extensors, hand interossei, iliopsoas, hamstrings, ankle dorsiflexors. Test
for a pronator drift. Test finger tapping, finger-to-nose, and heel-knee-shin
performance. Test tandem gait and walking on the heels.

4. Reflexes

Test plantar responses and biceps, triceps, patellar, and ankle reflexes
bilaterally.

5. Sensation

Test light touch sensation in all four distal limbs, including double simultaneous stimulation. Test vibration sense at the great toes.

Remember, this examination must be expanded when an asymmetry or
other abnormality is found. For example, if the triceps muscle is weak in
one arm, other muscles innervated by the radial nerve must be tested, as
well as other muscles in the distribution of the C7 nerve root. Patients'
specific symptoms and concerns may also compel modifications in the
examination. For example, patients reporting memory loss need thorough
mental status testing even if their performance on the screening examination is perfectly normal.

B. Video Examination

Technologic advances combined with issues of health care access and patient satisfaction motivated the development of techniques for providing medical care remotely, and the COVID-19 pandemic amplified that trend. Video interactions between patients and caregivers are now routine. Although some components of the neurologic examination require direct physical contact, much of the screening examination can be adapted to the video format using instructions like the following:

- "Hold up your right thumb at arm's length from your body. Do the same with your left thumb, about 18 inches away." [*or simply demonstrate this for the patient*] "Now close your left eye. With your right eye, look midway between your two thumbs. Can you still see both thumbs?"
- "Now open your left eye and close your right eye. Can you still see both thumbs?"
- "Now open both eyes and look at your left thumb. Without moving your head, move your eyes quickly to your right thumb. Now back to the left. Now the right. Now the left."
- "Turn your thumbs so they are horizontal and pointing toward each other. Keeping them at arm's length from your body, move them toward each other; when they reach each other, raise your right arm about 30° and lower your left arm about 30°." [*or simply demonstrate this for the patient*] "Without moving your head, move your eyes quickly to the top thumb. Now to the bottom. Now to the top. Now the bottom."
- "Lower your left arm. Keeping your right thumb at arm's length, slowly sweep it up and down while you follow it with your eyes without moving your head." [*or simply demonstrate this for the patient*]
- "Now hold your right arm horizontally with the thumb up and slowly sweep it from side to side while you follow it with your eyes without moving your head." [*or simply demonstrate this for the patient*]
- "Make a big smile."
- "Raise your eyebrows and wrinkle your forehead."
- "Close your eyes tightly."
- "Touch your left forehead briefly, then the right. Does it feel the same on the two sides?"
- "Do the same thing on your left and right cheek."
- "Do the same thing on the left and right sides of your chin."

- "Rub your fingers near your right ear—can you hear the rubbing? Do the same with your left ear."
- "Point the camera inside your mouth as you open it wide and say 'ah' or yawn."
- "Turn your head from side to side."
- "Shrug your shoulders."
- "Stick out your tongue. Move it from side to side."
- "Make a fist with your right hand. Open the thumb and index finger as far as they'll go. Now tap the tip of your index finger on the tip of your thumb over and over as quickly as you can." [or simply demonstrate this for the patient]
- "Now do the same thing with your left hand."
- "Hold up your left thumb at arm's length from your body. Touch the tip of the left thumb with your right index finger. Now touch your chin with your right index finger. Now keep moving your right index finger back and forth between your left thumb and your chin. Move your left thumb around as you do this." [or simply demonstrate this for the patient]
- "Now switch hands and do the same thing."
- "Hold your left hand in front of the camera with palm facing up. Slap your left palm with your right palm. Lift your right hand, flip it over, and slap your left palm with the back of your right hand. Lift your right hand again, flip it over, and slap your left palm with your right palm. Do this over and over as quickly as you can." [or simply demonstrate this for the patient]
- "Now switch hands and do the same thing."
- "Hold both arms stretched out in front of you with the palms facing the ceiling and then close your eyes for 10 seconds." [or simply demonstrate this for the patient]
- "Pick up a heavy book (such as a dictionary or bible) with one hand and with that same hand hold the book higher than the top of your head for 3 seconds." [or simply demonstrate this for the patient]
- "Now turn the book over so you're grasping it from above with the same hand." [or simply demonstrate this for the patient]
- "Do the same thing with the book in your other hand."
- "Stand up without using your hands."
- "Walk away from the camera. Now come back toward the camera walking on your heels, with your toes in the air. Now walk away from the

camera on your tiptoes. Now walk back toward the camera placing each foot directly in front of the other, like you're on a tightrope."

- "Stand with both feet together. Now close your eyes for 5 seconds."

- "Stand on your right leg. Now bend your right knee while still standing on only your right leg. Now straighten the leg and go up on your tiptoes, still standing on only your right leg."

- "Do the same thing on your left leg."

These instructions offer a good screen of the cranial nerve and motor portions of the exam (and patients who can perform all the tasks also must have good comprehension and lower extremity proprioception). Instructions for mental status testing are not included above because most of that testing is almost identical whether the interaction is remote or in person. Instructions for testing visual acuity, the pupillary light reflex, muscle tone, tendon reflexes, and limb sensation are not included because those functions are very difficult to test remotely.

Patients often need to be told how to adjust the lighting and their position relative to the camera so that the examiner can see the body part of interest, and they may need to arrange their room so that there is enough space to observe their gait. The instructions must be modified for patients who are unsteady on their feet, or generally weak—in fact, if the patient has trouble performing any portion of this video exam it may be necessary to schedule an in-person appointment for a more reliable exam. Like any screening exam, this video exam is most useful in documenting intact function and less helpful for evaluating deficits.

C. Examination of Patients with Altered Level of Consciousness

Many parts of the neurologic examination must be eliminated or modified when patients cannot answer questions or follow commands because of a depressed level of consciousness. Fortunately, the location of these patients' nervous system dysfunction is no mystery—it is in the brainstem or above. The neurologic examination is directed mainly at determining whether this pathology is due to a structural lesion or due to metabolic dysfunction (including drug effects). The basis for this determination is discussed in Chapter 11; the most pertinent examination findings are a consistent asymmetry between right- and left-sided responses or abnormal reflexes that indicate dysfunction in specific regions of the brainstem.

1. Mental status

For a patient in coma, the mental status examination is simply an assessment of the responses to visual, auditory, and noxious stimuli. The response to a noxious stimulus may be a reflex involving circuitry confined to the spinal cord, or it may reflect reflex pathways mediated by the brainstem. Two specific patterns of motor activity are classically described (Figure 2.7). *Decorticate posturing* consists of upper extremity adduction and flexion at the elbows, wrists, and fingers, together with lower extremity extension. *Decerebrate posturing* consists of upper extremity extension, adduction, and pronation together with lower extremity extension. This terminology reflects the analogy that has been drawn between these postures and the postures maintained by experimental animals after

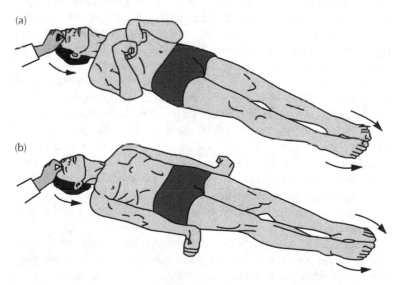

Fig. 2.7 a) Decorticate posturing (flexion and adduction of upper extremities, extension of lower extremities). b) Decerebrate posturing (pronation, adduction, and proximal extension of upper extremities, with wrist flexion; extension of lower extremities).

specific lesions, but in fact, these postures do not have reliable localizing value in human patients. In general, patients with decorticate posturing in response to pain have a better prognosis than those with decerebrate posturing.

2. Cranial nerves

In patients with impaired consciousness, visual field defects may sometimes be identified by assessing response to visual threat, such as a finger or small object introduced suddenly into the visual field. More precise assessments of visual fields and visual acuity are impossible. Pupillary reflexes can be tested in the same manner as in a conscious person.

Eye movements can be assessed by activating them using the *vestibulo-ocular reflex*. One way to test this reflex is with the *oculocephalic* maneuver, or *doll's eyes* maneuver. This is similar to the head thrust maneuver described in Part III, except that it does not require patient cooperation. Holding the patient's eyes open with one hand, turn the patient's head quickly to one side, and observe how the eyes move relative to the head. If there is any chance that there has been a traumatic injury to the cervical spine, plain films of the cervical spine must be obtained before performing this maneuver. Doll's eyes are considered to be positive (Figure 2.8) when the vestibulo-ocular reflex is intact: the eyes remain fixed on the same point in space during head rotation (i.e., they do not turn with the head; instead, they appear to be moving relative to the head in the direction opposite to the head movement). Absence of this response in a comatose patient indicates dysfunction somewhere in the vestibulo-ocular reflex pathway: in the afferent limb (from the labyrinth and vestibular nerve), the efferent limb (cranial nerves III and VI and the muscles they innervate), or the pathways connecting them in the midbrain, pons, and medulla. Technically, the oculocephalic maneuver also stimulates neck proprioceptors, so it is not a pure test of the vestibulo-ocular reflex, but in practice, this is not a major consideration.

Another maneuver that stimulates the vestibulo-ocular reflex more strongly is the *cold caloric* procedure. Place the patient in the supine position, with the head or upper body tilted forward so that the neck forms an angle of 30° with the horizontal. Fill a syringe with 50–100 mL of ice-cold water and attach a small catheter. Inject the water against the tympanic membrane (checking with an otoscope first to be sure the membrane is

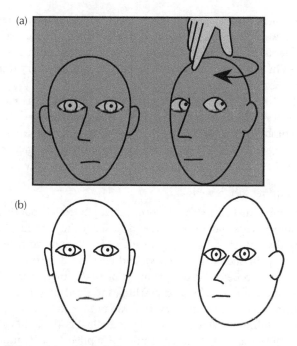

Fig. 2.8 a) Normal (positive) doll's eyes response: when the examiner rotates the patient's head in one direction, the patient's eyes stay fixed in space (as if the patient were trying to keep the eyes focused on a distant object)—thus, relative to the head, the eyes move in the opposite direction. b) Absent doll's eyes response: when the examiner rotates the patient's head in one direction, the patient's eyes rotate with the head—thus, relative to the head, the eyes remain fixed.

intact). In this position, cold water has the same effect on the horizontal semicircular canal as sustained turning of the head in the opposite direction; the result is sustained deviation of both eyes toward the ear being cooled. If the eyes remain stationary, there is a problem in the vestibulo-ocular reflex pathway—usually in the pons or medulla, but occasionally in the efferent or afferent limbs (cranial nerves III, VI, or VIII). In conscious subjects, the cold caloric procedure produces not only deviation of the eyes toward the cooled ear but also nystagmus, with the fast component away from the cooled ear. Caloric testing is usually not performed in conscious patients, however, because it can cause severe vertigo and nausea, and the same elements of the nervous system can be tested in much less noxious ways. Even in coma, the cold caloric procedure is unnecessary if the doll's eyes response is normal.

Cranial nerves V and VII can be assessed in unconscious patients by testing corneal reflexes and by observing facial grimacing in response to noxious stimulation (supraorbital pressure or nasal tickle, for example). Cranial nerves IX and X can be assessed by testing the gag reflex-but remember that the gag reflex may be absent in 20% of healthy subjects.

3. Motor and sensory systems

People in coma can't participate in formal strength testing, but their spontaneous movements should be observed to see if they are moving some limbs less than others. The strength with which they move each limb in response to pain should be assessed, and also the degree to which the movement is purposeful. Noxious stimulation of the lower extremity (produced by squeezing a nailbed or pinching the skin) may produce *triple flexion* (dorsiflexion of the ankle, with flexion of the knee and hip) purely as a local withdrawal reflex mediated by the spinal cord. To look for purposeful withdrawal, the stimulus should be applied in a location where triple flexion would be an inappropriate response, such as the anterior thigh: hip flexion would indicate purely reflex withdrawal, whereas hip extension would indicate a purposeful movement. In contrast, hip flexion in response to a noxious stimulus applied to the posterior thigh could be either a reflex or a purposeful response. In both upper and lower extremities, reflex withdrawal produces limb adduction, so to differentiate reflex withdrawal from purposeful movement, the noxious stimulus should be applied to the medial aspect of the limb.

Deep tendon reflexes and resistance to passive manipulation can still be tested in the usual manner. Pain sensation can be assessed by observing the response to noxious stimulation (and noting whether the response varies depending on which limb is stimulated). Other sensory modalities cannot be tested.

D. Inconsistent or Anomalous Examination Findings

When clinicians find exam abnormalities that don't match what would be expected with disorders of the nervous system, their first reaction should be to wonder whether those expectations are wrong. Maybe they remember the textbook incorrectly, or never completely understood it in the first place. Perhaps the textbook (even this one!) contains errors—many aspects of nervous system function remain poorly understood. The patient might have an anatomic variant or some other reason for atypical neurologic responses. There are many reasons clinicians should be humble.

Nonetheless, some anomalous exam findings have features that indicate something other than an incomplete understanding of how the nervous system works. Some findings defy the laws of physics; others violate the rules of logic. Some findings have been frequently observed in people whose symptoms developed at times of emotional stress and resolved when that stress disappeared. Examples of such findings are listed in Table 2.2; they are typical of the conditions often referred to as "functional disorders" discussed in Chapter 10, Part IV, Section E.

Many of the exam findings listed in Table 2.2 resemble what would be observed if someone were deliberately pretending to be impaired. Clinicians often can't help feeling as if the patient is "trying to trick" them. The exam becomes a trap to outwit the patient. This type of resentment is natural and understandable, but clinicians should be aware that most patients are not consciously trying to deceive them.

Anomalous or inconsistent exam findings do not mean the nervous system is normal—they just indicate that the nervous system is functioning at a higher level than the exam would otherwise suggest. There may or may not be neurologic deficits underlying the anomalous findings. I can imagine that if I had subtle sensory symptoms in one limb but I was still able to detect the sensory stimuli being applied by the examiner, I might try to help the examiner appreciate my deficits by "embellishing" them and reporting that I didn't feel stimuli in that limb at all. If I can imagine such embellishment at a conscious level, it is even easier to believe that patients might do this unconsciously. Thus, the most confident conclusion that can be drawn when patients have anomalous or inconsistent exam findings is that their examination is difficult to interpret.

VII. Supplementary Table for Reference

Table 2.2 Anomalous or Inconsistent Exam Findings

Apparent Deficit	Exam Maneuver	Anomalous or Inconsistent Finding	Explanation	Additional Comments
Reduced sensation on one side of the face	Place a vibrating tuning fork on the forehead a few millimeters to the left of the midline and ask if the patient feels the vibration; repeat with the tuning fork a few millimeters to the right of the midline.	The patient can't detect the vibration on the symptomatic side but detects it on the opposite side ("splitting the midline").	People who have complete loss of sensation on one side of the face should still be able to detect vibration on that side because the vibration will be transmitted by the frontal bone across the midline to the intact side.	Although people with loss of sensation on one side of the face will still be able to detect vibration there, it may feel less intense than when the tuning fork is placed on the intact side. I only find midline splitting useful when the patient reports a dramatic difference between the two sides.
Impaired abduction of one eye	Ask the patient to fixate on a target; without warning, turn their head quickly away from the eye with the deficit.	The eye with the deficit abducts.	If the head movement is performed suddenly and without warning, the patient doesn't suppress the vestibulo-ocular reflex.	
Weakness of eye closure	Ask the patient to try closing their eye while you hold their upper eyelid open.	The eye remains level.	Forceful activation of the orbicularis oculi muscle typically results in simultaneous activation of the superior rectus muscle, elevating the eye. This is known as the Bell phenomenon. Absence of the Bell phenomenon suggests that the patient was not trying their hardest to close the eye.	Although most people have a Bell phenomenon, not all do. Be cautious about drawing conclusions from an absent Bell phenomenon unless it is clearly present in the other eye.

Table 2.2 Continued

Apparent Deficit	Exam Maneuver	Anomalous or Inconsistent Finding	Explanation	Additional Comments
Hearing loss	During an unrelated section of the exam, with your back to the patient, use a very soft voice to ask the patient a question.	The patient answers the question.	The patient's hearing improves when not being explicitly tested.	
Hemiparesis	Test for pronator drift by having the patient hold their arms stretched out in front of them with the palms facing upward.	The weak arm drifts downward but doesn't pronate.	In the UMN pattern of weakness, forearm supinators are weaker than pronators.	I don't consider this finding very useful because it is present in some patients with a known CNS lesion.
Weak hip extension on one side	With the patient supine, place one hand behind the heel of the weak leg and ask the patient to dig the heel into the bed as you try to lift it. Leaving your hand in place, ask the patient to raise their opposite leg as you press down on it and simultaneously try to lift the weak heel.	You will be able to lift the heel on the weak side when the patient is asked to dig it into the bed, but not when the patient is asked to raise the opposite leg against resistance ("Hoover sign").	When flexing one hip against resistance, people forcefully extend their opposite hip for leverage.	This test can also be performed with the patient in a sitting position, lifting the weak leg behind the thigh rather than behind the heel.
Weak hip flexion on one side	With the patient supine, place one hand behind the heel of the unaffected leg and ask the patient to dig the heel into the bed as you try to lift it. Leaving your hand in place, ask the patient to raise their weak leg as you press down on it and simultaneously try to lift the heel on the unaffected side.	You will be able to lift the heel on the unaffected side when the patient is asked to raise the weak leg against resistance, but not when the patient is asked to dig the unaffected heel into the bed.	When flexing one hip against resistance, people forcefully extend their opposite hip for leverage. When they don't do that, it suggests incomplete effort.	This test can also be performed with the patient sitting rather than supine.

(continued)

Table 2.2 Continued

Apparent Deficit	Exam Maneuver	Anomalous or Inconsistent Finding	Explanation	Additional Comments
Weak elbow flexion on one side	Test strength of elbow flexion on the affected side. Then test strength of elbow extension on the unaffected side and simultaneously apply pressure against the elbow flexors on the affected side.	The elbow flexors on the affected side exert more force during testing of contralateral elbow extension than during direct testing.	When extending one elbow against resistance, people will forcefully flex their other elbow.	This test involves tricky positioning, and it requires that the patient be able to flex the affected arm to some degree.
Inability to move a limb or part of a limb	Raise the affected body part and support it for the patient. Ask the patient to lower it against your resistance. If you feel no downward pressure, gradually remove your support while asking the patient to keep pushing down.	The body part remains suspended in the air.	Instructing the patient to push down results in paradoxical activation of antigravity muscles that resist the intended movement (which requires only the force of gravity).	
Inability to move a limb or part of a limb	Observe how the patient uses the body part when strength is not explicitly being tested.	The patient has more trouble moving the body part during explicit strength testing than at other times (for example, they are unable to plantar flex their ankles when tested on the exam table but they can stand on their toes; or they move a body part smoothly while getting on or off the exam table but not during formal testing).	The patient's strength improves when not being explicitly tested.	Sometimes movements may not be equivalent even though they seem to be, because different body positions permit other muscles to perform supportive actions.

Table 2.2 Continued

Apparent Deficit	Exam Maneuver	Anomalous or Inconsistent Finding	Explanation	Additional Comments
Weakness (without total paralysis) of a muscle	Urge the patient to maintain maximum effort while you test the strength of the muscle; if you are overcoming the patient, intermittently reduce the force you're applying while continuing to encourage maximum effort.	The force in the muscle being tested suddenly falls to zero, even when you're applying negligible force ("breakaway weakness," "give-way weakness," "collapsing weakness").	When weakness is due to a CNS or PNS disorder, the muscle usually gives way smoothly and continuously, rather than suddenly.	Examiners should beware: it is very easy to over-call this finding. Whenever it is observed, the patient should be asked if the test was painful—pain is a common reason for patients to "give up" suddenly. Patients may also suddenly "cede defeat" when they conclude that they have no chance of overcoming the examiner; this is why it's important to keep encouraging the patient to give maximum effort even as you reduce the force you're applying.
Tremor in one limb	Ask the patient to perform a rhythmic movement with their contralateral limb.	The tremor frequency changes to match the frequency of the voluntary rhythmic movement ("entrainment") or the patient performs the requested movement with an irregular rhythm.	Tremor due to neurologic disease remains constant in frequency and doesn't affect contralateral movements.	

(continued)

Table 2.2 Continued

Apparent Deficit	Exam Maneuver	Anomalous or Inconsistent Finding	Explanation	Additional Comments
Impaired joint position sense (proprioception)	Test joint position sense in the normal way.	The patient says "up" each time the joint is moved down, and vice versa.	Someone with loss of vibration sense will answer correctly 50% of the time purely on the basis of chance. A 100% rate of incorrect responses indicates that information about joint position is being transmitted.	
Loss of light touch sensation in a body region	Ask the patient to say "yes" when they feel you touching them and "no" when they don't, and then lightly touch them repeatedly both within and outside the affected body region, taking care to avoid a rhythmic pattern.	The patient says "no" each time you touch them in the affected body region.	If the patient responds each time you touch them in the affected body region, some sensory information is being transmitted from that region.	
Loss of light touch or pain sensation on one side of the body	Carefully map the region of sensory loss on the trunk.	The region of sensory loss has a sharp margin at the midline ("splitting the midline").	There is overlap between the sensory maps of the two sides of the trunk, with each extending 1–2 cm beyond the midline, so sensory loss due to CNS or PNS dysfunction on one side does not extend all the way to the midline.	In my experience, this finding is not reliable enough to justify the time and patience required to map out the region of sensory loss this precisely.

VIII. Discussion of Localization Problems

Example 1. The magnitude of this patient's pupillary asymmetry is greatest in the dark. This is when the parasympathetic system—which constricts the pupils in response to light—is least active, so the sympathetic system is the one that is not functioning normally. In particular, it is not adequately dilating the left pupil, which is why it is smaller than the right pupil (see Figure 2.1A). Thus, this patient has a sympathetic lesion on the left, the left pupil (the smaller pupil) is abnormal, and mild left-sided ptosis would be expected.

Example 2. For a patient to have face, arm, and leg weakness all on the right side of the body, the lesion must be on the left side, at the level of the high pons or above (see Chapter 1, Speed Rule 6). Thus, this patient's facial weakness is due to a central lesion, not a peripheral lesion. A central lesion typically spares forehead muscles, because there is bilateral cortical input to the portion of the facial nerve nucleus controlling those muscles. This patient would be expected to have more weakness in the lower face than in the forehead.

Example 3. The L2-3 roots correspond to hip flexion, the L5-S1 roots to knee flexion, and the L4-5 roots to ankle dorsiflexion (see Figure 2.4). Thus, no single nerve root lesion could produce this pattern of weakness. No single peripheral nerve lesion could do so, either. This pattern is typical of an upper motor neuron (UMN) lesion, which usually produces more weakness in the flexors of the lower extremity than in the extensors.

Chapter 3

Diagnostic Reasoning: What's the Lesion? (Why We Localize)

James W. Albers and Douglas J. Gelb

I. Case Histories

For each of the following cases, answer the following questions:

1. Where's the lesion?
2. Is the lesion focal, multifocal, or diffuse?
3. Is this a mass lesion or a non-mass lesion?
4. What is the temporal profile?
5. What diagnostic category is most likely?

Case 1. A 55-year-old woman has been brought to the emergency department by her husband because she seems confused and is having progressively more difficulty expressing her thoughts. For at least the last 10 weeks, she has had increasing clumsiness and weakness in her right arm and leg, and she is bumping into objects in her home. On examination, she has aphasia, a right visual field defect (homonymous hemianopia), mild right hemiparesis (face, arm, leg), increased reflexes on the right side, and a right extensor plantar response (Babinski sign).

Case 2. A 72-year-old right-handed man noted the abrupt feeling of heaviness in his left arm while watching television. His left leg gave out when he tried to stand, and he fell to the floor. He called for help, and when his wife came into the room, she noted that the left corner of his mouth was sagging. He also seemed to be moving the left side of his face less than the right side. He could still speak. He had no symptoms other than the weakness of his entire left side. Over the next several hours he improved slightly.

Case 3. A 22-year-old patient was well until 2 days ago, when they developed fever, severe headache, nausea, and vomiting. They became progressively more obtunded over the next day. They had two generalized seizures in the morning and were brought to the emergency department, where examination revealed a fever and stiff neck. They were stuporous, and they had generalized hyperreflexia with bilateral Babinski signs.

Case 4. A 47-year-old man developed ringing in his right ear several years ago that has worsened over time. Over the same period, his hearing in that ear has gradually deteriorated, and he has developed weakness and loss of feeling on the right side of his face. Over the past few months, he has developed stiffness, weakness, and numbness of his left arm and leg.

Case 5. A 28-year-old accountant and part-time boxer has been brought to the urgent care clinic by his wife because he has become irritable and abusive. She reports that he has had intermittent headaches for 3 months, and the headaches have become more severe and constant in the past month. He has been unable to work for about a week because of excessive drowsiness, and he sleeps for up to 24 hours if not awakened.

On neurologic examination, he is drowsy and irritable but able to follow commands. The lower part of his face droops slightly on the left side. He has mild to moderate weakness in his left arm and leg, and a left pronator drift. Tendon reflexes are hyperactive on the left. There is a left Babinski response.

Case 6. A 21-year-old right-handed patient experienced a sensation of numbness and tingling over her abdomen and in her legs. The next day, her legs began to feel stiff and tight, and she had difficulty initiating her urinary stream. She also had the sense that her bladder wasn't emptying completely. As the day progressed, the numbness and tingling became more pronounced in her mid-abdomen and below, and she began to have trouble walking. She went to bed early that evening, and when she awoke the next morning she couldn't stand.

Case 7. A 69-year-old right-handed retired executive is seeing her internist for a routine checkup. Her husband mentions that she has undergone a marked personality change over the past several months. He also notes that she has been forgetful for about a year and keeps asking the same things over and over. She no longer seems interested in her personal appearance. The mental status examination confirms these observations. Her language output is fluent, but she frequently pauses because she can't think of a word. She has difficulty following complicated instructions. She can remember only one of three items after a 5-minute delay, and she recalls no current events. She is unable to subtract two-digit numbers in her head. The remainder of her examination is normal.

Case 8. A 44-year-old left-handed patient suddenly developed a severe bilateral temporal and occipital headache. He also said that his neck was stiff. When he tried to lie down, he experienced severe nausea and vomited twice. He was immediately taken to the hospital, where he was found to be somnolent but he responded appropriately to noxious stimulation, moving all four limbs with equal force. His level of consciousness deteriorated over the next 4 hours, to the point where he could not be aroused even with vigorous stimulation.

Case 9. A 57-year-old woman has come to the emergency department because in the middle of a business meeting earlier today she suddenly became dizzy and experienced nausea and vomiting. On examination, she is dysarthric and has weakness of the left side of her palate. She starts to cough when she tries to swallow water. She has ataxia of her left arm and leg and reduced pain sensation over the left side of her face and the right side of her body. Seven hours have passed, and there has been no progression or improvement.

Case 10. Over the course of a few days, a 30-year-old man with Hodgkin lymphoma began to experience severe pain in his back and encircling the left side of his chest in a band 3 cm wide just below his breast. The pain was very intense at first but subsided somewhat, coincident with a rash that appeared in precisely the same distribution. He is still having pain in that area two weeks later and notes diminished touch sensation in the region of pain.

Case 11. A patient reports pain on the left side of her chest that sounds very similar to the pain described by the patient in Case 10, but no rash is present. The pain has been getting worse over many months. It remains localized to a narrow and circumscribed area of her chest, making her think that it might be "heart trouble." In addition, she has developed difficulty walking and says that her left leg seems to be weak and stiff.

II. Beyond Localization

As noted in Chapter 1, the first step in addressing a problem is usually to figure out where it is. This is the rationale for emphasizing localization in

Chapters 1 and 2. For diagnosing medical problems, one particular feature of localization is paramount: is the problem focal or diffuse? Some disease processes characteristically affect only one region of an organ system. For example, a pulmonary embolus only affects the region of the lung that is normally supplied by the blocked blood vessel, and bacterial pneumonia or lung abscess is confined to the lobe of the lung where the organisms happen to take up residence. Other disease processes (especially metabolic and endocrine disorders) have no basis for favoring one region of an organ system more than another, and they affect the organ system diffusely; emphysema and idiopathic pulmonary fibrosis are examples. In the heart, mitral stenosis is focal, whereas hypertrophic cardiomyopathy is diffuse.

Disease processes also have characteristic temporal patterns. A pulmonary embolus or myocardial infarction occurs suddenly—a blood vessel becomes blocked and a previously perfused region of tissue is rapidly depleted of oxygen. Gunshot injuries and drug overdoses also happen abruptly. By comparison, many cancers grow very slowly. Osteoporosis, emphysema, and cataracts tend to develop gradually over many years.

These two features—the time course of a disease process and whether it is focal or diffuse—provide two separate axes for organizing categories of medical conditions. These axes are so fundamental that many clinicians don't often think about them even though they apply them routinely. They automatically exclude pulmonary embolism from the differential diagnosis of someone whose dyspnea has been present for years, just as they intuitively recognize that abnormal breath sounds in a single region of the chest are unlikely to be due to a systemic toxin. The purpose of this chapter is to make this type of reasoning more explicit and systematic. Many of the concepts and clinical vignettes in this chapter were adapted from material developed by neurologists at the Mayo Clinic. The approach is based on addressing the following three questions in order:

A. *Localization*: Where's the lesion?
B. *Temporal profile*: How did the symptoms begin, and how have they changed over time?
C. *Epidemiology*: Does the patient have risk factors for specific conditions?

A few terms must be defined before explaining how this information is used to draw conclusions about etiology.

A. Localization

The principles of localization were presented in Chapters 1 and 2. For clinical decision making, it is often sufficient to determine whether the lesion is supratentorial, in the posterior fossa, in the spinal cord, or in the peripheral nervous system. When considering potential etiologies, the most important question is whether the problem is focal, multifocal, or diffuse.

A *focal* process is confined to a single circumscribed area. Focal lesions are usually unilateral, but not always—a lesion that extends from one side to the other across the midline is also focal.

A *multifocal* process is made up of two or more focal lesions distributed randomly. These lesions may all be at the same level of the nervous system (for example, many different cortical lesions, or many lesions of individual peripheral nerves) or at different levels (for example, one in the spinal cord and one in the cerebral cortex).

A *diffuse* process involves symmetric parts of the nervous system without extending across the midline as a single circumscribed lesion. Diseases causing generalized dysfunction of neurons, or just of neurons in the basal ganglia, or just of peripheral nerves, or just of sensory nerves, or just of long nerves, would all be examples of diffuse processes.

B. Temporal Profile

The first consideration in describing the temporal profile is whether symptoms are transient or persistent. *Transient* symptoms resolve completely; *persistent* symptoms do not. Persistent conditions can be subdivided into three categories:

Static (stationary) symptoms reach maximum severity and then do not change.

Improving symptoms reach maximum severity and then begin to resolve.

Progressive symptoms continue to worsen.

These designations are mutually exclusive at any instant, but they are not immutable. For example, consider someone who develops symptoms that continue to get worse for a week, remain unchanged for a month, and then start to improve so that by 6 months they have completely resolved. If evaluated at 3 days, the symptoms would be considered progressive, but at 3 weeks they would be categorized as static, and at 3 months they would be classified as improving. For diagnostic purposes, the most important information about the temporal profile is the rapidity with which changes occur:

Acute symptoms evolve over minutes to hours.

Subacute symptoms evolve over days to weeks.

Chronic symptoms evolve over months to years.

These categories overlap, and they are intended as rough guidelines. Diseases that typically have a chronic time course may at times present acutely, conditions that ordinarily would be considered subacute sometimes evolve over years, and so forth. Nonetheless, these broad definitions turn out to be useful in most cases.

C. Epidemiology

Lesion localization and temporal profile are the most important factors in generating a list of potential etiologies. Epidemiologic considerations are used mainly to arrange the list in order of likelihood. For example, thyroid disease and brucellosis can both cause subacute diffuse processes, but a physician treating an affluent adult patient in an urban area would be much more concerned about thyroid disease because it is much more common in that setting. As another example, an elderly patient with a stroke is more likely to have atherosclerotic disease than an arterial dissection, but dissection becomes a serious consideration if the same patient has recently sustained trauma to the neck. The relevant epidemiologic factors vary depending on the disease, so they will not be discussed in detail in this chapter.

III. Etiology

Seven general categories of persistent neurologic disease can be distinguished, each with a characteristic spatial-temporal profile.

A. Degenerative Diseases

In degenerative disorders, one or more nervous system components begin to malfunction after functioning normally for many years. Once the deterioration begins, it doesn't stop. Two common examples are Alzheimer disease and Parkinson disease. Degenerative diseases are *diffuse*, *chronic*, and *progressive*.

B. Neoplastic Diseases

In practice, the term *neoplasm* is applied mainly to collections of cells that are multiplying uncontrollably because of some genetic transformation (i.e., cancer). The rules presented here apply to the more expansive, literal meaning of neoplasm, "new growth." Based on this definition, any new growing structural lesion (including a slowly enlarging hematoma or a herniating intervertebral disc) is classified as a neoplasm. This makes sense clinically, because when these processes are in the differential diagnosis, cancer is usually a possibility also, and it is appropriate to direct the diagnostic evaluation at the most serious potential diagnosis. Neoplastic diseases are characterized as *focal*, *chronic* (or, less often, *subacute*), and *progressive*.

C. Vascular Diseases

Disruption of the cerebrovascular system can produce either ischemia (resulting from obstructed blood vessels) or hemorrhage (resulting from ruptured blood vessels). Either way, the symptoms are almost always *acute*. Ischemic lesions are always *focal*. Hemorrhagic lesions may be either *focal* or *diffuse*, depending on whether the blood escapes into a freely interconnecting space (e.g., subarachnoid hemorrhage) or a confined space (e.g., subdural hematoma, parenchymal hemorrhage). Ischemic events can be *static*, *progressive*, or *improving*, largely depending on how much edema develops; hemorrhagic events are typically *progressive*.

D. Inflammatory Diseases

Inflammation in the nervous system is most often a response to an infection or some other insult. As with hemorrhage, an infection in a confined space (such as an abscess) results in a *focal* lesion, whereas in an unrestricted space the result is a *diffuse* lesion (e.g., meningitis or encephalitis). Either way, the time course is usually *subacute* and *progressive*. In some cases, the immune system appears to become activated even without external provocation (autoimmune diseases); *multifocal* or *diffuse* deficits typically result, with a *chronic* or *subacute* time course, usually *progressive*. Multiple sclerosis, vasculitis, and autoimmune encephalitis are examples.

E. Toxic and Metabolic Diseases

In one sense, all diseases are metabolic, because the only way to damage any organ is to interfere with cellular metabolism. For example, occlusive vascular disease deprives cells of oxygen and energy sources, ultimately terminating all cellular processes. This would not generally be considered a metabolic disease, however, because there is an underlying structural lesion: an obstructed blood vessel. The term metabolic disease is reserved for processes that disrupt cellular metabolism at a molecular level without any underlying structural lesion evident macroscopically. Diseases caused by toxic substances, both endogenous (e.g., uremia) and exogenous (e.g., drug overdose), are included in this category. Diabetes mellitus, thyroid disease, vitamin B12 deficiency, abnormal liver function, electrolyte abnormalities, and hypoxemia are some other metabolic disorders that commonly produce neurologic symptoms. Since structural lesions are excluded by definition, metabolic diseases are *diffuse*. Their time course can be *acute, subacute,* or *chronic*. They can be *static* or *progressive*.

F. Traumatic Diseases

The main feature distinguishing traumatic disease from vascular disease is an epidemiologic consideration: the onset in the setting of trauma. Traumatic disorders are always *acute* in onset. Non-hemorrhagic traumatic lesions are generally *static* or *improving*; they may be *diffuse* (concussion) or *focal* (contusion, encephalomalacia). Traumatic hemorrhage has the same spatial-temporal profile as nontraumatic hemorrhage: It is *progressive* and may be *diffuse* or *focal*.

G. Congenital and Developmental Diseases

Congenital and developmental disorders are conceptually very similar to degenerative diseases, except that the deterioration begins early in life. In some cases, the affected nervous system component never develops at all. Like degenerative disease, developmental disorders are characteristically *chronic* and *diffuse*. They may be *progressive* or (unlike degenerative disease) they may be *static*.

Table 3.1 summarizes the way in which these diagnostic categories can be distinguished based on focality and time course.

It is often helpful to distinguish between mass lesions and non-mass lesions. *Mass lesions* alter cellular function not only at the site of the lesion but also in the surrounding area, by compression or destruction of neighboring tissue. *Non-mass lesions* alter cellular function at the site of the lesion but spare adjacent tissue. Mass lesions cause *focal, progressive* symptoms. Diffuse processes, regardless of time course, are non-mass lesions; so are lesions that are focal but not progressive. The prototypical mass lesions are hemorrhages (parenchymal, subdural, and epidural), abscesses, and neoplasms.

The categories listed in Table 3.1 easily generalize to multifocal conditions. Thus, an acute multifocal process is still most likely vascular (and probably embolic) or traumatic. Just as subacute focal processes are generally inflammatory, so are subacute multifocal processes. Multiple sclerosis is the most common specific diagnosis when the lesions are all in the central nervous system. Other diagnoses in this category include vasculitis and endocarditis. When chronic symptoms are multifocal rather than focal, neoplastic disease remains the prime diagnostic consideration. Specifically, a metastatic tumor is the most likely diagnosis in this setting.

This approach is less useful for transient symptoms, where the distinction between acute, subacute, and chronic symptoms becomes less meaningful. Moreover, the symptoms often resolve so quickly that it is impossible to distinguish between multifocal and diffuse lesions. Even so, it may be possible to determine whether transient symptoms are focal or diffuse, especially when they recur episodically—over time, patients may learn to identify and describe their symptoms in detail. The three most common causes of focal transient symptoms are seizures, transient ischemic attacks, and migraines. Diffuse transient symptoms are typically caused by transient hypoperfusion (e.g., due to cardiac arrhythmia), seizures, or metabolic processes (e.g., hepatic encephalopathy, hypoglycemia, and intoxication).

Table 3.1 Characteristic Spatial-Temporal Profiles of Major Disease Process Categories

	Acute	Subacute	Chronic
Focal	1. Vascular (ischemic stroke; parenchymal hemorrhage) 2. Traumatic (parenchymal, subdural, or epidural hemorrhage; contusion)	Inflammatory (abscess)	Neoplastic
Diffuse	1. Vascular (subarachnoid hemorrhage) 2. Traumatic (concussion, subarachnoid hemorrhage) 3. Toxic-metabolic (including anoxic)	1. Inflammatory (meningitis, encephalitis) 2. Toxic-metabolic	1. Degenerative 2. Congenital-developmental 3. Toxic-metabolic

IV. Discussion of Case Histories

Case 1. The aphasia, right hemianopia, and right hemiparesis localize the lesion to the left cerebral cortex (if this is unclear, review Chapter 1). The lesion is therefore **focal**. It is also **progressive**, so it is a mass lesion. The time course is **chronic**, making a *neoplasm* most likely.

Comment: An appropriate summary note might read: "55-year-old woman with a 10-week history of progressive symptoms and neurologic findings suggestive of a left cortical mass lesion, likely neoplasm." In this case, magnetic resonance imaging (MRI) and biopsy confirmed the diagnosis of glioma. The patient was treated with radiation therapy and chemotherapy.

Case 2. Facial weakness ipsilateral to body weakness suggests a focal lesion in the high pons or above (see Speed Rule 6 in Chapter 1). There has been **no progression**, so this is not a mass lesion. The symptoms developed **acutely**. A focal lesion that develops acutely is usually *vascular* (unless there is a history of trauma); the rapid improvement would be more suggestive of an ischemic stroke than a hemorrhage.

Comment: A computed tomography (CT) scan demonstrated a small infarct in the right internal capsule. By the time he reached the emergency department, the patient was outside the time window for thrombolytic or intravascular therapy. He had his antihypertensive medications adjusted and was started on aspirin and atorvastatin.

Case 3. The altered level of consciousness indicates dysfunction in the brainstem, thalamus, or both cerebral hemispheres (see Speed Rule 11 in Chapter 1). The generalized seizures are indicative of bihemispheric disease. All of the abnormal neurologic findings (e.g., hyperreflexia and Babinski signs) are symmetric. Thus, the condition is **diffuse**. It follows that it is not a mass lesion. The symptoms developed over 2 days, making the onset **subacute**. A diffuse, subacute process could either be *toxic–metabolic* or *inflammatory* (meningitis or encephalitis). In this case, the fever and stiff neck make meningitis or encephalitis most likely.

Comment: The patient was empirically treated with ceftriaxone, vancomycin, acyclovir, and dexamethasone, and a lumbar puncture was performed immediately. Cerebrospinal fluid examination demonstrated greater than 200 white blood cells, predominantly lymphocytic. When cerebrospinal fluid cultures remained negative at 48 hours, the ceftriaxone and vancomycin were stopped and the acyclovir was continued. The patient gradually recovered, and polymerase chain reaction testing of the spinal fluid confirmed the diagnosis of herpes simplex encephalitis.

Case 4. The right facial numbness and left body numbness indicate a lesion on the right between the pons and the C2 level of the spinal cord (see Speed Rule 5 in Chapter 1). The right facial weakness and the tinnitus and hearing loss in the right ear localize the lesion further, to the right pons or pontomedullary junction. Such a precise unilateral localization implies a *focal* lesion. It is *progressive*, so it is a mass lesion. The progression has taken place over several years, making it *chronic*. A focal, chronic lesion is a *neoplasm*.

Comment: In this case, the neoplasm was a schwannoma—a benign tumor. It was resected, and the patient continues to do well 15 years later.

Case 5. As with Case 2, the weakness of the left face, arm, and leg implies a right-sided *focal* lesion at the level of the high pons or above. It is a mass lesion, because it is *progressive*. The time course is *chronic* (3 months). Again, a focal, chronic lesion signifies a *neoplasm*.

Comment: A CT scan demonstrated a right subdural hematoma. This shows how the rules are only approximations—if neoplasm is interpreted to mean malignancy, then the rules led us astray, but in fact, a subdural hematoma represents a "new growth" that slowly expands, so for practical purposes it behaves like a benign tumor. The patient had the hematoma evacuated, and he recovered fully.

Case 6. Even without information about the physical examination, the likely lesion localization can be inferred from this patient's history alone. The abnormal sensory and motor function below a level in the mid-abdomen implies a focal lesion in the spinal cord, at the thoracic level or above (see Speed Rule 3 in Chapter 1). A diffuse process involving peripheral nerves, plexus, or nerve roots could also result in sensory and motor symptoms throughout both lower extremities but would not cause a sensory level on the trunk. Since the symptoms are *focal* and *progressive*, this is a mass lesion. The time course is *subacute*. A focal, subacute lesion is typically *inflammatory*—specifically, an abscess.

Comment: An MRI scan of the cervical and thoracic spine failed to demonstrate an abscess, but it showed findings consistent with demyelination at the level of T7–T8 and a lumbar puncture revealed spinal fluid pleocytosis. All cultures were negative. This patient was thought to have myelitis, and her symptoms gradually resolved without treatment. The myelitis was thought to be autoimmune based on the negative cultures and the self-limited course. This is another example of how the rules can fail. In this case, they pointed to the correct diagnostic category (inflammatory) but the progressive time course suggested a mass lesion, especially an abscess. Even though the ultimate diagnosis was something different, the rules led to the correct diagnostic tests. It was appropriate to focus on the possibility of an abscess, which could not be excluded based on the clinical findings and would have required urgent treatment.

Case 7. This patient has personality changes and deficits in several different cognitive functions, including language comprehension, short-term and long-term memory, and calculations. This implies a *diffuse* cortical localization. Since it is diffuse, this is not a mass lesion. The deficits have *progressed* over several months, making this a *chronic* problem. A diffuse, chronic disorder can be a *degenerative* disease, a *congenital/developmental* problem, or a *toxic–metabolic* disorder. The patient is too old to be presenting with a congenital or developmental disease, and there is nothing to suggest any specific metabolic abnormality, so a degenerative disease is most likely.

Comment: Even though a degenerative disease is the most likely diagnosis, potential toxic-metabolic causes should be investigated. In fact, neoplasms can sometimes break the rules and produce a diffuse picture rather than a focal one (e.g., a CNS lymphoma). This patient had a head CT scan and a number of blood and urine tests to investigate these possibilities. All results were normal, and her subsequent course was consistent with Alzheimer disease.

Case 8. This case is similar to Case 3, except that the time course is *acute* rather than subacute. The lesion is *diffuse* (and therefore not a mass lesion), and it is *progressive*: This means it is either *vascular* (specifically, subarachnoid hemorrhage), *toxic-metabolic*, or *traumatic*. There is no history of trauma and no reason to suspect a toxic-metabolic disorder, so subarachnoid hemorrhage is the most likely diagnosis.

Comment: A head CT scan was normal, but a lumbar puncture showed subarachnoid blood. A cerebral angiogram demonstrated an aneurysm of the anterior communicating artery. The aneurysm was successfully coiled, and the patient has returned to his baseline level of function.

Case 9. The reduced pinprick sensation over the left side of the face and right side of the body implies a *focal* lesion on the left, between the pons and the C2 level of the spinal cord (see Speed Rule 5 in Chapter 1). The weakness of the left side of the palate confines the lesion to the medulla because only lower motor neuron lesions produce unilateral palatal weakness (see Chapter 2). Ataxia of the left arm and leg is also consistent with a focal lesion in this location because a lesion on the left side of the medulla can affect fibers traveling to the left cerebellar hemisphere via the left inferior cerebellar peduncle. The symptoms began *acutely* and have *not progressed*, so this is not a mass lesion. A focal, acute lesion is either *vascular* or *traumatic*, and there is no history of trauma. The fact that the symptoms have remained stable over 7 hours makes an ischemic stroke more likely than hemorrhage, but there is no way to be sure of this without an imaging study.

Comment: This patient had a normal noncontrast head CT scan, but an MRI revealed a small infarction in the left lateral medulla. Seven hours had passed since her symptoms began, so she was not eligible for intravenous thrombolysis, and vascular imaging showed no large vessel obstruction that would be amenable to clot retrieval. In the emergency department, she was found to have atrial fibrillation, which had never been noted before. The stroke was presumed to be embolic, so after 5 days anti-coagulant therapy was begun. Further evaluation revealed hyperthyroidism. She was converted to normal sinus rhythm, her hyperthyroidism was treated, and after 6 months the anticoagulation was stopped. By then, her symptoms had completely resolved except for minimal ataxia of the left arm.

Case 10. This patient has symptoms confined to the distribution of a single nerve root. This makes a lesion in the nerve root itself most likely, but, theoretically, the lesion could be anywhere from the level of the nerve root on up the sensory pathway to the cortex. Additional symptoms would be expected with any of these higher localizations, however. In any case, the lesion is *focal*. It is *not progressive*, so it is not a mass lesion. The time course is *subacute*, so the process is probably *inflammatory*.

Comment: Epidemiologic factors help diagnose the specific inflammatory disorder. A rash in a dermatomal distribution is very suggestive of herpes zoster reactivation, which can produce sensory symptoms (especially pain) in the same distribution. Immunocompromised individuals, including those receiving chemotherapy for cancer, have an increased risk of herpes zoster reactivation. The patient received famciclovir and pain treatment, and the symptoms gradually resolved.

Case 11. In addition to chest wall symptoms like those described by the patient in Case 10, this patient has left leg weakness, which could not be explained by a lesion in a thoracic nerve root. Instead, the most plausible localization is within the thoracic spinal cord on the left, in the one or two segments where the spinothalamic pathway has not yet crossed to the right side of the cord. This is a *focal* lesion, and since it is *progressive*, it is a mass lesion. The time course is *chronic*. A chronic focal lesion is a *neoplasm*.

Comment: An MRI scan revealed a meningioma compressing the left T4 nerve root and the spinal cord at that level. This benign tumor was resected, and the patient's only residual symptom was mild stiffness of the left leg.

II
Common Diseases

Chapter 4

Stroke

I. Case Histories

Case 1. A 65-year-old man drove himself to the emergency room at 9 a.m. after experiencing a 4-minute episode of word-finding difficulty and right hand weakness. He has experienced four similar episodes in the last 3 weeks. He had coronary bypass surgery for unstable angina a year ago, and he has a long history of hypertension and diabetes. He takes aspirin, propranolol, and glyburide daily. He is afebrile, his blood pressure is 140/80, his pulse is 85 per minute and regular, and the remainder of his examination (including neurologic examination) is normal.

Case 2. A 59-year-old woman came to the emergency room at her family's insistence at 9 p.m. after she mentioned that she had been having trouble seeing out of her left eye since awakening that morning. She has been in good health except for long-standing hypertension and occasional "rapid heartbeats." She denies previous visual symptoms or other episodic neurologic symptoms. She takes lisinopril. Her blood pressure is 170/95, her pulse is 130 per minute and irregular, and she has no murmurs or bruits. The only abnormality on neurologic exam is a left homonymous hemianopia.

Case 3. A 73-year-old man was brought to the emergency room by paramedics after he fell down on the way back from the bathroom and discovered that he could not move his left side. His symptoms have not progressed in the 90 minutes that have elapsed since the initial event. He has been hypertensive for 20 years and takes hydrochlorothiazide; he has also been taking lovastatin for a year because of hyperlipidemia. He denies previous episodes of focal neurologic symptoms. His blood pressure is 180/100 and his pulse is 80 per minute and regular. His examination is notable for a left visual field defect; a right gaze preference; weakness and reduced sensation in the left face, arm, and leg; and mild left-sided neglect.

Questions:

1. What are the causes of these patients' symptoms?
2. How would you manage these patients in the emergency room?
3. Would you admit these patients to the hospital?
4. What tests would you order?
5. What treatment would you initiate?

II. Approach to Stroke

In managing a patient who has suddenly developed neurologic symptoms, the first question is:

1. Are the symptoms due to vascular disease (ischemia, hemorrhage)?
   If the answer to this question is yes, three additional questions are fundamental:
2. If the patient has had an ischemic stroke, what can be done to restore blood flow?
3. What can be done to limit the damage?
4. What can be done to reduce the patient's risk of future strokes? Question 4 has two components:

   4a. What can be done to reduce the risk of cerebrovascular disease? In fact, this question applies to everyone with risk factors for vascular disease, even those who have never had neurologic symptoms. The term *primary prevention* refers to measures that can reduce the risk of stroke in patients who have never had one.
   4b. What can be done to reduce the risk of stroke in patients who have already had at least one stroke or TIA? These measures are referred to as *secondary prevention*—they are similar but not identical to things that are done for primary prevention.

   Question 1 is addressed in Part IV, Questions 2 and 3 in Part V, Question 4a in Part VIII, and Question 4b in Parts VI and VII. Part III presents some definitions and necessary background information.

III. Background Information

A. Definitions

stroke: cell death in a localized region of the central nervous system resulting from a disturbance of the local circulation, typically causing sudden
onset of a focal neurologic deficit

ischemic stroke: a stroke caused by inadequate blood flow (synonyms: cerebral infarction, or infarct)

hemorrhagic stroke: a stroke caused by bleeding through a ruptured blood
vessel wall; the location can be parenchymal, subarachnoid, subdural,
or epidural

transient ischemic attack (TIA): a transient episode of neurologic dysfunction caused by focal brain, spinal cord, or retinal ischemia, without
acute infarction

anterior circulation: the internal carotid arteries and all blood vessels
derived from them

posterior circulation: the vertebral and basilar arteries and all blood vessels
derived from them

B. Classification of Strokes by Etiology

About 80% of strokes are ischemic (also called infarctions or infarcts) and
20% are hemorrhagic. An ischemic stroke is usually due to obstruction of
an individual artery. In some cases the obstruction is caused by an embolus
that flowed downstream from the heart or some other proximal site in the
vascular tree and lodged in that artery. In other cases the blockage is due
to disease in the artery itself. The most common cause of local obstruction
is arteriolosclerosis (also called lipohyalinosis), a vasculopathy affecting
small arteries that penetrate the brain substance. It is most common in
patients with hypertension. Occlusion of a single penetrating artery to the
brain results in a small (less than 1.5 cm) subcortical infarct, often called
a *lacunar infarct,* or *lacune.* Atherosclerosis is another common cause of
local obstruction. Other potential causes include fibromuscular dysplasia,
arteritis, dissection of the arterial wall, migraine, and coagulopathies.

Strokes can also occur when there is thrombosis in a cerebral sinus
or vein, obstructing the venous drainage from a brain region. This most
commonly occurs in patients who have a coagulopathy, who are severely

dehydrated, or who are peripartum. COVID-19 infection and COVID-19 vaccination have both been implicated as risk factors in cerebral venous sinus thrombosis.

Ischemia damages not only the neurons and glial cells in the affected region but also the blood vessels in that region, rendering them more prone to rupture. This can result in "hemorrhagic transformation" (also referred to as "hemorrhagic conversion") of an infarct, which sometimes causes a recognizable deterioration in the patient's clinical condition, or smaller petechial hemorrhages that can be detected with imaging but may have no clinical consequences.

Hemorrhage into an infarct bed is distinguished from primary hemorrhage into the brain parenchyma, which is usually due to rupture of small dilatations of penetrating arteries in the brain. These dilatations are most common in patients with arteriolosclerosis, which is associated with chronic hypertension. Another cause of primary hemorrhage is cerebral amyloid angiopathy, a condition that is strongly associated with Alzheimer disease. In this condition, amyloid infiltrates the media and adventitia of small and medium-sized arterioles and capillaries of the cortex, weakening the arterial wall and leading to rupture. In contrast to primary hemorrhage associated with hypertension, which affects mostly deep structures, primary hemorrhage associated with amyloid angiopathy characteristically causes "lobar hemorrhage" involving both gray matter and the underlying white matter.

Hemorrhage into the subarachnoid space usually occurs after rupture of an arterial wall outpouching known as a *saccular (or "berry") aneurysm.* These are typically located at bifurcations of the major arteries in the circle of Willis. Rupture of a vascular malformation can result in either parenchymal or subarachnoid hemorrhage (or both). Vascular malformations are classified into four categories. *Arteriovenous malformations* (AVMs), consisting of direct communication between arteries and veins with no intervening capillary bed, are the ones most likely to produce hemorrhage. *Cavernous angiomas* (also known as *cavernous hemangiomas* or *cavernomas*) are small collections of closely packed, distended blood vessels of varying wall thickness without any intervening brain parenchyma; they are low pressure systems that are often clinically silent, but they may result in hemorrhage. *Venous angiomas* (also known as *developmental venous anomalies*) consist of one or more dilated veins, with no arterial component. They are very low-pressure systems that generally have no clinical significance. *Capillary telangiectasias* are made up of multiple small caliber, very thin-walled vessels within normal brain; they almost never bleed.

C. Pathophysiology

Ischemic stroke occurs when a localized area in the central nervous system is deprived of glucose and oxygen because of inadequate local blood flow. The severity of injury is a function of how much the blood flow has been reduced and for how long. In the center of a region of focal ischemia, blood flow is typically less than 20–30% of normal. If this degree of ischemia persists for more than an hour, all tissue elements in the region undergo complete necrosis. Surrounding this maximally affected zone is an area known as the ischemic penumbra, in which the blood flow reduction is less profound. Cells in this area revert to anaerobic glycolysis, triggering an *ischemic cascade*. Tissue lactate, hydrogen ions, and inorganic phosphate concentrations rise. Neurons lose their electrical excitability and their ability to regulate intracellular calcium. Calcium floods into the cells, precipitating the release of the excitatory amino acids glutamate and aspartate into the extracellular space. At high concentrations, these amino acids have a variety of harmful effects, including a further increase in intracellular calcium, which affects protein phosphorylation, leading to alterations in gene expression and protein synthesis. At the same time, the transmembrane ionic gradients begin to deteriorate and water flows passively into the neurons, resulting in cellular edema. Increased lipolysis leads to release of arachidonic acid and the production of free radicals, which are highly reactive species that damage proteins, DNA, and the fatty acids in cell membranes. These processes trigger specific derangements of genomic expression that result in apoptosis (programmed cell death).

If blood flow is restored early enough, the ischemic cascade can be terminated, but beyond a certain time window the destructive cycle becomes self-sustaining and cell death becomes inevitable. The duration of that time window depends on the extent to which blood flow is reduced—the more profound the reduction, the shorter the time window. The availability of collateral blood supply generally increases with increasing distance from the center of the stroke, so the time window for salvaging cells is usually longer in the periphery of the ischemic penumbra than in the more central regions.

The pathophysiology of ischemic stroke resulting from venous obstruction is less well understood, but most likely the obstruction in venous outflow produces a sudden mass effect in a localized region of brain, compressing the tiniest vessels in the arterial tree and compromising their ability to deliver oxygen to the brain tissue. This precipitates the same ischemic cascade that occurs when the disruption of blood supply is at the level of a larger, more proximal artery. The mechanism of cellular injury in hemorrhagic stroke is probably similar—a sudden increase in local pressure compresses all the end-arteries in the region, triggering the ischemic cascade—but this is less well established.

IV. Diagnosis

A. Clinical Features

In most cases, strokes can be diagnosed purely from history and examination. As discussed in Chapter 3, vascular disease presents with acute, focal symptoms. Focality is the key feature. For ischemic strokes, not only is the lesion focal, but also it lies within the territory of a single artery (see Figures 4.1, 4.2, and 4.3). Thus, recognition of ischemic stroke requires some knowledge of the typical syndromes produced by occlusion of the various arteries (Table 4.1).

Occlusion of the ophthalmic artery, the first branch of the internal carotid artery (ICA), results in loss of vision in the ipsilateral eye. The vision may go totally black, or it may just be dim, dark, or obscured. The episodes are usually transient, and patients sometimes describe the onset and resolution as "like a shade," first closing and later opening, but patients' descriptions vary widely. This symptom is often referred to as "amaurosis fugax."

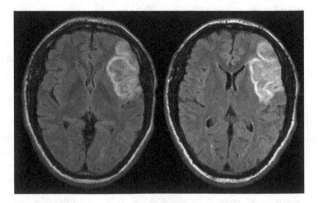

Fig. 4.1 MRI (FLAIR sequence, axial plane) images showing an ischemic stroke in the distribution of the superior division of the left middle cerebral artery (MCA). (*Source:* Preston DC, Shapiro BE. Neuroimaging in neurology: an interactive CD. Elsevier, 2007).

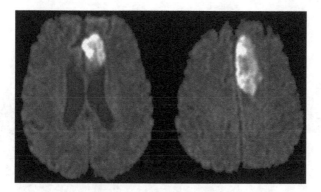

Fig. 4.2 MRI (diffusion-weighted sequence, axial plane) images showing an ischemic stroke in the distribution of the left anterior cerebral artery (ACA). Note that the diffusion-weighted sequences offer less spatial resolution than T1, T2, or FLAIR images, but they are more sensitive for identifying ischemia early in the course. (*Source:* Preston DC, Shapiro BE. Neuroimaging in neurology: an interactive CD. Elsevier, 2007).

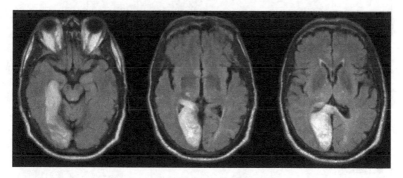

Fig. 4.3 MRI (FLAIR sequence, axial plane) images showing an ischemic stroke in the distribution of the right posterior cerebral artery (PCA). (*Source:* Preston DC, Shapiro BE. Neuroimaging in neurology: an interactive CD. Elsevier, 2007).

Occlusion of the middle cerebral artery (MCA) typically produces contralateral numbness and weakness affecting face and arm more than leg, a contralateral visual field deficit, and difficulty turning both eyes toward the weak side (i.e., toward the side contralateral to the occluded MCA). MCA occlusion on the dominant side can result in aphasia. MCA occlusion

Table 4.1 Clinical Features Associated with Ischemic Strokes in the Distribution of Major Cerebral Arteries

Artery	Weakness	Sensory Loss	Visual Field Deficit	Other
MCA	Contralateral face, arm > leg	Contralateral face, arm > leg	Contralateral hemifield	1. Impaired gaze in contralateral direction 2a. Dominant hemisphere MCA: aphasia 2b. Nondominant hemisphere MCA: visuospatial impairment 3. Contralateral hemineglect (especially with nondominant hemisphere MCA strokes)
ACA	Contralateral leg > arm	Contralateral leg > arm		Deficits of attention and/or motivation
PCA			Contralateral hemi field	Dominant hemisphere PCA: alexia without agraphia
Vertebrobasilar				
A. Lateral Medulla	Usually minimal	1. Ipsilateral face 2. Contralateral arm, leg, trunk		1. Ipsilateral Horner syndrome 2. Ipsilateral ataxia 3. Dysarthria, dysphagia 4. Nystagmus 5. Vertigo

Vertebrobasilar B. Medial Medulla	Contralateral arm, leg	Contralateral arm, leg (especially proprioception)	Ipsilateral tongue weakness
Vertebrobasilar C. Pons	1. Ipsilateral face 2. Contralateral arm, leg	1. Contralateral arm, leg, trunk 2. Ipsilateral face (sometimes contralateral or bilateral)	1. Impaired gaze in ipsilateral direction 2. Nystagmus 3. Ipsilateral Horner syndrome 4. Ataxia (ipsilateral or contralateral)
Vertebrobasilar D. Midbrain	Contralateral face, arm, leg		1. Ipsilateral third nerve palsy 2. Contralateral ataxia (in some cases)

on the nondominant side can produce visuospatial deficits; a distinctive example is difficulty dressing oneself ("dressing apraxia"). Contralateral neglect can result from MCA occlusion on either side, but it is usually more prominent with lesions on the nondominant side.

Anterior cerebral artery (ACA) occlusion typically produces numbness and weakness of the contralateral leg, with less involvement of the arm. ICA occlusion results in a combination of the MCA and ACA syndromes. Conversely, occlusion of a branch of the MCA or ACA produces only a portion of the full syndrome.

Posterior cerebral artery (PCA) occlusion produces a contralateral visual field defect. Some patients who have dominant hemisphere PCA occlusion that includes the splenium of the corpus callosum have alexia without agraphia—they can write but can't read (even things they just wrote themselves). Occlusions of the basilar or vertebral arteries or their branches produce infarcts in portions of the brainstem or cerebellum and corresponding clinical syndromes that reflect the cranial nerves in the affected territory, as well as the ascending and descending tracts passing through the infarcted region. One classic syndrome is the lateral medullary syndrome ("Wallenberg syndrome"), consisting of reduced pain and temperature sensation in the ipsilateral face and the contralateral limbs and trunk, an ipsilateral Horner syndrome, dysarthria, dysphagia, ataxia, vertigo, and nystagmus. Another classic syndrome is produced by infarction of the midbrain affecting the cerebral peduncle and the oculomotor nerve, resulting in an ipsilateral third nerve lesion and contralateral hemiparesis ("Weber syndrome").

Lacunar infarcts most frequently occur in the basal ganglia, thalamus, pons, or internal capsule, and they are associated with several classic clinical syndromes: pure motor (hemiparesis with no sensory deficit), pure sensory (numbness on one entire side of the body, but normal strength throughout), ataxic hemiparesis (ataxia and mild weakness on one side of the body), and "clumsy hand–dysarthria" (as the name implies). These *lacunar syndromes* are not specific, however. The same clinical syndromes can result from many other mechanisms, including large vessel occlusion, cardioembolism, vasculitis, and even compression from tumors or hematomas.

In some cases, ischemia resolves spontaneously before any permanent tissue damage occurs; this is called a transient ischemic attack, or TIA. By definition, the patient's neurologic examination reverts to baseline at the conclusion of a TIA, so TIAs are usually diagnosed purely on the basis of history (unless the patient can be examined while the event is still in progress). Some patients with complete resolution of their clinical symptoms nonetheless have evidence of permanent damage on MRI scans. In other words, their clinical presentation suggests a TIA, but their MRI scan proves that they've had a stroke. This discrepancy usually has no effect on management because the secondary prevention measures discussed in Part VI (and summarized in Table 4.2) are the same for TIAs and strokes.

Subarachnoid hemorrhage does not routinely invade the brain parenchyma, so unlike other types of stroke it does not typically present with focal symptoms and signs. The usual presenting symptoms are headache and meningeal signs, so it is discussed in Chapter 12. Venous infarcts are difficult to distinguish clinically from arterial ischemia, except that they need not conform to the distribution of an individual artery, and they typically occur in patients who are predisposed to coagulation disorders. Patients with venous infarcts often report headache. Recent head trauma is the main clue suggesting epidural or subdural hemorrhage. Parenchymal, subdural, and epidural hemorrhages usually produce greater mass effect than ischemic strokes do in the acute setting, so they are more likely to cause headache or a reduced level of consciousness. They can also produce signs and symptoms that overlap more than one arterial territory. At times, however, they can be indistinguishable from ischemic strokes—the only reliable way to differentiate ischemic stroke from parenchymal, subdural, or epidural hemorrhage is with imaging studies.

B. Imaging

Most acute infarctions are evident on the diffusion-weighted sequences of an MRI scan within minutes, but in most medical centers MRI scans are difficult to obtain acutely, during the time window in which immediate intervention is possible. CT scans are much more readily available in the acute setting, but acute infarctions are often undetectable on CT scans for hours or days after symptom onset. Parenchymal, subdural, and epidural hemorrhages are visible on CT scans immediately, however. Patients with these conditions may be clinically indistinguishable from patients with ischemic stroke, but the acute management is very different, so it is standard practice to obtain a non-contrast CT scan immediately in the setting of an acute stroke.

If the patient's clinical presentation is consistent with occlusion of a relatively large intracerebral artery, additional imaging studies are often necessary to guide decisions about mechanical clot retrieval (see Part V, Section A). When clot retrieval is a consideration, CT angiography (CTA) should be performed at the same time as the standard CT scan. In some situations, a CT perfusion (CTP) scan is helpful; this technique shows what part of the brain is receiving abnormally low blood flow and identifies the subset of that region where the damage is already irreversible. Magnetic resonance angiography (MRA) and magnetic resonance perfusion (MRP) scans provide analogous information, but they are less readily available.

In situations where venous infarcts are a consideration, magnetic resonance venography (MRV) or computed tomographic venography (CTV) can be performed. Carotid ultrasound, CTA, and MRA are all options for assessing the internal carotid arteries to inform decisions about carotid endarterectomy or stenting. Traditional intra-arterial (catheter) angiography is still considered the gold standard method for evaluating the extracranial and intracranial cerebral arteries, and it is necessary in some circumstances, but less invasive methods usually suffice.

V. Management of Acute Stroke

A. Restoration of Blood Flow in Ischemic Stroke

The primary goal of acute stroke treatment is to restore blood flow to the ischemic penumbra before the ischemic cascade reaches an irreversible stage. The two methods for restoring blood flow are administration of thrombolytic ("clot-busting") agents and endovascular mechanical clot retrieval. The standard thrombolytic agent used for stroke is recombinant tissue plasminogen activator (recombinant tPA, also called rtPA or simply tPA). Two formulations of tPA are available: alteplase and tenecteplase (TNK). Many centers in the United States have transitioned from alteplase to TNK because TNK is less costly and simpler to administer. Alteplase is administered as a bolus followed by a 1-hour infusion; TNK has a longer half-life, so it is given as a bolus without a subsequent infusion.

Unfortunately, when the ischemia persists beyond a certain point the brain tissue is no longer salvageable. At that point, restoration of blood flow can actually be harmful, because the sudden increase in perfusion pressure can overwhelm the already impaired blood vessels in the ischemic zone, resulting in hemorrhage. Hemorrhage is a particular concern when a thrombolytic agent is used. The result is that restoration of blood flow is beneficial only during a narrow time window.

The challenge is to determine when that window has closed. One approach is simply to calculate the amount of time that has elapsed since the onset of stroke symptoms. Patients who receive tPA intravenously within 4.5 hours of the onset of ischemic stroke symptoms are significantly more likely than untreated patients to have minimal or no neurologic deficit 3 months later. Although tPA treatment also increases the likelihood of intracerebral hemorrhage in the first 36 hours, the beneficial effect of the treatment outweighs the risk. Similarly, patients with occlusion of a relatively large intracerebral artery whose thrombus is removed using an endovascular stent retriever device ("mechanical thrombectomy") within 6 hours of the onset of stroke symptoms have a much higher likelihood of a good outcome than patients managed medically.

The time interval from stroke onset is an imprecise gauge of how much brain tissue can still be salvaged. The other approach to determining whether the window of opportunity for acute reperfusion therapy is still open is with imaging studies that identify brain regions that are underperfused and brain regions that are permanently damaged; CTP is the imaging modality typically used. When there is enough of a mismatch between ischemic core and penumbra (i.e., when a sufficiently large area of the underperfused region is not yet permanently damaged), then the benefits of mechanical thrombectomy often outweigh the risks, even out to 24 hours in some instances. This type of imaging evidence might also permit extension of the window for intravenous tPA. It remains unknown how much mismatch is necessary for the benefit of reperfusion treatment to outweigh the risk; some recent trials have suggested that reperfusion may be beneficial even when perfusion imaging shows a large ischemic core. Ongoing trials may expand the treatment window, patient eligibility criteria, or both.

The magnitude of benefit from mechanical thrombectomy, on average, is greater than the magnitude of benefit from intravenous tPA. For patients who are ultimately treated with mechanical thrombectomy, the evidence is mixed regarding whether prior administration of intravenous tPA improves outcomes. The current standard of care is to administer intravenous tPA to all patients who are eligible for it (see Table 4.3), even if they may also be a candidate for mechanical thrombectomy. Every effort should be made to start infusing the tPA as early as possible because the likelihood of benefit is time dependent. Because timing has such an impact on treatment decisions and outcomes, the goal of the initial neurologic examination is to get a general idea of the scope and severity of the patient's deficits as quickly as possible. The National Institutes of Health Stroke Scale, or NIHSS (Table 4.4), is often used for this purpose. The NIHSS provides only a rudimentary picture of the patient's condition. It is useful mainly because higher scores correlate with larger, more severe strokes. A high score does not necessarily mean that a patient has had a stroke, however. The clinical context is essential when interpreting the NIHSS, and a more thorough neurologic examination should be performed as soon as it's feasible.

In patients who have had a TIA or minor stroke who do not receive a thrombolytic agent, 3–4 weeks of combined treatment with aspirin and another antiplatelet agent (either clopidogrel or ticagrelor), started within 24 hours of symptom onset, reduces the risk of stroke recurrence. Aspirin administered within 48 hours of the onset of a stroke results in a small but statistically significant improvement in outcome.

Anticoagulation with low-molecular-weight heparin is recommended for patients with cerebral venous infarction, even when intracerebral hemorrhage is present. Patients whose condition continues to deteriorate are sometimes treated with thrombectomy or direct installation of a thrombolytic agent into the thrombus, but this has not been demonstrated to improve outcomes.

Although reperfusion therapy can have dramatic effects, there will always be situations in which the ischemic cascade reaches an irreversible stage before blood flow can be restored. The ideal would be to pair reperfusion therapy with treatments that can halt or even reverse the ischemic cascade. Attempts to limit free radical formation, excitatory amino acid release, trans-membrane ion shifts, or programmed cell death remain the subject of intense study, but every agent tried so far has been disappointing.

B. Limitation of Deficits

Even though the neuronal injury that results from a stroke cannot yet be treated successfully, factors that exacerbate the damage can be addressed. Both neurologic and systemic complications must be considered.

1. Neurologic complications

Strokes can produce significant edema, causing increased intracranial pressure that may result in mass effect on the brainstem, affecting level of consciousness and autonomic functions. This can be fatal. When clinical or radiologic findings suggest increased intracranial pressure, osmotic therapy and moderate hyperventilation (to a pCO_2 target of 30–34 mm Hg) are commonly used (see Chapter 11), although there is limited evidence that these measures are beneficial in the specific setting of stroke. Hemicraniectomy—removal of the lateral-coronal portion of the skull—can decompress a rapidly swelling cerebral hemisphere in patients with severely increased intracranial pressure due to large ischemic MCA strokes. Although this procedure may be lifesaving, it may also leave the patient with severe residual disability. Patients and families must be thoroughly informed of the risks and "best case" scenario before proceeding with this intervention. The best clinical outcomes have been reported with younger patients. Large ischemic strokes in the cerebellum can swell and compress the brainstem, and most clinicians agree (though the evidence is mainly anecdotal) that the appropriate treatment is urgent decompressive suboccipital craniotomy with removal of the necrotic tissue. Similarly, most clinicians advocate clot evacuation for patients who have a large parenchymal *hemorrhage* in the cerebellum, again based on anecdotal evidence. Clot evacuation has not been shown to be beneficial for supratentorial parenchymal hemorrhage, but studies with minimally invasive surgical techniques are ongoing.

Ischemic or hemorrhagic brain regions may serve as seizure foci. Seizures may even be the presenting symptom of infarction or hemorrhage on occasion. Patients who have seizures in the setting of a stroke should be loaded promptly with an antiseizure medication (ASM), because seizures produce a transient rise in intracranial pressure, and this can be particularly dangerous in stroke patients who already have increased intracranial pressure due to edema. Status epilepticus is even more ominous in that regard and requires urgent treatment (see Chapter 5). The consequences of a seizure may be particularly dire in patients who have had an intraparenchymal hemorrhage (who almost always have elevated intracranial pressure to some degree) or in patients who have had a subarachnoid hemorrhage (who are at high risk of rebleeding). For this reason, some clinicians begin prophylactic ASM treatment in these patients even if they have not had a seizure, but controlled trials have not been conducted, and current guidelines discourage the use of prophylactic ASMs. There is no evidence that prophylactic ASM treatment is beneficial after an ischemic stroke, and current guidelines discourage this practice, also.

Any patient with an intracranial lesion is at risk for hyponatremia, due to either SIADH (syndrome of inappropriate secretion of antidiuretic hormone) or cerebral salt wasting. Hyponatremia may in turn produce further neuronal injury, either directly or by provoking seizure activity. Serum sodium should be measured regularly, and appropriate testing and treatment undertaken if hyponatremia develops.

People who have suffered strokes (especially left hemisphere strokes) develop depression at a rate higher than would be predicted simply on the basis of a situational response to their deficits, suggesting that depression may be a direct manifestation of the brain injury. When severe, the depression may significantly impede clinical recovery from a stroke. Antidepressant medications may alleviate depression; it is unclear whether they affect overall post-stroke functional outcome.

2. Systemic factors

Hypoxia, hypotension, hyperthermia, hypoglycemia, and hyperglycemia may all exacerbate the neuronal injury that results from stroke. Patients should be monitored closely for the development of any of these conditions and treated promptly if they occur. One common mistake is to lower blood pressure too aggressively immediately after an acute stroke. In normal brain regions, autoregulatory mechanisms preserve a constant level of cerebral blood flow across a wide range of blood pressure, but these mechanisms are impaired in the ischemic penumbra, so a relatively small drop in blood pressure can reduce perfusion and convert a salvageable region to one that is irreversibly damaged. This can occur even at blood pressures that would typically be considered normal or high, because patients with long-standing hypertension often accommodate over time to their high baseline blood pressure, adjusting their autoregulatory mechanisms to a higher set point. Thus, although blood pressure control is an important long-term goal, high pressures do not necessarily require treatment in the acute setting. Extremely high blood pressure should be treated, however, especially in patients who received intravenous tPA.

People who have had a stroke often have impaired airway protection mechanisms and may need elective intubation to limit aspiration. A bedside evaluation of swallowing should be routine after stroke, and if the patient has problems, more extensive testing may be necessary. Some patients need feeding tubes until they can safely take in adequate nutrition by mouth.

Most patients should be mobilized as soon as possible after a stroke, but fall precautions are essential. Patients who are rendered nonambulatory by a stroke should be treated prophylactically to prevent deep venous thrombosis. They should also receive vigorous skin care to prevent skin breakdown and decubitus ulcers, and they should be monitored closely for the development of pneumonia or urinary tract infections.

C. Rehabilitation

Rehabilitation should be initiated soon after a stroke, with the intensity of therapy advancing over time. Patients should be trained to maximize their function based on their current abilities. Speech pathologists can teach patients strategies to improve communication skills. They can also evaluate patients' swallowing and suggest interventions to reduce the risk of aspiration. Physical therapists can teach patients exercises designed to increase range of motion and prevent contractures in weak muscles, as well as exercises to strengthen both the affected muscles and the unaffected muscles that may be required to compensate for the weak muscles. Constraint-induced movement therapy, in which patients are prevented from using their intact limbs and thereby forced to use their affected limbs, has shown promising results. Occupational therapists can also help to determine whether patients might benefit from facilitative or prosthetic devices.

VI. Secondary Prevention of Ischemic Stroke

Anyone who has had a TIA or stroke is at risk for future strokes, with potentially devastating consequences. The goal of secondary stroke prevention is to reduce that risk. In this context, strokes and TIAs are equivalent, because someone who has an ischemic event and recovers completely (i.e., someone who has a TIA) may not be so lucky with future ischemic events. When patients with TIAs are not treated, as many as 10–20% of them have strokes within 90 days, and half of those are within the first 48 hours.

Secondary stroke prevention resembles primary stroke prevention, which refers to measures that reduce the risk of stroke in people who have vascular risk factors, but who have never had a stroke or TIA. Although the elements of primary and secondary stroke prevention are similar, they are not identical. This is mainly because vascular risk factors may be mitigated by factors such as the development of collateral blood vessels or the presence of features that reduce the risk of plaque fragmentation and embolism. Because of those mitigating factors, a substantial subset of patients with stroke risk factors live to an advanced age without ever experiencing a stroke. People who have already had a TIA or stroke are clearly not in this subset, so risk/benefit calculations are different for them than for people who have never had a TIA or stroke. As a result, some interventions may result in benefits that outweigh the risks in the setting of secondary stroke prevention, but not in the context of primary prevention.

The major components of secondary stroke prevention are summarized in Table 4.2. An individual patient's specific clinical circumstances often introduce nuances that require interpretation and modifications, but in

Table 4.2 Principal Elements of Secondary Stroke Prevention

A. **Treat with a high-intensity statin** (atorvastatin 40 or 80 mg/day or rosuvastatin 20 or 40 mg/day). If LDL-C remains > 70 mg/dL, add ezetimibe (and, if necessary, a proprotein convertase subtilisein/kexin type 9 [PCSK9] inhibitor) [exceptions: (a) LDL-C < 70 mg/dL even without treatment (b) stroke/TIA was not due to atherosclerosis, e.g., from atrial fibrillation]

B. **Treat with an antiplatelet medication** (acceptable options: (a) aspirin, 50–325 mg/day; (b) clopidogrel, 75 mg/day; (c) extended-release dipyridamole/aspirin (200 mg/25 mg) twice a day). For TIA or small stroke, treat with aspirin plus clopidogrel or ticagrelor if treatment can be started within 24 hours of symptom onset; after 3–4 weeks, change to a single antiplatelet medication.

C. **Control blood pressure** (long-term outpatient goal: < 130/80 mm Hg) with a thiazide diuretic, angiotensin-converting enzyme inhibitor, or angiotensin II receptor blocker (or some combination)

D. **Continue (or initiate) all other primary prevention measures** (see Part VIII)

E. **In patients with atrial fibrillation or flutter:** *instead of* an antiplatelet medication, anticoagulate with apixaban, dabigatran, edoxaban, or rivaroxaban (warfarin is an acceptable alternative, and the preferred medication in patients who have a mechanical heart valve or moderate-to-severe mitral stenosis). In patients with contraindications to lifelong anticoagulation who can tolerate it for 45 days, consider percutaneous closure of the left atrial appendage.

F. **Patients whose TIA or stroke is in the territory of an ICA with severe (70–99%) extracranial stenosis should have carotid endarterectomy (or stenting in a subset of patients) as soon as it can be done safely**

most cases secondary prevention involves treating with a high-intensity HMG-CoA reductase inhibitor (statin) and an antiplatelet medication, addressing vascular risk factors (primary prevention measures), and evaluating for two specific conditions: severe ICA stenosis (if the stroke is in the territory of that ICA) and atrial fibrillation.

If the patient's stroke is in the ICA territory and the ICA hasn't already been evaluated in the course of making decisions about clot retrieval, the patient should have a carotid ultrasound, CTA, or MRA. To evaluate for atrial fibrillation, an ECG should be obtained for all patients with TIA or stroke, and cardiac telemetry monitoring should be performed while the patient is hospitalized. Another reason for telemetry is that strokes can cause serious arrhythmias. If atrial fibrillation hasn't been detected by the time of hospital discharge, the patient should have long-term (at least 2 weeks) outpatient rhythm monitoring. If the likelihood of paroxysmal atrial fibrillation is high enough, it may be reasonable to implant a loop recording device for even more prolonged monitoring. Unless the patient already has an indication for anticoagulation, an echocardiogram should be done to assess for thrombus, left atrial enlargement, reduced ejection fraction, or other features that could suggest a cardioembolic source. For some causes of cardioembolism, transesophageal echocardiography (TEE) is a more sensitive and specific test than conventional transthoracic echocardiography (TTE), but it is more invasive and has associated morbidity. In most circumstances, TTE is adequate; TEE findings change management in only a minority of patients.

Table 4.2 focuses on components of secondary stroke prevention for which the evidence is clear-cut. Even for those components, exceptions and modifications are necessary at times, especially for patients who would not have met the inclusion criteria for the relevant clinical trials. Some exceptions to the practices summarized in Table 4.2 are based on subgroup analyses of large clinical trials; others are based on clinical trials conducted on specialized patient populations; and others are based primarily on theoretical considerations. An introductory textbook is not the place to delve into all possible nuances, but it is worth exploring some of them in a little more detail.

A. Lipid Management

For people with no clinical evidence of atherosclerotic cardiovascular disease (ASCVD), lipid management involves estimation of the person's 10-year risk of ASCVD (see Part VIII). The guidelines for lipid management in *secondary* stroke prevention are more straightforward: people with ASCVD should be treated with a goal of low-density lipoprotein cholesterol (LDL-C) of less than 70 mg/dL. Initial therapy should be with a high-intensity statin if they can tolerate it. In addition to lowering lipid levels, statins may have other beneficial effects on atherosclerosis. High-intensity statins (atorvastatin 80 mg/day or 40 mg/day, or rosuvastatin 20 mg/day or 40 mg/day) reduce LDL-C levels by 50% or more. If the goal of LDL-C less than 70 mg/dL isn't reached with a statin, ezetimibe should be added; if the goal still isn't reached and the patient has another atherosclerotic disorder or multiple high-risk conditions, a proprotein convertase subtilisin/kexin type 9 (PCSK9) inhibitor should be added. These guidelines do not apply to people who have had a stroke or TIA that was thought to be cardioembolic, and who have no other clinical evidence of ASCVD.

B. Antiplatelet Medication

Unless they are taking warfarin, a factor Xa inhibitor, or a direct thrombin inhibitor, all patients who have had a TIA or ischemic stroke should receive antiplatelet therapy—aspirin (50–325 mg per day), clopidogrel (75 mg per day), or a combination of aspirin and extended-release dipyridamole (25 mg/200 mg twice a day). Although clopidogrel and combined aspirin/extended-release dipyridamole each showed statistically significant benefits when compared to aspirin in head-to-head trials, those results have been challenged. In general, any of the three antiplatelet medications is considered an acceptable choice for secondary stroke prevention, but aspirin is the one used most commonly because of its affordability, availability, and familiarity. The optimal dose has not been established, but because higher doses are associated with a greater risk of gastrointestinal hemorrhage, the recommended dose for secondary stroke prevention is 50–325 mg/day. It is conceivable that certain subgroups of patients respond differentially to the various antiplatelet medications, so if patients continue to have TIAs or strokes despite treatment with one antiplatelet agent one option is to try changing to a different one. For similar reasons, patients who continue to have TIAs or strokes while taking aspirin sometimes are told to take a higher dose. No definitive clinical trial evidence is available to support these practices.

There is no role for combining antiplatelet medications on a long-term basis, but dual therapy is beneficial in the first few weeks after a non-cardioembolic TIA or minor stroke: a combination of aspirin and either clopidogrel or ticagrelor should be started within 24 hours of symptom onset. Clopidogrel is generally preferred to ticagrelor because of a higher risk of serious bleeding complications with ticagrelor. After 3–4 weeks, one of the medications should be stopped, and the patient should remain on a single antiplatelet agent. Some studies have shown beneficial results when cilostazol is added to another antiplatelet agent, but further study is necessary.

C. Blood Pressure

Blood pressure management is just as important for secondary stroke prevention as it is for primary stroke prevention, and the goals and methods are the same (see Part VIII), with one exception: the initiation of treatment. As discussed in Part V, overaggressive treatment of blood pressure too soon after a stroke may expand the region of irreversible damage, but "overaggressive" and "too soon" are conceptual terms that have not been operationally defined. It is common to wait at least 24 hours before starting or resuming blood pressure therapy when someone has had an acute stroke, and during that time, to accept blood pressure readings that in other settings would be an indication to increase the dose of antihypertensive medication. This is referred to as permissive hypertension. Even when blood pressure treatment is started (or resumed), it should be done cautiously, slowly advancing the medication regimen as necessary.

Permissive hypertension has its limits. Patients with a systolic blood pressure greater than 185 mm Hg or a diastolic blood pressure greater than 110 mm Hg who are otherwise eligible for intravenous tPA (see Table 4.3) should be treated with medications to bring their blood pressure into the acceptable range so that they can receive thrombolytic treatment. This should be done with intravenous medications that can be rapidly titrated, such as labetalol, nicardipine, or clevidipine. The blood pressure should be maintained below 180/105 mm Hg for at least 24 hours after tPA treatment. Even patients who do not receive tPA should have their blood pressure treated if there is evidence of malignant hypertension causing damage to organs outside the brain. Blood pressures above 220/120 mm Hg are usually treated even in patients who did not receive tPA.

D. Other Risk Factors

In general, any risk factor modification that is effective for primary stroke prevention is also indicated for a patient who has already had a stroke or TIA. Patients who have experienced an episode of hemiparesis, aphasia, or some other dramatic deficit may be particularly amenable to major lifestyle changes (such as smoking cessation) that they had previously resisted. Clinicians should do everything possible to take advantage of the window of opportunity provided by this "wake-up call."

Nearly 40% of people who have had a stroke have moderate-to-severe obstructive sleep apnea, but many of them have never been diagnosed. As explained in Part VIII, obstructive sleep apnea is an independent risk factor for ASCVD. It remains unclear whether treating the sleep apnea affects the ASCVD, but given the other beneficial effects of treating sleep apnea, clinicians caring for patients who have had a TIA or stroke should have a low threshold for obtaining a polysomnogram.

E. Cardioembolic Disease

Atrial fibrillation commonly results in stagnant blood in the left atrial appendage, leading to thrombus formation and embolism. The risk from clinically apparent paroxysmal atrial fibrillation is similar to the risk from sustained atrial fibrillation. Patients who have had a TIA or stroke due to cardioembolism from atrial fibrillation should be treated with a factor Xa inhibitor (rivaroxaban, apixaban, or edoxaban), dabigatran (a direct thrombin inhibitor), or warfarin (a vitamin K antagonist)—any of these agents reduces the risk of subsequent stroke by a factor of 3. Dabigatran and the factor Xa inhibitors are referred to collectively as direct oral anticoagulants (DOACs). They are generally preferred to warfarin because they don't require frequent blood testing for dose adjustment and they are associated with a lower risk of intracranial hemorrhage. Apixaban appears to be less likely than the other DOACs to cause major gastrointestinal bleeding. DOACs are contra-indicated in patients with valvular atrial fibrillation (patients who have a mechanical heart valve or moderate-to-severe mitral stenosis) because of an increased risk of thromboembolism and bleeding, and they are contraindicated in patients with severe liver disease. Warfarin is the treatment of choice in these patients. Warfarin is also used in some cases because of economic or insurance considerations.

Antiplatelet agents also reduce the risk of stroke in patients with atrial fibrillation, but they are less effective than warfarin or DOACs. Percutaneous closure of the left atrial appendage is an option for patients who have contraindications to lifelong anticoagulation. It has been shown to be as effective as warfarin in reducing the risk of stroke in patients with atrial fibrillation. Unfortunately, it may not be an option for patients with a high risk of hemorrhagic complications because after the device is implanted patients are usually maintained on oral anticoagulation therapy for 45 days and on dual therapy with aspirin and clopidogrel for 4.5 months after that.

Patients who have a stroke or TIA due to an acute myocardial infarction, and who have a mural thrombus in their left ventricle, should also receive warfarin for at least 3 months. Similarly, patients with a stroke or TIA who have cardiomyopathy and thrombus in the left atrium or left ventricle should receive warfarin. When no thrombus is present, the choice between anticoagulation and antiplatelet therapy after a stroke or TIA in patients with acute myocardial infarction or cardiomyopathy is less clear. Patients with left ventricular assist devices (LVADs) are typically treated with both warfarin and aspirin. There is limited evidence regarding secondary prevention in patients who have valvular disease but neither atrial fibrillation nor a mechanical valve; antiplatelet agents are generally recommended for these patients. Because of a high risk of cerebral hemorrhage (see Chapter 10), bacterial endocarditis (in a patient without an artificial heart valve) is the one cardioembolic condition for which anticoagulation is generally considered to be contraindicated.

The management of *patent foramen ovale* (PFO) has been the subject of controversy. On the one hand, a PFO provides a potential route for thrombi in systemic veins to bypass the pulmonary circulation and travel directly into the left atrium and from there into the brain, and indeed, the incidence of PFO is higher in patients with stroke than in the general population. On the other hand, a PFO can be demonstrated on surface echocardiography in about 20% of healthy individuals, suggesting that most people with PFO are asymptomatic. For this reason, when PFOs are discovered in patients who have had a TIA or stroke and who have other conditions that predispose them to stroke (which tends to be the case in older patients), the PFOs are usually considered incidental findings and not the causes of the ischemia. In carefully selected patients, however—specifically, patients 18 to 60 years of age in whom thorough evaluation has failed to identify an alternative cause of stroke and in whom the PFO has certain anatomic features associated with an increased risk of embolism—studies have shown that percutaneous PFO closure modestly reduces subsequent stroke risk.

In patients who have just had a cardioembolic stroke, decisions regarding when to begin anticoagulation must balance two opposing risks. On the one hand, these patients are clearly at risk for recurrent stroke since the cardioembolic source is still present. On the other hand, the propensity for hemorrhagic transformation is particularly high after cardioembolic strokes. Current guidelines recommend initiating anticoagulation 2–14 days after a cardioembolic stroke; factors that influence the risk of hemorrhagic conversion, such as infarct size, should be considered when deciding whether to wait 2 days, 14 days, or an intermediate interval.

Anticoagulation should be maintained as long as the cardioembolic source remains; for many patients, this means lifelong anticoagulation. Patients taking warfarin need to be monitored regularly to maintain the correct degree of anticoagulation. An INR in the range of 2.0–3.0 is the usual goal, although a target range of 2.5–3.5 is indicated for some patients with mechanical heart valves (with details depending on the valve type and location).

F. Cervical Carotid Stenosis

Atherosclerotic plaques in the carotid artery can lead to strokes or TIAs in at least two ways. First, plaques can serve as a site of thrombus formation, and pieces of thrombus or plaque can subsequently break off and flow downstream until they reach a blood vessel too small to accommodate them, where they get stuck and block blood from flowing past them. Second, plaques (and associated thrombus) can grow in place within the carotid to the point where they reduce blood flow through the carotid below some critical level. It is usually difficult to determine which of these two mechanisms is more important in an individual patient, but either way, it would make sense that endarterectomy (surgical excision of the plaque and associated thrombus) could be beneficial. This procedure has risks, however. In fact, one risk is stroke, both because manipulation of the internal carotid artery during surgery can lead to embolism and because the artery must be temporarily occluded during surgery to prevent hemorrhage. Furthermore, endarterectomy might provide little or no benefit if the patient has already formed sufficient collateral blood vessels to compensate for the obstructed carotids. Of course, collateral blood vessels would not prevent pieces of plaque or thrombus from breaking off and lodging in smaller vessels downstream, but they could protect the region of brain supplied by those vessels by providing an alternate blood supply. Moreover, the likelihood of plaque fragmentation undoubtedly varies from one patient to another, influenced by such factors as the precise composition of the plaque, the degree of local turbulence, the systemic blood pressure, and so forth. Whether the benefit of endarterectomy outweighs the risk is ultimately an empiric question.

For patients who have had a TIA or stroke in the distribution of a carotid artery with a high-grade (70–99%) stenosis (*symptomatic* carotid stenosis), clinical trials have answered that question. Even with appropriate medical therapy, 26% of these patients will have another stroke on the same side within 2 years. Carotid endarterectomy reduces this risk significantly, as shown in Table 4.5. The statistics in Table 4.5 come from studies conducted in an era when statins were not yet used routinely and hypertension was treated less aggressively than it is now, so the specific numbers are probably not an accurate reflection of current risks and benefits. Nonetheless, the absolute risk reduction with carotid endarterectomy in patients with high-grade symptomatic stenosis is so great that the benefit almost always outweighs the risk.

The risk/benefit calculation is very different for patients who have had a TIA or stroke in the distribution of a carotid artery with only *moderate* carotid stenosis (50–69%). For these patients, carotid endarterectomy still results in a statistically significant reduction in the risk of subsequent stroke, but the risk is so low even in the group treated with medical therapy alone that the absolute risk reduction is much less dramatic than it is for patients with high-grade carotid stenosis (Table 4.5). In fact, for patients with 50–69% carotid stenosis, the absolute risk reduction is low enough that individual circumstances must be considered carefully in deciding whether to recommend the surgery. For example, the statistics in Table 4.5 come from a study that was done at centers selected for their high level of expertise. In centers with less experience, a higher complication rate could easily negate the small benefit of surgery. Similarly, patients with multiple medical problems may have a greater than average risk of surgical complications that would outweigh the benefit of the procedure.

The benefits of endarterectomy are greatest if the surgery is performed within 2 weeks of the onset of symptoms. There is some risk that restoration of blood flow soon after a stroke could lead to hemorrhagic conversion, because the blood vessels in the ischemic region are fragile, but this concern is counterbalanced by the high risk of recurrent stroke soon after an initial stroke.

Endovascular treatment (carotid angioplasty and stenting) is a less invasive alternative to endarterectomy. In the largest clinical trial comparing endovascular treatment to endarterectomy to date, patients randomized to receive endovascular treatment had fewer peri-procedural myocardial infarctions, but more strokes (with no statistically significant difference on a composite endpoint). Among patients who were younger than 70 years of age, the endovascular treatment group had a better composite outcome, whereas among patients who were 70 years of age or older the endarterectomy group had a better composite outcome. Endarterectomy remains the standard treatment for patients with symptomatic high-grade carotid stenosis, but angioplasty/stenting is a viable option in some cases, especially in younger patients or patients with comorbidities predisposing to complications from endarterectomy. Transcarotid artery revascularization (TCAR) is a newer stenting technique in which the direction of carotid blood flow is temporarily reversed by diverting it into the femoral vein and the stent is introduced directly into the carotid. Some evidence suggests that TCAR is associated with a lower risk of stroke than standard angioplasty/stenting, but no prospective trials have directly compared TCAR to traditional angioplasty/stenting or endarterectomy.

For patients who have had a TIA or stroke in the distribution of a carotid artery with less than 50% stenosis, neither endarterectomy nor endovascular therapy provides a significant benefit. No evidence supports endarterectomy or endovascular treatment of stenosis in cerebral blood vessels other than the internal carotid arteries.

G. Ischemic Stroke Mechanisms Other Than Cardioembolism and Cervical Carotid Stenosis

Unless they have a cardioembolic source that would be an indication for a DOAC or warfarin, patients who have had a TIA or ischemic stroke should be treated with antiplatelet medication. A few specific mechanisms merit further comment.

1. Occlusive disease of large intracranial arteries

The large intracranial arteries (such as the carotid siphon, middle cerebral artery, and basilar artery) are not accessible for endarterectomy, and no evidence supports the use of endovascular procedures (such as angioplasty with stenting). Current guidelines recommend considering dual antiplatelet therapy (specifically aspirin/clopidogrel, aspirin/ticagrelor, aspirin/cilostazol, or clopidogrel/cilostazol) in patients with a TIA or stroke thought to be due to severe stenosis of a large intracranial artery, but the evidence for this recommendation is not compelling. At one time, extracranial-intracranial bypass surgery was popular for intracranial disease in the anterior circulation, but studies have not shown any benefit for this procedure compared to medical management.

2. Penetrating artery disease

Neither endovascular techniques nor direct surgical approaches are feasible for treating occlusive disease of the penetrating arteries. Antiplatelet agents and statins are typically prescribed. Blood pressure control is paramount.

3. Vertebral artery stenosis

No evidence supports endarterectomy, vertebral artery transposition, or endovascular approaches for patients who have had a TIA or stroke due to stenosis of a vertebral artery. Antiplatelet agents and statins are considered the treatment of choice for secondary prevention.

4. Arterial dissection

With modern imaging techniques, arterial dissection is recognized much more often than in the past. It is most common in the setting of neck trauma, but the trauma may be surprisingly mild (such as an abrupt neck movement), and there is often no history of trauma at all. Clinical reports, and a few case–control studies, suggest that dissection can occur as a result of cervical manipulation (such as chiropractic treatment), but the incidence is probably low. Clinicians should be especially alert to the possibility of arterial dissection in younger patients without traditional risk factors for stroke. Patients are usually treated with either an antiplatelet agent or anticoagulation, but the risk of stroke recurrence is low, and the optimal management approach and duration of treatment have not been established.

5. Aortic arch disease

Atherosclerotic disease of the aortic arch is also increasingly recognized as a cause of stroke. Optimal treatment is unknown; current guidelines recommend antiplatelet medication and intensive lipid management for secondary stroke prevention in these patients.

6. Hematologic disorders, including coagulopathies

For patients with a predisposition to thrombosis, treatment is aimed at the underlying disorder. For example, patients with polycythemia vera are typically treated with phlebotomy and hemodilution, and patients with sickle cell disease should receive blood transfusions to maintain hemoglobin S levels that are less than 30% of total hemoglobin levels. Current guidelines recommend antiplatelet therapy for patients with a TIA or stroke who have resistance to activated protein C, elevated factor VIII levels, prothrombin 2021A mutations, or deficiencies of protein C, protein S, or antithrombin III, unless they have a history of other thrombotic events. Patients with a stroke or TIA who have elevated titers of antiphospholipid antibodies should be treated with antiplatelet agents unless they meet criteria for the antiphospholipid antibody syndrome, in which case they are typically anticoagulated.

H. Determining the Underlying Mechanism of Stroke

It can be difficult, and sometimes impossible, to identify the mechanism underlying a patient's stroke. Patients with risk factors for atherosclerosis often have vascular pathology at several different sites, and all may be equally plausible causes of stroke. For example, a patient may have both atrial fibrillation and carotid stenosis—which one was responsible for the stroke? In some cases, clinical or radiologic features help to narrow the list of possible stroke mechanisms. For example, penetrating artery disease cannot cause a dominant hemisphere MCA syndrome, with weakness, numbness, visual field defect, and aphasia, and it doesn't cause a lesion larger than 2 cm in diameter on imaging studies. Similarly, if a patient's clinical syndrome or imaging studies indicate a stroke in the posterior circulation (such as a lateral medullary syndrome), carotid disease was not the cause of the stroke (unless the patient has an anatomic variant of the cerebral blood vessels). Multiple acute cortical infarcts in different vascular territories are most suggestive of cardioembolism; rarer causes are diffuse atherosclerosis, coagulopathy, or vasculitis. Wedge-shaped cortical infarcts, particularly in the distribution of the middle cerebral artery, are usually caused by an embolic mechanism, whereas irregular, patchy infarcts in the border zones ("watershed areas") between the territories of the middle cerebral artery and the anterior cerebral artery or posterior cerebral artery are typically caused by low flow from carotid occlusive disease or global hypoperfusion.

Even when the clinical and imaging features are most consistent with a particular stroke mechanism, they usually are insufficient to exclude other potential mechanisms. Most patients require imaging of the carotid arteries and heart and cardiac rhythm monitoring. As already discussed, patients who have had a TIA or stroke should have a TTE or TEE unless they already have a known indication for anticoagulation and cardiac imaging would not change their management. Intra-arterial angiography is considered the gold standard for visualizing both extracranial and intracranial cerebral blood vessels, although MRA and computed tomographic angiography (CTA) are noninvasive and offer comparable resolution for many purposes. Duplex carotid ultrasound is a useful screening test for detecting carotid stenosis or occlusion. Normal carotid ultrasound results are usually reliable, but patients with abnormal carotid ultrasound results need further studies, because ultrasound estimates of the magnitude of stenosis are sometimes inaccurate, and a more detailed definition of the cerebral vascular anatomy may be needed if endarterectomy is a consideration. Transcranial Doppler is another technique for examining the intracranial circulation. The choice of vascular imaging modality depends on such factors as whether the patient has renal disease (which could be exacerbated by the use of contrast agents), whether the patient needs an MRI anyway (in which case it is usually relatively easy to include MRA as part of the study), and—most importantly—which information is likely to change patient management. For example, patients with ischemia in the posterior circulation often do not need imaging of their carotid arteries. As another example, management is often unaffected by determining the percentage stenosis of intracranial arteries.

In some cases, even after appropriate investigations, two or more mechanisms of stroke remain plausible. In those cases, it may be appropriate to treat for both. For example, if a patient with a stroke in the territory of the internal carotid artery has high-grade carotid stenosis on that side and also has atrial fibrillation, both endarterectomy and anticoagulation may be indicated. Conversely, when no stroke mechanism is identified—especially in young individuals with none of the common risk factors for stroke—it may be reasonable to test for relatively rare mechanisms, such as vasculitis, coagulopathy, other hematologic disorders, arterial dissection, connective tissue diseases, and certain infections (such as syphilis or herpes varicella-zoster). When patients have simultaneous strokes in both the anterior and posterior circulation, it might seem logical to conclude that the strokes were cardioembolic and treat with a DOAC or warfarin even when no cardioembolic source can be identified, but studies have not shown this strategy to be effective.

It can be even more difficult to determine the underlying mechanism in patients who have had a TIA than it is in patients who have had a stroke. By definition, TIAs resolve completely, and in many cases the patients have already returned to their baseline by the time of medical evaluation. As with strokes, the clinical features may narrow the list of possible mechanisms. For example, a detailed description of the event can make it very likely that it was in the distribution of the vertebrobasilar system, not the carotid. Identification of a single mechanism is often impossible, however, and it may be necessary to evaluate or even treat a patient for more than one plausible mechanism.

VII. Secondary Prevention of Cerebral Hemorrhage

The principal methods for avoiding recurrent subarachnoid hemorrhage from an aneurysm are to occlude the neck of the aneurysm at open surgery with a clip, or to introduce a coil into the aneurysm via endovascular catheter, with the intent of inducing thrombosis of the aneurysm. A randomized trial demonstrated a better outcome for coiling than for clipping at 1 year. Patients in the coiling group were more likely to require subsequent retreatment and had an increased risk of rebleeding, but even so, the risk of death within 5 years was lower in the coiling group than in the clipping group. Current guidelines recommend coiling rather than clipping when both are technically feasible. Not all aneurysms are amenable to coiling, so clipping is still indicated in certain cases. Newer endovascular techniques and devices, such as flow-diverting stents and web devices, are also available, but they have not been thoroughly evaluated. Regardless of the approach used, the ideal is to perform the intervention within 3 days of the initial hemorrhage, so that there will be less risk of rebleeding if pressors and fluids are required to treat vasospasm.

Techniques aimed at reducing the risk of recurrent hemorrhage from a vascular malformation include resection, embolization, and radiation. In patients with hypertension-related intraparenchymal hemorrhage, blood pressure control and avoidance of unnecessary antithrombotic medications are key to reducing the risk of recurrent hemorrhagic events.

VIII. Primary Prevention

The interventions discussed in Parts V, VI, and VII are aimed at optimizing the long-term outcome in patients who have had a stroke. Although these interventions are important, primary stroke prevention—which is aimed at preventing strokes from happening in the first place—has the potential for even greater impact. In fact, advances in primary stroke prevention are thought to be a major factor underlying a decline in the incidence of stroke that has occurred in high-income countries in recent decades. As explained in Part VI, primary and secondary prevention are very similar, but not identical. This is mainly because risk/benefit calculations in patients who have never had a TIA or stroke (who may have developed collateral blood supply or other mechanisms to neutralize their vascular risk factors) differ from the calculations in patients who have had a TIA or stroke (and who have thereby demonstrated that their body's protective adaptations have been at most partially effective). Because most people who have never had a TIA or stroke don't go to neurologists, primary stroke prevention is mainly in the domain of primary care providers.

A. Hypertension

Hypertension is a major risk factor for both ischemic and hemorrhagic stroke, and the higher the blood pressure, the greater the stroke risk. There is convincing evidence that control of hypertension substantially reduces the risk of stroke, even for mild hypertension. Lifestyle approaches to blood pressure control include salt restriction; a diet rich in fruits, vegetables, and low-fat dairy products; dietary potassium enhancement; moderation in alcohol intake; weight loss; and regular aerobic physical activity. People with an estimated 10-year ASCVD risk of 10% or more should be treated with antihypertensive medication if their average systolic blood pressure is 130 mm Hg or higher or their average diastolic blood pressure is 80 mm Hg or higher. Patients with an estimated 10-year ASCVD risk of less than 10% should be treated with antihypertensive medication if their systolic blood pressure is 140 mm Hg or higher or their diastolic BP is 90 mm Hg or higher. The long-term treatment goal should be a blood pressure consistently less than 130/80 mm Hg. The primary drug classes used for first-line treatment are thiazide diuretics, angiotensin converting enzyme (ACE) inhibitors, angiotensin receptor blockers (ARBs), and calcium channel blockers.

B. Smoking

Smoking also increases the risk of both ischemic and hemorrhagic stroke. The risk increases with the number of cigarettes smoked, and varies with stroke subtype, but the overall stroke risk is about twice that of nonsmokers. Smoking cessation is associated with a rapid reduction in stroke risk.

C. Diabetes

Patients with diabetes have an increased risk of stroke, independent of their other cardiovascular risk factors. It is not clear whether tight glycemic control modifies stroke risk (although it has other beneficial effects). Tight blood pressure control in diabetic patients reduces the risk of stroke, and it appears that angiotensin-converting enzyme (ACE) inhibitors and angiotensin receptor blockers may be particularly beneficial. Statins reduce the risk of stroke in patients with diabetes, especially those with at least one other vascular risk factor (hypertension, current tobacco use, retinopathy, or albuminuria), even if they do not have dyslipidemia.

D. Dyslipidemia

Most studies have found that dyslipidemia is associated with a reduced risk of hemorrhagic stroke and an increased risk of ischemic stroke. The guidelines for treatment depend on the patient's age, LDL-C level, whether they have diabetes, and their 10-year ASCVD risk. Several algorithms for calculating the 10-year ASCVD risk are available; the one that is most representative of the U.S. population is based on five prospective community-based studies, but it is best validated in non-Hispanic Blacks and non-Hispanic Whites 40 to 75 years of age. It is a complex algorithm that incorporates the patient's age, sex, race, total cholesterol level, HDL-C level, LDL-C level, systolic blood pressure, diastolic blood pressure, blood pressure treatment status, smoking status, use of a statin, use of aspirin, and whether the patient has diabetes. These variables can be entered into an online calculator available at https://tools.acc.org/ascvd-risk-estimator-plus/#!/calcul ate/estimate/. As noted in Part VI, Section A, this calculation is unnecessary in patients who already have established ASCVD (i.e., in the setting of secondary prevention). It is also unnecessary in people with diabetes and at least one other vascular risk factor and in people whose LDL-C is 190 mg/dL or higher. Patients in all these groups should be treated with a high-intensity statin. Patients who have diabetes and no other vascular risk factors should take a moderate-intensity statin.

E. Mechanical Heart Valves

Patients with mechanical heart valves have a very high risk of stroke and they should take warfarin. Treatment with warfarin reduces this risk by a factor of 4 or 5, whereas antiplatelet agents cut the risk of stroke roughly in half. DOACs are less safe than warfarin for patients with mechanical heart valves.

F. Atrial Fibrillation

Several scales have been developed to estimate the magnitude of stroke risk in patients with atrial fibrillation based on age and associated cardiovascular risk factors. The most commonly used instrument is the CHA_2DS_2-VASc scale, in which a patient receives points for each of the following risk factors: Congestive heart failure (1 point), Hypertension (1 point), Age 75 years or older (2 points), Diabetes (1 point), history of Stroke/TIA/thromboembolism (2 points), Vascular disease (1 point), Age 65–74 years (1 point), and Sex Category (1 point for females, 0 for males). In this formula, the term "Vascular disease" refers to prior myocardial infarction (MI), peripheral artery disease, or aortic plaque. Scales have also been developed to estimate the risk of bleeding associated with anticoagulation. Current guidelines recommend that patients with *nonvalvular* atrial fibrillation who have a CHA_2DS_2-VASc score of 2 or higher and acceptably low risk of hemorrhagic complications should receive antithrombotic therapy—either warfarin, with a target INR of 2.0 to 3.0, or a DOAC (recall that DOACs are contraindicated in patients with *valvular* atrial fibrillation, so warfarin is the treatment of choice in those patients). Patients who have already had a TIA or stroke have a CHA_2DS_2-VASc score of at least 2, which is why warfarin or a DOAC is always a feature of secondary stroke prevention for patients with atrial fibrillation (see Part VI, Section E). For patients with a CHA_2DS_2-VASc score of 2 or higher in whom anticoagulation is not an option, a combination of aspirin and clopidogrel (rather than aspirin alone) should be considered. Most patients with nonvalvular atrial fibrillation who have a CHA_2DS_2-VASc score of 0 do not need antithrombotic therapy. For patients with nonvalvular atrial fibrillation who have a CHA_2DS_2-VASc score of 1, warfarin, a DOAC, aspirin, or no antithrombotic treatment are all considered reasonable options, depending on the particular situation.

G. Cervical Carotid Stenosis

As explained in Part VI, Section F, patients who have had a TIA or stroke in the territory of an internal carotid artery with 70–99% stenosis have such a high likelihood of stroke recurrence that the benefits of carotid endarterectomy clearly outweigh the risks, whereas the risk/benefit comparison is much murkier with 50–69% stenosis because the likelihood of stroke recurrence is so much lower in the first place. The risk/benefit analysis in the setting of primary stroke prevention (asymptomatic carotid stenosis, i.e., cervical carotid stenosis in patients who have never had a TIA or stroke) is similar to the calculation for secondary prevention with 50–69% stenosis: in asymptomatic patients with internal carotid stenosis of 60% or more, carotid endarterectomy results in a statistically significant benefit, but the absolute risk reduction is only 1.2% per year (see Table 4.5). This is primarily because even without surgery the risk of stroke is so much lower in this context than in the context of secondary stroke prevention. This, in turn, is probably because many of the patients who have never had a TIA or stroke have plaque features associated with a lower risk of stroke or they have developed ample collateral circulation, whereas patients who have had a TIA or stroke have proven that they are in a higher risk group and their collateral circulation is imperfect. The result is that the benefit conferred by endarterectomy in the setting of *primary* stroke prevention could easily be negated in circumstances in which the surgical morbidity is less than ideal. Furthermore, as noted in Part VI, Section F, the studies summarized in Table 4.5 were conducted at a time when statins were not used routinely and hypertension was treated less aggressively than it is now, so clinical trials revisiting medical and surgical treatment for asymptomatic carotid stenosis are in progress.

The results with carotid angioplasty/stenting for primary stroke prevention mirror the results for secondary stroke prevention (see Part VI, Section F): compared to endarterectomy, angioplasty/stenting results in fewer peri-procedural myocardial infarctions but more strokes; patients who are younger than 70 years tend to do better with angioplasty/stenting, and older patients do better with endarterectomy. Thus, for patients with asymptomatic carotid stenosis of at least 60%, endarterectomy, angioplasty/stenting, and medical management (without performing any procedure to correct the blockage) are all reasonable options. The relative indications for the three alternative approaches remain uncertain, and as noted in the previous paragraph, this issue is the subject of active clinical trial investigation. For now, endarterectomy is currently standard for patients treated with a procedure, especially patients who are at low surgical risk, but angioplasty is a viable alternative, particularly in younger patients or patients with established cardiac disease or other major surgical risk factors.

In the context of primary stroke prevention, similar to secondary stroke prevention, no evidence supports endarterectomy or endovascular treatment of stenosis in cerebral blood vessels other than the cervical internal carotid arteries, or in a carotid artery with less than 60% stenosis.

H. Sickle Cell Disease

Stroke is very common in patients with homozygous sickle cell disease, and the highest rate of stroke is in early childhood. Patients with this disease should be screened starting at age 2 using transcranial Doppler (TCD) ultrasound, which can identify the patients at highest risk of stroke. Those patients should be treated with periodic blood transfusions, which can dramatically reduce the risk of stroke in this disease.

I. Other Factors

Dietary factors associated with a reduced risk of stroke include intake of fruits and vegetables, a Mediterranean diet supplemented with nuts or extra virgin olive oil, increased potassium intake, and reduced intake of sodium and saturated fats. Compared to abstinence, heavy alcohol intake is associated with an increased risk of all types of stroke, but intake of small to moderate amounts of alcohol is associated with a reduced risk of ischemic stroke. Elevated levels of homocysteine are associated with an increased risk of stroke, suggesting that administration of B-complex vitamins might reduce stroke risk, but trials have been disappointing. Similarly, most studies indicate that patients with high lipoprotein(a) levels have an increased risk of stroke, so it might be reasonable to use niacin to lower lipoprotein(a) levels in these patients, but this has not been proven. A sedentary lifestyle is associated with an increased risk of stroke, and regular exercise with a lower risk. Obesity appears to be associated with an increased risk of stroke, independent of other cardiovascular risk factors, but the results are not conclusive. Obstructive sleep apnea is an independent risk factor for stroke. Interventions to modify any or all of these risk factors could be beneficial, but at this point, such benefit is unproven. According to current guidelines, aspirin should not be used for primary prevention of cardiovascular disease in people age 60 years or older; low-dose (50–100 mg/day) aspirin can be considered in people age 40–59 with a 10-year ASCVD risk of 10% or more.

IX. Supplementary Tables for Reference

Table 4.3 Major Contraindications to Intravenous tPA Administration

1. Any of the following in the previous 3 months: stroke, significant head trauma, intracranial or intraspinal surgery

2. History of intracranial hemorrhage

3. Systolic BP > 185 mm Hg and/or diastolic BP > 110 mm Hg

4. Symptoms suggestive of subarachnoid hemorrhage (even if CT is negative)

5. Arterial puncture at noncompressible site in the previous 7 days

6. Any of the following risks for acute bleeding: (a) < 100,000 platelets; (b) INR > 1.7; (c) PT > 15 seconds or aPTT > 40 seconds; (d) use of direct thrombin inhibitors or direct factor Xa inhibitors within past 48 hours

7. Treatment dose of low-molecular-weight heparin within past 24 hours

8. Symptoms consistent with infective endocarditis

9. Known or suspected aortic arch dissection

10. Serum glucose < 50 mg/dL (but may be eligible if subsequently normalized)

11. Active internal bleeding

12. Intra-axial intracranial neoplasm

Table 4.4 National Institutes of Health Stroke Scale (NIHSS)

1a. Level of consciousness
0 = alert
1 = not alert, but arousable with minor stimulation
2 = not alert, responds only to repeated or painful stimulation
3 = no response to stimulation other than reflex responses

1b. level of consciousness questions ("What month is it?"; "How old are you?")
0 = answers both correctly
1 = answers one correctly
2 = answers neither correctly

1c. level of consciousness commands ("Open and close your eyes"; "Grip and release with your hand"—use a different 1-step command if hands can't be used)
0 = performs both correctly
1 = performs one correctly
2 = performs neither correctly

2. horizontal gaze
0 = normal
1 = partial gaze palsy
2 = total gaze palsy or forced deviation

3. vision
0 = no vision loss
1 = partial hemianopia
2 = complete hemianopia
3 = bilateral hemianopia

4. face movement
0 = normal
1 = minor weakness
2 = partial paralysis
3 = complete paralysis (of one or both sides)

5a. left arm strength (palms down; extended to 90 degrees if sitting, 45 degrees if supine)
5b. right arm strength (palms down; extended to 90 degrees if sitting, 45 degrees if supine)
0 = maintains for 10 seconds with no drift
1 = drifts down before 10 seconds but doesn't hit bed or other support
2 = some effort against gravity, but drifts down and hits bed or other support before 10 seconds
3 = no effort against gravity
4 = no movement
x = unable to test

Table 4.4 Continued

6a. left leg strength (raised to 30 degrees while supine)
6b. right leg strength (raised to 30 degrees while supine)
0 = maintains for 5 seconds with no drift
1 = drifts down before 5 seconds but doesn't hit bed
2 = some effort against gravity, but drifts down and hits bed before 5 seconds
3 = no effort against gravity, falls to bed immediately
4 = no movement
x = unable to test

7. limb ataxia
0 = absent
1 = present in one limb
2 = present in two or more limbs
x = unable to test

8. sensory
0 = normal
1 = mild-to-moderate sensory loss
2 = severe-to-total sensory loss

9. language
0 = no aphasia
1 = mild-to-moderate aphasia
2 = severe aphasia
3 = mute

10. speech articulation
0 = normal
1 = mild-to-moderate dysarthria
2 = severe dysarthria (unintelligible)
x = unable to test (e.g., intubated)

11. neglect/inattention
0 = no neglect
1 = extinguishes visual or tactile stimuli on double simultaneous stimulation
2 = extinguishes both visual and tactile stimuli on double simultaneous stimulation

Source: National Institute of Neurological Disorders. 2023. "NIH Stroke Scale." Last modified June 12, 2023. https://www.ninds.nih.gov/health-information/public-education/know-stroke/health-professionals/nih-stroke-scale

Table 4.5 Internal Carotid Endarterectomy Statistics: Proportion of Patients with Stroke Ipsilateral to Stenotic ICA

	Medical Treatment Alone	Endarterectomy Plus Medical Treatment	Absolute Risk Reduction
≥70% stenosis, symptomatic (secondary prevention)	26% at 2 years	9% at 2 years	17% at 2 years = 8.5% per year
50–69% stenosis, symptomatic (secondary prevention)	22% at 5 years	16% at 5 years	6.5% at 5 years = 1.3% per year
>60% stenosis, asymptomatic (primary prevention)	11% at 5 years	5% at 5 years	6% at 5 years = 1.2% per year

X. Discussion of Case Histories

Case 1. This patient's right hand weakness and word-finding difficulty localize to the left cerebral cortex (which is dominant for language in most people, and almost all right-handed people). Thus, this man's episodes are focal. As discussed in Chapter 3, the most common causes of focal, transient symptoms are seizures, TIAs, and migraines. The time course of his symptoms would not be typical of seizures or migraines, and he has multiple vascular risk factors, so his spells most likely represent TIAs. In particular, the spells are consistent with the clinical syndrome produced by ischemia in the dominant MCA territory.

The normal neurologic exam suggests that the patient has had a TIA, not a stroke. Between 5% and 10% of patients who have had a TIA will have a stroke within the next 48 hours if no preventive treatment is initiated, and 10–20% of patients who have had a TIA will have a stroke at some point in the 3 months following the TIA, so this is the ideal time to intervene. The patient should be rapidly evaluated to facilitate preventive treatment. If he proceeds to have a stroke while this evaluation is in progress, he should be treated with intravenous thrombolytic therapy and endovascular clot retrieval as indicated. During this time, hypotension should be avoided, and he should be well hydrated. A structural lesion, such as a hematoma or brain tumor, can sometimes precipitate TIAs, so he should have brain imaging to be sure he doesn't have a structural lesion. He needs evaluation for carotid stenosis and for a potential cardioembolic source.

Comment: A CT scan of the head was normal and a carotid ultrasound suggested greater than 80% stenosis of the left internal carotid artery. An echocardiogram was normal. The carotid ultrasound result was replicated on CT angiography, and the patient had a carotid endarterectomy 2 days after admission. The surgery went well and the patient was discharged 2 days later. In addition to the medications he was taking on admission, he was discharged on atorvastatin, 80 mg/day, because of his symptomatic vascular disease (both cardiac and cerebrovascular). He reported no new symptoms at a follow-up visit 6 weeks later.

Case 2. Patients with homonymous hemianopia frequently think their visual loss is monocular. Covering one eye at a time will often reveal the binocular visual loss to the patient. This patient has an acute, focal lesion with no history of trauma. This suggests a vascular etiology, and the specific syndrome (left homonymous hemianopia with no other deficits) is consistent with ischemia in the right PCA territory. The irregular heartbeat suggests the possibility of atrial fibrillation and, therefore, a cardioembolic mechanism. The presence of a potential cardioembolic source doesn't exclude the possibility that her stroke was caused by some other mechanism, but it makes it less likely. In any case, her stroke was not in the distribution of the internal carotid artery, so endarterectomy is not a consideration and there is no need to image the carotid arteries.

This patient is not a candidate for thrombolysis or mechanical thrombectomy because her stroke could have occurred at any time after she fell asleep last night, nearly 24 hours ago. Although anticoagulation is clearly indicated for long-term stroke prophylaxis in patients with chronic atrial fibrillation who have had a stroke, early initiation of anticoagulation could increase the risk that the infarct will undergo hemorrhagic transformation. Current guidelines recommend initiating anticoagulation 2–14 days after a cardioembolic stroke.

Comment: A non-contrast CT scan of the head was obtained in the emergency department to rule out hemorrhage. It was normal. Infarctions may not be evident on CT scan for 24–48 hours. The patient's mildly elevated blood pressure was left untreated to avoid relative hypotension and diminished cerebral perfusion. An EKG confirmed that she had atrial fibrillation and suggested a prior myocardial infarction, but no acute cardiac ischemia, and cardiac enzymes were normal. She had normal thyroid function. Diltiazem was started for rate control, and aspirin was initiated. Because her clinical syndrome suggested a relatively small infarction, her CT scan showed no edema or hemorrhage, and her blood pressure was only mildly elevated, she was deemed to have a low risk of hemorrhagic conversion, so apixaban was started 2 days after her admission to the hospital and aspirin was stopped. Her blood pressure had normalized (without any specific intervention) by then. She had persistent hemianopia but no new deficits. She was discharged the next day on captopril, diltiazem, atorvastatin, and apixaban, with arrangements for outpatient cardiology evaluation for her coronary artery disease. Because of her visual field deficit, she was instructed not to drive.

Case 3. The patient's left hemiparesis suggests a right-sided lesion at the level of the pons or above. The reduced sensation on the left side of the body, left visual field defect, right gaze preference, and left-sided neglect narrow the possible localizations even further, to the right frontoparietal cortex. An acute, focal lesion is most likely vascular, and this patient's deficits are all consistent with an ischemic stroke in the territory of the right MCA, but intracranial hemorrhage is also possible. Either way, the sudden onset of left hemiparesis could have caused his fall. Another possibility is that he fell for some unrelated reason and experienced a traumatic brain lesion, which can also result in an acute, focal lesion. The patient reached medical attention within 90 minutes of symptom onset, and his blood pressure, though high, is less than the 185/110 cutoff, so he is a candidate to receive intravenous tPA (and possibly mechanical thrombectomy) if his deficits are, in fact, due to ischemia.

Comment: A non-contrast head CT scan showed an old, small (1 cm) basal ganglia infarct on the left, but no lesion correlating with his current symptoms. This is not surprising, because ischemic strokes may not be evident on CT scans for 24–48 hours. A CTA was also performed, and it showed occlusion of the proximal right MCA. There was no evidence of hemorrhage on the CT scan, the patient had a normal serum glucose, and he had no history of coagulopathy or recent stroke or surgery, so intravenous tPA was administered while arrangements were made for mechanical thrombectomy, which was successfully completed 3 hours after symptom onset. The patient was admitted to the neurology service, and his blood pressure was monitored in an intensive care unit for the next 24 hours, following an institutional protocol. By the time the patient was transferred out of the intensive care unit, he had recovered to the point where he only had mild weakness of the intrinsic muscles of his left hand. An echocardiogram performed the next day was normal, and the CTA had not shown high-grade carotid stenosis on either side. An MRI scan of the brain 2 days after admission showed a small (2 cm) sub-acute infarct in the right MCA territory and the previously noted chronic left basal ganglia infarct. The patient was started on aspirin, and an ACE inhibitor was prescribed in addition to the diuretic for better long-term blood pressure control. His stroke qualified as clinical atherosclerotic cardiovascular disease, so he was changed from lovastatin to high-intensity therapy (in this case, atorvastatin was selected, 80 mg/day).

The current standard of care is to administer intravenous tPA to patients who are eligible for it, even if they will be undergoing mechanical thrombectomy, although whether this provides added benefit is still uncertain. The MRI scan reassured the clinicians managing this patient that their diagnosis was correct, but did not change management, so it was not really necessary. With no evidence of carotid disease or a cardio-embolic source, long-term stroke prophylaxis in this patient consisted of more aggressive blood pressure control together with the atorvastatin and an antiplatelet medication. When the available antiplatelet drugs were reviewed with the patient, he requested aspirin because he could obtain it at very low cost, whereas he had a high copay for prescription medications.

Chapter 5

Seizures

I. Case Histories

Case 1. A 7-year-old boy has been noted by his teacher to be intermittently inattentive in the classroom. He stares with a blank expression on his face for several seconds at a time. During these staring spells, he doesn't respond when his name is called and he sometimes has rapid fluttering movements of his eyelids. Once the staring stops, he immediately returns to what he was doing and seems no different from usual. His pediatrician is able to provoke one of the spells by having the boy hyperventilate in the office.

Questions:

1. What is the most likely diagnosis in this patient?
2. What other diagnoses need to be considered?
3. What is the drug of choice in this syndrome?

Case 2. A 27-year-old patient in the second trimester of her first pregnancy has been referred to the epilepsy clinic from the high-risk obstetrics clinic. She had her first generalized tonic-clonic seizure when she was 21 years old, while studying for a final exam. She had three more seizures during her early 20s, each beginning with an unpleasant sensation in her abdomen, followed on one occasion by staring and picking at the buttons of her sweater before progressing into a generalized tonic-clonic seizure. She was the product of a normal pregnancy and delivery with normal developmental milestones. At age 15 months she experienced two prolonged seizures with high fever, both lasting approximately 25 minutes and associated with transient paralysis of her right arm. She continued to develop normally and was successful in her classes and in sports. Since age 24 years she has been taking phenytoin, 200 mg twice a day, and has had no seizures. Her only other medications are prenatal vitamins and supplemental folate, 1 mg a day.

Questions:

1. What type of seizures does this patient have?
2. What diagnostic tests does this patient need?
3. What are the drugs of choice for this patient?
4. How should this patient be managed:
   a. through the rest of her pregnancy?
   b. thereafter?

Case 3. A 55-year-old patient had a generalized tonic-clonic seizure while grocery shopping one afternoon. They had been experiencing moderately severe headaches early each morning for about a week, but they had been well previously. When the emergency medical service arrived, the patient was having a second generalized tonic-clonic seizure. A witness reported generalized stiffening of all four extremities followed by clonic movements associated with cyanosis, frothing at the mouth, and urinary incontinence. The patient had two more seizures without recovering consciousness before reaching a local emergency room. The emergency room physicians diagnosed convulsive status epilepticus.

Questions:

1. Do you agree with the emergency room doctors' diagnosis?
2. How should this patient be managed in the emergency room?
3. What tests should be done after the seizures are controlled?

II. Approach to Seizures

Four questions must be addressed in someone who has had a seizure:

1. Is the diagnosis correct?
2. Is urgent treatment necessary?
3. Why did the person have a seizure?
4. What long-term treatment (if any) is indicated?

Question 1 is addressed in Part IV. The one situation in which treatment of seizure activity is truly urgent is status epilepticus, which is covered in Part VII. Question 3 is addressed in Part V, and Question 4 in Part VI. Part III presents some definitions and necessary background information.

III. Background Information

A. Definitions

epilepsy: a brain disorder characterized by the occurrence of at least one seizure, and an enduring predisposition to generate seizures

NOTE: This definition is conceptual, not official. To minimize ambiguity, the International League Against Epilepsy (ILAE) has approved the following official definition:

epilepsy: "a disease of the brain that meets any of the following conditions:

(1) at least two unprovoked seizures occurring more than 24 hours apart (this includes reflex seizures, such as seizures that occur in response to photic stimuli)

(2) one unprovoked (or reflex) seizure and a probability of further seizures similar to the general recurrence risk after two unprovoked seizures, occurring over the next 10 years (a risk of at least 60% over the next 10 years)

(3) diagnosis of a specific epilepsy syndrome"

resolved epilepsy: a term that applies to individuals who had an age-dependent epilepsy syndrome but are now past the applicable age, or individuals who have remained seizure-free for the last 10 years, with no seizure medicines for at least the last 5 years

seizure: a transient occurrence of signs and/or symptoms due to abnormal excessive or synchronous neuronal activity in the brain

focal-onset seizure ("focal seizure"): a seizure that originates within networks limited to one hemisphere; these networks may be discretely localized or more widely distributed, and they may be located in subcortical structures

focal aware seizure: a focal seizure during which consciousness is intact throughout

focal impaired awareness seizure: a focal seizure in which consciousness is impaired for any portion of the seizure

generalized-onset seizure ("generalized seizure"): a seizure that originates at some point within, and rapidly engaging, bilaterally distributed networks; these networks can include cortical and subcortical structures, but they do not necessarily include the entire cortex

tonic activity: sustained muscular contraction lasting a few seconds to minutes and resulting in rigid extension or flexion

clonic activity: rhythmic jerking of muscles

seizure disorder: epilepsy

status epilepticus: a state of abnormally prolonged seizure activity; for generalized convulsive activity, this is operationally defined as 5 minutes or more of continuous seizure or two or more discrete seizures with failure to return to a baseline level of alertness between the seizures

NOTE: The official ILAE definition is a little more complicated:

status epilepticus: "a condition resulting either from the failure of the mechanisms responsible for seizure termination or from the initiation of mechanisms which lead to abnormally prolonged seizures (after time point t1). It is a condition that can have long-term consequences (after time point t2), including neuronal death, neuronal injury, and alteration of neuronal networks, depending on the type and duration of seizures."

Older terms that are now discouraged include: *partial seizure* (roughly synonymous with focal seizure), *simple partial seizure* (roughly synonymous with focal aware seizure), *complex partial seizure* (roughly synonymous with focal impaired awareness seizure), and *partial seizure with secondary generalization* (a focal—i.e., partial—seizure that evolves into bilateral convulsive activity.

B. Clinical Characteristics of Seizures

The clinical manifestations of a seizure depend on where the abnormal neuronal activity starts (the seizure focus) and how it spreads.

1. Focal onset seizures

Any seizure that begins in a localized region in one cerebral hemisphere is called a *focal onset seizure* (or, more informally, a focal seizure), even if the electrical activity subsequently spreads bilaterally and produces bilateral clinical manifestations. Focal seizures were previously called "partial" seizures but that term is now discouraged. When the focus is in the primary motor area, the seizure typically consists of rhythmic jerking (clonic movements) of the body part represented in that region of the brain. Rigid posturing (tonic activity) of a body part may occur with a seizure focus in the supplemental motor area. A seizure focus in the prefrontal cortex often produces more complex patterns of motor activity and can result in unusual posturing. Seizures that begin in the primary sensory cortex generally consist of localized paresthesias or numbness. A seizure focus in the occipital lobe may cause visual illusions (distorted perception of real visual stimuli) or hallucinations (visual perception unrelated to actual visual stimuli). As a general rule, seizures produce "positive phenomena" (shaking of a limb, visual, auditory, or olfactory hallucinations, tingling, etc.) whereas transient ischemic attacks (TIAs) and strokes typically produce "negative phenomena" (inability to move a limb, loss of vision, numbness, etc.). Foci in the medial temporal lobes commonly produce a rising sense of epigastric discomfort or nausea. Other common manifestations of foci in or near the temporal lobe include fear, olfactory symptoms, auditory illusions or hallucinations, and distortions of memory including déjà vu (a strong sense of having had an experience previously) and jamais vu (a sense of unfamiliarity with previous experiences).

Focal seizures can remain confined to the original focus, or they can spread. One classic, but rare, example of spread is a "jacksonian march" across the motor or sensory cortex (or both cortices), with corresponding motor (or sensory, or both) activity that spreads from one body part to an adjacent body part and from there to another, progressively involving one entire side of the body. When the spread of electrical hyperactivity stays in one hemisphere and spares neuronal networks that are important for consciousness, patients may remain aware of external stimuli and respond normally during a seizure; such seizures are called "focal aware" seizures (previously called "simple partial" seizures).

Focal seizures that *do* affect neuronal networks important for consciousness are called "focal impaired awareness" seizures (previously called "complex partial" seizures). During these seizures people often exhibit a motionless stare during which they don't respond to external stimuli, and they may manifest involuntary, stereotyped, automatic motor behaviors known as automatisms. For example, they may smack their lips, make chewing movements, wring their hands, pick at clothes, rearrange objects, walk in circles, or utter short, stereotyped phrases. Patients usually can't remember what happened during these seizures, so observers' reports are crucial. When the initial symptoms of a focal seizure are purely subjective and not evident to observers, that portion of the seizure is called the *aura*. Patients may sometimes have auras that do not spread—these are still focal seizures, but they can't be recognized by observers.

2. Generalized onset seizures

Some seizures have no apparent focus—from the very beginning, they seem to involve neuronal networks spread throughout both cerebral hemispheres. These are called *generalized onset seizures* (or generalized seizures). Generalized seizures usually result in impairment of consciousness, often at the onset, although some generalized seizures (especially myoclonic seizures) may be so brief that impaired consciousness can't be detected. The term *generalized seizure* applies to a variety of seizure types.

Absence seizures are characterized by sudden interruption of activity associated with unresponsiveness and a blank stare, sometimes with fluttering of the eyelids. They usually last less than 10 seconds, followed by immediate resumption of the interrupted activity. Absence seizures can often be precipitated by hyperventilation.

Generalized tonic-clonic seizures begin with a sudden, tonic contraction of limb and axial muscles accompanied by upward eye deviation, pupillary dilatation, and loss of consciousness. Contraction of the respiratory muscles and larynx often produces a forced expiration resulting in an "epileptic cry" or gasp, and the patient may become cyanotic. This is followed by jerking (*clonic*) movements that gradually increase in amplitude while the frequency gradually falls to the point where there are discrete pauses between the jerks, and then the jerking stops completely, with relaxation of all muscles. This relaxation includes respiratory muscles and sphincter muscles, so urinary (and, rarely, fecal) incontinence may occur at this point. People may bite their tongue or inner cheek during either the tonic or the clonic phase. The clonic phase usually ends within 60 seconds, and the entire period of involuntary muscle activity usually lasts 90–120 seconds, at which point patients resume breathing but usually remain unresponsive for minutes to hours. On return to consciousness, they are often confused or sleepy for several hours or longer, and they may have a headache, sore mouth, or generalized aching or stiffness.

Less commonly, generalized seizures can proceed in a different sequence, such as a tonic phase with no clonic component, or a clonic phase with no tonic component, or a clonic phase followed by a tonic phase followed by a clonic phase.

Atonic seizures consist of a sudden decrease in muscle tone leading to a loss of postural control without loss of consciousness. The loss of postural control can be localized (such as a head drop) or generalized. When it is generalized, patients may fall; these are often called drop attacks. The spells typically last 1–2 seconds, after which the person immediately returns to baseline, except for whatever injuries might have been sustained during the fall.

Infantile spasms are characterized by sudden, rapid flexion of the neck and trunk, adduction of the shoulders and outstretched arms, and variable flexion of the lower extremities. Some children exhibit fragments of the full-fledged movement. Infantile spasms tend to occur upon awakening and with feeding. They often occur in clusters that can consist of more than

100 seizures. Infantile spasms usually present between the ages of 3 and 11 months, and almost always before the age of 2 years; they tend to stop by the age of 5 years.

Myoclonic seizures consist of nonrhythmic, rapid, jerking movements that can be local or widespread. Nonepileptic forms of myoclonus also exist; the most common example is the isolated limb jerk that often occurs in healthy individuals as they fall asleep. Some patients exhibit diffuse, severe nonepileptic myoclonus after anoxic brain injury.

3. Seizures of unknown onset

In some cases, the information available from history, direct observation, and supplementary testing is insufficient to draw conclusions about whether the seizure onset is focal or generalized, so the seizures are classified as unknown onset. With further information, it is sometimes possible to reclassify these seizures into one of the other two categories.

C. Seizures vs. Epilepsy

Someone who has had a seizure does not necessarily have epilepsy. Hypoxia, hyponatremia, hyperglycemia, hypoglycemia, hypocalcemia, hypomagnesemia, uremia, hepatic failure, fever, cerebral edema, a variety of prescription and recreational drugs, and other metabolic and physical insults can all provoke seizures in normal individuals. As long as the precipitating factor can be identified and treated effectively, these people are no more likely than the general population to have recurrent seizures. Even when someone has a seizure and *no* precipitating trigger can be found, they do not necessarily have a predisposition to seizures. In fact, about 50% of people who have an unprovoked seizure never have another one. It is not clear why this should be the case, but presumably, some rare constellation of metabolic factors (e.g., electrolyte concentrations, glucocorticoid levels, body temperature) and neuronal activation patterns may combine in just the right way to result in a seizure, and that combination may never recur in the person's lifetime. In contrast, people who have had *two* unprovoked seizures have a 60–90% chance of subsequent seizures. These people probably have a brain abnormality predisposing to recurrent seizures (i.e., they have epilepsy and require medication).

Factors that increase the likelihood that someone who has had a single seizure will subsequently have recurrent seizures include an abnormal neurologic examination, abnormal brain imaging, certain findings on electroencephalogram (EEG; see Section E), a previous brain insult that was likely to have caused the seizure, and occurrence of the seizure during sleep. When these factors are judged to increase the likelihood of recurrent seizures to a level as high as it is in people who have had two unprovoked seizures (at least 60%), epilepsy may be diagnosed. One other situation in which epilepsy can be reliably diagnosed without waiting for a second seizure is when the individual has features that are characteristic of a known epilepsy syndrome, especially if a causative mutation for a genetic syndrome can be identified.

D. Epilepsy Classification

The current International League Against Epilepsy (ILAE) system of epilepsy classification includes four epilepsy types: focal, generalized, combined generalized and focal, and unknown. People with generalized epilepsy have seizures that are all generalized in onset, and people with focal epilepsy have seizures that are all focal in onset, although individuals in either category may have a range of seizure types. For example, someone with generalized epilepsy may have any combination of absence, myoclonic, atonic, tonic, and tonic-clonic seizures. People who have some seizures that are focal and others that are generalized are classified as having combined generalized and focal epilepsy, and people who have seizures with unknown onset are classified as unknown. The determination of epilepsy type, like seizure type, is based mainly on clinical features, supported by EEG findings and sometimes other test results.

Some people with epilepsy can be classified as having an epilepsy syndrome. These are characterized by clusters of clinical features, EEG findings, and imaging abnormalities that tend to occur together, often with typical age-dependent features (such as age of onset or remission) and comorbidities. Many epilepsy syndromes are associated with specific underlying causes, such as a structural, genetic, infectious, metabolic, or immune disorder. Of course, the same types of conditions can be the cause of epilepsy even when it does not conform to a recognized syndrome. Identification of an epilepsy syndrome often has implications for treatment and prognosis. It is beyond the scope of this textbook to cover all of the epilepsy syndromes, but a few representative examples are discussed in Part V, Section B.

E. Electroencephalography

An electroencephalogram (EEG) is a test in which electrodes are placed at standard positions on the scalp to record extracellular electric currents that are produced by transmembrane ion flow resulting from activity in the apical dendrites of the radially oriented pyramidal cells in layers III and V of the cerebral cortex. The electric activity detected by one electrode reflects the summated activity of roughly 100 million neurons. The EEG, in effect, compares the sum of this activity in the vicinity of one electrode to the sum of activity surrounding an adjacent electrode. Because each of these electrodes summates the activity of neurons participating in multiple circuits with diverse functions, the EEG can only provide information about large pools of neurons. In particular, the frequency spectrum of the summated activity is relatively consistent across normal individuals, and brain damage can distort that frequency distribution. During a seizure, the hypersynchronous activity of large networks of neurons can result in distinctive, abnormal patterns of EEG activity. Thus, an EEG recorded during a clinical spell (referred to as an *ictal* EEG) can be used to determine whether or not the spell is a seizure, if the abnormal electrical activity involves a large enough area of cortex.

Although an EEG recorded between spells (termed an *interictal EEG*) can't be used to determine whether a particular spell was a seizure, an interictal EEG can reveal characteristic "epileptiform" abnormalities that are more common in people with epilepsy than in the general population. The particular characteristics of the epileptiform activity on EEG may provide clues regarding the nature of the underlying epilepsy syndrome. For example, absence seizures characteristically are associated with a pattern described as regular spike-and-wave activity at a frequency of 3 Hz.

Interictal EEGs are neither completely specific nor completely sensitive. About 2–3% of people with interictal abnormalities on EEG never have any symptoms consistent with a seizure, and about 10–20% of people with clinically unequivocal epilepsy have consistently normal interictal EEGs. A single interictal EEG will show epileptiform activity in 50–70% of people with epilepsy. The yield can be increased by obtaining more than one interictal EEG or with activation procedures such as hyperventilation (especially useful for provoking absence seizures) or sleep deprivation. Some EEG abnormalities are more informative than others, and interpretation requires specialized training and expertise.

In some circumstances, it is desirable to characterize seizures as carefully as possible. This requires continuous EEG monitoring and concurrent video recording of the patient, with the goal of recording their actual spells (rather than just interictal activity). This is only practical if they have spells fairly frequently. For patients in whom long-term monitoring is feasible, the details of what the person does during the seizure and the specific changes seen on EEG during the seizure can be very helpful in identifying an epilepsy syndrome. Spells that involve definite alteration of consciousness or responsiveness with no associated EEG change are not seizures (with rare exceptions). Of course, the patient could have *other* spells that *are* seizures—some people with epilepsy also have nonepileptic spells of psychogenic origin.

F. Pathophysiology of Seizures and Epilepsy

The fundamental mechanisms underlying seizure onset, propagation, and termination remain obscure, and the mechanisms may differ depending on the type of epilepsy. Two key conditions are required for seizures to occur: (1) excessive neuronal excitability and (2) a pattern of synaptic connections between neurons that permits hypersynchrony. Many different cellular processes contribute to these conditions, notably the activity of voltage-gated ion channels (which, in turn, affects the neuron's resting potential and electrical excitability), the distribution and activity of inhibitory (predominantly GABA-ergic) synapses, and the distribution and activity of excitatory (especially glutamatergic) synapses. Glial cells and features of the extracellular space can also affect neuronal excitability and synaptic organization. Experimental manipulation of any of these processes in laboratory animals can cause seizures, and it seems likely that perturbations in neuronal excitability and synaptic connections can produce seizures in humans, also.

The mechanisms underlying epilepsy (as opposed to individual seizures) are also obscure. It is not clear what factors make one region of brain more likely than another to serve as a seizure focus. The formation of positive feedback (recurrent excitatory) circuits is probably important. In mesial temporal sclerosis, a condition commonly associated with epilepsy, the mossy fibers of the hippocampus sprout collateral branches that could serve as the substrate for such circuits. A similar process has been implicated in the formation of neuronal connections during memory storage. Indeed, one reason so many patients have a seizure focus in the temporal lobe may be that plasticity and synaptic remodeling occur routinely in the normal hippocampus. There is evidence that seizures themselves may induce collateral sprouting, and thus contribute to recurrent excitatory circuits. This increases the likelihood of further seizures, leading to additional sprouting, and so forth.

Thalamocortical circuits seem to be critical in many cases of recurrent generalized seizures. The normal thalamus enters an oscillatory or "burst" mode during drowsiness or sleep, and these inherent rhythm-generating mechanisms may serve as the substrate for abnormal rhythmic activity when the circuits are damaged. There is evidence for this mechanism in animal models of generalized absence epilepsy.

IV. Diagnosis

When people present with transient symptoms that might represent a seizure, the diagnostic process involves two steps. The first is to characterize the presenting spell, and to determine if it is likely to be a seizure or some other condition. If a seizure is likely, the second step is to try to identify the cause. Although these two steps are conceptually distinct, they are entwined in practice. Complete and accurate characterization of a seizure often suggests the cause, especially when patients have a recognized epilepsy syndrome. Conversely, identification of a likely cause of epilepsy increases the likelihood that the presenting spell was, in fact, a seizure. Thus, the distinction between these two diagnostic steps is somewhat artificial information pertinent to one is also relevant to the other—but for purposes of exposition it is useful to discuss them separately. To minimize redundancy, procedures (such as blood tests, MRI, and EEG) that are important in identifying the underlying cause of seizures are discussed in Part V, whereas the current discussion focuses on features of the spells themselves.

A. Characterizing the Presenting Spell

Seizures, like TIAs, are transient. Patients have usually returned to baseline by the time they receive medical attention, so the history is typically more useful than the neurologic examination. People with focal aware seizures may be able to provide an accurate description of their spells, but you should also be sure to talk to an independent witness, even if you have to track them down by phone. People with focal impaired awareness seizures or generalized seizures usually have little or no recollection of the spell, so witnesses' accounts are especially important.

Typical manifestations of seizures were reviewed in Part III. Many of these features can be dramatic and distinctive, but some can be very subtle. Patients and witnesses often overlook important details and misinterpret others (such as generalized tremulousness, which is a very nonspecific phenomenon). You should begin by asking open-ended questions (e.g., "What was the first thing you noticed that seemed abnormal today?"; "Did you have a warning?"; "What's the next thing you remember?"; "How did you feel when you regained consciousness?"; "Were you immediately able to resume what you had been doing before the spell?"), but be prepared to follow up with focused questions (e.g., "Did you smell anything unusual?"; "Was one side of your body different from the other?"; "When you regained consciousness, was there any sign that you had bitten your tongue?"; "Had you wet yourself or soiled yourself?"). If they bit their tongue, ask whether it was the tip of the tongue (which can occur with any fall) or on the side of the tongue (which is relatively specific for a seizure). Try to obtain as detailed a description as possible of everything the patient experienced—or witnesses observed—before, during, and after the spell, including the exact sequence of events and how long each stage lasted. Ask what the patient was doing just before the episode and earlier that day, especially anything different from their usual routine. Pay special attention to features that would help determine whether the onset was focal or generalized. Ask if the patient had any persistent focal deficits after the spell ended, because such deficits are more common with focal seizures.

B. Identifying Prior Spells

Unless patients spontaneously mention previous spells, you should ask them direct, pointed questions to determine if they have previously experienced characteristic seizure symptoms ("Do you ever smell things that aren't there?"; "Have you ever had the sense that you were outside your body looking down?"). In many cases, you can obtain more useful diagnostic information by concentrating on subtle or minor spells that patients have experienced in the past than you can by trying to characterize the more dramatic spell that brought them to medical attention. If you don't ask about these symptoms explicitly, patients may not volunteer them, because they consider them too insignificant, or too strange, or too embarrassing. People may also be too embarrassed to mention incontinence until you ask them about it explicitly.

C. Recognizing Spells That Are Not Seizures

In addition to questions regarding typical manifestations of seizures, ask about features that might indicate some other disorder. A variety of non-epileptic conditions produce recurrent spells that can be confused with seizures.

1. Spells involving loss of consciousness

The most common cause of temporary loss of consciousness is syncope, which occurs when a transient reduction in cardiac output produces generalized cerebral ischemia. Many different conditions can produce syncope, including cardiac arrhythmia, obstructed cardiac outflow (such as occurs with aortic stenosis), sudden cardiac failure from a large myocardial infarction, or impaired autonomic reflexes (e.g., orthostatic hypotension). Excessive parasympathetic tone, often called vasovagal syncope or vasodepressor syncope, is the most common cause. It occurs when there is excessive parasympathetic response to a sudden increase in sympathetic activity, most often in the setting of stress or excitement. Excessive parasympathetic responses may also be responsible for micturition syncope and defecation syncope.

Most episodes of syncope are preceded by a premonitory state known as presyncope, consisting of light-headedness and sometimes nausea, diaphoresis, tinnitus, fading of vision, and change in skin color. These premonitory symptoms may be helpful in distinguishing a syncopal spell from a seizure, but not always—some people with syncope lose consciousness suddenly, without warning, and others describe presyncopal symptoms that are similar to what people with focal seizures sometimes report. Another useful distinguishing feature may be the setting in which the spells occur. For example, people who lose consciousness when having their blood drawn probably have vasovagal syncope, and a common setting for orthostatic syncope is during a religious service, when a person suddenly stands after prolonged sitting or kneeling that resulted in venous pooling in the legs. After syncope, people are usually only briefly confused, if at all; more prolonged postictal confusion would suggest a seizure. Asymmetric symptoms after the spell are more typical of seizure than syncope. Incontinence is also more common with seizures, though it can occur with syncope. Spells that include rhythmic motor activity are usually seizures, but myoclonic jerks may occur with restitution of blood flow after a syncopal episode, making distinction from a seizure difficult in some cases. This is called convulsive syncope.

Transient metabolic disturbances, such as hypoglycemia, can produce symptoms that resemble syncope or seizures. People with excessive daytime somnolence from any cause can experience "sleep attacks," in which they suddenly fall asleep with hardly any warning. These episodes are not associated with any of the other typical features of seizures, so they are usually not hard to distinguish as long as reliable witnesses are available.

2. Spells without loss of consciousness

Both TIAs and migraines may produce transient neurologic symptoms that spread in a manner similar to a focal seizure (see Chapters 4 and 12). Accompanying headache helps to distinguish migraine from seizure, but some people with otherwise typical migraine never experience headache (so-called migraine equivalents), and some people who have seizures have severe headaches afterward. The motor or sensory symptoms that occur with migraine tend to evolve more slowly than the symptoms of a seizure, which, in turn, tend to develop more slowly than the symptoms of a TIA. The sensory and motor manifestations of TIAs tend to be "negative" phenomena, such as numbness or weakness, whereas seizures are more likely to produce "positive" symptoms, such as paresthesias or jerking movements.

Cataplexy—a sudden loss of muscle tone most commonly seen in people with narcolepsy (see Chapter 9)—is sometimes mistaken for a seizure. A variety of other abnormal movements or behaviors can occur with sleep disorders, and sometimes the only way to distinguish these from seizures is to perform EEG monitoring while the person sleeps.

3. Spells of psychogenic origin

Psychological conditions can result in spells that resemble seizures; they are often referred to as psychogenic nonepileptic spells (PNES) or psychogenic nonepileptic events (PNEE). Features that may suggest this possibility include a long period of motionless unresponsiveness, forced eye closure, asynchronous limb movements, side-to-side ("no-no") shaking of the head, dramatic bilateral limb movements while talking, and crying shortly after the spell. Spells that vary substantially from one episode to another (such as spells that involve one limb on one day and a different limb the next, or visual symptoms on some occasions and auditory symptoms on other occasions, or spells lasting 2 minutes at times and 2 days at other times) would all be atypical of epilepsy and suggestive of a non-neurologic disorder. If the spells occur only when the person is in a psychologically stressful situation, this may also be a clue that the condition is psychogenic. There are exceptions to all these generalizations, however. For example, seizures that originate in the prefrontal cortex sometimes result in bilateral limb movements without alteration of consciousness. Spells should not be assumed to have a psychogenic origin simply because they are unusual or seem inconsistent. All fields of medicine abound with examples of conditions that were erroneously considered psychogenic.

V. Determining the Cause of Seizures

Once you have determined that someone has had a seizure, or that it is at least a realistic consideration, management depends on the underlying cause. People who present with seizures can be grouped into three broad categories: (1) those whose seizures are precipitated by clearly identified systemic factors, (2) those with epilepsy, and (3) those who experience a single unprovoked seizure with no evidence of predisposition to recurrent seizures. People in the first category are managed by treating whatever precipitating factors are identified. People with epilepsy are treated with antiseizure medications (ASMs) or the other modalities discussed in Part VI. People with single unprovoked seizures are usually followed conservatively.

A. Provoked Seizures

The most common endogenous metabolic causes of seizures are hypoxia, hyponatremia, hyperglycemia, hypoglycemia, hypocalcemia, and hypomagnesemia. Seizures may also occur with acute uremia or hepatic failure. Prescription drugs and recreational drugs are common causes of seizures, especially antidepressants and antipsychotic medications (particularly when doses are increased too rapidly), aminophylline and other methylxanthines, lidocaine, penicillins, narcotic analgesics, cocaine, heroin, methylenedioxymethamphetamine (MDMA, or "ecstasy"), phencyclidine, and alcohol. Withdrawal from alcohol may produce seizures, usually after 6–48 hours of abstinence. Withdrawal seizures may also occur in people who have been taking barbiturates or benzodiazepines regularly.

Fever is a common precipitating factor in children. About 2–4% of children have a febrile seizure, usually within the first 3 years of life. About a third of children who have a febrile seizure will have one or more recurrences. Febrile seizures typically occur during the rising phase of the temperature curve; they do not correlate with the severity of the fever. They are almost always generalized, and they usually last less than 15 minutes. The incidence of subsequent epilepsy is significantly higher in children who have febrile seizures than in the general population, but the rate is still lower than 5%. Factors associated with a higher likelihood of subsequent epilepsy are seizure duration longer than 15 minutes, seizure recurrence within 24 hours, focal features to the seizure, a history of abnormal neurologic development, an abnormal neurologic examination, and a family history of epilepsy. Children with none of these factors have a <1% risk of developing epilepsy subsequently. Febrile seizures do not require treatment other than trying to control subsequent fevers promptly with antipyretic medication and sponge baths.

B. Epilepsy

Recognition of a defined epilepsy syndrome (based on clinical characteristics and diagnostic test results) may provide prognostic information or facilitate management decisions. It is beyond the range of this book to review all of the known epilepsy syndromes, but it is worth mentioning a few representative examples.

Childhood absence epilepsy is characterized by absence seizures that typically begin in children ages 4–8 years old and usually (in two thirds of patients) resolve before adulthood. Ethosuximide is the drug of choice for this syndrome. *Juvenile myoclonic epilepsy* is characterized by myoclonic jerks of the shoulders and arms, usually occurring soon after awakening. More than 90% of people with this syndrome have generalized tonic-clonic seizures, and about 25% also have absence seizures. The myoclonic jerks precede the generalized tonic-clonic seizures by a year or more in about half the patients. The typical age of onset is 12–18 years. This condition usually responds very well to appropriate medications, but life-long medication is often necessary. People with *self-limited epilepsy with centrotemporal spikes* (SeLECTS, previously known as "benign epilepsy with centrotemporal spikes," "BECTS," or "benign rolandic epilepsy") have focal seizures characterized by unilateral movements of the lips, tongue, cheek, pharynx, or larynx, often with abnormal sensations in the same regions, associated with excessive salivation and drooling. The patients are fully conscious, but they may be unable to speak when the focus is in the dominant hemisphere. There may be spread to the arm and leg on the same side or sometimes to the entire body. The seizures usually occur during sleep. They typically present at ages 5–10 years, and almost always resolve spontaneously by age 18 years.

Lennox-Gastaut syndrome is a particularly severe condition that typically manifests between ages 2 and 8 years. It is characterized by the triad of cognitive disability, a diffuse slow spike-and-wave pattern on EEG, and multiple types of generalized seizures, including atonic seizures, tonic seizures, myoclonic seizures, and atypical absence seizures. Status epilepticus is common in children with this syndrome. A variety of underlying brain disorders can cause this syndrome. In about a third of patients, the underlying cause is not identified.

C. The Diagnostic Evaluation

The process of obtaining a detailed description of the episode (and previous episodes, if any) was discussed in Part IV. Your history should also focus on features that would increase the likelihood that the patient has an underlying brain disorder that could predispose to seizures (such as a family history of epilepsy or a history of premature birth, developmental delay, febrile seizures with poor prognostic indicators, head trauma, stroke, meningitis, or encephalitis). You should also take a thorough medical history because the patient might already be known to have one or more conditions that predispose to seizures. You should perform a full neurologic examination—abnormal findings obviously increase the likelihood of underlying brain dysfunction.

If you are seeing a patient soon after a spell that sounds like it could have been a seizure, and the person has no prior history of seizures, you should check serum electrolytes (including calcium and magnesium, which are not routinely included in some screening blood panels), glucose, blood urea nitrogen, creatinine, liver enzymes, and blood counts. People who present acutely with seizures should be evaluated for systemic infection, and if the clinical presentation is at all suggestive of meningitis or encephalitis a lumbar puncture should be performed. A urine toxin screen should be obtained. The yield of this testing is usually low.

People who present with the first seizure of their lives should have an imaging study. An MRI scan performed with and without gadolinium using a specific protocol and sequences for epilepsy is the imaging procedure of choice. In the acute setting, this is often unavailable, so patients often have a noncontrast head CT scan in the emergency department to exclude lesions that would require urgent treatment, such as intracranial hemorrhage or a tumor producing significant mass effect. They can then be scheduled to have an MRI scan as an outpatient within the next few weeks.

Patients should also be scheduled for an outpatient EEG in the same time frame. The patient will probably not be obliging enough to have a spell during the EEG, so it will most likely be an interictal recording. As discussed in Part III, some interictal EEG abnormalities correlate with a predisposition to generate seizures, and interictal EEG findings can sometimes provide information regarding the specific epilepsy syndrome. In certain circumstances, genetic testing may also be indicated.

Before these investigations, patients should be advised that the evaluation often fails to identify a specific underlying reason for seizures, so they should not be distressed if the search is unrevealing.

VI. Management of Seizures and Epilepsy

A. People with Seizures But No Proven Epilepsy

For people with provoked seizures, management usually involves correction of the precipitating condition. For example, seizures occurring in the setting of severe hyperglycemia or uremia are best addressed by treating the underlying metabolic abnormality, and seizures related to drug toxicity or alcohol withdrawal require management of the underlying substance use disorder. Treatment directed at the seizure itself is generally unnecessary. The main exception is status epilepticus due to an underlying toxic/metabolic disorder, for which antiseizure medications (ASMs) may be required acutely until the underlying abnormality can be corrected (see Part VII, Section A).

For people who have experienced an isolated, unprovoked seizure, management decisions are complicated. About half of these individuals do not have epilepsy and will never have another seizure, so the benefit of prompt initiation of treatment in a patient who needs it must be balanced against the risk of prolonged ASM use when it is not necessary. Initiation of an ASM after a single unprovoked seizure reduces the risk of recurrence within the next 2 years by about 35%, but does not affect long-term prognosis. Thus, when there is no evidence of a brain disorder predisposing to seizures, it is reasonable to follow patients conservatively and only prescribe an ASM if they have a second seizure. Only 20–30% of people who have a normal neurologic examination, EEG, and brain MRI scan will have recurrent seizures, so for these patients ASMs are almost never recommended. In contrast, certain abnormalities on neurologic examination, imaging studies, or EEG can signify an underlying condition that predisposes to seizures and warrants treatment after a single episode.

B. People with Epilepsy

1. Antiseizure medications (ASMs)

A few people have seizures very infrequently, perhaps once every few years, and they would rather live with these rare seizures than take medication on a regular basis. Because there is no proof that such rare seizures produce any long-term adverse consequences, this choice can be reasonable for some patients. This situation is quite rare, however. Most people with epilepsy have more than one seizure a year. Even people whose seizures are infrequent often find them so disturbing that they will go to great lengths to avoid them. Thus, almost all people with epilepsy receive ASMs.

ASMs suppress seizures by altering the electrical properties of neurons, typically via effects on membrane ion channels or receptors, but they have not been shown to induce any permanent change in the neuron's electrical properties or in the pattern of neuronal connections. Thus, there is no reason to think that they change the underlying predisposition to have seizures—i.e., the epilepsy. Nonetheless, many people who have been seizure-free for a number of years while taking ASMs are able to discontinue the medications and their seizures do not return. It is not clear why this is so. Most likely, it is due to spontaneous reorganization of the underlying synaptic connections. Given that spontaneous remission is rare in untreated people with epilepsy, it seems likely that recurrent seizures reinforce the connections responsible for the seizure circuit, and by suppressing those seizures, ASMs may eliminate that reinforcement. In other words, ASMs do not directly cure epilepsy, but they may provide an environment that allows the epileptic brain to "heal itself."

Decisions regarding which ASM to use for the initial treatment of a person with epilepsy are based on what types of seizures the individual has (and especially whether they are focal or generalized), whether the person has a specific epilepsy syndrome, the person's comorbidities, their preferences regarding dosing schedule and potential side effects, and financial considerations. Table 5.1 lists the most commonly used ASMs and their side effects. Table 5.2 shows which ASMs the U.S. Food and Drug Administration (FDA) has approved for particular seizure types and epilepsy syndromes, as well as other ASMs that may be effective and ASMs to avoid in patients with those seizure types or syndromes. When someone has several types of seizures, the goal is to use a single medication that is effective against all the varieties of seizures the patient experiences. The most commonly used "broad-spectrum" ASMs (ASMs that are effective for both focal-onset and generalized-onset seizures) are lamotrigine, levetiracetam, topiramate, and valproic acid. Brivaracetam and zonisamide are also in this category.

Once an ASM is selected, it should be introduced slowly to allow the metabolism to "ramp up" to a steady state and to give the patient time to adjust to the sometimes troubling initial symptoms such as sleepiness and a slight reduction in mental sharpness. The dose should be increased gradually until seizure control is achieved or the patient can't tolerate any further increase because of toxic symptoms. Serum drug levels should not be the principal basis for making dose adjustments. The published "therapeutic range" for any drug is based on a population average. There is considerable variability in individual's responses to these drugs. Some people achieve complete seizure control with levels below the published therapeutic range, whereas others require levels higher than the upper limit of the range. Some people experience unacceptable toxic effects at the lowest possible doses of a medication, whereas others have no problems at levels above the therapeutic range. Drug levels thus provide only approximate guidelines for therapy. They are useful for monitoring adherence to the medication regimen, and they may also be helpful in determining why someone who was previously well controlled has resumed having seizures. If there is a record of the drug level during the period of good control, it can be compared to the current drug level. Superimposed medical illnesses or drug-drug interactions may cause changes in ASM levels despite a stable dosing regimen.

If a person's seizures can only be controlled at doses that cause intolerable side effects, the medication dosage should be reduced slightly to the highest dose the patient can tolerate, while adding a second ASM at a low dose. Drug-drug interactions must be reviewed when doing this. The dose of this second medication should be gradually increased as necessary for seizure control. If seizures are not controlled even after increasing the dose of the second medication as high as the person can tolerate, then one of the two medications (whichever one seems to be less effective for them or harder for them to tolerate) should be gradually withdrawn and replaced with a third agent. This maneuver should be repeated (up to a point—see the discussion of surgical resection for refractory epilepsy below) until a medication pair is found that controls the patient's seizures without producing unacceptable side effects. When this has been accomplished, it is usually prudent to leave the person on both medications for a while, but if they remain seizure-free, at some point it is reasonable to consider whether the most recently added medication would be sufficient to control the patient's seizures all by itself. The main way to answer this question is to withdraw the other medication gradually. If seizures recur, the dose can be increased back to the previously effective dose and the patient can remain on the combination regimen. Only occasionally do patients need to use more than two ASMs at one time.

Decreased bone density can occur in people who take phenytoin, valproic acid, phenobarbital, or primidone on a chronic basis. Carbamazepine may also affect bone metabolism, but the evidence is conflicting. ASMs that do not induce liver enzymes do not appear to affect bone metabolism. Patients must be educated about strict medication adherence and possible side effects. For certain drugs, periodic laboratory testing is necessary to monitor for potential toxicity (such as bone marrow suppression, liver damage, or osteopenia). These laboratory tests should also be checked before starting the patient on the medication so that a baseline is available for comparison.

When seizure control is achieved, patients should be informed that they must remain on the ASM until instructed otherwise by their physician. For people with some epilepsy syndromes, such as juvenile myoclonic epilepsy, the likelihood of seizure recurrence after ASM withdrawal is so high that lifelong medication may be necessary. For people with other epilepsy syndromes, it is often reasonable to attempt to withdraw ASMs after the seizures have been completely controlled for 2 years or more, but this should always be done under the close supervision of a physician. The medication taper should be gradual (over approximately 3–6 months). Seizures are most likely to recur within the first year after drug withdrawal. Factors that favor successful withdrawal from ASMs include a longer period of being seizure-free, a low lifelong number of seizures, a normal neurologic examination, normal EEG, and normal MRI.

2. Surgical resection of the seizure focus

When seizure control is not achieved after an adequate trial of two or three ASMs, the likelihood of success with subsequent ASMs is very low. About one third of people with epilepsy have seizures that cannot be fully controlled with medications, and about half of these patients may be candidates for surgical resection of the seizure focus. To establish that someone is a surgical candidate, it is necessary to prove that their spells are definitely seizures, that the majority of the seizures originate from a single focus, and that the focus is in a region of brain that can be removed safely. To identify the site of seizure onset as precisely as possible, patients are typically hospitalized for long-term video/EEG recording of ictal activity, sometimes using invasive recording with depth or subdural electrodes. Detailed structural imaging and functional imaging studies of cerebral metabolic activity or blood flow at baseline and immediately after a seizure are also used. Other investigations are aimed at determining whether the portion of brain where the seizures originate may be safely removed without causing serious neurologic deficits (such as severe memory loss, language disturbance, or major motor deficits). In carefully selected groups of patients, resective surgery may produce complete seizure resolution in up to 80% of patients in whom medical therapy has failed.

3. Other ablative surgery

In addition to resection of the seizure focus, other surgical approaches are sometimes pursued. Hemispherectomies may be an option in young children with widely distributed epileptic disturbances over one hemisphere, especially when there is a contralateral hemiparesis. Section of the corpus callosum can be of benefit in a small number of people with refractory seizures characterized by frequent falls and sometimes other seizure types. Such people may achieve elimination of one seizure type but generally do not become seizure free. Another disconnection procedure that can be effective in select patients is to perform multiple subpial transections.

4. Vagus nerve stimulation

Vagus nerve stimulation is another surgical approach that can be tried in people who are refractory to medical therapy; its mechanism of action is not well understood. Two helical electrode coils are wrapped around the left vagus nerve in the carotid sheath and connected to an infraclavicular pulse generator. The generator is then programmed to deliver pulses of a specified duration, frequency, and amplitude. Patients treated in this way initially average a 25–30% reduction in seizure frequency, and 25–30% of people have at least a 50% reduction in seizure frequency. The benefit seems to increase with the duration of stimulation, so that over several years more than 50% of patients experience a 50% reduction in seizure frequency. Patients also have the option of using an external magnet to activate the device when they start to experience a seizure; for some people, this can abort the seizure or reduce its severity. For individuals who have tachycardia at the start of seizures, the device can be programmed to deliver stimulus pulses when it detects a heart rate above a predetermined level.

5. Deep brain stimulation

Deep brain stimulation is similar to vagus nerve stimulation except that the stimulation is delivered to the anterior nuclei of the thalamus; again, the mechanism of action is not well understood. This treatment is usually reserved for patients with multifocal or poorly localized epilepsy.

6. Responsive brain stimulation

Responsive (closed-loop) stimulation is another surgical option for people with refractory focal seizures who have one or two seizure-onset zones. In this approach, a cranially implanted programmable stimulator is connected to electrodes that continually monitor electrical activity in the (previously identified) seizure-onset zone (or zones). The stimulator is programmed to detect specific patterns of electric activity and deliver brief stimulus pulses when those patterns occur. The median reduction in seizure frequency with this device is about 50%.

7. Ketogenic diet

In people with epilepsy whose seizures cannot be controlled with medications (or who require such high doses of medication that the side effects are unacceptable), a high-fat, adequate-protein, low-carbohydrate diet can produce a significant reduction in seizure frequency. The mechanism is not known. The benefit of this approach (known as the ketogenic diet because it mimics a starvation state and results in increased production of ketone bodies) does not appear to depend on seizure type or EEG pattern. Many people have trouble adhering to this diet. Constipation and gastroesophageal reflux are common. Other potential adverse effects include growth retardation, renal stones, and hypercholesterolemia.

C. Patient Education (for People with Isolated Seizures or Epilepsy)

Certain issues are such a frequent source of confusion or concern for patients and their family members that physicians should make a point of discussing them explicitly. Good resources can be found online at the website http://www.epilepsy.com.

1. Reassurance regarding the nature of seizures

Seizures can be very frightening for patients and observers alike. You should reassure patients and their family members that seizures are a common, well-described phenomenon. Explain that if the person has another seizure, bystanders should try to get the patient into a position that limits the risk of a dangerous fall, but they do not need to intervene in any other way as long as the seizure resolves quickly.

2. Diagnostic evaluation in the Emergency Department

Explain that you will be ordering blood tests, urine tests, a brain CT scan, and possibly a lumbar puncture to look for anything that might have provoked the seizure, but that you will not be surprised if all the results are normal—in many people with seizures, no underlying cause is identified. Similarly, you will be arranging for the patient to have an EEG and MRI at some point in the next few weeks, but it will not be surprising if those results are normal or nonspecific, also.

3. Rationale for not starting an ASM

Explain to the patient that a single seizure is often an isolated event that never recurs, and for this reason, antiseizure medication is not usually recommended after a single seizure. Go into as much detail as the patient requires regarding the relative risks of an unnecessary medication vs. an untreated seizure. When patients insist that they would prefer to be on medication, and you are convinced that they understand the relevant issues and risks, it may be appropriate to prescribe one.

4. Reassurance regarding epilepsy

People who ultimately prove to have epilepsy often require reassurance that they can still lead normal and productive lives. Many prominent people in the worlds of art, literature, music, politics, and sport have had epilepsy. The stigma that traditionally surrounded epilepsy was misguided.

5. ASM risks and benefits

When you prescribe an ASM, explain how you plan to adjust the dose and review the potential side effects. Be sure the patient understands that there is no single medication that is effective for everyone with a given type of epilepsy, and that for any given medication the effective dose varies from one person to another, so an element of trial and error is unavoidable. While the medication is being titrated, people may experience additional seizures, which can cause them and their family members considerable distress, but you should urge them not to overreact. Ultimately, the goal is to eliminate seizures entirely, but some seizures along the way may be unavoidable. Although you should try to avoid unnecessary delays, you should also avoid making changes too quickly. A seizure that occurs shortly after increasing the medication dose may not be a true reflection of the effects of the higher dose. Likewise, it may take several weeks for a side effect to resolve after reducing the dose. By making sure that patients have realistic expectations and a clear understanding of how they are supposed to take their medications, you can increase the likelihood that they will adhere to the plan.

, with 6 months being a common requirement). Other states apply more flexible restrictions, sometimes influenced by the recommendations of the treating physician. Some states require physicians to report people who have had a seizure, but most states don't. Individual state driving restrictions are available at https://www.epilepsy.com/driving-laws.

Other common-sense restrictions also apply. Nobody who has epilepsy should swim alone. People with epilepsy should use a shower rather than a bathtub, as it is possible to drown in just a few inches of water. They should avoid situations that might put them at risk if they were to have a seizure, such as working at heights or using power equipment. They should also be informed of a rare complication known as sudden unexplained death in epilepsy (SUDEP); the biologic basis for SUDEP is not known, but it is most common in people with uncontrolled bilateral tonic-clonic seizures.

VII. Special Clinical Problems

A. Status Epilepticus

Status epilepticus is defined in Part III. It is a medical emergency with significant mortality (10–20% in adults and 2–5% in children) and major morbidity. The prognosis is closely related to the cause. The most common cause is insufficient medication in people previously diagnosed with epilepsy, often because of inadequate adherence to the medication regimen. In people with no history of epilepsy, the most common causes are stroke, hypoxia, toxic-metabolic disorders, and infection. When status epilepticus is due to insufficient medication, it usually responds to supplementation (or reinstitution) of ASMs and the prognosis is better than it is for people with status epilepticus and no history of epilepsy. The longer a person is in status, the worse the outcome. This is partly because the duration is more likely to be prolonged in people with more severe underlying disease, but there is also considerable experimental evidence that status epilepticus itself damages the brain and that the degree of damage is a function of duration. Current guidelines state that treatment for status epilepticus should be started at 5 minutes for tonic-clonic seizures, 10 minutes for focal seizures with impaired consciousness, and 10–15 minutes for absence seizures.

The management of status epilepticus involves cardiorespiratory stabilization, correction of metabolic abnormalities, and treatment with ASMs. Benzodiazepines are the preferred ASMs for initial treatment of status epilepticus, but they have short half-lives, so they are usually followed with a second agent. Table 5.3 lists the ASM options for a status epilepticus treatment protocol. Each phase of treatment should be initiated as soon as the previous phase is completed unless the status epilepticus has resolved. There are several ASM options at each phase, with no compelling evidence to favor one of them over the others, so physicians (or institutions) should decide on a standard protocol that they follow routinely to avoid wasting valuable moments trying to decide which agent to use or where to find it. Animal and human studies indicate that the efficacy of treatment decreases the longer the seizures have been present.

If the motor manifestations of status epilepticus resolve, but the patient's mental status does not normalize, an EEG should be obtained to determine if electrographic seizures are still present. Ongoing electrographic seizure activity without any motor manifestation is termed nonconvulsive status epilepticus. If this condition is present, it should be treated as aggressively as if motor activity were still evident (convulsive status epilepticus).

In contrast to the situation in which nonconvulsive status epilepticus evolves from convulsive status epilepticus, some people with focal seizures or absence seizures present with status epilepticus that is nonconvulsive from the outset. People with focal seizures can also develop convulsive status epilepticus that only affects one region of the body; this is known as epilepsia partialis continua. In general, these forms of status epilepticus have a better prognosis than generalized convulsive status epilepticus, and a less aggressive management protocol is often applied.

B. Seizures and Pregnancy

Pregnancy presents some difficult management issues for people with epilepsy. Seizures pose a risk to the fetus, and so does ASM exposure. Although no controlled trials have directly compared these risks, most experts agree that the risk to the fetus from uncontrolled convulsive seizures outweighs the risk from ASM exposure, and that complete ASM withdrawal is not a reasonable or safe option for most patients who are pregnant. The goal should be to identify the medications that pose the lowest risk, and to determine the safest ways to administer them.

Valproic acid should be avoided during pregnancy—and, in fact, it should only rarely be prescribed to anyone with childbearing potential—because it is the ASM associated with the highest unadjusted prevalence of major congenital malformations (9.3%). Lamotrigine, levetiracetam, and oxcarbazepine are the ASMs associated with the lowest prevalence (about 3% for each, as compared to the unadjusted prevalence of major congenital malformations among children born to individuals without epilepsy, which is about 2.5%). Phenobarbital should be avoided during pregnancy to reduce the risk of cardiac malformations, and topiramate should be avoided to reduce the risk of the child being born small for gestational age. Some of the ASMs have also been associated with increased risk of adverse perinatal outcomes or neurodevelopmental outcomes. All of these risks must be weighed against other considerations that are specific to each patient. For example, valproic acid may be the only ASM that results in good seizure control for some people with both generalized tonic-clonic and myoclonic seizures, and they are likely to experience seizure recurrence if switched to a different ASM. Regardless of which ASM is prescribed, the goal is to maintain the lowest dose that is effective. Physiologic changes during pregnancy can alter the metabolism, clearance, and protein binding of ASMs, resulting in fluctuations in total and free drug levels that are difficult to predict. Ideally, a free drug level should be measured before conception during a time when seizures are well controlled, and free drug levels should be monitored during pregnancy so that the ASM dose can be adjusted to maintain the preconception level. In the general population, folic acid supplementation reduces the risk of major congenital malformations, especially neural tube defects. This benefit has not been specifically demonstrated in people with epilepsy, but some evidence suggests that folic acid supplementation may improve neurodevelopmental outcomes; the current recommendation is to take at least 0.4 mg a day before conception and during pregnancy, and some clinicians recommend doses as high as 5 mg per day in high-risk groups, such as patients who must take high doses of valproic acid.

These topics should be discussed with anyone with childbearing potential soon after the diagnosis of epilepsy is established, so that they can make informed decisions far in advance of a pregnancy. Some patients whose most recent seizure was at least 2 years ago might even elect to taper off ASMs before trying to conceive.

There are many potential interactions between ASMs and oral contraceptive drugs. Clinicians should be sure to review these before starting or stopping any medication. Hormonal therapies used in assisted reproductive technology may exacerbate seizures; ASM use does not appear to affect the likelihood of successful treatment with assisted reproductive technology.

C. Refractory Seizures

When seizures fail to respond to medications, the treating physician should review the following points: Was the original diagnosis of epilepsy accurate? If so, was the correct type of epilepsy identified and were the appropriate ASMs used? If so, is the patient truly adhering to the medication regimen, as determined by adequate ASM levels? Does their lifestyle require modification? Were the medications pushed to the highest doses the patient could tolerate? Were combination regimens attempted? People who continue to be refractory to medical management should be referred to a major epilepsy center where experimental ASMs or epilepsy surgery may be available.

VIII. Supplementary Tables for Reference

Table 5.1 Commonly Used Antiseizure Medications (ASMs)

Generic Name	Trade Names	Side Effects
Brivaracetam	Briviact	Somnolence, dizziness, fatigue
Cannabidiol	Epidiolex	Sedation, fatigue, decreased appetite, diarrhea, elevated liver enzymes, elevated creatinine
Carbamazepine	Tegretol, Carbatrol, Epitol	Dizziness, nausea, sedation, ataxia, nystagmus, diplopia, hyponatremia, leukopenia, hepatotoxicity, osteopenia, rash[1]
Cenobamate	Xcopri	Somnolence, dizziness, fatigue, rash[2]
Clobazam	Onfi	Somnolence, fever, rash, incoordination, dysarthria
Clonazepam	Klonopin	Somnolence, cognitive dysfunction, incoordination
Eslicarbazepine	Aptiom	Dizziness, somnolence, headache, nausea, diplopia, fatigue, hyponatremia, rash

Table 5.1 Continued

Generic Name	Trade Names	Side Effects
Ethosuximide	Zarontin	Nausea, sedation, bone marrow suppression, rash
Gabapentin	Neurontin	Somnolence, edema, weight gain, fatigue, ataxia, dizziness, nausea, tremor
Lacosamide	Vimpat	Dizziness, ataxia, headache, nausea, diplopia, prolonged PR interval
Lamotrigine	Lamictal	Rash,[3] dizziness, sedation, diplopia, headache, nausea
Levetiracetam	Keppra	Somnolence, dizziness, lack of energy, anxiety, irritability, hostility
Oxcarbazepine	Trileptal	Dizziness, ataxia, diplopia, somnolence, headache, fatigue, hyponatremia, rash
Perampanel	Fycompa	Dizziness, somnolence, headache, fatigue, blurred vision, irritability, aggression
Phenobarbital	Luminal	Sedation, dizziness, ataxia, osteopenia, behavior disturbance in children
Phenytoin	Dilantin, Phenytek	Ataxia, dizziness, nystagmus, sedation, rash, gingival hyperplasia, hirsutism, leukopenia, hepatotoxicity, osteopenia, lymphadenopathy
Pregabalin	Lyrica	Weight gain, edema, somnolence, dizziness, ataxia, tremor
Primidone	Mysoline	Sedation, dizziness, ataxia, osteopenia, behavior disturbance in children
Rufinamide	Banzel	Dizziness, headache, nausea, ataxia, somnolence, shortened QT interval, anemia, leukopenia
Tiagabine	Gabitril	Dizziness, somnolence, cognitive disturbance, irritability, tremor
Topiramate	Topamax, Trokendi	Cognitive disturbance, somnolence, paresthesias, ataxia, dizziness, weight loss, kidney stones, metabolic acidosis, impaired sweating, hyperthermia, emotional lability, glaucoma

(Continued)

Table 5.1 Continued

Generic Name	Trade Names	Side Effects
Valproic acid	Depakote, Depakene, Depacon	Tremor, weight gain, nausea, sedation, hepatotoxicity, hyperammonemia, thrombocytopenia, hair loss, pancreatitis
Vigabatrin	Sabril	Irreversible visual field constriction, headache, somnolence, dizziness, ataxia, weight gain
Zonisamide	Zonegran	Somnolence, cognitive disturbance, ataxia, kidney stones, weight loss, rash, impaired sweating, hyperthermia

[1] Including Stevens-Johnson syndrome; FDA requires HLA-B1502 genotyping in people of Chinese ancestry to minimize rash risk.

[2] DRESS (drug rash with eosinophilia and systemic symptoms) syndrome; risk minimized by titrating dose slowly.

[3] Including Stevens-Johnson syndrome; to reduce risk, dose must be titrated very slowly (and even more slowly in people taking valproate).

Table 5.2 Seizure Types/Epilepsy Syndromes and the Antiseizure Medications (ASMs) That Are Effective for Them

Seizure Type	FDA-Approved ASMs	Other Potentially Effective ASMs	ASMs That May Exacerbate
1. Focal onset	- Brivaracetam (M, A)	- Clobazam	
	- Carbamazepine (M, A)	- Rufinamide	
	- Cenobamate (M, A)	- Vigabatrin	
	- Eslicarbazepine (M, A)		
	- Gabapentin (A)		
	- Lacosamide (M, A)		
	- Lamotrigine (M when converting from another ASM; A)		
	- Levetiracetam (M, A)		
	- Oxcarbazepine (M, A)		
	- Perampanel (M, A)		
	- Phenobarbital (M, A)[1]		
	- Phenytoin (M, A)		

Table 5.2 Continued

Seizure Type	FDA-Approved ASMs	Other Potentially Effective ASMs	ASMs That May Exacerbate
	- Pregabalin (A) - Primidone (M, A)[1] - Tiagabine (A) - Topiramate (M, A) - Valproic acid (M, A) - Vigabatrin (for patients refractory to several other ASMs; A) - Zonisamide (A)		
2. Generalized			
a. Generalized tonic-clonic	- Carbamazepine (M, A) - Lacosamide (A) - Lamotrigine (A) - Levetiracetam (A) - Perampanel (A) - Phenobarbital (M, A)[1] - Phenytoin (M, A) - Primidone (M, A)[1] - Topiramate (M, A) - Valproic acid (A)[2]	- Brivaracetam - Clobazam - Zonisamide	
b. Absence	- Clonazepam (for patients refractory to ethosuximide: M, A) - Ethosuximide (M, A) - Valproic acid (M, A)	- Clobazam - Lamotrigine (less effective than ethosuzimide and valproic acid)	- Carbamazepine - Eslicarbazepine - Gabapentin - Oxcarbazepine - Phenobarbital - Phenytoin - Pregabalin - Tiagabine - Vigabatrin

(Continued)

Table 5.2 Continued

Seizure Type	FDA-Approved ASMs	Other Potentially Effective ASMs	ASMs That May Exacerbate
c. Myoclonic	- Valproic acid (A)[2]	- Brivaracetam - Clobazam - Lamotrigine (but may exacerbate in some patients) - Levetiracetam (class I evidence) - Perampanel - Primidone - Topiramate	- Carbamazepine - Eslicarbazepine - Gabapentin - Lamotrigine (but may be effective in some patients) - Oxcarbazepine - Phenytoin - Pregabalin - Tiagabine - Vigabatrin
d. Infantile spasms	- Vigabatrin (M)		
e. Atonic	- Valproic acid (A)[2]		- Carbamazepine
Epilepsy Syndrome			
1. Juvenile myoclonic epilepsy	- Levetiracetam (A)	- Brivaracetam - Valproic acid	
2. Lennox-Gastaut syndrome	- Cannabidiol (M, A) - Clobazam (A) - Lamotrigine (A) - Rufinamide (A) - Topiramate (A)		

M = FDA-approved as monotherapy; A = FDA approved as adjunctive therapy (NOTE: for ethical reasons, most new ASMs are initially studied as adjunctive therapy, and that is the basis for FDA approval. Many of these drugs are subsequently used as monotherapy, even if they haven't been submitted to the FDA for this indication.)

[1] FDA indications for phenobarbital and primidone are vaguely worded.

[2] FDA indication: "adjunctive therapy in patients with multiple seizure types that include absence seizures."

Table 5.3 Antiseizure Medications (ASMs) for Status Epilepticus

Treatment Phase	ASM Options
Phase 1 Within: 5 minutes for tonic-clonic seizures 10 minutes for focal seizures with impaired awareness 10–15 minutes for absence seizures	Choose one of the following 3 first-line options: (1) Intramuscular midazolam (10 mg for > 40 kg; 5 mg for 13–40 kg); single dose (2) Intravenous lorazepam (0.1 mg/kg, max dose 4 mg); may repeat once (3) Intravenous diazepam (0.15–0.2 mg/kg, max dose 10 mg); may repeat once If none of the 3 first-line options possible, choose one of the following: (a) Intravenous phenobarbital (15 mg/kg); single dose (b) Rectal diazepam (0.2-0.5 mg/kg, max dose 20 mg); single dose (c) Intranasal or buccal midazolam
Phase 2 Immediately after Phase 1 unless status epilepticus has resolved	Choose one of the following intravenous medications (single dose): (1) Fosphenytoin (20 mg PE/kg, max dose 1500 mg PE) (2) Valproic acid (40 mg/kg, max dose 3000 mg) (3) Levetiracetam (60 mg/kg, max dose 4500 mg) If none of the above three options available, give one of the following intravenous medications (single dose): (a) Lacosamide (400 mg) (b) Phenytoin (20 mg/kg) if fosphenytoin not already given (c) Phenobarbital, 15 mg/kg, if not given already

(Continued)

Table 5.3 Continued

Treatment Phase	ASM Options
Phase 3 Immediately after Phase 2 unless status epilepticus has resolved	One of the following: (1) One of the options from Phase 2 that hasn't been tried already (2) Intubate (if not already intubated), connect to continuous EEG monitor (if not already done), and administer anesthetic doses of midazolam, propofol, pentobarbital, or thiopental, with target of "burst suppression" pattern on EEG
Phase 4 Immediately after Phase 3 unless status epilepticus has resolved	If not already done: intubate, connect to continuous EEG monitor, and administer anesthetic doses of midazolam, propofol, pentobarbital, or thiopental, with target of "burst suppression" pattern on EEG. Ketamine may also be considered.

PE = phenytoin equivalents.

IX. Discussion of Case Histories

Case 1: This history is typical of absence seizures. The provocation of the attacks by hyperventilation is also characteristic. Other entities to be considered in the differential diagnosis include focal seizures (which can also be associated with motionless staring with no other symptoms, but are less readily provoked by hyperventilation), attention deficit disorder, or some other form of behavioral disturbance.

Comment: An EEG showed bursts of generalized 3-Hz spike-and-wave activity occurring spontaneously and provoked by hyperventilation. In view of the normal neurologic examination and the generalized nature of the child's EEG discharges, no imaging studies are indicated. This child was treated with ethosuximide, introduced slowly and built up to a dose of 750 mg (25 mg/kg for this 30 kg boy) per day. This drug is well tolerated and eliminates both the seizure activity and the EEG discharges in almost all cases. The outlook for normal neurologic and intellectual development in this patient is excellent.

Case 2: Based on her history, this patient has focal seizures that progress to result in alteration of consciousness and then to generalized tonic-clonic activity. Of note, she had a higher than average risk of developing epilepsy because the febrile convulsions when she was age 15 months were prolonged and associated with focal abnormalities on neurologic examination, but this was still not sufficient reason to start treatment until she actually experienced seizures later in life. She should have an EEG (if it has not already been done), looking for focal slowing and interictal epileptiform activity that could indicate the site of her seizure focus. She should also have a brain MRI scan (with epilepsy protocol) looking for a structural abnormality underlying her epilepsy, but it can be delayed until after delivery because the long history excludes a rapidly evolving mass lesion. Similarly, a search for a toxic-metabolic cause of seizures is unnecessary given the long history.

Teratogenic effects of ASMs occur during the first trimester. Because this patient is in her second trimester, it would be prudent to continue drug therapy at the current dose. The patient should be seen frequently during the remainder of her pregnancy. Free levels of phenytoin should be checked regularly, and the dose should be adjusted to maintain a stable free level. She should continue to take at least 0.4 mg of folate a day throughout the pregnancy.

She has been seizure-free for 4 years, so she might be a candidate for ASM withdrawal, but this should be deferred until she is in a relatively stable physiologic state. She is likely to be sleep deprived for at least several months after delivery, and sleep deprivation is a common precipitant of seizures in predisposed people.

After delivery, she should return to her pre-pregnancy phenytoin dose by the first month postpartum. An MRI scan should be obtained, as mentioned above, and regular follow-up under the supervision of a neurologist should be arranged. About 6 months after delivery, when her metabolism has returned to baseline and her child's sleep schedule has been established, her physician can discuss the advantages and disadvantages of ASM withdrawal with her. She will have to weigh the inconvenience of taking daily medications, and the potential side effects (including teratogenic risk if she becomes pregnant again in the future), against the risk of having a seizure while caring for a young child and the inconvenience of refraining from driving while tapering her medication and for some months thereafter. She must ultimately decide which of these considerations are most important to her; she should be reassured that the physician will support her decision either way. If she chooses to remain on an ASM, she should continue to take folic acid, at least 0.4 mg daily, to reduce the risk of major teratogenic side effects in the event of future pregnancy.

Comment: She delivered a healthy boy at term, with no complications. Although she was happy to learn that she might someday be able to come off medication, she said that it would be impractical for her to stop driving, especially now that she had a new baby. She also said that she thought she would probably try to get pregnant again in 2–3 years, and wanted to know if any other antiseizure medications had less teratogenic potential. After further discussion, she and her neurologist decided to transition from phenytoin to levetiracetam, and she continued to be seizure-free.

Case 3: The emergency room physicians' diagnosis of convulsive status epilepticus is correct. This patient had four tonic-clonic seizures with failure to return to normal consciousness in between, which certainly satisfies the definition of status epilepticus. Emergency management of the patient should proceed as outlined in Table 5.3 and Part VII, Section A. Even if seizures cease rapidly, anyone who has just been treated for status epilepticus should be admitted to an intensive care unit for at least 24 hours of close observation. An epileptic disorder presenting de novo as status epilepticus requires immediate investigation. In this patient, the likelihood of finding a significant underlying problem is high, especially given the history of headaches for the past week.

Comment: An MRI scan in this patient revealed multiple areas of signal abnormality that enhanced with contrast. The patient proved to have multiple small cerebral metastases from a primary tumor that was never identified.

Chapter 6

Neuromuscular Disorders

Mark B. Bromberg and
Douglas J. Gelb

I. Case Histories

Case 1. A 45-year-old woman began having trouble standing up from low chairs about 3 months ago, and the problem has progressed to the point that she now must use her arms to push off from any chair. She recently started having difficulty holding up her arms to set her hair. Her weakness is symmetric. Her head and neck muscles are strong, and she has no shortness of breath. She has no pain or sensory disturbance. There is no family history of neurologic disorders. She has no relevant past medical issues and is taking no medication.

On examination, she has normal mental status and cranial nerve function. Muscle bulk and tone are normal. Neck flexor strength is grade 4 on the 5-point Medical Research Council scale. Shoulder abduction is grade 4 and hip flexion is grade 3, in a symmetric distribution. She must be helped to a standing position and cannot perform a deep knee bend. Tendon reflexes, plantar responses, and sensory examination are normal.

Questions:

1. Does this localize to the peripheral nervous system? If so, is the problem at the level of nerve, neuromuscular junction, or muscle?

2. What tests would you order to confirm the suspected localization? Is this likely to be a treatable condition?

Case 2. A 55-year-old man has been experiencing double vision, mild limb weakness, and rapid fatigability with routine activities. He first noted double vision 6 months ago. It resolved after several days but reappeared 2 weeks ago, and at the same time he began having trouble climbing stairs. His endurance has decreased markedly, to the point where he now must rest after walking a short distance. He has no pain or sensory loss. He has no history of previous medical problems, and no family history of neurologic disease. He takes no medications.

On examination, he has normal mental status and cranial nerve function except for weakness in the distribution of the right third and sixth cranial nerves, mild right ptosis, and bilateral eye closure weakness. Shoulder abduction and hip flexion are strong on initial testing, but quickly fatigue after several repetitions of muscle activation. Tendon reflexes, plantar responses, and sensory examination are normal.

Questions:

1. What are the important differences between this and the first case? Is the lesion at the same site?
2. What tests, if any, would distinguish between the two conditions?
3. How should this patient be managed?

Case 3. A 60-year-old man fell 1 year ago and fractured his left ankle. After the cast was removed, he noted weakness and atrophy of his calf. Prolonged physical therapy did not help. Six months ago he began having trouble unscrewing the tops of jars and turning off the bath faucet completely, and when he tried hard he would get muscle cramps. All his symptoms have continued to get worse. He is constantly fatigued and has lost 30 lb. His wife says she "can see his muscles working."

On examination, the man has normal mental status and cranial nerves. He is thin and has frequent muscle twitching (fasciculations) in his trunk and all four limbs. The intrinsic muscles of both hands are atrophic, and atrophy is also prominent in anterior and posterior muscles in the left leg. A clasp-knife phenomenon (spasticity) is evident with passive manipulation of all limbs. Strength is markedly reduced in distal upper extremity muscles and in his left foot, which he cannot move voluntarily. He has mild weakness in all other muscles. Deep tendon reflexes are hyperactive, and he has a right extensor plantar (Babinski) response. Sensory examination is normal.

Questions:

1. How does this pattern of weakness differ from the patterns in Cases 1 and 2?
2. Where does this localize in the nervous system?
3. How should this patient be managed?

Case 4. A 45-year-old woman has difficulty walking and numbness of her legs. She noted tingling in her toes 6 months ago, and it spread over several weeks to include much of her legs. Her fingers have recently developed a similar tingling. She notes difficulty standing from a chair and complains of unsteadiness when she walks. She had similar problems a year ago, but they were less severe, and they resolved without medical consultation.

On examination, her mental status and cranial nerves are normal. She has mild weakness throughout her lower extremities and in the distal muscles of her upper extremities. Tendon reflexes are absent. Her gait is very unsteady, and she cannot maintain her balance with her eyes closed. Vibratory perception is absent in the feet and reduced at the fingers.

Questions:

1. What components of the nervous system are involved? How do they differ from those in Case 3?

2. How would electrodiagnostic tests help distinguish between Cases 3 and 4?

3. How should this patient be managed?

II. Approach to Neuromuscular Diseases

Unlike the central nervous system, where a single structural lesion may produce widespread effects because of disruption of ascending and descending fiber tracts, a single structural lesion in the peripheral nervous system produces symptoms in a narrowly localized region, usually in a single limb. Many diseases affect the peripheral nervous system diffusely, however, and can't be localized to a single lesion site. While the localization approach described in Chapter 1 is still valid for multifocal and diffuse diseases, it is generally most useful to characterize these diseases by determining which *components* of the peripheral nervous system are affected. For example, some diseases affect peripheral nerves and not muscles, whereas other diseases do the converse. In managing patients with neuromuscular disease, four questions are fundamental:

1. Which components of the peripheral nervous system are involved?
2. What is the specific disease?
3. Is urgent treatment necessary?

    3a. Is the person's disease one that is associated with *autonomic instability* or *respiratory failure*? (These are the only two complications of neuromuscular disease that represent true emergencies.)

3b. If so, how rapidly is the patient's condition deteriorating?

4. What long-term management is indicated?

Question 1 implies that you have already determined that the patient does not have a lesion in the central nervous system, based on the localization reasoning process discussed in Chapter 1 and the examination features discussed in Chapter 2. Additional features useful in localizing the disorder to specific components of the nervous system are discussed in Part III. Questions 2, 3a, and 4 are covered in Part IV. Question 3b is addressed in Part V, along with other management issues common to neuromuscular diseases in general.

III. Background Information

A. Functional Divisions of the Peripheral Nervous System and Associated Symptoms

The peripheral nervous system can be divided into the autonomic and somatic nervous systems. The somatic system is further subdivided into sensory and motor nerves. Motor nerves activate muscles through the neuromuscular junction. The autonomic, somatic sensory, and somatic motor nerves are physically intermingled at some levels of the nervous system and separated at others, but it is useful to conceptualize them as distinct pathways. Each can be associated with a variety of symptoms.

Lesions of the autonomic system can produce dysfunction of practically any visceral organ. Some of the more prominent symptoms include postural hypotension, sphincter dysfunction, impotence, and sweating abnormalities. Lesions of sensory pathways can produce negative symptoms or positive symptoms. Negative symptoms include hypesthesia (reduced sensation) and anesthesia (absence of sensation). Positive symptoms include pain, paresthesias (abnormal, unpleasant sensations that typically occur spontaneously and are often likened to "pins and needles"), and dysesthesias (abnormal or unfamiliar sensations that occur in response to an external stimulus, usually but not always unpleasant and typically having a burning or electric quality). Pain receptors, also called nociceptors, are usually free nerve terminals that respond to stimuli severe enough to cause tissue damage; this is referred to as nociceptive pain. Neuropathic pain is the term for pain that results from dysfunction of nerves in the pain pathways (nociceptive pathways). Neuropathic pain can result in hyperalgesia (more intense pain in response to a noxious stimulus than would be expected) or allodynia (pain in response to a stimulus that would normally be innocuous). Hyperesthesia is another term for allodynia. Lesions of the peripheral motor system can also produce both negative symptoms (e.g., weakness and muscle atrophy) and positive symptoms (e.g., fasciculations and muscle cramps).

B. Proximal-to-Distal Organization of the Peripheral Nervous System

Disorders of the neuromuscular system can be viewed in a proximal-to-distal anatomic pattern, with different clinical syndromes corresponding to each level of peripheral nervous system involvement. The peripheral nervous system portion of the motor pathway originates in the *anterior horn cells*. Conditions that affect anterior horn cells are known as *motor neuron diseases*. The principal clues that suggest a motor neuron disease are (1) motor signs and symptoms (both positive and negative) in the absence of sensory abnormalities and (2) a patchy distribution, often asymmetric, with no consistent pattern of proximal versus distal muscle involvement.

The cell bodies of peripheral sensory neurons are located in the dorsal root ganglia. Conditions that affect these cell bodies can be thought of as the sensory correlates of motor neuron diseases. They are known as sensory neuronopathies, or ganglionopathies. These conditions can affect any type of sensory neuron, so any sensory modality can be impaired; early involvement of proprioceptive neurons is common, often resulting in poor coordination ("pseudoataxia") and even involuntary writhing movements ("pseudoathetosis") that improve when the patient looks at their limbs. Clues suggestive of a sensory neuronopathy are (1) sensory signs and symptoms (both positive and negative) in the absence of weakness and (2) a patchy distribution, often asymmetric, with no consistent pattern of proximal versus distal involvement.

Lesions affecting dorsal and ventral *roots*, or the spinal roots that they form, are called *radiculopathies*. If more than one nerve root is involved, the term *polyradiculopathy* is often used. Structural abnormalities can impinge on a single unilateral nerve root, bilateral nerve roots at a single level, or nerve roots at several contiguous levels. Metabolic, inflammatory, and neoplastic disorders can also affect one or more roots. Radiculopathies may be mild and asymptomatic, or they may be associated with severe pain in the back or limbs. People with radiculopathies usually have both sensory and motor symptoms, though one or the other may predominate. The main clue that someone has a radiculopathy is that all of the sensory and motor symptoms and signs are consistent with the known distribution of one or several nerve roots.

Before forming peripheral nerves, some fibers exiting the nerve roots undergo a complex crossing and regrouping to form the brachial plexus and lumbosacral plexus. When someone has symptoms and signs that would suggest a polyradiculopathy but the pattern does not conform to the distribution of any individual nerve root or combination of nerve roots, or to the distribution of any individual peripheral nerve or combination of peripheral nerves, *plexopathy* is likely.

Moving another step distally, peripheral nerve lesions take the form of *polyneuropathies* when involvement is diffuse or mononeuropathies when a single nerve is involved. Polyneuropathies frequently affect both sensory and motor nerves, though there are exceptions that involve only one type of nerve. Sensory nerves have a peripheral and a central axon, and both may be affected. Most polyneuropathies affect the longest nerves in the body earliest, so symptoms and signs occur in the feet first and progress proximally. When signs and symptoms reach approximately knee level, nerves to the fingers become involved. This is referred to as a stocking-glove distribution. Length-dependent polyneuropathies are usually symmetric.

The next step going from proximal to distal is the neuromuscular junction. In *disorders of the neuromuscular junction*, the most prominent weakness typically occurs in muscles that move the eyes, face, pharynx, and proximal limbs. A prominent feature of the most common neuromuscular junction disease, myasthenia gravis, is the rapid onset of fatigue after even just a few minutes of activity. Disorders of the neuromuscular junction do not affect sensation.

The most distal component of the motor pathway is the *muscle*. As with disorders of the neuromuscular junction, primary muscle disorders produce no sensory symptoms, and usually (but not always) result in a proximal distribution of limb weakness. With some exceptions, primary muscle diseases usually spare muscles innervated by cranial nerves, so symptoms like diplopia, dysarthria, and dysphagia are rare, in contrast to neuromuscular junction disorders. Some hereditary abnormalities of membrane ion channels produce weakness that is episodic, and some result in a phenomenon known as myotonia, which is a prolonged muscle contraction after voluntary activation or percussion of the muscle.

Figure 6.1 summarizes a general way to recognize that someone might have a diffuse neuromuscular disorder and to identify the level of the peripheral nervous system that is most likely involved. This approach is not foolproof (e.g., some myopathies *do* cause diplopia, dysarthria, or

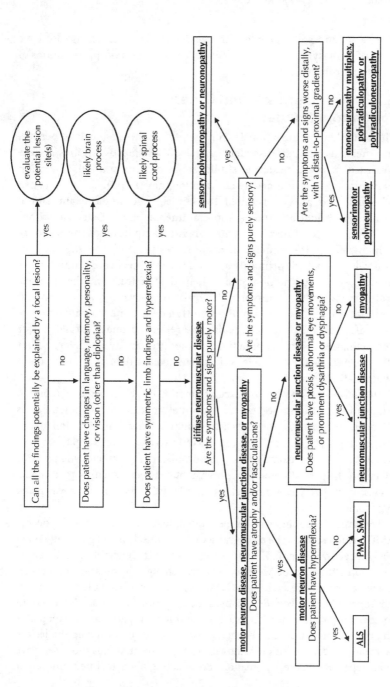

Fig. 6.1 A flowchart for identifying and categorizing diffuse neuromuscular disorders.

dysphagia, and some people with neuromuscular junction disease have none of those symptoms), but it reliably categorizes most presentations of diffuse neuromuscular disease.

C. Electrodiagnostic and Other Laboratory Studies

The tests that are most consistently helpful in the diagnosis of peripheral nervous system disorders are electrodiagnostic studies. These consist of nerve conduction studies, tests of neuromuscular junction transmission, and the needle electromyogram (EMG). These tests can be considered an extension of the clinical neurologic examination. In nerve conduction studies, the examiner applies an electric stimulus to a peripheral nerve and measures the amplitude of the response (which reflects the number of nerve fibers present) and the conduction velocity (which primarily assesses the myelin sheath around nerve fibers). Nerve conduction studies help demonstrate whether peripheral nerve function is impaired. By evaluating several sensory and several motor nerves, the examiner can often determine which nerves are most affected and whether the damage reflects primary axonal loss or demyelination. Nerve conductions studies principally assess large-fiber somatic nerves; they are relatively insensitive for detecting dysfunction of small-fiber nerves.

The integrity of the neuromuscular junction can be assessed by repeated stimulation of the motor nerve: A normal neuromuscular junction has adequate reserve to ensure that each stimulus will result in an action potential in the muscle fiber, whereas synaptic transmission sometimes fails when there is a neuromuscular junction disorder. Characteristic patterns of failure help to differentiate postsynaptic defects, such as myasthenia gravis, from presynaptic defects, such as the Lambert-Eaton myasthenic syndrome.

The third component of an electrodiagnostic evaluation is the needle EMG, which records the electrical activity of muscle fibers preceding muscle contraction. Needle EMG is very sensitive to denervation and can be used to distinguish between *neuropathic* changes in muscle (due to primary nerve damage such as radiculopathy, motor neuron disease, or polyneuropathy) and *myopathic* changes (due to primary muscle disorders). In focal neuropathic conditions, such as a mononeuropathy or radiculopathy, the pattern of muscle involvement is often useful in localizing the lesion. A variant of this technique, known as single fiber EMG, is more sensitive than repetitive nerve stimulation for detecting abnormal neuromuscular transmission, but it is a technically involved procedure that requires a great deal of cooperation from the patient.

Supplementary diagnostic tests include nerve, skin, and muscle biopsies. A nerve biopsy can be useful in determining whether the underlying nerve pathology is primary axon damage or primary demyelination, or it may provide evidence of a vasculitis affecting the small arterioles supplying the nerve. The most common biopsy site is the sural nerve at the ankle. Processes that primarily affect small-fiber nerves produce changes in intraepidermal nerve fiber density and morphology on skin biopsy. These small-fiber neuropathies—most common in diabetes—are often extremely painful, and as noted above, they may not be evident on traditional electrodiagnostic studies. Muscle biopsies help distinguish among dystrophies, congenital myopathies, metabolic myopathies, and inflammatory myopathies. Common muscle biopsy sites are vastus lateralis and biceps brachii muscles. Another informative test is determination of the serum creatine kinase (CK) level. This enzyme is found in highest concentration in skeletal muscle, and an elevated serum level can be an indication of muscle damage. For certain neuromuscular diseases, antibody assays and genetic tests are extremely useful, and often definitive. When the clinical evidence suggests a focal process, such as a mononeuropathy, plexopathy, radiculopathy, or myopathy, imaging studies of the affected structure can be helpful.

IV. Specific Neuromuscular Diseases

A. Motor Neuron Diseases

The most common form of motor neuron disease in adults is amyotrophic lateral sclerosis (ALS), which involves both lower motor neurons (LMNs) and upper motor neurons (UMNs). LMN involvement predominates in some patients and UMN involvement predominates in others. In an individual patient, the pattern of involvement may change over time. For example, some people initially present with primarily LMN involvement and only later develop UMN symptoms and signs.

ALS may begin at any adult age but it is more common with increasing age. It is generally thought that symptoms only appear after the disease has been present for a considerable length of time, and that as many as 50% of the motor neurons are lost before weakness is detected. The initial symptom is usually weakness in a focal area, which gradually spreads to contiguous muscles in the same region of the body. Most often, the initial weakness is in an arm. It can occasionally be confined to the distribution of a single nerve or nerve root, leading to potential diagnostic confusion, but it usually includes muscles that are innervated by more than one nerve or nerve root. The lack of sensory involvement helps to differentiate early ALS from mononeuropathy or radiculopathy. Typical symptoms of hand weakness include difficulty turning a key, opening a bottle or jar, buttoning, or turning a door knob. Typical symptoms of lower extremity weakness include unstable gait, falling, fatigue when walking, or foot drop. In about 25% of patients, the initial weakness is confined to muscles innervated by cranial nerves, leading to disorders of speech or swallowing. These patients may be difficult to differentiate from people with myasthenia gravis or from people who have brainstem mass lesions or infiltrative processes (such as tuberculous meningitis or sarcoidosis). All of these conditions can present with dysarthria, hoarseness, or dysphagia, but over time their clinical course diverges from that of ALS: people with brainstem lesions eventually develop nonmotor symptoms or signs, and people with myasthenia gravis usually don't have the inexorable progression of weakness over months that is typical of ALS. Other useful diagnostic features are that people with ALS may also display emotional incontinence, inappropriate crying or laughing, or excessive forced yawning.

Fasciculations occur in all individuals, including healthy control subjects, but they are especially profuse and continuous in people with ALS, because of extensive damage to lower motor neurons. Although fasciculations are not prominent when the disease first presents, almost all patients develop fasciculations soon after disease onset. Cramps are also common in denervated muscles. These are often most distressful when lying in bed, to the point where they may interfere with sleep. As the disease continues to progress, muscle atrophy occurs. This is often exacerbated by generalized cachexia in people whose dysphagia prevents adequate caloric intake. Symptoms of UMN involvement include muscle spasms and stiffness, and UMN examination findings include spasticity, hyperreflexia, and Babinski signs (see Chapter 2).

The disease characteristically begins in one upper extremity, then spreads to the contralateral upper extremity, then the ipsilateral lower extremity, then the contralateral lower extremity, and then the bulbar muscles. Any pattern of progression is possible, however. For example, the disease sometimes begins in one lower extremity, spreads to the contralateral limb, and then to the upper extremities. When the initial symptoms are in bulbar muscles, they tend to spread to distal upper extremities first, then the thoracic region, and then the lower extremities. For some reason, extraocular muscles are spared throughout most of the disease course, and so are bladder and bowel sphincter muscles. The disease is relentlessly progressive, but the rate of progression varies considerably between patients. Although many individuals rapidly become disabled and die within several years, others may experience much more gradual progression over 10 years or more. Bulbar onset is typically associated with more rapid progression. Bulbar muscles are eventually affected in more than 90% of patients, leading to inadequate airway protection and increased risk of aspiration, and at the same time producing progressive weakness of respiratory muscles. Respiratory failure and pneumonia are the most common causes of death. The mean survival from the time of symptom onset is 27 to 43 months. About 25% of patients survive 5 years, and 8–16% survive 10 years.

A substantial percentage of people (20–40%) with ALS have cognitive impairment, with clinical and neuroimaging features that are consistent with frontotemporal dementia (FTD), a condition covered in Chapter 7. A similar percentage of people presenting with FTD meet clinical criteria for the diagnosis of ALS.

ALS is diagnosed based on clinical evidence of combined UMN and LMN abnormalities starting focally and progressing. Before making the diagnosis of ALS, all potentially treatable conditions must be excluded. In particular, structural causes of the UMN and LMN abnormalities should be considered. The most common source of confusion is degenerative disease of the cervical spine, which may produce UMN signs in the lower extremities on the basis of spinal cord compression and LMN signs in the upper extremities because of compression of multiple cervical nerve roots. The diagnosis can usually be clarified using the distribution of findings, the presence or absence of sensory abnormalities, and the results of imaging studies and electrodiagnostic tests, but occasionally the situation remains unclear.

The cause of ALS is not known. Most people with ALS have ubiquitinated cytoplasmic inclusions in many (but not all) motor neurons. These inclusions contain a protein called TAR (transactivation response) DNA binding protein of 43 kDa, or TDP-43, leading to the proposal that impaired protein processing is a factor in the pathogenesis of ALS. TDP-43 is also associated with FTD, which may help to explain why so many people have clinical features of both. Epidemiologic evidence suggests that environmental toxins may contribute to ALS, although no specific causative toxins have been identified. Most cases of ALS are sporadic, but familial forms also exist. Among the familial forms, more than 50 associated genes have been identified (with genes not yet identified in about 20% of families). Mis-sense mutations in the gene coding for TDP-43 have been found in some cases of familial and sporadic ALS; curiously, most of the people with these mutations had no dementia. Expanded hexanucleotide repeats in the *chromosome 9 open reading frame 72* (*C9ORF72*) are the most common mutations associated with familial ALS, accounting for up to 40% of familial cases (the exact percentage depends on the population). It has been suggested that these mutations result in impaired membrane trafficking or RNA processing. Expanded repeats in *C9ORF72* are also the mutations most commonly identified in familial FTD. The second most commonly mutated gene in familial ALS is the gene for superoxide dismutase (SOD), accounting for about 20% of cases. SOD is an antioxidant enzyme, suggesting that free radical toxicity and oxidative stress may contribute to neuronal death in ALS. Other factors that may be involved in the pathogenesis of ALS include impaired axonal transport, mitochondrial dysfunction, altered calcium homeostasis, inflammation and immune dysregulation, reduced neurotrophic support, glial cell abnormalities, and glutamate excitotoxicity. Glutamate is the principal excitatory neurotransmitter in the nervous system, including motor neurons, but excess levels of glutamate are toxic to neurons.

Riluzole, a drug that modulates glutamatergic neurotransmission, results in a modest prolongation of survival in people who have ALS. A combination of sodium phenylbutyrate (which affects protein folding and aggregation) and taurursodiol (which affects apoptosis pathways) has also been approved for ALS based on evidence that it slows progression, although the evidence of its efficacy has been challenged. Edaravone, a free radical scavenger, has also been approved based on evidence that it slows progression and prolongs survival, but the effect is modest. In patients who have mutations in the gene for SOD, tofersen (an antisense oligonucleotide targeting the RNA produced by the mutated gene) may slow disease progression.

A major focus of treatment is the management of such symptoms as spasticity, cramps, excessive secretions, aspiration, communication difficulty, reduced mobility, and difficulty breathing. The use of bilevel positive airway pressure (BiPAP) may prolong survival and increase quality of life, although this is based on mostly observational studies and one randomized controlled trial. The combination of dextromethorphan hydrobromide and quinidine sulfate can reduce the symptoms of emotional incontinence (also known as pseudobulbar affect). In patients with severe dysphagia who develop clinically significant weight loss resulting in depletion of fat and protein stores, percutaneous endoscopic gastrostomy (PEG) tubes or other types of feeding tubes may also prolong survival and increase quality of life.

Primary lateral sclerosis is a very rare form of motor neuron disease that affects only UMNs; the progression is usually very slow, over the course of decades. About 10% of people with motor neuron disease have purely LMN involvement; this is called *progressive muscular atrophy* (PMA). The true prevalence of this condition is difficult to establish because many people initially diagnosed with PMA ultimately develop UMN features—i.e., they prove to have ALS. Some viral infections preferentially target motor neurons. The classic example is poliovirus, but many other enteroviruses can produce the same clinical syndrome: a flu-like illness followed by fulminant focal or multifocal weakness with LMN characteristics. In particular, West Nile virus can produce this syndrome.

Spinal muscular atrophy (SMA) is a genetic disorder affecting LMNs, caused by mutations in a gene called the *survival motor neuron 1* (*SMN1*) gene. There are five phenotypes, Types 0 (fewer than 5% of people with SMA), 1 (about 45%), 2 (about 20%), 3 (about 30%), and 4 (fewer than 5%). The specific phenotype is determined by the copy number of a neighboring gene, *SMN2*, which is almost identical to *SMN1*—it differs by only five nucleotides, but this difference disrupts a splice modulator. As a result, 90% of the transcript from *SMN2* lacks exon 7 and it is rapidly degraded. People with SMA have mutations in the *SMN1* gene that render it non-functional, so the only normal protein their cells produce is derived from the 10% of *SMN2* transcript that includes exon 7. The more copies of the *SMN2* gene they have, the greater the quantity of normal protein and the less severe the clinical syndrome. People with Type 1 SMA have two copies of the *SMN2* gene. They have severe hypotonia and generalized weakness at or before birth or within the first 6 months of life. They typically have respiratory distress and no head control. If untreated, the disease progresses rapidly, and death usually occurs by age 2 years due to respiratory failure or pneumonia. Most people with Type 2 SMA have three copies of the *SMN2* gene. They begin having hypotonia and generalized weakness between the ages of 6 and 18 months. Most of them eventually achieve the milestones of rolling over and sitting unsupported, but they rarely manage to walk independently, and as they age they may lose the ability to sit independently. Their swallowing and respiratory function decline as they grow older, and they are vulnerable to respiratory infections. Most people with Type 3 SMA have three or four copies of the *SMN2* gene. Their symptoms typically begin between the ages of 5 and 15 years. They are able to walk independently, but their gait gradually deteriorates as they grow older, with a waddling quality and exaggerated lumbar lordosis. They have a normal life span. People with Type 0 SMA usually have only one copy of the *SMN2* gene; their symptoms begin prenatally, and they have respiratory failure at birth. They are unable to breathe independently, and they do not usually survive beyond 6 months. On the other end of the spectrum, people with Type 4 SMA usually have more than 4 copies of the *SMN2* gene, with minimal if any symptoms and a normal life span.

The outlook for people with SMA has improved dramatically in recent years. Nusinersen is an anti-sense oligonucleotide designed to alter splicing of *SMN2* pre-messenger RNA, resulting in increased transcription of the normal SMN protein. Onasemnogene abeparvovec-xioi is an adeno-associated, virus-delivered gene replacement therapy. Risdiplam is a small molecule that modifies *SMN2* pre-messenger RNA. With each of these treatments, children with SMA have managed to achieve motor milestones that would never have been possible in the past. The benefit is greatest when the treatment is administered early in the disease course.

B. Nerve Root Disorders (Radiculopathies)

The most common cause of radiculopathy is degenerative disease of the spinal column, involving the vertebral bodies, the facet joints, or the discs. Other structural lesions, including tumors and abscesses, may also compress the nerve roots. The diagnostic and management considerations for these structural causes of radiculopathy are discussed in Chapter 15.

Nerve roots may also be involved by many of the same processes that produce neuropathies, including vasculitis, infections, metabolic abnormalities, and inflammatory demyelination. Usually the radiculopathy and neuropathy coexist; the evaluation and management is discussed in Section D. On occasion, the radiculopathy occurs without a significant neuropathy; this is most often seen in people who have diabetes. This is especially common in the thoracic nerve roots. These individuals should be evaluated for a structural cause (especially neoplastic) before concluding that the radiculopathy is due to metabolic disease.

Herpes varicella-zoster virus produces a radiculopathy that may be excruciatingly painful; it is usually straightforward to diagnose because of the accompanying skin lesions in the distribution of the affected root, but they are occasionally absent. Zoster is discussed in further detail in Chapter 10. Lyme disease and cytomegalovirus both may produce a polyradiculopathy; treatment is directed at the underlying infection.

C. Plexus Disorders (Plexopathies)

Common causes of *plexopathies* are cancer, radiation therapy, metabolic disorders such as diabetes mellitus, or trauma. There are also idiopathic plexopathies; although the cause is not known, they are thought to be auto-immune. For some reason, diabetes affects the lumbosacral plexus much more frequently than the brachial plexus, whereas the converse is true of autoimmune plexopathies. Plexus disorders are diagnosed by establishing relevant details of the history (e.g., a history of radiation therapy or recent immunization), performing electrodiagnostic tests to confirm the localiza-tion, and—if the cause is not clear from the history—imaging the plexus to exclude a structural lesion. Treatment is directed at the underlying cause. Only supportive therapy (mainly pain control and physical therapy) is available for idiopathic plexopathies, but fortunately, the outcome is gener-ally favorable.

D. Peripheral Nerve Disorders (Neuropathies)

People with peripheral nerve disorders may have an isolated abnormality of a single peripheral nerve (*mononeuropathy*), a combination of several mononeuropathies (*mononeuropathy multiplex*; Figure 6.2), or a more gen-eralized process involving peripheral nerves (*polyneuropathy*; Figure 6.3). Using the terminology defined in Chapter 3, polyneuropathy is a diffuse process, whereas mononeuropathy multiplex is multifocal. Unless other-wise qualified, the term *neuropathy* is usually used interchangeably with the term *polyneuropathy*.

The most common cause of mononeuropathy is compression, espe-cially at a site where the nerve is particularly confined and subject to trauma (such as the median nerve at the carpal tunnel, the ulnar nerve at the elbow, or the common peroneal nerve—also known as the com-mon fibular nerve—at the knee). In typical cases, diagnostic testing may be unnecessary; when there are atypical features, electrodiagnostic stud-ies usually clarify the diagnosis. Imaging studies are sometimes helpful. Compression mononeuropathies (also called entrapment mononeuropa-thies) often respond to stabilization of the joint with a splint or protection with a pad. Local steroid injections can also be helpful. When the response to these treatments is unsatisfactory, or when the compression is already moderately severe by the time the person seeks medical attention, surgical decompression of the nerve is indicated.

Unlike peripheral nerves elsewhere in the body, cranial nerves are gener-ally well insulated from external pressure, so compression injury to cranial

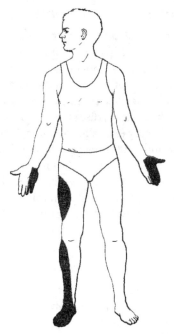

Mononeuropathy multiplex

Fig. 6.2 The regions of sensory involvement in someone with mononeuropathy multiplex. This is a multifocal process affecting several discrete peripheral nerves (in this case, the left median nerve, right ulnar nerve, right lateral cutaneous nerve of the thigh, and right peroneal nerve). The involved areas are not confluent or symmetric.

nerves is usually due to pressure from within the nervous system itself. Mass lesions such as tumors or aneurysms or even tortuosities in the vertebral or basilar arteries can compress cranial nerves directly. Cranial nerves may also be compressed as a result of increased intracranial pressure caused by distant mass lesions. A lesion of cranial nerve III due to transtentorial herniation is the most notorious example (see Chapter 11). Trauma can damage cranial nerves either directly or by producing shear injury. Cranial nerves I and IV are at particular risk for shear injury. Isolated cranial nerve palsies often result from ischemic disease of penetrating arteries, especially in people who have diabetes or hypertension. Inflammatory disease, both infectious and noninfectious, can cause cranial neuropathies. Neoplastic spread to the meninges can do so also.

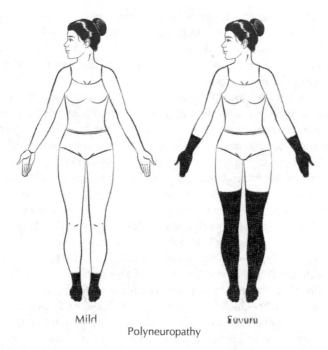

Mild   Severe
Polyneuropathy

Fig. 6.3 "Stocking-glove" distribution of sensory loss typical of polyneuropathy. This is a diffuse process in which involvement is confluent and symmetric. With mild disease (the figure on the left), only the distal lower extremities are involved. With more severe disease (the figure on the right), there is proximal extension in the lower extremities, and the distal upper extremities are also involved.

Bell palsy, or idiopathic facial nerve palsy, deserves special mention because it usually has a benign course, in contrast to stroke (with which it is sometimes confused). It has been associated with a variety of viruses, especially herpes simplex. The distinctive feature of Bell palsy is a LMN pattern of unilateral facial weakness, including the forehead muscles (see Chapter 2). There is often associated pain, especially in the ear, and there may be changes in hearing or taste. Patients may also have sensory symptoms. Almost all patients recover to some extent within 3 months, and the recovery is complete in 55–90% of them. Complete facial weakness at the peak of the episode (present in roughly 50% of patients), non-ear pain, and older age are associated with a poorer prognosis. Several well-designed trials have demonstrated that a 10-day course of prednisolone, started within 3 days of symptom onset, improves outcome. Acyclovir or valacyclovir is often used in conjunction with prednisolone, but the evidence for this practice is much less compelling; it is typically recommended only when the weakness is severe.

People who have multiple cranial neuropathies without involvement of the brainstem parenchyma itself should be evaluated for inflammatory diseases or carcinomatous involvement of the meninges (see Chapter 10). People who have multiple mononeuropathies in the limbs may simply have several entrapment mononeuropathies, especially if they engage in activities that involve forceful, repetitive movements. Obesity, diabetes, and thyroid disease are independent risk factors for compression mononeuropathies. There is also a rare familial condition, hereditary neuropathy with liability to pressure palsies, which should be considered even when there is no apparent family history. When patients have none of these predisposing factors, or when mononeuropathies occur at sites where entrapment is unusual, the most likely cause of mononeuropathy multiplex is vasculitis. Vasculitis produces nerve damage by affecting nutrient vessels to the nerve, so the onset is typically sudden. It can be associated with a more widespread collagen vascular disorder, or it can occur as an isolated process restricted to the blood vessels supplying peripheral nerves while sparing other blood vessels and other organ systems.

When mononeuropathy multiplex is severe, the nerve involvement can become confluent, resembling polyneuropathy. In such cases, the most reliable way to distinguish mononeuropathy multiplex from polyneuropathy is to inquire about the onset of the disease. Mononeuropathy multiplex affects first one nerve and then another in an unpredictable sequence, whereas polyneuropathy affects nerves in a systematic pattern that is evident throughout the course of the disease.

Polyneuropathy typically affects the longest nerves in the body first and progressively shorter nerves become involved as the condition progresses, resulting in a "stocking-glove" distribution of symptoms. Some polyneuropathies may exhibit variations or deviate from this pattern. In some cases, only myelinated nerves are affected; in others, only small, unmyelinated nerves are involved. Some patients report only sensory symptoms. Many of these people actually have a mild sensorimotor polyneuropathy but they are unaware of the motor involvement; it is evident only on clinical testing or electrophysiologic testing. Some polyneuropathies really do affect only sensory nerves, however. In one condition (leprosy), it is said that the coldest (i.e., the most exposed) nerves are involved. In general, if the pattern of nerve involvement cannot be expressed in a rule that makes some physiologic sense, a polyneuropathy is unlikely. For example, it is hard to imagine a plausible rule that would result in involvement of the right median nerve but not the left, or of the left median and radial nerves but not the left ulnar nerve. These would be examples of mononeuropathy multiplex, not polyneuropathy. People with either of these patterns of nerve involvement from mononeuropathy multiplex might progress to have involvement of the median, ulnar, and radial nerves bilaterally, as well as nerves throughout the lower extremities, at which point the pattern of nerve involvement would resemble that seen with a polyneuropathy. As noted in the previous paragraph, a detailed history of the onset and progression of the symptoms is the most reliable way to distinguish polyneuropathy from advanced mononeuropathy multiplex.

There are many causes of polyneuropathy. A frequently used mnemonic is **DANG THERAPIST**:

D   iabetes

A   lcohol

N   utritional (deficiencies of vitamins B12, B1 [thiamine], B6, and E)

G   uillain-Barré (acute inflammatory demyelinating polyradiculoneuropathy [AIDP])

T   oxic (lead, arsenic, other metals, excessive vitamin B6, many medications)

HE   reditary

R   ecurrent (chronic inflammatory demyelinating polyradiculoneuropathy [CIDP])

A   myloid

P   orphyria

I   nfectious (leprosy, human immunodeficiency virus [HIV], Lyme disease, diphtheria, mononucleosis)

S   ystemic (uremia, hypothyroidism, lupus, Sjögren, granulomatosis with polyangiitis)

T   umors (paraneoplastic; also CIDP associated with myeloma)

The first two diagnoses in this list merit special comment. Diabetes is the most common cause of polyneuropathy in the United States, and probably the world. There are several patterns of diabetic polyneuropathy, including a painless loss of sensation with weakness (resulting in unnoticed foot injury and ulcers) and a painful loss of distal leg sensation. People with prediabetes (fasting glucose of 100–125 mg/dL, hemoglobin

A1c of 5.7–6.4%, or 2-hour glucose tolerance test in the impaired tolerance range) also have an increased incidence of primarily painful sensory neuropathies. This is probably due to a combination of an inherent susceptibility and the episodic spikes in glucose levels that occur in impaired glucose tolerance. Prediabetes is frequently a component of the metabolic syndrome that includes hypertension, hyperlipidemia, and increased waist circumference, so there may be a combination of factors contributing to the polyneuropathy.

The polyneuropathy associated with alcohol use appears to be due to a combination of direct toxic effects and other factors, including malnutrition (particularly reduced thiamine intake and thiamine absorption). People with neuropathy who have a history of alcohol use should be evaluated for other potential causes of neuropathy, rather than automatically attributing their condition to alcohol.

A detailed history may help to identify specific conditions from the above list that are particularly likely in an individual patient. The pattern of nerve involvement can be helpful, since different "rules" are followed by different causes of polyneuropathy, as already mentioned. For example, Table 6.1 lists some conditions that can be associated with polyneuropathies that primarily affect small sensory fibers, typically resulting in spontaneous paresthesias, burning pain, and reduced ability to sense painful stimuli; Table 6.2 lists some conditions that can cause polyneuropathies primarily affecting large sensory fibers or sensory neuron cell bodies in the dorsal root ganglia, typically resulting in ataxia and reduced position sense. Determining whether the process is demyelinating or axonal may also narrow the differential diagnosis of a polyneuropathy. Demyelinating neuropathies primarily affect the myelin sheath or nodes of Ranvier, resulting in slowed conduction in myelinated nerves. Axonal neuropathies primarily involve the underlying axons; both myelinated and unmyelinated fibers are affected. Demyelinating and axonal neuropathies can usually be distinguished based on the results of nerve conduction studies: Demyelinating neuropathies result in abnormal nerve conduction velocities with relatively normal amplitudes, whereas axonal neuropathies produce the opposite pattern. Most metabolic and systemic diseases produce axonal polyneuropathies.

The most common demyelinating polyneuropathies are the *inflammatory demyelinating polyradiculoneuropathies*. They are characterized by inflammation of the myelin sheath both proximally at the root and distally along peripheral nerves. Examples include *acute* forms (including *AIDP*, the most common subtype of the clinical condition known as *Guillain-Barré syndrome*) and *chronic* forms (such as CIDP). Because the pathology involves both peripheral nerves and roots, proximal symptoms and signs are often apparent (along with distal symptoms) early in the course, and areflexia is a prominent early finding. The weakness peaks within 4 weeks in people with AIDP, whereas the characteristic course of CIDP is slowly progressive over more than 2 months or relapsing and remitting. Note that despite the word "acute" in its name, the time course of AIDP is subacute. People who have AIDP or CIDP usually have an elevated spinal fluid protein, with a normal cell count. Table 6.3 contains additional information about AIDP and some of the other subtypes of Guillain-Barré syndrome.

Hereditary neuropathies are usually very slowly progressive and may go unnoticed in affected family members. The most common forms of hereditary neuropathy fall into the general category of hereditary motor sensory neuropathy, or Charcot-Marie-Tooth (CMT) disease (based on the names of the first clinical observers). CMT disease encompasses a group of neuropathies that are distinguished, in part, on the basis of clinical and electrodiagnostic criteria (such as whether nerve conduction velocities are slow or normal). Further distinction of different forms of CMT is based on genetic testing. Causal mutations have been identified in more than 100 different genes, associated with a variety of functions including formation and compaction of myelin, response to growth factors, mitochondrial processes, protein synthesis and degradation, axonal transport, transfer of ions and small molecules between cells, and signal transduction.

Treatment of neuropathies depends on the underlying cause. For example, polyneuropathy due to nutritional deficiency is treated with dietary replacement and polyneuropathy due to a toxin is treated by removing the causative agent. For polyneuropathy associated with diabetes or prediabetes, the only available treatment is exercise and tight glucose control. AIDP and CIDP are believed to include a humorally mediated component, and they respond to plasma exchange (also called plasma apheresis, or plasmapheresis). This is a procedure in which units of whole blood are removed from the body and separated into the red cell and plasma fractions. The red cells are reinfused, while the plasma, which contains the antibodies, is discarded. Intravenous immunoglobulin (IVIg) administration is also effective for both AIDP and CIDP. Prednisone is effective for CIDP, but not for AIDP. Other immunosuppressive agents are also used to treat CIDP. Other autoimmune neuropathies are also treated with IVIg, plasma exchange, or immunosuppressive medications. There are no specific treatments for hereditary neuropathies. The treatment options for other neuropathies are a function of the underlying cause and the degree to which it can be treated. In some cases, no underlying cause is found, and symptom management is the only option.

E. Neuromuscular Junction Disorders

Some disorders of neuromuscular transmission affect the postsynaptic membrane; myasthenia gravis is the prototypical example. Others, such as botulism and Lambert-Eaton myasthenic syndrome (LEMS), affect the presynaptic terminal. Myasthenia gravis is much more common than LEMS. Other disorders of the neuromuscular junction (including botulism) are extremely rare.

Myasthenia gravis and LEMS are both autoimmune diseases. In myasthenia gravis, antibodies bind to a component of the postsynaptic end plate region, activating complement through a T-cell dependent process. This results in injury to the postsynaptic membrane, and its usually highly folded pattern becomes simplified, with reduced number and density of acetylcholine receptors. The most common antibodies associated with myasthenia gravis are antibodies to the acetylcholine receptor. In addition to their immunologic effects, they may also block acetylcholine from binding to the receptors, and they may induce cross-linking of receptors, prompting endocytosis and degradation of the receptors. About a third of the patients with myasthenia who do not have antibodies to the acetylcholine receptor have antibodies to a protein called muscle-specific kinase, or MuSK, which is part of a transmembrane protein complex located near the acetylcholine receptor. Antibodies to other proteins in that complex, low-density lipoprotein-related protein 4 (LRP4) and agrin, are present in rare cases.

About 15% of people with myasthenia have thymomas, and 65–70% of those without tumors have hyperplastic changes in the thymus. The precise role of the thymus in pathogenesis is not known, but the thymus is involved in induction of tolerance against self-antigens, and it contains myoid cells that share epitopes with the acetylcholine receptor; it is thought that in people with myasthenia, these myoid cells and nearby dendritic cells present antigens that result in autosensitization to the acetylcholine receptor. Some people who receive immune checkpoint inhibitors develop a form of myasthenia (others develop an inflammatory myopathy, as discussed below, and some patients develop a combination).

LEMS is associated with an immune-mediated reduction in the voltage-gated calcium channels on presynaptic motor nerve terminals. In normal subjects, these channels open in response to an action potential, causing calcium to enter the nerve terminal and stimulate the mobilization of acetylcholine. In LEMS, this mobilization is impaired, so that the action potential triggers the release of fewer quanta of acetylcholine than normal.

Myasthenia gravis can begin suddenly or gradually. Patients usually present with ptosis, diplopia, or both. Problems with speech, swallowing, or chewing are also common early in the course. In about 25% of patients, the weakness remains restricted to lid, eye, and bulbar muscles, but most people subsequently develop limb weakness. In many patients, the limb weakness is relatively mild, and it may only be evident on formal testing. It generally affects proximal muscles more than distal muscles. People with myasthenia gravis associated with anti-MuSK antibodies tend to have prominent weakness of the neck, shoulder, and respiratory muscles, with less limb weakness and rare ocular involvement.

One characteristic feature of myasthenia gravis is fatigability—with repeated muscle use, more neuromuscular junctions fail to transmit impulses, and weakness rapidly becomes apparent as a sense of fatigue. Transmission improves when the muscle is rested. As a result, the symptoms typically get worse as the day progresses or with prolonged activity. For example, jaw weakness tends to get worse when chewing tough meats or chewy candy. Speech can deteriorate markedly after a few sentences but recover when the patient pauses to listen to other people speak. The symptoms also fluctuate from day to day.

The peak age of onset is between 20 and 30 years in women and between 50 and 60 years in men. The course of the disease is extremely variable. Even in untreated individuals, the weakness may improve spontaneously, but the improvement is typically followed by a relapse. In treated patients, most relapses are associated with reductions in the dose of medication. As a general rule, people with myasthenia gravis experience their maximal degree of weakness within 2 to 5 years. This means that if their disease is restricted to ocular weakness during the first 5 years, they are unlikely to experience limb weakness at a later date. Conversely, those who experience weakness of limbs and respiratory muscles early in the course can develop severe exacerbations that may include respiratory failure. Eventually, if left untreated, the weakness becomes progressive, although in rare cases the symptoms resolve. Even optimally treated patients may develop fixed weakness in the muscles of the eyes and face, and rarely in limb muscles. Before the advent of effective treatment for the underlying disease, and before the introduction of intensive care units, mechanical ventilation, and other treatments for respiratory failure, the prognosis for this disease could be grim (hence the name "gravis"). With treatment, most patients do well, and those with respiratory failure can be treated and weaned.

Several clinical features distinguish the different disorders of neuromuscular transmission. In addition to affecting the neuromuscular junction, LEMS and botulism disrupt transmission in autonomic ganglia, causing symptoms such as dry mouth and impotence. Although the reasons are not clear, neuromuscular junction transmission abnormalities in botulism and myasthenia gravis frequently affect a combination of extraocular and lid levator muscles, while these muscles are less involved in LEMS. In some people with LEMS, strength improves during brief exercise (and then declines as the exertion is sustained). This can be demonstrated when testing tendon reflexes—they will be depressed or absent in the rest state due to failed transmission, but if the patient activates the tested muscle for about 10 seconds, neuromuscular transmission briefly improves and the tendon reflex can be elicited.

As noted in Part III, Section C, neuromuscular junction disorders cause a decrement in the compound motor action potential on repetitive nerve stimulation because synaptic transmission fails in progressively more fibers as the stimulation is maintained. Detailed electrodiagnostic testing can help differentiate between the various neuromuscular junction disorders. Serologic testing is also helpful in diagnosis. Antibodies to the acetylcholine receptor are present in the serum in 80–85% of people with generalized myasthenia and in 55% of people with myasthenia whose clinical manifestations are restricted to the extra-ocular muscles. When acetylcholine receptor antibodies are not found in someone whose clinical presentation is suggestive of myasthenia gravis, anti-MuSK antibodies should be assayed. Low-affinity acetylcholine receptor antibodies are present in many people who are seronegative for MuSK and acetylcholine receptor antibodies using conventional assays. Antibodies to voltage-gated calcium channels are present in the serum of almost all people who have LEMS. All of these antibody tests are very specific; false-positive results are very rare. Disease severity does not correlate with antibody titers in either myasthenia or LEMS.

One traditional test for myasthenia gravis involves intravenous administration of edrophonium (Tensilon), a short-acting acetylcholinesterase inhibitor. In people with myasthenia gravis, the weakness briefly improves. This test is no longer performed very often because it can be difficult to standardize and can cause bradycardia. A similar test that can be easily performed at the bedside in people with prominent ptosis is to apply an ice pack to the eye for 2 minutes. Again, the ptosis briefly improves in people with myasthenia gravis.

All people with newly diagnosed myasthenia should have a CT scan of the chest to look for thymoma. About 50% of people with LEMS have an underlying malignancy, and about 80% of these have small cell lung cancer. The cancer is often subclinical and may be so small that it can take several years to grow to sufficient size for detection on imaging studies. Those who do not have cancer often have immune-mediated diseases or organ-specific auto-antibodies in their serum, further supporting an immune mechanism. People who have LEMS should be evaluated for these underlying conditions, and even if the evaluation is unrevealing, they should be monitored for cancer for several years.

There are three approaches to treating myasthenia gravis: acetylcholinesterase inhibitors, immunomodulation, and thymectomy. Acetylcholinesterase inhibitors, such as the oral drug pyridostigmine (Mestinon), provide a purely symptomatic benefit. These agents slow the enzymatic degradation of acetylcholine, thereby prolonging its availability at the postsynaptic receptor on the muscle membrane.

Although pyridostigmine can be very effective, it does not treat the underlying autoimmune process. For this reason, immunosuppressive medications (such as prednisone, azathioprine, cyclosporine, mycophenolate, eculizumab, ravulizumab, efgartigimod, rozanolixizumab-noli, or zilucoplan) are used. Some of these medications are less effective in people with MuSK antibodies; these people are sometimes treated with rituximab. The most rapidly acting treatments are intravenous immunoglobulin (IVIg) or plasma exchange, which are often very effective, but the effects are temporary. Patients with severe myasthenia gravis may require a combination of all these treatment modalities.

Thymectomy is indicated for people who have a thymoma because total resection is possible if the thymoma has not grown to invade surrounding structures. Even when a thymoma is not present, thymectomy has been shown to improve outcomes in people with myasthenia who are age 65 years or younger.

Many medications, including aminoglycosides, fluoroquinolones, some anti-arrhythmics, and magnesium, affect neuromuscular transmission and can exacerbate myasthenia gravis. Before prescribing any medication to someone with myasthenia gravis, look it up to see whether it is safe.

People with LEMS sometimes respond to acetylcholinesterase inhibitors, plasma exchange, or IVIg, but the results are not as consistent as in myasthenia. Symptoms may improve with 3,4-diaminopyridine, which blocks potassium channels and thereby prolongs the presynaptic action potentials, thus increasing the amount of acetylcholine released by motor nerve terminals with each action potential. People with botulism who receive intensive medical support, especially respiratory support, usually do well, although recovery can be very slow. Antitoxin administration is controversial because of a high incidence of side effects and a lack of consistent benefit.

F. Muscle Disorders (Myopathies)

As with neuropathies, the differential diagnosis for myopathy is very broad, encompassing both hereditary and acquired disorders. The *muscular dystrophies* are hereditary diseases caused by mutations that affect structural proteins that maintain muscle membrane stability. These disorders most often present early in life, but some forms only become symptomatic in middle age or later. The progression is gradual. Duchenne muscular dystrophy is an X-linked disorder that typically presents in the first few years of life with a waddling gait, frequent falling, inability to jump, and difficulty climbing stairs or getting up from the floor. This condition is caused by mutations in the gene for dystrophin, a protein that is part of a glycoprotein complex that links the extracellular matrix with the cytoskeleton inside the muscle fiber. The gene that encodes dystrophin is the largest gene in the human genome (about 10 times larger than the next largest gene and 90 times larger than the average gene) and therefore subject to a high rate of spontaneous mutations. Genetic therapy is available, but the clinical effects are modest. Steroids slow the rate of progression. Becker muscular dystrophy is caused by dystrophin gene mutations that preserve the open reading frame. The clinical manifestations are similar to those of Duchenne muscular dystrophy, but milder, with onset later in childhood.

Other muscular dystrophies result from mutations in other genes, including the genes for many of the other proteins in the dystrophin-glycoprotein complex. The muscular dystrophies have characteristic patterns of muscle involvement, age of onset, and associated symptoms, but there is considerable overlap, so they are usually diagnosed by genetic testing. The most common muscular dystrophy is myotonic dystrophy type 1. In addition to weakness, patients with this condition experience delayed muscle relaxation, or myotonia. A related disease, myotonic dystrophy type 2, typically results in a different distribution of muscle involvement, but the most reliable way to make the diagnosis is with genetic testing. Both myotonic dystrophy type 1 and type 2 are inherited in an autosomal dominant fashion and associated with multisystem abnormalities that can include early cataracts, impaired glucose tolerance, cardiac conduction defects and arrhythmias, testicular atrophy, early male baldness, and mild cognitive delay.

Other hereditary myopathies result from biochemical defects that interfere with the mobilization of energy sources (typically, abnormalities of glycogen metabolism or of lipid metabolism), resulting in exercise intolerance. Some of these defects, such as myophosphorylase deficiency (McArdle disease), prevent the rapid breakdown of glycogen to glucose. People with this condition are often relatively asymptomatic at rest, but they experience pain, cramping, and fatigue within the first few minutes of forceful exertion. They can sometimes experience a "second wind" as their muscles convert to increased utilization of free fatty acids. In contrast, carnitine palmitoyltransferase (CPT) deficiency causes defective utilization of fatty acids, so patients develop pain, cramps, and weakness after prolonged exercise, and they do not experience a second-wind phenomenon. They can perform short, intense exercise without symptoms. Disorders that interfere with the ability of mitochondria to generate usable energy for cellular processes also produce myopathies.

Acquired myopathies can be caused by endocrine disorders, such as hypothyroidism, hyperthyroidism, hyperparathyroidism, and Cushing syndrome. Some other systemic illnesses, such as sarcoidosis, cysticercosis, and trichinosis, can cause myopathy. A variety of medications can cause myopathy, notably exogenous steroid therapy and statins. Chronic alcohol use can also cause myopathy.

Acquired myopathy can also be due to intrinsic muscle inflammation, not due to infection or systemic inflammation. The most common inflammatory myopathies are dermatomyositis, antisynthetase syndrome, overlap myositis, and immune-mediated necrotizing myopathy. Polymyositis was previously thought to be a common form of inflammatory myopathy, but it is now thought that most patients diagnosed with polymyositis actually have a different inflammatory myopathy or even a muscular dystrophy with inflammation; some authorities even question whether polymyositis is a distinct condition. Dermatomyositis is the most common form of inflammatory myopathy throughout childhood and through middle adult life. As the name implies, the muscle involvement is often—but not always—accompanied by a characteristic violet rash that has a predilection for the upper eyelids, anterior chest (in a V shape), back and shoulders (in a shawl configuration), and extensor surfaces of the metacarpophalangeal, elbow, and knee joints. People with antisynthetase syndrome often have interstitial lung disease, arthritis, fever, Raynaud syndrome, and "mechanic's hands" (thickened, dry, cracked skin on the fingers and palms) in addition to the myopathy. Overlap myositis is the term used when someone with a well-defined systemic autoimmune condition (such as systemic lupus erythematosus, rheumatoid arthritis, Sjögren syndrome, or systemic sclerosis) develops an inflammatory myopathy. Some people who receive immune checkpoint inhibitors develop an inflammatory myopathy (others develop a form of myasthenia, as discussed above, and some patients develop a combination). Immune-mediated necrotizing myopathy is often triggered by statin use but progresses even after discontinuation of the statin (unlike the less severe, self-limited, noninflammatory myopathy that can occur during statin use). It can also occur in people who have never taken a statin.

All of these conditions cause symmetric, proximal muscle wasting and weakness. The course is gradual, typically progressing over weeks in dermatomyositis and over months in antisynthetase syndrome, overlap myositis, and immune-mediated necrotizing myopathy. Muscle pain occurs more commonly with inflammatory myopathies than with other myopathies, but the pain is usually mild, and the disease is painless in a substantial proportion of people with inflammatory myopathy.

Serum CK levels are typically abnormal in inflammatory myopathies, but the results usually do not distinguish between these disorders and other primary muscle diseases. The exception is immune-mediated necrotizing myopathy, in which CK levels are usually markedly elevated. Serum levels of other muscle enzymes, such as aldolase, lactate dehydrogenase (LDH), aspartate transaminase (AST), and alanine transaminase (ALT), are often abnormal in inflammatory myopathies, also, but these results are also non-specific. Some EMG features are characteristic of inflammatory myopathy, but for the most part the EMG findings resemble those seen in noninflammatory myopathies. Serum antibodies that can aid in diagnosis—and sometimes prognosis—are summarized in Table 6.4. Muscle biopsy is the most reliable diagnostic test for inflammatory myopathy.

The risk of systemic malignancy is increased in people with dermatomyositis, especially in the presence of some particular antibodies. People with immune-mediated necrotizing myopathy and negative antibody testing also have an increased risk of systemic malignancy.

All of the inflammatory myopathies are treated with immunosuppression. Corticosteroids are the standard first-line agents, but relapses sometimes occur when a prednisone taper is attempted, necessitating long-term steroid use that can itself cause myopathy (as well as many other side effects, including diabetes mellitus, osteoporosis, high blood pressure, promotion of cataracts, and bleeding gastric ulcers). For patients who do not respond to prednisone or who experience relapses whenever withdrawal from prednisone is attempted, a variety of other immunosuppressive treatments are sometimes used. People with immune-mediated necrotizing myopathy usually require intense immunosuppressive therapy.

Inclusion body myositis (IBM) is the most common acquired myopathy after age 50. The characteristic histopathologic features are intramuscular rimmed vacuoles and focal inflammation. Antibodies to cytosolic 5'-nucleotidase 1A (cN1A) are present in 40–60% of people with IBM. Because of the inflammatory changes and the associated antibodies, IBM has traditionally been classified as an inflammatory myopathy, but it does not respond to immunosuppressive treatment and the vacuoles contain a variety of molecules typically associated with degenerative dementing illnesses (including beta amyloid, hyperphosphorylated tau, and TDP-43; see Chapter 7), suggesting that IBM may be primarily a degenerative disease and the inflammation may be reactive. People with IBM often have a distinctive pattern of weakness, with prominent involvement of knee extensor, deep finger flexor, and forearm flexor muscles. The muscle involvement is often asymmetric. Dysphagia is also common in IBM, and there may be mild involvement of facial muscles. The weakness typically progresses over years. There is no known treatment.

V. Symptomatic Treatment

Disease-targeted treatments are available for some neuromuscular disorders (such as myasthenia gravis, inflammatory myopathies, and spinal muscular atrophy) but not for others (such as hereditary neuropathy and IBM). Either way, treatment directed at symptoms rather than at the underlying disease process may be beneficial.

A. Emergency Measures

Anyone who has a rapidly progressive condition with the potential to affect muscles of respiration should be hospitalized for observation until it is clear that the clinical situation is stable. These patients should be monitored with daily (and sometimes more frequent) bedside respiratory testing of forced vital capacity (FVC) and negative inspiratory force. Individuals whose FVC falls below 10–12 mL/kg require elective intubation. Those with a rapidly deteriorating negative inspiratory force or FVC should be intubated even sooner, when the FVC falls to 15 mL/kg.

When someone has a condition that can produce autonomic insufficiency (particularly AIDP), continuous electrocardiogram monitoring and frequent assessment of vital signs are necessary until the clinical situation has stabilized. Significant hypotension and arrhythmias should be treated with medications as needed; in some cases, temporary or permanent cardiac pacing may be required.

B. Non-Urgent Measures: Motor Symptoms

Whether or not there is a treatment for the underlying cause of a patient's weakness, efforts should be made to prevent unnecessary deterioration and to take full advantage of the strength that remains. Physical therapists can teach patients exercises to this effect, and occupational therapists can recommend facilitative devices and environmental modifications to improve function. Speech pathologists have a crucial role in both the assessment and management of dysarthria and dysphagia. For some patients, simple strategies may be sufficient, whereas others may require augmentative communication systems or a temporary or permanent feeding tube.

People who have progressive, irreversible diseases such as motor neuron disease should be encouraged at a relatively early stage in their illness to consider whether they want to be intubated when their respiratory function fails. They should express their wishes clearly to family members and take formal legal measures such as writing a living will or designating a durable power of attorney for medical issues.

C. Non-Urgent Measures: Sensory Symptoms

Neuropathic pain and dysesthesia often respond to symptomatic treatment with tricyclic antidepressant medications, selective serotonin and norepinephrine reuptake inhibitors, or certain antiseizure medications, notably carbamazepine, gabapentin, pregabalin, topiramate, and phenytoin. The necessary doses are often much lower than those required to treat depression or seizures. Because these medications have many potential side effects and the treatment will not change the underlying condition, they should be started at low doses and titrated up slowly. An alternative treatment is capsaicin cream, a medication that binds to specific receptors on pain-sensitive neurons. It often produces initial irritation, so some advocate applying a topical lidocaine preparation before applying the capsaicin.

There is no reliable treatment for numbness or paresthesias, but if the patient reports significant discomfort, tricyclic antidepressants or gabapentin may be tried.

VI. Supplementary Tables for Reference

Table 6.1 Conditions Associated with Small-Fiber Sensory Neuropathy

General Category	Specific Conditions
Metabolic	Diabetes, prediabetes
Autoimmune	Sarcoidosis, systemic lupus erythematosus, Sjögren syndrome, celiac disease, paraneoplastic
Infectious	Leprosy; HIV; hepatitis C
Genetic	Familial amyloidosis; Fabry disease; hemochromatosis
Other	Sporadic amyloidosis; various medications

Table 6.2 Conditions Associated with Large-Fiber Sensory Neuropathy or Neuronopathy

General Category	Specific Conditions
Nutritional deficiency	Cyanocobalamin (B12); thiamine (B1); folate; alpha-tocopherol (E); copper
Toxic	Pyridoxine (B6); nitrous oxide; platinum-based chemotherapy (cisplatin, oxaliplatin)
Autoimmune	Systemic lupus erythematosus; Sjögren syndrome; Guillain-Barré syndrome; distal acquired demyelinating symmetric neuropathy (DADS); chronic ataxic neuropathy, ophthalmoplegia, M protein, agglutination with disialosyl antibodies (CANOMAD); paraneoplastic (anti-Hu, anti-CV2/CRMP5)
Genetic	Friedreich ataxia; cerebellar ataxia, neuropathy, vestibular areflexia syndrome (CANVAS); neuropathy, ataxia, retinitis pigmentosa (NARP)

Table 6.3 Subtypes of Guillain-Barré Syndrome

Syndrome	Common Features
Acute inflammatory demyelinating polyradiculoneuropathy (AIDP)	- Limb weakness - Reduced sensation - Hyporeflexia or areflexia - Pain in back or limbs - Autonomic involvement - Cranial nerve involvement in > 50% (facial weakness, impaired eye movements, dysphagia) - Respiratory weakness (25–30%)
Acute motor axonal neuropathy (AMAN)	- Limb weakness - Hyporeflexia or areflexia - Weakness of cranial nerve–innervated muscles - Often associated with anti-GM_1, GD_{1a}, Ga1NAc-GD_{1a}, or GM_{1b} antibodies
Acute motor-sensory axonal neuropathy (AMSAN)	- Similar to AIDP, usually severe
Miller Fisher syndrome	- Impaired eye movements - Ataxia - Areflexia - More than 80% associated with anti-GQ_{1b} antibodies

Table 6.4 Antibodies Associated with Inflammatory Myopathies

Syndrome	Target Antigen	Other Organ Involvement	Comments
Dermatomyositis			
	Mi-2	Skin	Good prognosis
	TIF-1γ	Skin	Strong association with cancer
	NXP-2	Skin	Increased risk of cancer
	MDA-5	Skin, lungs	Rapidly progressive interstitial lung disease; poor prognosis
	SAE	Skin	May have little or no myopathy
Antisynthetase syndrome			
	Jo-1	Skin, lungs	Progressive interstitial lung disease, "mechanic's hands"
	PL-7	Lung	Severe interstitial lung disease
	PL-12	Lung	Severe interstitial lung disease; may have little or no myopathy
	EJ, OJ, or KS	Lung	Interstitial lung disease
Immune-mediated necrotizing myopathy			
	HMG-CoA reductase (hydroxymethylglutaryl coenzyme A reductase)		Severe myopathy; history of statin use in 70% of patients
	SRP (signal recognition particle)	Lung (occasionally)	Severe myopathy

VII. Discussion of Case Histories

Cases 1 and 2: The patients in both Case 1 and Case 2 have weakness in all four limbs, so if their symptoms were due to a single focal lesion it would have to be in the high cervical spine or above. Lesions in these locations would typically result in hyperreflexia, which is not present in either of these patients. A focal cortical lesion extensive enough to cause weakness in all four limbs would typically cause sensory symptoms and cognitive manifestations. A focal brainstem lesion causing weakness in all four limbs would typically cause cranial nerve problems. Although the person in Case 2 has some eye movement abnormalities, they can't all be explained on the basis of a single focal lesion. All of the patient's symptoms and examination findings in Case 1 are symmetric, suggesting that her condition is diffuse. The patient in Case 2 has some asymmetric abnormalities, suggesting a multifocal process. The absence of upper motor neuron findings in either case suggests a peripheral nervous system localization. The absence of sensory symptoms suggests a primary muscle disease, a neuromuscular junction disorder, or a disease exclusively of motor neurons. In both patients, the limb weakness appears to involve mainly proximal musculature, which is typical of a primary muscle disease or a neuromuscular junction disease (but not motor neuron disease). The prominence of diplopia in Case 2 makes a defect in neuromuscular junction transmission most likely, and the fatigability is characteristic of myasthenia gravis. The symptoms and signs in Case 1 are typical of a myopathy—a primary disorder of muscle—and the time course is typical of an inflammatory myopathy.

The course of myasthenia gravis fluctuates, accounting for the initial episode of diplopia in Case 2. Myopathies, whether inflammatory or non-inflammatory, do not fluctuate in this manner.

In both cases, nerve conduction studies were normal for both sensory and motor nerves. This provided additional evidence that these patients did not have a disorder of the peripheral nerves. In Case 1, the EMG was consistent with myopathic damage, but it is difficult to distinguish by EMG between several of the primary muscle diseases, including inflammatory muscle disease (such as dermatomyositis, antisynthetase syndrome, or immune-mediated necrotizing myopathy), IBM, muscular dystrophy, and congenital myopathy. Serum antibody panels, which can sometimes be helpful in diagnosing inflammatory myopathies and IBM, were negative. The best test to distinguish among the primary muscle diseases is muscle biopsy, which in this case showed characteristic findings of dermatomyo-sitis. This woman was treated with steroids, and her symptoms gradually resolved. The steroids were successfully tapered.

In Case 2, tests of neuromuscular transmission showed abnormalities consistent with those seen in myasthenia gravis, and ruled out the other main diagnostic consideration, Lambert-Eaton myasthenic syndrome. This man was also found to have acetylcholine receptor antibodies in his serum. He was treated with pyridostigmine, with marked improvement. His symptoms did not resolve, however, and prednisone was eventually added. A CT scan of the chest showed no thymoma. The patient is sched-uled to have a thymectomy.

Cases 3 and 4: As with the patients in Cases 1 and 2, the patients in Cases 3 and 4 have symptoms and signs that can't be explained on the basis of a single focal lesion in the nervous system. Both patients show evidence of LMN dysfunction: weakness, fasciculations, and atrophy in Case 3, and weakness with areflexia in Case 4. In Case 4, there is also sensory disturbance, so the site of pathology must be at the level of nerve roots, plexus, or peripheral nerves. This woman's sensory symptoms fit a "stocking-glove" distribution, as is typically seen in a peripheral polyneu-ropathy, but she has both distal and proximal weakness, which would be unusual early in the course of a polyneuropathy. In most neuropathies, the longest nerves in the body are affected first, and the disability pro-gresses from distal to proximal. In contrast, when there is a polyradicular component, roots going to proximal muscles as well as distal muscles are affected, causing proximal and distal weakness. Thus, the pattern of this woman's symptoms suggests a combined polyradiculopathy and poly-neuropathy. The patient in Case 3 has no sensory problems, making radic-ulopathy, plexopathy, and neuropathy less likely. In addition to the LMN involvement, this man has signs of UMN involvement, with spasticity, brisk reflexes, and an extensor plantar response. This pattern of both UMN and LMN involvement is characteristic of ALS. Although structural lesions can sometimes affect both UMNs and LMNs, a structural lesion causing LMN findings in the legs (such as this man's leg muscle atrophy and fasciculations) would have to be located in the lumbosacral spinal cord or distally, and such a lesion could never cause UMN findings in the arms (such as this patient's arm hyperreflexia and spasticity). LMN loss is widespread in ALS, resulting in diffuse atrophy that can explain the weight loss and the general level of fatigue. The initial fall could have been the result of leg weakness that the man didn't recognize at the time.

Electrodiagnostic studies confirmed these impressions. The patient in Case 3 had normal nerve conduction studies, but needle EMG showed widespread denervation, consistent with the clinical diagnosis of motor neuron disease. He received physical therapy and appropriate counseling and was treated with riluzole and BiPAP. His weakness continued to progress, and he developed an aspiration pneumonia 18 months later. His respiratory status declined precipitously, and in accordance with his previously expressed wishes, he was not intubated or resuscitated.

The patient in Case 4 had a nerve conduction study that showed markedly reduced conduction velocities implying an element of demyelination. Based on these results, together with the clinical history, the findings on physical examination, and an elevated spinal fluid protein, the diagnosis of CIDP was made. In this case, an initial episode remitted spontaneously, while the recurrence took place over 6 months. This woman declined a course of steroids but accepted treatment with intravenous immunoglobulin, and her symptoms stabilized.

Chapter 7

Dementing Illnesses

Linda M. Selwa and Douglas J. Gelb

I. Case Histories

Case 1. A 78-year-old woman with a history of hypertension has been brought to the emergency room by her daughter, who says, "She's been getting worse for 6 months, but I hoped it wouldn't come to this." Her decline began with stomach troubles, which prompted her first visit to a doctor in years, and ranitidine (Zantac) was prescribed. She was started on metoprolol (Toprol XL) because her blood pressure was noted to be high, and when her blood pressure failed to normalize, lisinopril (Zestril) was added. She began calling her daughter late at night to complain that she couldn't sleep and that she was scared to be alone. She was given a prescription for flurazepam (Dalmane) to treat her insomnia. Her gait became unsteady, and she fell and hurt her hip 1 week ago. She has been taking pain medicine ever since. When her daughter went to check on her late this afternoon, she was lying in bed and the sheets were soaked with urine. She did not recognize her daughter at first, and when she did, asked her, "Who are all those little men with you?"

On examination, the patient is alert, but agitated and inattentive. Her language output is fluent, but the things she says are often tangential or irrelevant. She follows simple commands but becomes irritated with complicated ones. She is disoriented to time and thinks she has been brought to "the precinct house." She states her name correctly, except that she gives her maiden name rather than her married name. She recalls two of four words after five minutes of distraction and can spell "world" forward, but not backwards. When asked to name the president, she becomes angry. She can name all five of her siblings but can't remember where they each live. The rest of her examination is normal, except that her reflexes are slightly more brisk on the right than on the left. She has a high serum white blood count, pyuria, normal electrolytes, and normal renal and hepatic function. A head CT scan and lumbar puncture are normal.

Questions:

1. Is this woman likely to have Alzheimer disease (AD)?
2. How would you evaluate her in the emergency room?
3. What underlying illnesses are possible?
4. How would you direct her subsequent evaluation and treatment?

Case 2. An 81-year-old man has come to see his family doctor because his wife "thinks I need to be checked out." The man says that nothing is wrong with him and that his wife has always had a tendency to overreact. His wife reminds him that he has had trouble driving recently, getting lost on several familiar streets, and that at a recent reunion he had been unable to recognize some old friends. She says that her husband has forgotten to pay several bills over the past year, and they hired an accountant 2 years ago because her husband said that the finances were "just too complex." She notes that her husband has not been taking his usual care in dressing. The patient responds that she is "making mountains out of anthills." He says that she would do better to worry about the recent burglary in their house. When his wife asks, "What burglary?" the patient says he had not wanted to worry her, but ever since they returned from a recent trip, "things were missing" around the house and new scratches had appeared on their antique furniture. He had concluded that the home was burglarized and might still be "under watch."

Except for a long history of gout and an ulcer many years ago, the patient has no history of medical problems. He takes no medications. His general physical examination is normal. He is very outgoing and speaks fluently, repeatedly joking about his age. He makes frequent paraphasic errors (i.e., he uses incorrect words) and sometimes makes up his own words. He cannot recall any of three words after five minutes of distraction and says, "That was much too long ago." He is aware of the clinic name but not the town and says it is "fallish" in 1982 or 1992. He cannot name the current president, but when told the answer, he says, "I knew that. I thought you asked if I had ever met him." He is able to tell you the names of only three of his five children. He has considerable difficulty drawing a clock. The remainder of his examination is normal.

Questions:

1. Does this man have Alzheimer disease (AD)?
2. What tests would be appropriate in his evaluation?
3. What other questions about his daily life would be important in management?
4. Would it be appropriate to discuss a durable power of attorney?

Case 3. A 64-year-old woman was brought in for evaluation because she has been "acting strangely" for several months. At first, she just seemed to be having occasional "senior moments" in which she would forget where she put something or struggle to think of a word, but she has become increasingly forgetful to the point where she can no longer perform her job as a reference librarian. In fact, her supervisor has told her that she can't return to work until she gets a medical evaluation. Her son says that over the past 2 weeks she has been very lethargic, and when she isn't asleep she seems to be responding to stimuli that aren't actually present. She has a history of irritable bowel syndrome, but no other medical problems. She takes no medications, and she only drinks an occasional glass of wine. She doesn't smoke cigarettes or use recreational drugs.

Her general physical examination is normal, except that her weight is 15 kg less than at her most recent appointment (6 months ago). She is alert at times but at other times tends to doze off. During the intervals when she is alert, she speaks fluently, with normal comprehension, repetition, and naming abilities. She can spell "world" forward, but has difficulty spelling it backward. She can only recall two of four words after five minutes of distraction. She is not oriented to place. She can name only three of her seven grandchildren, and her son says she would have been able to name all seven without hesitation in the past. She is able to calculate the number of nickels in a dollar, but not in $1.35; again, her son says this is very different from her baseline. On several occasions during the examination, she stops talking, looks off to her left, looks fearful, and doesn't respond to questions; after about 30 seconds, she blinks, looks around, and becomes responsive again. The remainder of her neurologic examination is normal.

Questions:

1. Is this woman likely to have Alzheimer disease (AD)?
2. What further evaluation is necessary?
3. What is the best plan for follow-up and treatment?

II. Approach to Dementing Illnesses

Patients with symptoms of cognitive impairment should be evaluated systematically by addressing the following questions:

1. Are the symptoms truly abnormal?
2. Are there any potentially reversible components?
3. Do the history, examination, and test results suggest a specific primary dementing illness, especially Alzheimer disease (AD), dementia with Lewy bodies (DLB), frontotemporal dementia (FTD), vascular cognitive impairment, or limbic-predominant age-related TDP-43 encephalopathy (LATE)?

The following discussion expands on each of these questions and their significance.

A. Is It Abnormal?

Most people experience occasional cognitive lapses, such as difficulty remembering the name of an acquaintance, misplacing something, forgetting to pay a bill, or missing an appointment. The boundary between normal and abnormal is often indistinct, and it becomes more blurred with increasing age. Even in people with no evidence of neurologic disease, cognitive functions decline with age. In fact, as early as the third or fourth decade of life, sophisticated testing reveals slight slowing of some cognitive processes. This deterioration becomes more prominent with increasing age, but the rate of decline varies from person to person. Because of this variable rate of decline and the wide variation even in baseline cognitive abilities, it is often difficult to define the precise point at which cognitive deficits are severe enough to be considered pathologic. Even young adults frequently worry about the fact that they have trouble thinking of words or remembering facts. People who have watched close associates or family members struggle with Alzheimer disease (AD) may be especially anxious when they perceive themselves having similar difficulties. They become very self-conscious, as any slight mistake serves to confirm their worst fears. The more they fixate on minor errors, the more anxious and self-conscious they become. This affects their ability to focus their attention, resulting in problems with memory consolidation and retrieval that engender additional mistakes—which makes them even more anxious, further diminishing their ability to attend, leading to more mistakes, and so forth in a "vicious cycle." Dementia is an inherently terrifying prospect to most people, because it affects functions that are integral to their personality and sense of self. The physician's task is to identify those patients in whom there is a legitimate suspicion of dementia and reassure the rest.

A common misconception is that people with dementia are either incapable of recognizing their deficits or unwilling to acknowledge them, so people who say they are worried that they might have dementia probably don't have it. Although this is true in some cases, many people with dementia recognize that they have a problem and are distressed by it. A more reliable generalization is that people who report specific incidents of memory impairment that happened on specific days—and proceed to describe all the details of exactly what they could do and what they couldn't, and how they felt about it—are unlikely to have a dementing illness. People with dementia typically have trouble providing specific examples of their deficits. They may say they have problems remembering names, or trouble at work, or trouble remembering where they left items around the house, but they usually express these concerns in fairly general terms and turn to family members for help when asked to provide specific examples.

Another fairly reliable generalization is that cognitive lapses or changes in personality or behavior that are so severe or frequent that they affect someone's function at home or at work usually signify a serious condition, or at least a condition that needs to be thoroughly evaluated. Examples include problems with routine cooking or other chores at home, trouble using appliances, poor financial decisions, episodes of disorientation while driving in areas that should be familiar, new obsessions or compulsions, reduced motivation for activities that previously brought satisfaction, or a decline in job performance to the point where employers or colleagues express concern. People with sustained cognitive deficits so severe that they interfere with daily function are considered to have dementia. When people with cognitive deficits are still able to perform their daily activities, the situation is not as clear—a substantial subset of them are experiencing the early stages of a degenerative dementing illness, but others never develop dementia. In explaining the situation to these people and their families, it is helpful to have a relatively brief term that means, essentially, "cognitive deficits that are more extensive or more severe than usual, but not severe enough to interfere with social or occupational function, and therefore not severe enough to be considered dementia." A shorthand term is also useful for research—people in this category have been the subject of extensive investigation aimed at identifying the subgroup who will eventually progress to dementia and determining what can be done to prevent, delay, or lessen the severity of dementia in this subgroup. Many terms have been proposed, and the one that has become most prevalent is *mild cognitive impairment* (MCI). Patients with MCI can be further subdivided into those with *amnestic* MCI and those with *nonamnestic* MCI based on whether memory disturbance is their predominant cognitive deficit. About 10–15% of people with amnestic MCI will have symptoms severe enough to be categorized as dementia within 2 years. The term *MCI due to Alzheimer disease* (or *MCI due to AD*) is used to signify the symptomatic pre-dementia phase of AD, thereby distinguishing this group from people with MCI who will never develop AD, either because they will turn out to have some other dementing illness or—most often—because they will never develop dementia at all.

References to MCI in the popular press (and sometimes in the medical literature) often make it seem as if it is a well-defined condition, whereas it is really just a convenient way to refer to a heterogeneous group of patients. Some patients with MCI eventually progress to the point where they clearly have dementia. Other patients with MCI never reach that level of severity—it may be that they are simply at one extreme of the normal "bell-shaped curve" with respect to the cognitive decline that occurs with aging. Others may have unrecognized depression or some other stable condition. When diagnosing MCI, you should inform patients that the situation is ambiguous, and that you will need to follow them over time to see if they eventually develop dementia. Formal neuropsychological testing is often useful, because it provides quantitative measures that can be monitored for progression. Several cerebrospinal fluid (CSF), serum, and imaging biomarkers are associated with a significantly higher risk of progression to dementia and—if an autopsy is eventually performed—the diagnosis of AD, but their utility in routine clinical practice is not yet established. It might seem reasonable to treat MCI using one of the medications typically prescribed for people with dementia consistent with AD, but controlled trials of those medications in patients with MCI have failed to demonstrate a convincing long-term benefit.

B. Are There Any Potentially Reversible Components?

Dementia is defined as an *acquired, persistent decline of intellectual function that causes impaired performance of daily activities, without clouding of the sensorium or underlying psychiatric disease. The decline must involve at least two of the following domains: (a) ability to learn and remember new information, (b) reasoning and judgment, (c) visuospatial perception,*

(d) language function, and (e) personality and behavior. This definition explicitly excludes some important categories of disease, which must be considered before concluding that someone has dementia.

Delirium is defined as an *acute, transient, fluctuating confusional state characterized by impairment in maintaining and shifting attention, often associated with sensory misperception or disorganized thinking.* Delirium is often due to a toxin or a metabolic disturbance, so it is frequently reversible. The evaluation and management of delirium are discussed in Chapter 11.

Differentiation between *dementia* and *depression* may be extremely difficult at times. A "chicken and egg" problem arises: Many people with dementia are depressed, partly because they are upset by their decline, and partly because the underlying brain degeneration can affect the neural circuitry involved in mood. Conversely, primary depression may result in so much slowing of thought and speech and such limited motivation that it resembles dementia. This has been called the *pseudodementia* of depression. If the person has vegetative signs, such as changes in eating or sleeping patterns, or if the cognitive decline began after the death of a spouse or some other emotional trauma, depression is a major consideration. These clues are not always reliable, however. Symptoms of dementia may go unnoticed until the death of a spouse who had previously been "covering for" the patient's deficits. Furthermore, people with primary dementia can develop changes in eating or sleeping patterns that resemble the vegetative signs of depression. Various diagnostic tests have been suggested for differentiating dementia and depression, but none is completely reliable. At times, an empiric trial of antidepressant medication is necessary. If the primary disorder is depression, the cognitive deficits may resolve, and even if the primary disorder is dementia, treatment of secondary depression may improve function and quality of life, even though it doesn't eliminate the cognitive deficits.

Dementia is sometimes just one component of a more generalized disease process. Some of these processes, such as vitamin B12 deficiency, may be relatively subtle. Others, such as hematologic diseases, systemic infections, and disorders of electrolytes, glucose, renal, or hepatic function, are unlikely to be the underlying cause of dementia without producing delirium or obvious systemic symptoms. Even so, screening for these conditions is important because dementia from any cause may be exacerbated by systemic illness, and treatment of the systemic disease may result in meaningful improvement of cognitive function even when the underlying dementing illness is irreversible. Furthermore, someone with dementia may fail to report symptoms that would otherwise make a systemic illness obvious. Thus, patients with dementia should be tested for thyroid disease and vitamin B12 deficiency as well as renal disease, liver disease, electrolyte abnormalities, diabetes, chronic infections, and common tumors. In patients for whom a history of syphilis exposure is a realistic possibility, serum FTA (fluorescent treponemal antibody) or MHA-TP (microhemagglutination–*Treponema pallidum*) should be tested. VDRL and RPR (rapid plasma reagin) are not sufficient in this context, because they convert back to normal in a substantial fraction of individuals with late stages of syphilis.

Hearing loss—which is present in about 65% of people older than 60 years—is a risk factor for dementia. The reason is unknown, but many potential explanations have been proposed. Likewise, it has not been established whether treatment of hearing loss (typically with hearing aids) slows the progression of dementia or reduces the likelihood of developing it, but it can enhance function.

On rare occasions, dementia is due to a mass lesion in the brain, such as a primary or metastatic brain tumor, an abscess, or a subdural hematoma. This usually produces focal abnormalities on neurologic examination, but not always (especially if the disease affects both hemispheres equally), so patients with progressive dementia should have a brain CT or MRI scan. An imaging study is also helpful in determining the likelihood of a multi-infarct state or amyloid angiopathy (see Chapter 4), and the pattern of atrophy on an imaging study sometimes provides evidence for or against specific dementing illnesses.

In addition to direct pressure on the nearby brain parenchyma, mass lesions sometimes press on the ventricular system and obstruct outflow, causing CSF to accumulate at increased pressure in all portions of the ventricular system proximal to the obstruction. This condition, called obstructive hydrocephalus, is associated with cognitive deterioration, gait disturbance, and incontinence, together with symptoms and signs of increased intracranial pressure. Treatment is directed at removing the obstruction, if possible, and draining the enlarged ventricular system.

Normal pressure hydrocephalus (NPH) is an analogous syndrome, except that the ventricular enlargement occurs without an increase in intracranial pressure, and there is no structural obstruction to outflow. Imaging studies show little or no sulcal enlargement, except possibly in the inferior subarachnoid spaces, around the lateral fissures. Some of these patients have a history of previous meningeal irritation (e.g., from meningitis or subarachnoid hemorrhage), presumably resulting in impaired CSF absorption at the level of the arachnoid granulations. In other patients no cause can be identified. In any event, NPH is a syndrome characterized by the clinical triad of dementia, gait disturbance, and incontinence; enlargement of the ventricular system on brain imaging studies; and clinical improvement in response to ventricular shunting procedures. These procedures are usually straightforward; the main risks are infection and subdural hematoma.

NPH is a controversial diagnosis, and the literature is difficult to evaluate because of variability in diagnostic criteria and outcome measures. The presence of the clinical triad does not guarantee a response to a shunt. Conversely, shunting may be effective for some patients who have only one or two components of the triad. There is no consensus on which clinical, radiologic, or other diagnostic test findings correlate with a favorable response to shunting. Some authors challenge the diagnosis of NPH entirely. These issues should be discussed thoroughly with patients and their families.

In people with dementia that has progressed rapidly, the evaluation should include HIV testing, a search for a systemic cancer (either a whole-body positron emission tomography (PET) scan or a CT of the chest, abdomen, and pelvis), an autoimmune encephalitis antibody panel, and spinal fluid analysis for chronic meningitis or other inflammatory conditions. Systemic inflammatory diseases such as systemic lupus erythematosus or giant cell (temporal) arteritis may present with dementia, and a sedimentation rate can be used as a screen.

To summarize, specialized testing may be indicated in selected patients, especially young patients or those with a particularly rapid decline, but for most patients the following battery of tests will suffice to screen for potentially reversible causes of dementia:

Serum: electrolytes, blood urea nitrogen, creatinine, glucose, calcium, liver enzymes, complete blood cell count, differential, sedimentation rate, vitamin B12, thyroid-stimulating hormone
Imaging: head CT or MRI

C. Which Primary Degenerative Dementing Illness Is Most Likely?

Striking loss of short- and long-term memory with preserved immediate recall and relatively preserved remote memory occurs in Korsakoff syndrome, a condition caused by chronic thiamine deficiency, most commonly in people with long-standing alcohol use disorder. Patients who have experienced an episode of brain dysfunction from a wide variety of causes, such as anoxia, encephalitis (especially herpes simplex), head trauma, surgical procedures, electroconvulsive therapy, radiation therapy, meningoencephalitis, status epilepticus, or subarachnoid hemorrhage, may be left with significantly impaired cognitive function that subsequently remains stable or improves. These nonprogressive dementing conditions do not present the same diagnostic or management issues as the degenerative dementias and are not considered further here.

Progressive dementia is most often due to a primary degenerative disease of the brain. There are no completely reliable diagnostic tests for the most common primary dementing illnesses, and systemic or structural causes of dementia can sometimes mimic them fairly closely, so it is important to look for causes that might be reversible, but patients and families should be warned in advance that the blood, urine, and brain imaging studies discussed in Section B will probably have a low yield.

Definitive diagnosis of one of the primary dementing illnesses usually requires neuropathologic confirmation, but clinical features permit an accurate diagnosis during life in most patients. The diagnosis is based on how closely a patient's history, examination, and test results match the typical pattern of one of these conditions. The most common pattern is a memory-predominant syndrome. This typically begins with the type of mild memory lapses that are difficult to distinguish from normal aging. These gradually become more frequent and more severe, and changes in other cognitive domains (such as language function, judgment, visuospatial skills, mathematical abilities, personality, and behavior) start to appear. With time, the patient develops widespread cognitive deficits, which gradually progress.

In some people with a primary dementing illness, the initial symptoms are restricted to language function, with sparing of memory and other cognitive domains. This is called primary progressive aphasia (PPA), and it is subdivided into three subtypes: nonfluent/agrammatic, semantic variant, and logopenic variant. Characteristic features of these three subtypes are summarized in Table 7.1. In brief, the nonfluent/agrammatic subtype resembles the traditional Broca aphasia, and the pathology primarily involves the anterior portion of the dorsal language stream discussed in Chapter 1. The logopenic variant is notable for difficulty processing the phonologic content of speech, and therefore particular difficulty with repetition, with preserved ability to understand the meaning of individual words; the pathologic changes are concentrated in the posterior region of the dorsal language stream. The semantic variant is characterized by profound difficulty processing the meaning of individual words with relative preservation of the ability to recognize and reproduce the component sounds of those words, and the pathology primarily resides in the ventral language stream. All three of these subtypes tend to become increasingly similar to each other as they progress, and patients eventually develop problems in cognitive domains beyond language processing.

Some people with a primary dementing illness present with visual symptoms; this is known as posterior cortical atrophy. They typically have normal visual acuity and normal results on a standard ophthalmologic examination, but they have difficulty processing what they see. Three subtypes of posterior cortical atrophy have been described, although some question whether they are truly distinct syndromes; Table 7.2 summarizes their features. The table mentions "Balint syndrome," which is a condition in which people can recognize items that are present in individual small regions of a scene, but they have difficulty synthesizing them—it is as if they are viewing the world through a narrow tube that they have trouble maneuvering, so they can only see one fragment of the scene at a time, in no systematic order. The acute onset of Balint syndrome is usually due to bilateral parieto-occipital strokes; a subacute or chronic onset is usually due to posterior cortical atrophy (with the same localization). As with PPA, posterior cortical atrophy eventually becomes more generalized and involves other aspects of cognition.

Some people with a primary dementing illness present with a behavioral syndrome, characterized by marked changes in personality that can include disinhibited conduct; changes in eating, dressing, or hygiene; inappropriate sexual behavior; difficulty with anger management; or other problems with control of emotions. Others present with a dysexecutive syndrome, characterized by apathy, blunted affect, difficulty maintaining and directing attention, poor planning, and impaired judgment. There is also a syndrome called progressive apraxia of speech that is analogous to PPA, but it manifests with progressive impairment of the motor production of speech rather than language difficulty. Affected individuals struggle to pronounce words correctly or produce them with a normal rhythm, but they have no trouble thinking of words or understanding them, and they can read and write without difficulty.

The treatment options for all of the primary dementing illnesses are limited, so it might seem that differentiating between them isn't worth the effort, but most patients and families are eager for a specific diagnosis. They appreciate knowing what to expect, and what to watch for, and this differs depending on the underlying disorder. You should be open with patients and families about the diagnosis or potential diagnoses. Some physicians avoid using terms like dementia or Alzheimer disease because they are reluctant to frighten or depress patients, but they should realize that the possibility will not come as a surprise to most patients and families.

III. Primary Dementing Illnesses

A. Alzheimer Disease (AD)

1. Epidemiology, pathology, and etiology

Alzheimer disease (AD) is the most common cause of progressive dementia in adults, accounting for about 60% of cases of dementia. Age is the strongest risk factor for AD. As a rough guideline, the prevalence of AD is about 1% among 60-year-old people, and doubles every 5 years thereafter up until age 85, at which point the prevalence remains constant or declines.

Both genetic and nongenetic factors contribute to the development of AD. In addition to advancing age, female sex, vascular disease and vascular risk factors, history of head trauma, low level of education, stress, depression, and low levels of physical and intellectual activity are associated with an increased risk of AD. Numerous susceptibility genes—associated with an increased likelihood of developing AD, but not a 100% correlation—have been identified. The strongest association is with the gene for apolipoprotein E (ApoE). There are three common alleles of the ApoE gene: E2, E3, and E4. The E2 allele is less common than the other alleles in people with AD, whereas the frequency of the E4 allele in people with late-onset sporadic AD is approximately double the frequency found in control groups. Moreover, the age of symptom onset correlates with the number of E4 alleles: it is considerably lower in homozygotes for E4 than in heterozygotes, and highest of all in people with no copies of the E4 allele. Even so, some homozygotes never develop the disease, and a substantial fraction of people with AD have no E4 allele. It remains unclear how ApoE and other genes influence pathogenesis. A tiny minority (1% or less) of cases of AD are inherited in an autosomal dominant pattern with nearly complete penetrance (and usually an onset before age 65 years). Three causative genes have been identified, and all are involved in the processing of Aβ-peptide, which is a prominent feature of AD pathology.

The characteristic pathologic findings in AD are loss of neurons, loss of synapses, shrinkage of large cortical neurons and their dendritic arbors, amyloid plaques, and neurofibrillary tangles. At autopsy, cell loss is most prominent in the temporal and parietal lobes, although the brain regions affected earliest (based on functional imaging studies during life) are the posterior cingulate cortex and other areas that coincide with the "default mode network," a set of interconnected brain regions that tend to be active when normal subjects are instructed to relax and avoid cognitive tasks. The pathophysiologic significance of this overlap between the default mode network and the areas of earliest dysfunction in AD is not known. The typical pathologic findings of AD sometimes coexist with pathologic features of other degenerative dementias or strokes; this is increasingly common with advancing age. A number of neurochemical abnormalities have been described in AD, including loss of choline acetyltransferase in neurons with cell bodies in the nucleus basalis of Meynert, the major source of cholinergic input to the cerebral cortex.

Neurofibrillary tangles are cytoplasmic inclusions located in the axon hillock of neurons. They are composed of filaments twisted around each other in a helical structure, called paired helical filaments. The filaments, in turn, are composed of hyperphosphorylated forms of the microtubule-associated tau protein, which stabilizes microtubules. In the normal brain, phosphate groups are rapidly removed from tau protein by phosphatases, whereas the tau protein in the paired helical filaments in the brains of people with AD is relatively resistant to dephosphorylation. The excess phosphorylation presumably interferes with the function of the microtubule-binding regions, leading to destabilization of microtubules and abnormal cellular transport mechanisms.

Neuritic amyloid plaques are extracellular proteinaceous deposits that are composed mainly of a peptide known as beta amyloid, or Aβ-peptide, surrounded by degenerating or dystrophic nerve endings (neurites). Diffuse amyloid plaques consist of accumulated Aβ-peptide without dystrophic neurites. Aβ-peptide is a fragment of a larger protein, called beta amyloid precursor protein (APP), which is a transmembrane protein found in normal cells. It is expressed in both neural and non-neural tissue and its function is not known. The primary metabolic pathway for APP in normal cells involves an enzyme known as α-secretase, which cleaves the extracellular portion of the APP just above the surface of the membrane and produces a large fragment, soluble APP. An alternative APP processing pathway, which normal cells use much less often than the primary pathway, involves cleavage further from the membrane by an enzyme known as β-secretase, followed by cleavage at a site in the intramembranous portion of APP by an enzyme known as γ-secretase. This results in the production of Aβ-peptide (see Figure 7.1). The cleavage site for α-secretase (the primary processing pathway) lies within the Aβ-peptide domain, because it is closer to the cell membrane than the cleavage site for β-secretase. Thus,

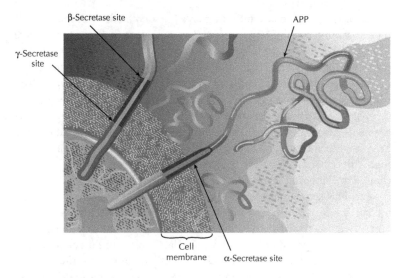

Fig. 7.1 Sites of action of α-secretase, β-secretase, and γ-secretase. The APP protein spans the cell membrane. The β-secretase cleavage site is outside the membrane, and the γ-secretase site is within the membrane; the fragment of APP produced by their combined action is the Aβ-peptide (in the figure, the two dark regions that have one end within the membrane and the other end outside the cell). The α-secretase cleavage site is outside the cell membrane but not as far out as the β-secretase site, so it lies within the Aβ-peptide domain. Thus, α-secretase activity prevents Aβ-peptide formation.

in normal circumstances α-secretase ensures that only small amounts of Aβ-peptide are produced, but in AD there is increased production of Aβ-peptide, which aggregates as insoluble β-pleated sheets that form the basis of the amyloid plaque.

The most common gene responsible for autosomal dominant, early-onset AD is *presenilin-1*, which codes for a component of the γ-secretase complex. The second most common causative gene is *APP* itself. The third gene, *presenilin-2*, encodes a protease homologous to presenilin-1 but located on a different chromosome. Transgenic mice that express mutant *presenilin-1* or *APP* genes (or both) display behavioral and neuropathologic features that are analogous to human AD, so abnormal APP processing appears to be integral to the development of AD, at least in some cases. Researchers have also produced mouse models of AD by manipulating the expression of tau protein.

The accumulation of Aβ-peptide begins many years or decades before symptoms begin, and the rate of Aβ-peptide accumulation predicts the onset of tau accumulation. The distribution of neuronal loss parallels the location of tangles, and the severity of dementia correlates more closely with the extent of tangle formation than it does with the extent of plaque formation. These and other lines of evidence have led many researchers to propose the "amyloid cascade hypothesis," which holds that the initial step in AD pathogenesis is deposition and spread of Aβ-peptide, which somehow triggers the propagation of hyperphosphorylated tau pathology through the neocortex, which in turn results in synaptic loss, neurodegeneration, and ultimately cognitive decline. Some proponents of the amyloid cascade hypothesis have suggested that Aβ-peptide may spread by inducing the pathologic transformation of normal protein, analogous to the propagation of prions (see Section F). Other processes thought to contribute to the cell damage that results from the amyloid cascade include inflammation, excitotoxicity (toxic effects of excessive levels of the excitatory amino acids, glutamate and aspartate), and oxidative stress (toxic effects of free radicals). Although the amyloid cascade hypothesis is the most widely held theory of AD pathogenesis, it is neither definitively proven nor universally accepted.

2. Clinical features

The most common clinical presentation of AD is the memory-predominant syndrome discussed in Part II, Section C, but AD occasionally presents as posterior cortical atrophy, logopenic variant PPA, behavioral syndrome, or dysexecutive syndrome. Regardless of the initial presentation, additional cognitive deficits gradually appear. The order in which they appear and the rate of progression are highly variable, so there is no "typical" pattern of deficits. The disease eventually progresses to the point of severe impairment in all cognitive domains.

Cognitive deficits are usually the only neurologic abnormalities in early AD, but additional problems commonly develop over time. About 20–40% of people with AD eventually develop bradykinesia and rigidity, which are called parkinsonian features (or parkinsonism) because they are typical of Parkinson disease (PD; see Chapter 8). This can lead to diagnostic uncertainty, because many people with PD have dementia; in fact, up to 80% may have some manifestations of dementia by the time of death. Dementia with Lewy bodies (DLB; see Section B) is also characterized by a combination of cognitive impairment and parkinsonism. Thus, patients who have both dementia and parkinsonism could have any combination of the typical neuropathologic features of AD, PD, or DLB. Some investigators view

PD and DLB, and possibly even AD, as different points along a spectrum of a single underlying process, or possibly separate pathologic conditions that can affect variable brain regions, with different clinical manifestations in each individual depending on which regions are most involved. Nonetheless, AD, PD, and DLB are distinct enough in most cases to consider them different diseases. In particular, the parkinsonian features are less prominent and develop later than the cognitive deficits in most people with AD, but exceptions occur.

Myoclonus is common in advanced AD, but it is rarely present at the onset of cognitive impairment. Seizures occur in up to 10% of patients, especially late in the course. Focal seizures can be quite subtle in people with dementia, so this possibility should be considered whenever episodes of unresponsiveness are reported. People with AD may also develop spasticity, dysarthria, and dysphagia. Incontinence is unusual early in the course but is much more common later, and it is often one of the most difficult issues caretakers confront. Another difficult management problem is posed by psychiatric manifestations. When these are prominent early in the course, an alternative diagnosis—especially DLB—should be considered, but psychiatric symptoms eventually occur in about 50% of people with AD. Delusions, agitation, and depression are common. Hallucinations are less common but also occur. Wandering behavior and sleep disturbances can also present management challenges.

The course of AD is extremely variable, so it is very difficult to predict exactly when individual patients will lose specific functions. The average length of survival after the onset of symptoms is 8–10 years but can range up to 20 years. Patients and family members should be told that the disease is invariably progressive—at some point, patients will have to restrict their activities, and other people will have to handle finances, cook, or do home repairs. People with AD will eventually develop deficits in reading, reasoning, or visual perception that make it unsafe for them to drive. At later stages, they will lose the ability to maintain personal hygiene. They may become progressively more agitated to the point of violence, or progressively more withdrawn to the point of akinesia. They will eventually lose the ability to recognize even spouses and children. Death usually results from infection, most often due to aspiration pneumonia or urosepsis.

3. Diagnostic tests

The diagnosis of AD is usually based primarily on clinical evidence. Patients whose history and mental status examination (and sometimes formal neuropsychologic testing, which can augment the bedside mental status examination and characterize the cognitive deficits in more detail) are consistent with AD, with nothing suggesting an alternative explanation for cognitive decline (after completing a physical examination and the serum and imaging studies listed at the end of Part II, Section B), are usually presumed to have AD. When autopsies are conducted on such patients, about 85% have typical pathologic features of AD.

A variety of diagnostic tests for AD have been developed in an effort to improve diagnostic accuracy or to allow diagnosis earlier in the course—ideally, before the cognitive deficits have progressed to the point where they are impairing performance of daily activities (that is, at the stage of MCI rather than dementia, or even at a presymptomatic stage). Quantitative analysis of the volume of specific brain regions on MRI—especially when repeated a year later to measure the rate of regional atrophy—can help distinguish between dementia and MCI, but it will not necessarily identify the specific dementing illness. AD is associated with a typical pattern of reduced temporoparietal metabolism and blood flow on functional imaging studies (fluorodeoxyglucose-positron emission tomography [FDG-PET] or single photon emission tomography [SPECT]), but when functional imaging is performed in people with MCI both the sensitivity and specificity of these results for the ultimate diagnosis of AD are in the 75–85% range. Posterior cingulate and precuneus involvement increase the likelihood of AD. PET scans using an amyloid-binding agent also show characteristic abnormalities in people who are ultimately diagnosed with AD. Similar abnormalities are present in some people with MCI and may help to identify those patients with MCI who will ultimately develop AD, but with increasing age there is increasing likelihood of finding incidental deposition of Aβ-peptide that is not the primary cause of symptoms. The reliability of this imaging technique in general clinical practice remains to be established. It is expensive, and most insurance companies will not pay for it. PET ligands that bind to tau are also available, and studies suggest that PET imaging for tau may be useful in differentiating AD from other degenerative dementing illnesses, but further research is needed.

The CSF of patients with AD contains lower than normal levels of Aβ-peptide and higher than normal levels of both total tau protein and phosphorylated tau protein. Furthermore, among patients with MCI, high CSF levels of tau and low levels of Aβ-peptide correlate with an increased likelihood of eventually developing dementia (with typical pathologic features of AD if an autopsy is ultimately performed). Technological advances have led to improved sensitivity of serum assays for Aβ-peptide and tau. A commercially available blood test is based on the ratio of the 42-amino acid and 40-amino acid forms of Aβ-peptide, combined with age and ApoE genotype, but it is not covered by most health insurance companies. Other blood tests are in development. The best use of these blood tests, CSF assays, and imaging modalities in clinical practice remains to be determined.

4. Treatment

Three acetylcholinesterase inhibitors—donepezil (Aricept), rivastigmine (Exelon), and galantamine (Razadyne)—are FDA approved and currently marketed for use in patients who are thought to have AD. The rationale for their use is that the neuronal cell loss that occurs in AD disproportionately involves cholinergic neurons. Memantine (Namenda), an antagonist of the NMDA (N-methyl-d-aspartate) subclass of glutamate receptors, is also FDA approved for dementia attributed to AD, based on the rationale that excitotoxicity has been implicated in the pathogenesis of AD. All of these medications result in symptomatic improvement, but they have not been shown to alter the course of AD, probably because both neuronal cell loss and excitotoxicity occur at relatively late stages of pathogenesis. Each of these medications has been shown to produce a modest, but statistically significant, improvement on neuropsychological measures and on clinician and family ratings of symptom severity. The amount of improvement is roughly equivalent to the amount an average patient deteriorates in 6 months, so the effect of treatment can be likened to "setting the clock back" by 6 months. The duration of the beneficial effect is unknown—most of the controlled trials lasted 6 months, but follow-up studies suggest that the cholinesterase inhibitors continue to be beneficial for at least 2 years. There is no evidence that any one of the cholinesterase inhibitors is more effective than another, so selection of a specific drug is based mainly on side effects, cost, and convenience. In people with moderate or severe dementia attributed to AD, simultaneous treatment with both memantine and donepezil results in better cognitive performance than treatment with donepezil alone, but the difference is not dramatic. A common approach is to begin treatment with one of the cholinesterase inhibitors when the dementia is first diagnosed, and to add memantine when it becomes moderately severe.

Evidence that oxidative stress contributes to the pathophysiology of AD has prompted studies of antioxidant medication. Two placebo-controlled studies have found that alpha tocopherol (vitamin E) delays clinical progression of dementia attributed to AD, but it was not found to be helpful for patients with MCI. The doses used (2000 IU per day) have been found (in other studies) to increase cardiovascular risk.

Numerous approaches targeted at blocking the formation, limiting the aggregation, or increasing the clearance of Aβ-peptide (including active immunization, passive immunization, inhibition of γ-secretase or β-secretase) have been studied or are currently being studied. Some of these treatments have resulted in substantial reduction of Aβ-peptide on amyloid-PET scans, but the clinical results have been disappointing. Some people cite this as evidence that the amyloid cascade hypothesis is incorrect; others contend that because the patients enrolled in these trials already had cognitive symptoms, the amyloid cascade may have been too far advanced for the treatment to stop it—in effect, that reducing the Aβ-peptide burden after cognitive symptoms have already developed is analogous to trying to stop a raging forest fire by blowing out the match that started it. This type of reasoning has led investigators to design trials focused on patients who are at an earlier stage in the amyloid cascade, such as patients who have amyloid-PET or CSF biomarker results typical of AD, but minimal or no symptoms. Two antibodies to Aβ-peptide that were investigated using this type of trial design, aducanumab and lecanemab, have been approved by the FDA for the treatment of mild dementia or MCI due to AD (based on amyloid imaging). Aducanumab's approval was very controversial, because even though trials demonstrated striking reduction of Aβ-peptide deposits on PET imaging, the evidence of a clinical benefit was unconvincing. Furthermore, about 40% of study participants developed MRI findings that have been labeled amyloid-related imaging abnormalities (ARIA), consisting of microhemorrhages and/or edema that can sometimes be dramatic. For these reasons, as well as high cost, aducanumab has not been broadly adopted in clinical practice. In the lecanemab trials, fewer participants developed ARIA, and there was more consistent evidence of clinical benefit, although the magnitude of the benefit was modest. It remains unknown whether treatment even earlier in the disease course would result in more clinically meaningful benefit, but such a strategy would have major economic and ethical implications. Another Aβ-peptide antibody that showed a clinical benefit, donanemab, is under FDA review. Other approaches to treating AD, focused on inflammation, excitotoxicity, tau protein production and polymerization, microtubule stabilization, glial function, neurotransmitter modulation, and ion channel function, are under investigation.

The current standard for managing patients who are thought to have AD consists of a cholinesterase inhibitor (with or without vitamin E), eventual addition of memantine, and symptomatic treatment. Patients who develop new symptoms—even symptoms that commonly occur as dementia progresses—should be evaluated for non-neurologic causes of those symptoms. For example, males who develop urinary incontinence should be evaluated for prostatic hypertrophy before automatically attributing the incontinence to their dementing illness. When non-neurologic causes are not identified, nonpharmacologic management approaches should usually be tried first, because many of the medications commonly used for urinary incontinence have anticholinergic properties that can exacerbate confusion. Regularly scheduled bathroom breaks may be sufficient treatment in early stages of incontinence; protective pads or diapers may eventually be necessary.

Agitation should be treated with reassurance and redirection, but when the agitation is severe enough to be potentially dangerous to the patient or others, selective serotonin reuptake inhibitors (SSRIs) or antipsychotic agents may be necessary. The newer antipsychotic medications are less likely to exacerbate confusion or cause parkinsonism than the older drugs, but they are also associated with increased cardiac mortality. "Sundowning" and sleep disorders sometimes respond to light therapy. Safety issues are important, and access to stoves, power tools, driving, and even unsupervised walks should be individually discussed and monitored. Firearms should be stored securely.

Measures to ease the burden on caregivers are also critical. Families should be advised of community resources such as senior apartment complexes, home health aides, day care activities, visiting nurses, temporary respite programs, and (for more debilitated patients) full-time nursing care or nursing home placement. The availability of these resources depends on the community and the family's financial situation and insurance coverage, and families may wish to consult a social worker.

Patients should be encouraged to issue advance directives while they are still competent. Advance directives are documents expressing a person's wishes regarding medical, legal, and financial decisions. The two most common forms of advance directive are the living will and durable power of attorney. In a living will, an individual expresses personal preferences regarding specific situations (such as when they would want to be put on mechanical ventilation, if ever). With durable power of attorney, a person designates a surrogate who has the authority to make these decisions when the person is not competent to do so. Only people who are legally competent can create a living will or designate power of attorney, so these measures should not be deferred for too long. People who are legally competent can change or revoke these documents at any time.

B. Dementia with Lewy Bodies (DLB)

Lewy bodies are eosinophilic intracytoplasmic neuronal inclusions that were originally described in the substantia nigra and other subcortical locations in patients with Parkinson disease (PD), which is discussed at length in Chapter 8. Forty years after Lewy bodies were described in PD, they were found in the cortex of many patients with dementia. When researchers retrospectively reviewed the medical records of patients with these neuropathologic findings, they realized that these patients often exhibited clinical features that were not typical of AD. They concluded that the patients had a different disease, which is now called *dementia with Lewy bodies*, or DLB. Features that are characteristic of DLB and uncommon in AD are (1) recurrent visual hallucinations (typically well formed and detailed, often representing family members or other people they know) early in the course; (2) marked fluctuations in cognition or alertness; (3) REM sleep behavior disorder (see Chapter 9); and (4) parkinsonian features (see Chapter 8), especially rigidity and bradykinesia. Other features that are suggestive of DLB include (1) extreme sensitivity to antipsychotic medications; (2) repeated episodes of falling or loss of consciousness; (3) severe autonomic dysfunction; (4) systematized delusions or tactile or olfactory hallucinations; and (5) prominent depression. DLB appears to progress a little more rapidly than AD, but the pattern and time course of progression are variable.

In some cases, the diagnosis can be fairly straightforward, but at times DLB can be difficult to distinguish from AD or from PD, especially because many people with AD have parkinsonian features and many people with PD have dementia. Compared to people with AD, people with DLB tend to have less severe memory deficits and more severe impairment of visuospatial and executive functions. Whereas people with PD usually do not develop dementia until their disease has progressed to moderate or severe stages, people with DLB either present with dementia or develop it within a year of symptom onset. These distinctions are not always reliable, however. In fact, as discussed in Section A, some investigators believe that PD and DLB are just gradations along a spectrum of a single underlying disease process, or possibly the result of separate pathologic conditions whose clinical manifestations vary depending on which brain regions are most affected. Dopamine transporter (DAT) scans may be useful for differentiating AD and DLB, because basal ganglia uptake is typically reduced in DLB and normal in AD, but DAT scans don't distinguish between DLB and PD or other diseases that cause parkinsonism. Certain abnormalities on nuclear medicine scans of the heart are also characteristic of DLB.

The neurochemical abnormalities in DLB resemble a composite of those that occur in AD and PD. There is a dopaminergic deficit in cortical and subcortical areas due to loss of substantia nigra neurons, and a severe cortical cholinergic deficit related to loss of neurons in the nucleus basalis of Meynert. The cause of DLB is unknown, but Lewy bodies are obvious candidates for investigation. Biological characteristics of Lewy bodies and their principal component, the protein α-synuclein, are discussed in Chapter 8.

Cholinesterase inhibitors can produce some cognitive improvement in patients with DLB, and they are sometimes effective for hallucinations and delusions in these patients. Small studies have also found memantine to be modestly effective. Levodopa and dopamine agonists are much less reliably effective in DLB than in PD, and the magnitude of benefit is usually less dramatic, but it is still reasonable to try them when parkinsonian features interfere with the patient's function. One study found that a low dose of the antiseizure medication zonisamide was effective as an adjunct to levodopa. The same symptomatic treatment modalities used for AD also are used for DLB, except that if at all possible antipsychotic agents should be avoided because of the risk of severe sensitivity. If these medications are unavoidable, it is probably best to use one of the agents with fewer extrapyramidal side effects, such as clozapine (Clozaril), quetiapine (Seroquel), olanzapine (Zyprexa), or pimavanserin (Nuplazid), and to start with very low doses. Sleep disorders should be managed as they would be in other patients.

C. Frontotemporal Dementia (FTD)

Frontotemporal dementia (FTD), as the name implies, is characterized by degeneration that predominantly involves the frontal and temporal lobes, in contrast with the predominant temporal and parietal lobe involvement in AD. The age of onset tends to be younger than for AD, but it can also begin at older ages. About two thirds of people with FTD present with a behavioral syndrome, and one third with PPA (20% with the nonfluent/agrammatic subtype and 12% with the semantic subtype). These syndromes are discussed above (Part II, Section C) and in Table 7.1. Typical features of the behavioral syndrome are behavioral disinhibition, apathy/

inertia, reduced sympathy or empathy, perseveration, hyperorality/dietary changes, and reduced executive function; the pathology begins primarily in paralimbic structures and gradually spreads anteriorly toward the dorsolateral prefrontal cortex and posteriorly toward the anterior and lateral temporal lobes bilaterally. As discussed in Chapter 6, many people with ALS develop cognitive and behavioral symptoms suggestive of FTD, and many people with FTD develop features of motor neuron disease. FTD can also overlap two movement disorders discussed in Chapter 8, progressive supranuclear palsy (PSP) and corticobasal degeneration (CBD).

The characteristic pathologic findings of FTD are atrophy within the frontal and temporal lobes, with neuronal loss, gliosis, dystrophic neurites, and ubiquitinated protein inclusions. Ubiquitin is a component of the principal cellular mechanism for degrading and eliminating proteins that have become unfolded or misfolded. Just as the clinical manifestations of FTD are heterogeneous, so are the microscopic findings—in particular, the specific proteins that are ubiquitinated vary. In the largest subgroup of patients, the inclusions contain transactivation response DNA binding protein of 43 kDa, or TDP-43. In the second largest subgroup, they contain tau protein. In most of the remaining patients, the inclusions contain the "fused in sarcoma" (FUS) protein. As discussed in Chapter 6, TDP-43 inclusions are also present in the motor neurons of most patients with ALS, and in the muscle fibers of patients with inclusion body myositis. As discussed in Section A, tau protein is found in the neurofibrillary tangles of AD. Tau protein also accumulates in two of the movement disorders discussed in Chapter 8, PSP and CBD. The term "Pick disease" refers to a subgroup of people with the behavioral syndrome presentation of FTD in whom the tau protein is located in neuronal inclusions known as Pick bodies, and the atrophic regions of brain contain swollen neurons. The swollen neurons in Pick disease are similar to those seen in CBD, which is also characterized by accumulation of tau protein (see Chapter 8).

Although most cases of FTD are sporadic, some are familial, usually with an autosomal dominant inheritance pattern. Expanded hexanucleotide repeats in the chromosome 9 open reading frame 72 (C9ORF72) are commonly associated with familial FTD, just as they are with familial ALS (see Chapter 6). Most of the remaining cases of familial FTD are associated with mutations in the gene encoding tau protein or in the gene encoding a protein known as progranulin. Patients with mutations in C9ORF72 or the gene for progranulin have inclusions containing TDP-43, and patients with mutations in the gene for tau have inclusions containing the tau protein.

Mutations in other genes (including the genes encoding TDP-43 and FUS/ TLS, which have also been associated with some cases of familial ALS) are rare causes of FTD.

Some clinicopathologic correlations have emerged. Manifestations of ALS occur primarily in patients with TDP-43 inclusions and sometimes in patients with FUS inclusions, but not in patients with tau inclusions. Patients with the semantic subtype of PPA most often have TDP-43 inclusions and rarely have tau inclusions, whereas the nonfluent agrammatic subtype is generally associated with tau inclusions (but not necessarily with FTD—patients with this subtype of PPA are more likely to have pathologic findings of PSP or CBD, two movement disorders characterized by tau inclusions, than they are to have findings of FTD). Any of the three types of inclusion can be found in patients with the behavioral subtype of FTD.

The diagnosis of FTD is based primarily on the clinical presentation and the exclusion of other diseases that can produce a similar pattern (such as herpes simplex encephalitis, brain tumors, or chronic subdural hematomas). Neuroimaging studies show a frontotemporal distribution of atrophy and hypometabolism, with a distinct pattern for each of the three major clinical subtypes. The Centers for Medicare and Medicaid Services will reimburse FDG-PET studies when obtained to distinguish FTD from dementia due to AD, but not all insurance carriers will do so.

FTD is steadily progressive. On average, it progresses more rapidly than AD, but the rate of progression varies. The course is most rapid in patients with associated features of ALS. No specific treatment is available for FTD. There is no indication that cholinesterase inhibitors are beneficial. Behavioral management is often the most prominent practical issue.

D. Vascular Cognitive Impairment

The term *vascular cognitive impairment* encompasses a broad range of conditions. Individual strokes often result in cognitive deficits, whether the stroke is ischemic or hemorrhagic, and regardless of whether the underlying pathology is arteriolosclerosis, atherosclerosis, or amyloid angiopathy (see Chapter 4). When people have multiple strokes, the cognitive deficits can accumulate, leading to clinical syndromes that can range from mild cognitive impairment to dementia. In some cases, the contribution of vascular disease to the cognitive syndrome is clear-cut; for example, a person might develop right hemiparesis and aphasia with imaging that confirms a stroke in the territory of the left MCA, and a few years later develop left hemiparesis, left-sided neglect, and visuospatial impairment with imaging showing a stroke in the territory of the right MCA, and a few years after that develop a right visual field defect and worsening language and visuospatial function with imaging showing a stroke in the territory of the left PCA. In other cases, the role of vascular disease is more speculative. For example, some people have cognitive deficits that began abruptly and accumulated in a stepwise manner and they have focal abnormalities on neurologic examination or brain imaging studies, but their episodes of cognitive decline were never accompanied by focal neurologic symptoms. The relationship between cognitive symptoms and vascular disease is also tenuous when people have a clear history of strokes, but the progression of their dementia does not correspond to the timing of the strokes. The strokes may be the cause of the dementia, or they may be coincidental. The strokes could also be exacerbating an underlying (possibly unrecognized) dementia from some other cause, such as AD. At autopsy, many patients have pathologic features of both AD and strokes. Similar diagnostic uncertainty results when people with dementia have radiologic findings that suggest chronic ischemic changes, but there is no evidence of clinical strokes on history or neurologic examination. In many cases, a definitive diagnosis of vascular cognitive impairment is impossible, and clinicians can only draw conclusions about its relative likelihood. Factors that increase the likelihood that vascular disease is contributing to a patient's cognitive deficits include: a history of clinically recognizable strokes, focal abnormalities on the neurologic examination, a history of stroke risk factors, abrupt onset and stepwise progression of the cognitive impairment, and brain imaging studies that suggest multiple ischemic lesions. To further complicate the issue, evidence suggests that vascular disease and vascular risk factors may be involved in the pathogenesis of AD, even in the absence of strokes.

The clinical features of vascular cognitive impairment are extremely variable and depend on the timing, location, and size of the strokes. In principle, progression can be halted completely if future strokes can be prevented, so these patients are candidates for all of the primary and secondary stroke prevention measures discussed in Chapter 4, as appropriate. Endarterectomy or stenting for more than 70% cervical carotid stenosis should only be considered in individuals who have experienced a clinically recognizable stroke in the territory of that carotid in the previous 6 months (i.e., the same recommendation as for people without vascular cognitive impairment).

Randomized controlled trials of cholinesterase inhibitors have shown that their use results in modest cognitive improvement in patients with dementia attributed to vascular cognitive impairment, so it is usually reasonable to try one of these medications. Otherwise, most treatment is symptomatic. The same considerations that apply to AD in that regard are relevant to patients with vascular dementia.

E. Limbic-Predominant Age-Related TDP-43 Encephalopathy (LATE)

Some older patients with a memory-predominant presentation of dementia are found at autopsy to have TDP-43 aggregates similar to those that occur in FTD or ALS, but they are concentrated in limbic regions, especially the amygdala, hippocampus, and middle frontal gyrus. Many of these people also have hippocampal sclerosis (profound neuron loss and gliosis). This condition is called limbic-predominant age-related TDP-43 encephalopathy (LATE). It mainly occurs in people older than 80 years, and in that age range it is present in 20–40% of people with dementia. Many of these people also have pathologic findings of AD. It is impossible to distinguish between pure AD, pure LATE, and mixed AD/LATE based on clinical features. The absence of Aβ-peptide accumulation on imaging or corresponding CSF findings in someone with memory-predominant dementia who is older than 80 years would be evidence for pure LATE, but it is unclear that this determination is necessary because there is no known treatment for LATE. An alternative approach would be to treat patients empirically as if they had AD. Retrospective review of the clinical course of people who had diagnoses established at autopsy indicates that the rate of cognitive decline is faster in people with pure AD than it is in people with pure LATE, but fastest of all in people with mixed AD/LATE.

F. Creutzfeldt-Jakob Disease (CJD)

Creutzfeldt-Jakob disease (CJD) is an extremely rare condition that is of interest principally because of its public health implications and its distinctive molecular and cellular features. It is characterized by a rapidly progressive dementia that leads to death within months to a year (average: 7 months). It usually affects people in the age range 50–70 years. During the first few weeks to months, patients typically have discrete neurologic or psychiatric symptoms, such as change in appetite, altered sleep pattern, loss of libido, loss of energy, memory problems, difficulty concentrating, poor problem solving, inappropriate behavior, emotional lability, or self-neglect. Over the next few months, cognitive function deteriorates rapidly, and most people develop frequent myoclonic jerks. Many also demonstrate signs of cerebellar dysfunction such as ataxia and dysarthria, and about a third have significant behavioral disturbance or psychosis. In the final stages, patients become progressively more withdrawn and ultimately enter a state of akinetic mutism. In one variant of the disease, cerebellar symptoms are prominent early in the course. In another variant, visual symptoms predominate and may be the only symptoms at first. Another variant is marked by early muscle wasting and fasciculations that can mimic motor neuron disease. The typical neuropathologic findings are widespread neuronal loss and vacuolation, producing a spongy appearance, so CJD is often referred to as a *spongiform encephalopathy*.

CJD is usually sporadic, but 5–15% of cases are familial. Under certain rare conditions, the disease can be transmitted. The transmissible pathogen is a protein known as a prion (derived from the phrase "proteinaceous infectious particle"). The unique feature of this pathogen is that, unlike a virus or any other previously described infectious agent, it contains no nucleic acid. The prion protein is actually a misfolded form of a protein (referred to as PrP^C) that is located on the outer surface of cells in healthy individuals. The pathogenic form of this protein (referred to as PrP^{Sc}) has the same amino acid sequence but a different conformation, resulting in a dramatic change in physical-chemical properties, including increased resistance to proteinases, reduced solubility in detergents, and increased tendency to polymerize and aggregate to produce amyloid. The physiologic role of the normal cellular prion protein, PrP^C, is not known. For all three modes of transmission (hereditary, sporadic, and transmitted), a critical feature of disease propagation is that PrP^{Sc} has the ability to bind to PrP^C and induce it to change conformation and convert to PrP^{Sc}. Similar induction by misfolded proteins has been proposed as a mechanism of disease propagation for a variety of degenerative diseases, including AD, FTD, PD, and ALS (see Sections A and C, and also Chapters 6 and 8).

It is not clear what triggers the sporadic forms of CJD. The hereditary forms are caused by mutations in the gene encoding the prion protein (thus, unlike the sporadic forms of CJD, in which the pathogenic protein has the same amino acid sequence as the normal protein, in the hereditary forms of CJD the pathogenic protein differs from the normal protein by one amino acid). Most of the documented cases of human transmission of prion diseases have involved situations in which individuals were exposed to high concentrations of substances derived from the nervous systems of affected individuals. Kuru, a prion disease (with clinical manifestations similar to those of CJD) that was once endemic among the Fore tribe of Papua, New Guinea, was ultimately linked to cannibalism. Other cases have been attributed to human growth hormone derived from pooled pituitary tissue from cadavers, corneal transplants, contaminated surgical instruments, implanted EEG electrodes, and dural grafts.

The propagation of PrP^{Sc} often involves interactions with prion-associated proteins. These proteins differ between species, so transmission between species is even less common than transmission within species. Nonetheless, the species barrier is not insurmountable. In experimental animals, distinct patterns of disease are produced depending on the prion isolate used. A variant form of CJD that was first reported in Great Britain in 1996, affecting younger patients (mean age of onset: 28 years), with more prominent psychiatric manifestations and a longer survival time, is thought to be related to the ingestion of beef derived from cattle infected with bovine spongiform encephalopathy (BSE, so-called mad cow disease), a prion disease of cattle. Fortunately, the incidence of both BSE and variant CJD has declined dramatically since a peak in 2000. Four cases of likely transmission of variant CJD through blood transfusion have been documented; blood-borne transmission has never been proven for any other form of CJD.

Even though CJD is rare, it should be considered when a patient presents with very rapid progression of dementia, or with prominent myoclonus or ataxia early in the disease course (although myoclonus also occurs in other dementing illnesses). The most reliable diagnostic test is a CSF assay called real-time quaking-induced conversion (RT-QuIC), which has more than 90% sensitivity and nearly complete specificity. In this test, a sample of the patient's CSF is seeded with recombinant PrP^C; if there is PrP^{Sc} present in the CSF, it will induce conversion of the PrP^C into PrP^{Sc}, which polymerizes into amyloid fibrils that are detected with an ultrasensitive fluorescence assay. Certain MRI scan findings (cortical or basal ganglia hyperintensities that are typically more prominent on diffusion-weighted sequences than on FLAIR sequences) have more than 90% sensitivity and specificity for sporadic CJD when the scans are interpreted by experienced neuroradiologists. Other tests that can be informative include EEG (which shows periodic complexes occurring about once a second in about two thirds of individuals with sporadic CJD) and CSF levels of tau protein, 14-3-3 protein (a protein found in the cytoplasm of central nervous system neurons and thought to have a chaperone function in intracellular signal transduction pathways), and a protein called neuron-specific enolase, but these tests are less sensitive and specific than RT-QuIC and MRI. The MRI, EEG, and CSF tau, 14-3-3, and neuron-specific enolase abnormalities that are typical of sporadic CJD are much less common in the inherited or transmitted forms of CJD. One MRI finding known as the pulvinar sign is typical of variant CJD, but it is neither specific nor entirely sensitive. When test results are unclear, a brain biopsy (or autopsy) may be necessary; special precautions are required in performing these procedures and handling the specimens, to minimize risk of transmission. There is no known treatment for CJD, but if the diagnosis can be established, important prognostic information can be delivered to the family.

Some of the autoimmune encephalopathies and paraneoplastic syndromes discussed in Chapter 10 (Part III, Section A) can be very difficult to distinguish from CJD. Because those conditions respond to treatment and CJD is rapidly fatal regardless of treatment, it is sometimes reasonable to try an empiric course of immunosuppressive therapy even when CJD is the most likely diagnosis.

G. Other Neurologic Diseases That Produce Dementia

Dementia is common in PD, as discussed earlier. Some other movement disorders that typically produce dementia are discussed in Chapter 8. In addition to the strong connections between FTD and motor neuron disease, other neuromuscular disorders—including some forms of muscular dystrophy and some myopathies—are sometimes associated with dementia. Dementia can also occur with multiple sclerosis, other inflammatory diseases of the nervous system, and some epileptic syndromes. In most cases, the diagnosis is apparent from the constellation of neurologic abnormalities, and the underlying disease process dictates management.

IV. Supplementary Tables for Reference

Table 7.1 Primary Progressive Aphasia (PPA) Subtypes

	Nonfluent/ Agrammatic	Logopenic Variant	Semantic Variant
Fluency	Severely impaired	Mildly impaired (mainly due to word-finding pauses)	Intact
Grammar	Simplified	Normal	Normal
Naming errors	-Phonemic paraphasias -More trouble with verbs than nouns	Phonemic paraphasias	-Semantic paraphasias -Circumlocutions -More trouble with nouns than verbs
Repetition	Mildly/moderately impaired	-Severely impaired -Intact for single words	Intact
Auditory comprehension	-Intact for single words and simple sentences -Impaired for complex syntax	-Intact for single words -Impaired for some complex constructions	Difficulty with single words, especially less frequently encountered ones (e.g., leopard)
Reading/spelling	Intact	Difficulty with irregular words and pseudowords	Patients read (and spell) irregular words phonetically
Localization	-Left posterior and inferior frontal -Left insula -Left premotor cortex -Left supplementary motor area	-Left temporoparietal junction -Left posterior perisylvian	Bilateral (left > right) ventrolateral anterior temporal lobes
Pathology	Most often tau accumulation (PSP or CBD; see Chapter 8)	Most often AD (plaques and tangles)	-Most often TDP-43 accumulation (FTD) -Sometimes AD -Sometimes tau accumulation (FTD)

Table 7.2 Posterior Cortical Atrophy Subtypes

	Dorsal Variant	Ventral Variant	Caudal Variant
Characteristic clinical features	-Balint syndrome -Apraxia -Difficulty with calculation -Difficulty writing -Left/right disorientation	-Difficulty reading (dyslexia) -Difficulty recognizing faces (prosopagnosia)	Visual field defects
Localization	-Bilateral superior parietal lobule -Sometimes left angular gyrus -Sometimes right lateral parietal lobe	-Bilateral occipitotemporal	-Occipital
Pathology	Most often AD	Most often AD	Most often AD

Table 7.3 Characteristic Protein Aggregates, Mutations Causing Familial Forms, and Clinical Presentations of Dementing Illnesses

	Aggregated Protein	Mutations When Familial	Clinical Presentations
Alzheimer disease (AD)	-Aβ-peptide (in plaques) -Tau (in tangles)	-*Presenilin 1* (encodes a γ-secretase component) -Gene for amyloid precursor protein (*APP*) -*Presenilin 2* (encodes a γ-secretase component)	-Memory-predominant syndrome (most common) -Posterior cortical atrophy -PPA, logopenic variant -Behavioral syndrome -Dysexecutive syndrome
Dementia with Lewy bodies (DLB)	α-Synuclein (in Lewy bodies; see Chapter 8)	N.A.	-Dysexecutive syndrome, vision deficits, memory problems, parkinsonism, hallucinations, REM-sleep behavior disorder

(continued)

Table 7.3 Continued

	Aggregated Protein	Mutations When Familial	Clinical Presentations
Frontotemporal dementia (FTD)	TDP-43	-C9ORF72 -Gene for progranulin	-PPA, semantic variant; sometimes with ALS features
	Tau (in Pick bodies)	Gene for tau	Behavioral syndrome
	Tau (without Pick bodies)	Gene for tau	-Behavioral syndrome -PPA, nonfluent/ agrammatic
	FUS	N.A. (not familial)	PPA, semantic variant; sometimes with ALS features
Limbic-predominant age-related TDP-43 encephalopathy (LATE)	TDP-43	N.A.	Memory-predominant syndrome
Creutzfeldt-Jakob disease (CJD)	PrP^{Sc}	Gene for PrP^{C}	Rapidly progressive amnestic and behavioral syndromes; sometimes with predominant ataxia initially; sometimes with posterior cortical atrophy symptoms initially

V. Discussion of Case Histories

Case 1: This woman's presentation suggests a toxic delirium, rather than dementia. She is irritable, inattentive, and disoriented. She was apparently hallucinating when her daughter found her. Although people with dementia are at particular risk for delirium, many people with delirium have no underlying dementia. Until the delirium has been effectively managed, and the woman's sensorium is no longer clouded, it is impossible to determine whether she has dementia. Patients with delirium most often have a toxic or metabolic problem. Initial evaluation should include electrolytes, a search for underlying infection, and a drug screen to evaluate for opiates/opioids or other contributing agents.

In this case, medications are probably a major component of her delirium. Elderly people are very susceptible to the cognitive effects of a number of drugs, including opiates/opioids, H2-blockers, anticholinergics, tricyclic antidepressants, and phenothiazines. They are quite sensitive to benzodiazepines, particularly those with longer half-lives, like flurazepam. Besides taking flurazepam and pain medication, this woman is taking an H2-blocker, a beta-blocker, and another antihypertensive medication. She also has a urinary tract infection, which can cause fairly severe confusion in the geriatric population.

If this woman has residual cognitive deficits after simplifying her medication regimen and treating her urinary tract infection, she may need further evaluation for dementia. Vascular cognitive impairment is a particular consideration in view of her asymmetric reflexes and history of hypertension, so an MRI scan would be appropriate, in addition to blood tests for thyroid disease and vitamin B12 deficiency. She has already been tested for other potentially reversible causes of dementia. Baseline neuropsychological testing might be helpful in monitoring for future progression.

Comment: All of the woman's medications were stopped and she was managed with calcium channel blockers and nonsteroidals. Her urinary tract infection was treated with a single dose of trimethoprim/sulfamethoxazole. Her mental status cleared completely, and no further tests were performed. She continued to have normal cognitive function at her subsequent clinic visits.

Case 2: This man has a typical history of moderately advanced dementia due to AD. He has a prominent memory disturbance with associated language disturbance, visuospatial deficits, and delusions. Social skills remain relatively intact. Although the delusions raise the possibility of DLB or FTD, he has no parkinsonian features, personality changes, or disproportionate language dysfunction. Formal neuropsychological testing might be useful to demonstrate to him that there is objective evidence of cognitive impairment and that his wife is not just "making mountains out of anthills." Such testing could also identify his areas of relative strength. An imaging study is important to look for structural lesions, but these are unlikely given his history and nonfocal examination. This patient should have the standard laboratory tests to look for a potentially reversible cause of dementia. Hearing should also be assessed to see if it is contributing to problems understanding spoken language. Assuming no other cause of dementia is identified, he most likely has AD and should begin taking a cholinesterase inhibitor. Once it is clear that he is tolerating the cholinesterase inhibitor, memantine should be added.

Other issues that must be addressed in patients with progressive dementia include safety, behavior problems, and family support. The patient should have a formal assessment of his driving ability. Consideration should be given to whether he should operate tools, cook, or handle any financial matters. The wife's ability to care for the patient and meet her own needs in this situation should be tactfully assessed and support offered. The patient and family should be educated about the illness, and advance directives should be discussed.

Case 3: As with the patient in Case 1, this woman's presentation suggests a subacute delirium rather than dementia. The salient features are intermittent sleepiness, disorientation, and poor processing of new material. Again, as with the patient in Case 1, it is impossible to determine if this patient has an underlying dementia until her clouded sensorium has been successfully treated. In any patient who has delirium, primary considerations are metabolic abnormalities (especially drug-related) and infectious or inflammatory processes.

Comment: This woman had no history of previous medical problems, medication use, or substance use that might have provided clues to the cause of her current delirium, and screening lab tests (comprehensive metabolic profile, complete blood count, and differential) were normal. A brain MRI scan was also normal. Because of the concern that her episodes of unresponsiveness might be seizures, she had long-term EEG monitoring. This confirmed that she was, in fact, having seizures, so levetiracetam was started. Her delirium cleared—she was no longer sleepy and the spells of unresponsiveness resolved—but her memory continued to get worse. The rapidly progressive dementia, the occurrence of seizures early in the course, and the 15-kg weight loss prompted her physicians to evaluate her for a paraneoplastic syndrome (see Chapter 10, Part III, Section A). A lumbar puncture was notable for elevated spinal fluid protein, a serum antibody panel was positive for antineuronal nuclear antibody-1 (ANNA-1), and a chest CT revealed small-cell carcinoma of the lung. Her memory improved with treatment of the underlying tumor but did not return to baseline.

Chapter 8

Movement Disorders

Linda M. Selwa and Douglas J. Gelb

I. Case Histories

Case 1. A 70-year-old woman being seen for health care maintenance says that she has been experiencing "shakiness" in her left hand for about 6 months. She also says that she has lost a lot of her previous energy and motivation. She no longer attends conferences that once occupied much of her time and energy, and she has limited her gardening activities significantly this year. She tells you, "It's no fun getting old." She takes no medications. Her general physical examination is normal. She presents her history clearly and concisely and responds appropriately to questions and instructions. Her cranial nerves are normal except for a rather expressionless face, with no clear facial weakness. She has a slight stoop, but no postural instability. Her stride is normal. She has decreased arm swing on the left, and she turns en bloc in four steps. Her finger movements are slow but normally coordinated. She has a prominent rest tremor in the left arm that improves with volitional movement. There is some cogwheel rigidity on the left. She has normal strength, reflexes, and sensation.

Questions:

1. What would you tell this woman about her diagnosis?
2. What potential complications should be addressed at this stage?
3. What therapy is appropriate?

Case 2. A 59-year-old woman has been experiencing generalized weakness and bilateral upper extremity tremor for the last 3 months. She has fallen twice but thinks this was just because she tripped. She reports abdominal bloating and weight loss. She has diabetes that has been difficult to manage. She also has numbness in her feet and wonders whether

her foot problem is causing some of her unsteadiness. Medications include thyroid hormone replacement, insulin, metoclopramide (Reglan), and diltiazem (Cardizem). On examination, she has normal mental status and cranial nerves, though her face is expressionless. Her gait is festinating and slow, with reduced arm swing bilaterally. There is mild postural instability. She has marked bradykinesia, rigidity, and a mild bilateral rest tremor. There is full strength in all muscle groups. Her reflexes are normal in the upper extremities and at the knees but can only be elicited at the ankles with reinforcement. Except for some mild reduction of vibration sense at the toes bilaterally, she has normal sensation throughout.

Questions:

1. How would you proceed with the evaluation?
2. Does she need evaluation for peripheral polyneuropathy?
3. What is the most appropriate treatment for this woman?

II. Approach to Movement Disorders

The term *movement disorder* refers to a heterogeneous group of conditions that result in abnormal form or timing of voluntary movement in individuals with normal strength and sensation. Appropriate management of a patient with a movement disorder depends on the answers to five questions:

1. How can the movements be characterized?
2. Are the movements due to a potentially reversible systemic cause, such as an endocrine disorder, a rheumatologic condition, or medication toxicity?
3. Do the abnormal movements and accompanying abnormalities conform to a recognized condition?
4. What oral medications are likely to help this condition?
5. If the patient's condition can't be controlled adequately with oral medications, are injections or surgical interventions feasible?

Question 1 is addressed in Part III. Questions 2, 3, 4, and 5 are addressed in Part IV.

III. Background Information

A. Anatomic Definitions

Basal ganglia: caudate, putamen, globus pallidus, substantia nigra, and subthalamic nucleus

Corpus striatum: caudate, putamen, and globus pallidus [this term is rarely used by clinicians]
Lentiform nucleus (also called the *lenticular nucleus*): putamen plus globus pallidus
Striatum: caudate and putamen (synonym: *neostriatum*)

B. Clinical Definitions

action tremor: a tremor that is most prominent on voluntary contraction of a muscle; this encompasses both postural tremor and kinetic tremor
akinesia: lack of voluntary movements

ataxia: incoordination or awkwardness in the performance of a voluntary motor task, resulting in misdirected or poorly timed movements

athetosis: slow, sinuous writhing of the distal parts of limbs—may accompany chorea, and is probably another point on the spectrum of clinical manifestations of the same pathophysiologic mechanism

ballism: large-amplitude, involuntary flinging movements of the proximal parts of limbs—probably another point on the spectrum (with chorea and athetosis) of clinical manifestations of a single pathophysiologic mechanism

bradykinesia: reduced spontaneity, amplitude, and speed of voluntary movements; sometimes referred to as *hypokinesia*

chorea: rapid, irregular, unpredictable, often jerky involuntary movements appearing in various body parts, sometimes seeming to "flow" from one region to another. See *athetosis* and *ballism*

cogwheeling: ratchet-like, rhythmic interruptions in resistance to passive manipulation

decrement: a progressive decline in the amplitude of a sustained or repetitive movement (such as finger tapping)

dystonia: involuntary, tonically or intermittently sustained muscle contractions often having a preferred direction, resulting in maintenance of an abnormal posture or repetitive movements that are typically patterned and twisting and may be tremulous

festination: an involuntary tendency for a movement to accelerate as it decreases in amplitude; usually applied to gait

intention tremor: a kinetic tremor that is most prominent on approaching the target of a goal-directed movement (i.e., a *terminal kinetic tremor*)

kinetic tremor: an action tremor that is present during guided voluntary movement (such as handwriting or touching finger to nose). Kinetic tremor can be subdivided into *initial tremor* (occurring predominantly at the initiation of movement), *transition tremor* (predominantly during the movement), or *terminal tremor* (predominantly at the termination of movement). See *intention tremor*

myoclonus: rapid shock-like muscle jerks similar to chorea, but more discrete (less likely to blend into one another) and more likely to be localized

parkinsonism: some combination of bradykinesia, rigidity, and rest tremor; typical of idiopathic Parkinson disease, also present in many other conditions

postural tremor: an action tremor that is most prominent when the body part is maintained in a non-resting posture (such as keeping the arms extended parallel to the floor), less prominent when the body part is completely relaxed

rest tremor: tremor that is most prominent when the body part is in complete repose and not working against gravity, less prominent with movement or maintenance of a posture (also called *resting tremor*)

rigidity: increased resistance to passive manipulation throughout the range of movement, equal in flexors and extensors, and independent of the velocity of movement

task-specific tremor: kinetic tremor that appears or is exacerbated during certain tasks, such as writing, but is absent or attenuated when not engaged in those tasks

tics: abrupt, transient, stereotyped, coordinated movements or vocalizations that are associated with a premonitory urge; they can often be voluntarily suppressed but at the expense of a buildup of inner tension that is relieved when the suppression ends

tremor: involuntary rhythmic oscillation of a body part, produced by either alternating or synchronous contractions of reciprocally innervated antagonist muscles

C. Classification of Movement Disorders

Movement disorders are closely associated with dysfunction of the cerebellum and basal ganglia, which can be thought of as a brain system devoted to the implementation of motor plans developed in the cortex. The basal ganglia consist of the striatum (the caudate and putamen), the globus pallidus, the substantia nigra, and the subthalamic nucleus. Movement disorders can be grouped into three general categories, *hypokinetic, hyperkinetic,* and *ataxic.*

The hallmark of hypokinetic movement disorders is parkinsonism, which is characterized by bradykinesia, rigidity, and rest tremor. It correlates with disruption of striatal dopaminergic transmission, improves with enhancement of dopamine transmission, and worsens in response to dopamine antagonism.

Hyperkinetic movement disorders are characterized by involuntary movements that intrude into the normal flow of motor acts. Chorea, athetosis, and ballism may all represent points on a spectrum of clinical manifestations of the same underlying pathophysiologic mechanism. These movements correlate with dysfunction within the striatum or the subthalamic nucleus. They are suppressed by dopamine antagonism and exacerbated by increased dopaminergic transmission. Postural and kinetic tremors may be due to abnormalities of cerebellar outflow to the thalamus. Dystonia is marked by twisting and repetitive movements or sustained abnormal postures, often with a preferred direction. Dystonia is classified as focal (involving specific, localized muscle groups), segmental (involving two or more contiguous areas of the body), multifocal (involving two or more noncontiguous areas), hemidystonia (involving one side of the body), or generalized (involving the entire body). Dystonia is thought to be due to dysfunction in the basal ganglia-sensorimotor network and the cerebellothalamocortical pathway. No drug consistently improves or exacerbates dystonia. Tics are also classified as hyperkinetic movement disorders.

Ataxic movement disorders are characterized by irregularities of speed and accuracy when performing acts requiring the smoothly coordinated activity of several muscles. Typical features include dysmetria (inaccurate trajectory of a body part during active movements), dysrhythmokinesis (inability to move a body part in a regular rhythm), dysdiadochokinesis (impaired speed, precision, and rhythm when performing rapidly alternating movements), difficulty correcting for perturbations of body position, unstable gait, and dysarthria (characterized by irregular variations in the rate, volume, and pitch of speech). These abnormalities correlate with dysfunction of the cerebellum or its connections. As mentioned above, abnormalities of cerebellar outflow are also associated with tremor.

IV. Specific Movement Disorders

A. Essential Tremor

Essential tremor is a common movement disorder characterized by action tremor—usually both postural and kinetic—of both upper extremities without other neurologic abnormalities such as parkinsonism, dystonia, or ataxia (current criteria stipulate that the tremor must have been present for at least 3 years before essential tremor can be diagnosed to ensure that these other neurologic abnormalities are truly absent). The tremor may be asymmetric, and at onset it may be unilateral. With time, there may be an associated tremor of the jaw, head, voice, or lower extremities (but tremor of the head, jaw, or voice without arm tremor is *not* consistent with essential tremor; instead, it is most often a manifestation of dystonia). Many cases are familial. Generally, symptoms are mild and associated with only minor progression over decades, but in some cases the condition is disabling enough to interfere with writing, dressing, and eating. Essential tremor often responds transiently to ethanol consumption.

Postmortem studies suggest that the pathophysiologic processes underlying essential tremor involve the cerebellum, especially the Purkinje cells, basket cells, and climbing fibers, but the abnormalities are not visible on standard diagnostic imaging. The diagnosis of essential tremor is established primarily on the basis of a typical history and examination and the absence of other causes of tremor. Before diagnosing essential tremor, hyperthyroidism should be excluded. Beta-adrenergic agonists, lithium, valproic acid, cyclosporine, tacrolimus, tamoxifen, amiodarone, and thyroxine commonly cause action tremor. Selective serotonin reuptake inhibitors and tricyclic antidepressant medications can also cause tremor. Caffeine, amphetamines, nicotine, and cocaine can all cause postural or kinetic tremor.

Once they have been reassured that the condition is not life-threatening (and that they do not have Parkinson disease), many patients say that the tremor is tolerable and they do not need treatment. When the tremor causes significant embarrassment or interferes with their daily activities, medication should be prescribed. Beta-adrenergic blockers (particularly propranolol) and primidone are the most consistently effective agents. Topiramate was also found to be beneficial in controlled trials; the evidence is more limited for other beta-blockers, gabapentin, benzodiazepines, and botulinum toxin injections. For severe, refractory essential tremor, surgical implantation of a deep brain stimulator in the ventral intermediate nucleus of the thalamus contralateral to the affected limb produces dramatic improvement in approximately 85% of patients. The mechanism by which high-frequency stimulation reduces tremor is unclear. Ablative surgery of the same site is also effective, but less commonly used. Promising results have also been reported with magnetic resonance–guided focused ultrasound to the same site.

B. Parkinson Disease (PD)

1. Clinical features

The cardinal signs of Parkinson disease (PD) are bradykinesia, rest tremor, rigidity, and (eventually) postural instability. These combine to produce characteristic manifestations. One is *decrement*, a tendency toward progressively decreasing amplitude when carrying out a sustained motor activity. This may be accompanied by a rise in rate, called *festination*, as if the person is trying to compensate for the reduced amplitude by increasing the frequency. This term is most often used to describe a distinctive gait in which the steps get smaller and smaller and faster and faster until the patient is practically running in place (anyone who has ever hit the accelerator of a car stuck in snow, only to find the wheels spinning ineffectively, can relate to this phenomenon). Similarly, people with PD often have *micrographia*, or small handwriting, which gets progressively smaller toward the end of a writing sample. The motor control of speech is also subject to this phenomenon—people with PD typically speak at low volumes, with their speech growing progressively softer and more rapid the longer they talk. This type of *dysarthria* is classified as hypokinetic. Another typical manifestation is reduced facial expression and blinking rate (a *masked face*). As the disease progresses, the postural instability and rigidity may cause patients to *turn en bloc* when walking: rather than pivot 180 degrees in a single step, they make many small angular adjustments while standing in one place, as if they are standing on a small, raised platform surrounded by water. In advanced stages of the disease, patients often have particular difficulty initiating movement, appearing totally "frozen," but after intense effort they set themselves in motion and then proceed to carry out the movement almost normally. Sometimes the initiation of movement can be facilitated by placing an obstacle in their way; it can be quite striking to watch a patient fixed in one spot suddenly begin walking normally when asked to step over the examiner's foot. A similar phenomenon is described in a sudden emergency, such as a fire, in which patients have even been observed to run. Unfortunately, this type of facilitation is only temporary; Before long, the steps become smaller and faster, and the patient often gets stuck again.

The characteristic tremor of PD is a rest tremor with a frequency of 4–6 Hz, and in the hands there is classically a "pill-rolling" character. The tremor usually becomes less prominent with voluntary movement, but a "re-emergent" tremor often appears about 5–10 seconds after adopting a new posture. In contrast, some people with PD have a low-amplitude postural or kinetic tremor of 7–8 Hz. Some people with PD have both of these types of tremor. Either type of tremor may fluctuate dramatically from one moment to the next, independent of medication regimen. The tremor, rigidity, and bradykinesia often begin in a single limb, gradually progressing to involve the other limb on the same side, and eventually to the other side of the body.

As discussed in Chapter 7, the majority of people with PD who survive long enough eventually develop dementia (often with a prodrome of MCI). Depending on when they present, it can be difficult to distinguish someone who has dementia as a result of PD from someone who has DLB or even from someone with AD who also has parkinsonian features. Up to 60% of people with PD experience delusions or hallucinations at some point in the course. These are often related to drug therapy; they sometimes occur in untreated patients, but this should prompt consideration of DLB. Depression occurs in up to 50% of people with PD. It appears to be a direct manifestation of the underlying neuropathologic changes, and not just a reaction to the disabling symptoms. Pain is often an early feature of PD, and so is olfactory dysfunction. Sleep disorders and some degree of autonomic dysfunction are very common. In fact, REM sleep behavior disorder (see Chapter 9) may precede other manifestations of PD by many years. Constipation is frequently present in the years prior to diagnosis, also. PD is uncommon below the age of 50 years, but it affects about 1% of individuals above that age; the incidence is slightly higher in males than in females (1.5:1).

2. Pathology and etiology
Pathologically, PD is characterized by diffuse loss of pigmented neurons in the pars compacta of the substantia nigra, associated with a deficit of dopamine production in the nigrostriatal pathway. Surviving neurons often contain characteristic inclusions known as Lewy bodies, which are also present in the locus ceruleus and several other discrete nuclei. The principal component of Lewy bodies is α-synuclein, a protein that helps to maintain the integrity of neurotransmitter-bearing vesicles and facilitates their transport. Several other proteins are present in Lewy bodies, including ubiquitin. As explained in Chapter 7 (in the discussion of FTD), the ubiquitin-proteasome system

is the principal cellular mechanism for degrading and eliminating proteins that have become unfolded or misfolded. A popular hypothesis, for which the evidence is suggestive but not definitive, holds that α-synuclein initially accumulates in the periphery, possibly in the enteric nervous system, and that the pathology then spreads to the medulla and olfactory bulb before ascending to the substantia nigra and eventually the cortex. Some researchers have suggested that this spread may be mediated by abnormal α-synuclein molecules inducing transformational change in nearby α-synuclein molecules, analogous to the propagation of prions (see Chapter 7).

The pathophysiology of PD is only partly understood. Both genetic and environmental factors play a role. Causative genes have been identified, but they account for only a small fraction of the incidence of PD. Numerous susceptibility genes influence the risk of developing sporadic PD. Environmental factors associated with an increased risk of developing PD include rural living, lifetime exposure to well water, head trauma, manganese, lead, and some pesticides and herbicides. In contrast, cigarette smoking and caffeine consumption are associated with a reduced risk of developing PD (this is one of the few health benefits ever attributed to smoking by anyone outside the tobacco industry). Diets high in fruits, vegetables, and fish; diets resulting in high serum urate levels; exercise; use of nonsteroidal anti-inflammatory drugs; and use of calcium channel blockers have also been reported to be associated with a reduced risk of developing PD, but the evidence is less conclusive. Based on these environmental associations, together with the products encoded by the causative genes and susceptibility genes, several factors appear to be important in the pathogenesis of Parkinson disease: impaired clearance of unwanted proteins (especially α-synuclein) by the ubiquitin-proteasome system, mitochondrial dysfunction, defective intracellular trafficking, abnormal calcium homeostasis, oxidative stress, excitotoxicity, and inflammation. Each of these factors could precipitate or exacerbate any of the others, and it is not clear if any one factor is more fundamental than the others.

3. Differential diagnosis

Drug-induced parkinsonism must be carefully considered in anyone thought to have PD, especially when symptom onset is acute or subacute. Early withdrawal of the offending agent is important. Parkinsonism is a frequent side effect of antipsychotic medications (including phenothiazines and butyrophenones) and antiemetic medications (such as metoclopramide, prochlorperazine, and promethazine). Less commonly, parkinsonism may be caused by reserpine, tetrabenazine and other catecholamine-depleting agents, some calcium channel blockers, valproic acid, amiodarone, and some immunosuppressants; it can also occur after manganese poisoning or exposure to carbon monoxide.

Parkinsonian signs can sometimes be present in patients with cirrhosis. Patients who have had multiple strokes may develop clinical features that resemble PD, and occasionally this can occur after a single subcortical stroke. There are also several syndromes in which parkinsonism accompanies other neurologic abnormalities. The clinical and neuropathologic findings that distinguish these illnesses are reviewed in Section C. Many of the distinctive clinical features may not appear until later in the course of the disease, making it hard to differentiate them from PD initially. In general, people with other parkinsonian syndromes are less likely than people with PD to respond to dopaminergic therapy, and in those who do respond the benefit may be only partial and temporary.

The most common diagnostic question that arises in the context of PD is whether a patient simply has essential tremor. Classically, essential tremor has different characteristics from the tremor of PD, but people with PD do not always exhibit the "classic" tremor, so differentiation from essential tremor on this basis is sometimes difficult. The most reliable way to distinguish the two disorders is on the basis of accompanying rigidity or bradykinesia, but these may be quite subtle, especially early in the course. At times, a patient must be observed for months to years before the diagnosis is clear.

Even when experienced clinicians diagnose PD, the diagnosis is confirmed at autopsy in only 75–85% of patients. Nonetheless, when patients with typical clinical features experience a substantial and sustained response to dopaminergic therapy, and several "Parkinson mimics" have been eliminated, the diagnosis is usually straightforward. In more confusing cases, single photon emission computerized tomography (SPECT) to visualize dopamine transmitter (DAT) may be helpful. In healthy subjects, the DAT scan shows a symmetric, homogeneous comma pattern in the striatum bilaterally. This pattern is not present in PD, but unfortunately, it is also absent in other degenerative diseases with parkinsonian features. A DAT scan is most useful in differentiating people with PD from healthy subjects or people with essential tremor. Promising results have been reported with RT-QuIC assays for α-synuclein in the CSF or other sources (analogous to the PrP^{Sc} RT-QuIC assay for CJD), but these assays are not available for clinical use.

4. Treatment of motor manifestations

Levodopa (L-dihydroxyphenylalanine, or L-dopa) is the cornerstone of therapy. Dopamine itself does not cross the blood-brain barrier and causes systemic side effects, but levodopa crosses the blood-brain barrier and is converted to dopamine within neurons by the enzyme aromatic L-amino acid decarboxylase (AADC). Levodopa is administered orally in combination with a drug called carbidopa, which blocks peripheral AADC, resulting in reduced conversion to dopamine peripherally and thereby minimizing systemic side effects and increasing the amount of levodopa entering the brain. The levodopa/carbidopa formulation that is typically used for initial treatment of PD is marketed as Sinemet; Table 8.1 lists other formulations, with a range of half-lives and modes of administration, that are sometimes used later in the disease course.

Levodopa is generally started once symptoms interfere with a patient's activities, often as a result of gait difficulty. Most people improve substantially even on very low doses of medication, and almost everyone with PD improves to some degree if high enough doses are used. In fact, levodopa and dopamine agonists are so consistently effective that a failure to respond should prompt the clinician to reconsider the diagnosis. As the disease progresses, the initially effective dose gradually becomes inadequate. At first, this can be addressed by increasing the levodopa dose or shortening the time interval between doses, but eventually, many patients develop unpredictable fluctuations between an "on" state in which the medication is effective and an "off " state in which they may be nearly immobile. In the "on" state, some patients develop frequent or continuous involuntary movements, or dyskinesia, to the point where they spend the bulk of their time unable to function because they are either in the "off" state or severely dyskinetic.

When these adverse motor phenomena can't be managed by adjusting levodopa dose and timing, additional medications are often introduced. The options (Table 8.1) include dopamine receptor agonists, catechol O-methyltransferase (COMT) inhibitors, monoamine oxidase type B (MAO-B) inhibitors, anticholinergic (specifically, antimuscarinic) agents, an adenosine A_{2A} receptor antagonist, and amantadine (an antagonist of glutamate, specifically NMDA). In principle, an advantage of dopamine agonists is that they act directly on the postsynaptic dopamine receptors, so they do not require processing by the presynaptic dopaminergic cells (which gradually die off as the disease progresses). Levodopa has the advantage of acting via presynaptic cells, so the timing of release is coordinated with motor activity and the profile of dopamine receptor subtype activation is physiologic. The rationale for using COMT inhibitors is to block another route of levodopa metabolism in peripheral tissue that makes less levodopa available for entry into the brain. MAO-B is one of the enzymes that metabolizes dopamine within neurons, so MAO-B inhibitors increase intraneuronal dopamine levels. Acetylcholine and adenosine A_{2A} receptors are present on neurons that counteract the actions of dopamine in basal ganglia circuits, providing the rationale for treating PD with antagonists to these receptors. Some studies suggest that cholinesterase inhibitors can improve gait stability in people with PD. Various exercise regimens have been shown to be beneficial; tai chi, in particular, has been associated with improved balance. Dancing and boxing are other activities for which there is anecdotal evidence.

For some severely affected patients who can no longer be managed effectively with medications, surgical intervention may be beneficial. The goal of ablative procedures, including pallidotomy and thalamotomy, is to counteract an imbalance in the circuitry connecting basal ganglia, thalamus, and cortex. These procedures are effective, but they have been largely supplanted by the technique of stereotactic implantation of a stimulating electrode in the subthalamic nucleus or the internal segment of the globus pallidus. Although the precise mechanism is debated, deep brain stimulation disrupts the basal ganglia circuitry without producing a permanent anatomic lesion. It produces enduring improvement in bradykinesia, rigidity, and gait disturbance, but only in patients whose symptoms respond to levodopa. The degree of improvement is generally comparable to the level of improvement the patient experiences when in the best levodopa "on" state. Unlike the other parkinsonian features, tremor may respond to deep brain stimulation even when it is refractory to medication. Another way in which tremor differs from other parkinsonian features is that it responds not only to stimulator placement in the subthalamic nucleus or the internal segment of the globus pallidus, but also to stimulation of the ventral intermediate nucleus of the thalamus (the same site typically targeted in patients with essential tremor). Deep brain stimulation should not be considered in patients who have dementia. Magnetic resonance-guided, high-intensity focused ultrasound is an alternative to deep brain stimulation but it has only been approved for unilateral treatment and offers no opportunity for adjusting treatment parameters. Trials of cell-based therapies, including transplantation of adrenal or fetal tissue into the brain, have not demonstrated a consistent benefit.

5. Treatment of nonmotor manifestations

Unfortunately, many antipsychotic medications can exacerbate the motor features of PD. When patients experience hallucinations that are nonthreatening and nondisruptive, it may not be necessary to treat them at all. When they are severe enough to require treatment, pimavanserin, quetiapine, and clozapine are the antipsychotic medications least likely to exacerbate the motor symptoms (clozapine is used less than the others because it requires frequent monitoring for potential hematologic and cardiac toxicity). Depression responds to standard treatment; MAO-B inhibitors and some dopamine agonists also have antidepressant effects. People with PD and dementia are typically treated with cholinesterase inhibitors; anticholinergic medications should be avoided (or at least minimized). Cholinesterase inhibitors are also sometimes used to treat delusions or hallucinations, but they have not been proven to be effective for these manifestations. Sleep disorders are very common in people with PD; they should be evaluated and managed in the standard fashion (see Chapter 9). Those with severe daytime somnolence should discontinue dopamine agonists, which can cause this problem. Orthostatic hypotension can also occur in PD. In some cases, it is medication-induced, and manipulation of the medication regimen can be helpful. In other cases, it is due to the underlying disease process and treated with the same measures used in multiple system atrophy (see Section C); droxidopa (Northera), a norepinephrine prodrug, is also used, although patients must be monitored for supine hypertension.

C. Other Parkinsonian Syndromes

Several diseases are characterized by parkinsonism in association with additional neurologic abnormalities. These conditions share many clinical and pathologic features, so they can be difficult to differentiate. Some conditions that were previously thought to be distinct are now known to overlap substantially, and some conditions are more heterogeneous than previously suspected. Many of these diagnostic categories are still in flux.

The accumulation of abnormal protein is a common feature of many conditions that result in progressive dementia, parkinsonism, or both. It is thought that the particular proteins involved, and the specific abnormalities those proteins contain, may determine the nature and distribution of pathology. Thus, these conditions can be roughly categorized into three groups, based on whether the abnormal protein accumulation consists of Aβ-peptide (in amyloid plaques), tau protein, or α-synuclein (see Table 8.2).

1. Dementia with Lewy bodies (DLB)

DLB is discussed in greater detail in Chapter 7. This condition results in cognitive deficits (which may fluctuate dramatically), parkinsonism, REM sleep behavior disorder, and hallucinations. These symptoms can develop in any order, but the dementia usually appears relatively early in the course, so the standard convention is to diagnose DLB only when the dementia precedes the parkinsonism or develops within a year of the onset of the parkinsonism. Patients who have motor manifestations of parkinsonism for more than a year before developing any symptoms of dementia are classified as having PD with dementia.

2. Progressive supranuclear palsy (PSP)

The earliest symptoms of progressive supranuclear palsy (PSP) often resemble typical PD, but patients eventually develop characteristic eye movement abnormalities. Downgaze palsy is often the initial abnormality. Patients next develop an upgaze palsy and then difficulty with voluntary horizontal gaze. The vestibulo-ocular reflex is intact, indicating that the gaze palsy is supranuclear (see Chapter 2). Other features that help distinguish PSP from PD are that in PSP, prominent gait disturbances and falls occur earlier in the illness, tremor is less common, and response to levodopa is less consistent. Neck dystonia and axial (trunk and head) rigidity are often present in PSP. Dysphagia develops early in the course and can be a severely limiting feature, and dysarthria is also prominent. Cognitive deficits consist primarily of "executive" or "frontal lobe" features such as personality changes, poor judgment, impulsiveness, perseveration, concrete thinking, and difficulty maintaining or focusing attention. Communication is generally disrupted much more by the dysarthria than by the dementia. Current criteria for diagnosing PSP are based on characterizing the patient's degree of impairment in four core domains: ocular motor dysfunction, postural instability, akinesia, and cognitive dysfunction. Depending on the relative severity in these domains, patients are categorized into one of eight clinical predominance types, or variants, with different levels of diagnostic certainty. For example, nonfluent/agrammatic PPA is prominent in one variant, whereas a behavioral syndrome is the hallmark of another variant. The most common variant is characterized by marked postural instability early in the disease course. Some patients whose ultimate pathologic diagnosis is PSP present with a clinical syndrome similar to corticobasal degeneration (see the next section). Neurofibrillary tangles and other deposits of tau protein are characteristic histopathologic features of PSP, but the specific tau isoforms differ from those that are present in the neurofibrillary tangles of AD.

A trial of levodopa is usually warranted in patients with PSP, because some patients experience substantial benefit, at least transiently. Positive results have been reported in occasional patients with dopamine agonists or tricyclic antidepressant agents, but most patients do not respond to these medications. Although cholinergic systems show widespread degeneration in PSP, results with cholinesterase inhibitors have been disappointing. Regardless of treatment, the disease is relentlessly progressive and typically results in severe impairment within a few years, primarily due to gait disturbance, dysphagia, and dysarthria.

3. Corticobasal degeneration (CBD)

Corticobasal degeneration (CBD; also called corticobasal ganglionic degeneration)presents almost exclusively after age 50 years. It typically begins with clumsiness, stiffness, or jerking of one arm (or, less often, one leg) and usually spreads to involve the ipsilateral limb before it affects the other side of the body. Patients often have dystonic posturing and apraxia on one side of their body, leading at times to an "alien limb" phenomenon in which patients report that the limb seems to float about their body or grab objects, independent of voluntary control. Some patients develop sensory neglect of one side of the body. The primary parkinsonian features are rigidity and bradykinesia. Postural tremor and kinetic tremor are common, but rest tremor is rare. Myoclonic jerks are often prominent, especially in response to external stimuli. Global cognitive deficits are usually mild to moderate, but some patients develop nonfluent/agrammatic PPA and some exhibit a behavioral syndrome or dysexecutive syndrome. Dysarthria and dysphagia are also common later in the course. As mentioned in Chapter 7, histopathologic characteristics of this condition overlap those seen in patients with FTD; tau-positive deposits and distinctive swollen neurons occur in both. Levodopa helps some of these patients.

Unfortunately, the clinical features described in the previous paragraph are not specific for CBD. They can also occur in patients whose ultimate pathologic diagnosis is PSP, FTD, or even AD. Because of this lack of specificity, many clinicians use the term *corticobasal syndrome* to refer to the clinical features and reserve the term *corticobasal degeneration* for patients in whom there is pathologic confirmation of the diagnosis.

4. Multiple system atrophy (MSA)

Multiple system atrophy (MSA) is characterized by any combination of parkinsonism, cerebellar dysfunction, and autonomic impairment. Patients may also have spasticity, dystonia, cranial nerve abnormalities, anterior horn cell dysfunction, or peripheral polyneuropathy in any combination. At least two thirds of patients have REM sleep behavior disorder (discussed in Chapter 9) at some point in the course, often before any other symptoms. In later stages of the disease, patients may also develop obstructive sleep apnea, central sleep apnea, or both. The clinical findings and presentation vary widely, but the course is gradually progressive. The term MSA-C is used when cerebellar dysfunction predominates, and MSA-P is applied when the predominant clinical feature is parkinsonism, but this distinction can be difficult because the symptoms often overlap, especially later in the course. An older term for the combination of parkinsonism and autonomic insufficiency is Shy-Drager syndrome. Early in the clinical course, people with MSA-P are often hard to distinguish from people with PD, except that they are less likely to have rest tremor and they tend to be more refractory to levodopa. Eventually, they develop one or more symptoms of autonomic insufficiency (orthostatic hypotension, urinary retention or incontinence, impotence, constipation, or thermoregulatory abnormalities), or ataxia of limbs, gait, or speech. Dopaminergic medication itself can cause orthostatic hypotension, so if a patient previously diagnosed with PD begins to develop severe orthostatic hypotension, MSA should only be diagnosed if the orthostatic hypotension persists after withdrawing the medication or if the patient develops other signs of autonomic dysfunction. A thin rim of increased signal in the lateral putamen on the MRI fluid attenuated inversion recovery (FLAIR) sequence is highly specific for MSA, but not sensitive. The "hot cross bun" sign, a characteristic MRI finding in the pons, is less specific and has low sensitivity.

Pathologic changes include widespread but variable neuronal loss in the striatum, brainstem, cerebellum, and spinal cord nuclei, with special stains revealing prominent glial cytoplasmic inclusions and less prominent neuronal cytoplasmic and nuclear inclusions, all of which contain α-synuclein. Between one third and one half of patients with MSA-P respond to levodopa, but the response is usually only partial and transient, and dyskinesias or worsened hypotension can be limiting side effects. Otherwise, treatment is symptomatic. Supportive therapy for gait disturbance or dysphagia may be helpful. Drinking a bolus of 350 cc of water first thing in the morning can be helpful for orthostatic hypotension; it also helps to drink boluses before standing up at other times of the day. Other nonpharmacologic measures include support stockings, abdominal binders, increased salt intake, and elevation of the head of the bed. Medications for orthostatic hypotension include mineralocorticoids such as fludrocortisone (Florinef), α-adrenergic agonists (e.g., midodrine or—less often—clonidine), droxidopa (which is metabolized to norepinephrine), indomethacin, and cholinesterase inhibitors (pyridostigmine).

D. Hereditary Ataxias

1. Friedreich ataxia
Friedreich ataxia presents early in adolescence with progressive gait difficulty, and it eventually affects coordination of the arms. Neurologic examination typically reveals profound loss of position and vibration sense in the lower extremities, absent tendon reflexes in the lower extremities and often in the upper extremities, ataxic gait, ataxic speech, and extensor plantar responses (Babinski signs). About 50% of patients have skeletal deformities such as scoliosis or pes cavus, and about 60% have a hypertrophic cardiomyopathy. Less frequent complications include optic atrophy, deafness, and diabetes mellitus. Pathologic hallmarks are demyelination and degeneration in the posterior column, pyramidal and spinocerebellar tracts of the spinal cord, and cell loss and demyelination in the cerebellar dentate nuclei, Clarke's column, dorsal root ganglia, and peripheral nerves. Disability usually occurs within 15 years. Life expectancy after onset is 35–40 years.

Friedreich ataxia has an autosomal recessive inheritance pattern. It is caused by an unstable expansion of a GAA trinucleotide repeat in the gene coding for frataxin, a protein that appears to be involved in making iron available for several mitochondrial processes. Homozygotes for this mutation have partial deficiency of frataxin, leading to mitochondrial overload, impaired utilization of iron for synthesis of iron-sulfur clusters, decline of mitochondrial respiratory activity, and increased production of free radicals.

The diagnosis of Friedreich ataxia is established by demonstration of the trinucleotide repeat expansion on a blood test that is commercially available. Omaveloxolone improves function slightly, and it has FDA approval for Friedreich ataxia in people age 16 years or older; otherwise, therapy is supportive.

2. Ataxia telangiectasia

Ataxia telangiectasia usually becomes symptomatic in the first decade of life, within a few years of learning to walk. The child develops an ataxic gait, followed by upper extremity ataxia and ataxic speech. Many patients also develop choreoathetosis or dystonia, and they have a characteristic difficulty initiating saccadic eye movements ("oculomotor apraxia") that requires them to thrust their heads in the intended direction of gaze. Mild intellectual decline may occur by the end of the first decade of life, and by adolescence most patients lose the ability to walk independently. Patients usually have hyporeflexia and hypotonia on examination. Telangiectasias appear after the onset of ataxia, usually in the second half of the first decade of life. They most frequently occur in the conjunctivae, ears, bridge of the nose, and antecubital fossa. About 60% of patients have immunodeficiency and experience recurrent sinopulmonary infections. Patients also have an increased risk of malignancies, particularly lymphoma.

Ataxia telangiectasia has an autosomal recessive inheritance pattern. It is caused by mutations in the *ATM* (ataxia telangiectasia mutated) gene, which codes for the first protein in a protein kinase cascade that senses breaks in double-stranded DNA. *ATM* and a related gene, *ATR*, form the core of the DNA damage repair system, and they are involved in multiple aspects of cell cycle control and DNA damage surveillance. Heterozygous carriers of the mutation that causes ataxia telangiectasia have an increased risk of early death, primarily due to cancer and ischemic heart disease.

Diagnosis can be difficult early in childhood before telangiectasias develop, but once telangiectasias are visualized the clinical features are diagnostic. Patients consistently have elevated levels of α-fetoprotein, also. No additional testing is usually required. When the diagnosis is ambiguous, other tests that can be performed include immunoblotting for the ATM protein and genetic sequence analysis. Other than treatment of infections and malignancies, therapy is supportive.

3. Spinocerebellar ataxias (SCAs)

The spinocerebellar ataxias (SCAs) are dominantly inherited disorders characterized by progressive ataxia. The ataxia usually begins in adolescence or later, and the progression is generally slow. More than 40 SCAs have been identified. Ataxia of gait, limb movements, and speech are common in all of the SCAs, but some of the SCAs are associated with additional neurologic abnormalities such as restricted eye movements, vision loss, hyporeflexia, spasticity and hyperreflexia, choreoathetosis, parkinsonism, dystonia, myoclonus, sensory loss, seizures, developmental delay, intellectual disability, and dementia. The clinical features of the SCAs overlap considerably, so diagnosis of the specific SCA usually requires genetic testing. Therapy is supportive.

The mutations that cause SCA can be classified into three broad categories. The most common are expanded regions of trinucleotide repeats in the coding region of a gene, which are thought to lead to proteins with abnormal folding patterns that form toxic aggregates. The second category of SCA-related mutations consists of repeat expansions in the noncoding region of a gene; these are thought to result in RNA interference. The third category consists of conventional mutations (deletions, mis-sense, nonsense, and splice site mutations). The underlying pathophysiology is not known, but many of these mutations disrupt ion channel function either directly or indirectly.

4. Episodic ataxias

The episodic ataxias are characterized by transient episodes of ataxia. The episodes last seconds to minutes in some of these conditions and hours to days in others. Between the attacks, patients have relatively normal neurologic function, although some of these conditions are associated with slowly progressive ataxia, seizures, migraine, or other manifestations between the bouts of ataxia. Nine subtypes of episodic ataxia have been identified. All of the subtypes have an autosomal dominant inheritance pattern and genetic testing is necessary to establish the diagnosis; most of the known causative mutations are in genes coding for ion channel subunits. Acetazolamide is beneficial in some of these disorders, but not all.

5. Fragile X-associated tremor/ataxia syndrome (FXTAS)

The maternal grandfathers of boys with fragile X syndrome sometimes develop a syndrome that begins after the age of 55 years and is characterized by slowly progressive ataxia, kinetic tremor, parkinsonism, and polyneuropathy. This has been labeled the fragile X-associated tremor/ataxia syndrome (FXTAS). The gene responsible for fragile X syndrome has a trinucleotide repeat region that contains 6–50 repeats in unaffected individuals, 55–200 repeats in people with FXTAS, and more than 200 repeats in people with fragile X syndrome. The protein coded by that gene is absent or nearly absent in people with fragile X syndrome, but it is present at normal or mildly reduced levels in patients with FXTAS. Thus, whereas very long expansions result in a loss of gene function and lead to fragile X syndrome, intermediate-length expansions are thought to have a toxic effect, leading to sequestration of certain nuclear proteins. Female carriers of the mutation may also develop symptoms, but they are usually milder, because females have an additional, normal X chromosome, and random inactivation of either the normal or abnormal chromosome leads to phenotypic variability. No specific treatment is available.

E. Huntington Disease

Huntington disease is a genetic condition with progressive symptoms that typically begin in the late third or fourth decade of life. The predominant symptoms are chorea and changes in cognition and behavior. The cognitive disturbances begin as personality changes and evolve to more global intellectual decline. Slowed saccadic eye movements and slowed distal fine finger movements can usually be detected on examination even before the involuntary movements become apparent. The chorea is often difficult to detect early in the illness. When it is relatively mild, the person may just seem "fidgety." Patients are characteristically unaware of their chorea until it is moderate or severe. They sometimes incorporate the chorea into normal voluntary actions; for example, they may quickly reach up to smooth their hair when their arm flexes involuntarily. The chorea grows progressively more severe over time, but it may attenuate in later disease stages. Patients often manifest varying degrees of athetosis, dystonia, or bradykinesia, and these features may come to predominate. Dysarthria and dysphagia worsen throughout the course. Gait abnormalities and falls are extremely common and eventually become disabling. Depression is very common, and a variety of other psychiatric disorders may also occur.

In approximately 10% of people with Huntington disease, clinical symptoms begin before age 20 years; this juvenile form is often characterized by prominent parkinsonism rather than chorea, and myoclonus is very common. Seizures are also common in juvenile-onset Huntington disease, and rare in adult-onset disease.

When someone with a positive family history of Huntington disease develops the characteristic movement disorder, the diagnosis is clear; no additional testing is necessary. In the absence of abnormal movements, in contrast, the psychiatric or behavioral manifestations of Huntington disease are not specific enough to establish the diagnosis, even when there is a positive family history. In those circumstances, or when people have typical clinical manifestations of Huntington disease but no family history, the diagnosis can be established by testing for the Huntington mutation.

Huntington disease is inherited in an autosomal dominant pattern. It is caused by an expanded CAG trinucleotide repeat that codes for an elongated polyglutamine chain in the tail of a protein that has been named huntingtin. Anyone who has 40 or more repeats develops Huntington disease, and nobody with fewer than 27 repeats develops it; people who have 27–39 repeats may or may not develop the disease. Repeat lengths above 26 are unstable and may expand when transmitted from parent to offspring. Higher repeat numbers correlate with greater penetrance, younger age of symptom onset, and more rapid progression. Marked expansion of the repeat length appears to be more common in spermatogenesis than in oogenesis, which probably explains why most children with juvenile-onset disease inherited it from their father. Huntingtin is widely expressed both within the nervous system and outside it; its function is unknown. The pathology in Huntington disease is thought to result from a gain of function in the elongated mutant protein (as opposed to a loss of the normal protein's function, which is the situation in most recessively inherited conditions). Mitochondrial dysfunction, free radical toxicity, glutamate excitotoxicity, and caspase-mediated programmed cell death are all thought to play a role in the resultant pathologic process.

Pathologic examination reveals marked atrophy with loss of selective subsets of cells in the striatum, particularly at the head of the caudate. Neuronal loss is also described in the globus pallidus, thalamus, and cerebral cortex. Characteristic changes in neurotransmitters and receptors (especially GABA [gamma-aminobutyric acid], enkephalin, benzodiazepine, acetylcholine, and excitatory amino acids) have been described.

Treatments aimed at disease modification, and many attempts at gene therapy, are the focus of research, but for now the only available treatments are directed at symptoms. When the chorea is mild and doesn't impair function, it may not require treatment. Table 8.3 lists medications that may be useful when chorea is more severe, as well as medications used to treat behavior disorders. Swallowing problems and gait difficulty should be addressed with education and therapy. Dysphagia, immobility, and dementia usually lead to death within 15–25 years of symptom onset.

Difficult psychosocial and ethical issues arise from the ability to screen for a genetic condition that does not produce clinical manifestations until midlife and for which only limited symptomatic treatment is available. Individuals at risk for Huntington disease should receive extensive counseling to ensure that they understand how the disease is transmitted and to help them decide whether to be tested.

F. Tardive Dyskinesia

About 20% of patients chronically taking dopamine receptor-blocking antipsychotic or antiemetic medications develop hyperkinetic movement disorders, especially dyskinetic movements or dystonic postures. These often appear late in the course of therapy, especially after reducing the medication dose or stopping it entirely. The incidence increases in proportion to the duration of exposure and is highest in the elderly. The most common dyskinesias are repetitive, stereotyped oro-bucco-lingual movements, but in many patients, the trunk and distal extremities are involved as well. Other examples of tardive dyskinesia include repetitive rocking of the body, leg crossing, or even intrusive respirations. The pathophysiologic mechanism is uncertain. Proposed mechanisms include supersensitivity of postsynaptic striatal dopamine receptors, oxidative stress, GABA-ergic striatal dysfunction, and excess glutamatergic activity. Treatment consists of titrating to the lowest doses of medication needed to control psychotic symptoms (or nausea) and, ideally, eliminating the offending medication entirely—if necessary, substituting ondansetron for nausea or treating psychosis with clozapine or quetiapine (atypical antipsychotic medications that rarely cause tardive dyskinesia, although clozapine requires frequent monitoring because of potential hematologic and cardiac toxicity). Dyskinesias may or may not resolve after discontinuation of the offending agents; improvement may take weeks to months. For disabling persistent movements, Table 8.3 lists medications that may be of benefit. Positive results have also been reported with pallidotomy or pallidal deep brain stimulation, but the evidence is limited.

G. Dystonias

Many different movement disorders (as well as a number of other neurologic diseases and systemic problems) can produce dystonia. Dystonia can also occur as an isolated problem. Although any pattern of muscle activity may be seen, the most common examples of isolated dystonia in adults are the focal syndromes of cervical dystonia (torticollis), blepharospasm, and writer's cramp. In cervical dystonia, the patient's head may be turned to one side, flexed, extended, or tilted; the resultant posture depends on which muscle or muscles are most active. The head may be maintained in a fixed position, or there may be superimposed jerking movements or tremor. In blepharospasm, there is involuntary, bilateral eye closure, often exacerbated by bright light or other environmental stimuli. In writer's cramp, the hand assumes an involuntary, often twisted posture when the patient attempts to write. Many analogous task-specific forms of isolated dystonia also exist. In addition to the inconvenience and embarrassment resulting from these conditions, the sustained muscle contractions often cause considerable pain. The severity of focal dystonia typically fluctuates widely and can be influenced both by the individual's emotional state and by environmental stimuli. The underlying pathogenesis of focal dystonia is not known. Hemidystonia is usually associated with structural damage in the contralateral basal ganglia. Psychiatric conditions can result in postures that can be difficult to distinguish from dystonia. The difficulty is compounded by the fact that many people with psychiatric illness are treated with antipsychotic medications, which can themselves produce dystonia.

Isolated dystonia that begins in adulthood is usually focal or segmental, whereas approximately 50% of cases of childhood-onset isolated dystonia are generalized. The most common form of early-onset generalized dystonia, DYT-*TORIA* dystonia (formerly termed DYT1 dystonia, or dystonia musculorum deformans), is inherited as an autosomal dominant trait with relatively low penetrance. It presents in the first decade of life in about 50% of patients. It usually begins in one limb and spreads to the rest of the body over 1 to 10 years. DYT-*TORIA* dystonia is caused by a deletion in the gene for a protein that has been named torsin A, whose function is unknown, but it is homologous to the adenosine triphosphatases and heat-shock proteins, and it is thought that mutant forms may interfere with endoplasmic reticulum function, intracellular trafficking, vesicular release, or processing of misfolded protein.

Dopa-responsive dystonia (DYT/PARK-*GCHI* dystonia, previously referred to as DYT5 dystonia), is a rare form of childhood-onset generalized dystonia that is notable for marked diurnal variation. Children with this condition may have normal or nearly normal motor function in the morning, but over the course of the day they have progressively increasing dystonia, parkinsonism, and hyperreflexia. They have a dramatic and sustained response to relatively low doses of levodopa, and even after prolonged levodopa use they usually do not develop hallucinations, autonomic dysfunction, motor fluctuations, or dyskinesias. This is presumably related to the fact that this condition (unlike PD) only affects dopamine synthesis, not the integrity of the dopaminergic neurons themselves. Anticholinergic drugs may also be helpful. More than 75 mutations in the gene for guanosine triphosphate cyclohydrolase-1 (GCH1)—an enzyme involved in the synthesis of tetrahydrobiopterin, which is a cofactor in dopamine synthesis—have been implicated in this condition. It is usually dominantly inherited with incomplete penetrance, and females are preferentially affected. Another levodopa-responsive condition, DYT/PARK-*TH* dystonia, is an autosomal recessive disorder caused by mutations in the gene for tyrosine hydroxylase.

In most adults with isolated dystonia, the diagnosis is based on clinical features. Patients should generally be tested for Wilson disease, which may present with focal or segmental dystonia. Single-gene testing is available for children (and sometimes adults) who have features that are highly suggestive of a specific genetic condition, such as DYT-*TORIA* dystonia; dystonia gene panels are also available when the presentation is less distinctive.

Table 8.3 lists medications that may be helpful for dystonia. Focal dystonias can be treated with local injections of botulinum toxin to weaken the overactive muscles. Although this approach does not directly address the abnormal motor programming responsible for the disorder, it can produce significant symptomatic relief. The effect is temporary, so the injections must be repeated every few months. Botulinum toxin injections can at best provide regional relief to patients with DYT-*TORIA* dystonia, who eventually develop severe disability in most cases. DYT-*TORIA* dystonia often responds to a deep brain stimulator placed in the internal segment of the globus pallidus, so this is an option in patients who are refractory to medications. The response is less predictable than in patients with essential tremor or PD and may not be apparent until several months have elapsed. This treatment can also be effective for patients with other forms of dystonia, including cervical dystonia refractory to other management approaches. The subthalamic nucleus also appears to be an effective target for deep brain stimulation in the treatment of dystonia, but it has been studied less extensively.

H. Wilson Disease

Wilson disease is a disorder of copper metabolism characterized by progressive—but often reversible—dysarthria, dystonia, gait disturbance, tremor, parkinsonism, choreoathetosis, dysphagia, psychiatric symptoms, and cognitive deterioration. These manifestations may occur in any combination and in any temporal sequence. The dystonia can be focal, segmental, multifocal, or generalized. The tremor can be a rest tremor, a postural tremor, or a kinetic tremor. Clinically significant hepatic involvement is common, and other organ systems may also be affected. In general, patients who present with liver abnormalities usually do so between the ages of 8 and 16 years, whereas those who present with neurologic symptoms usually do so after puberty.

Histopathologic examination reveals excess copper deposition in the liver and throughout the brain, with prominent degeneration of the putamen, globus pallidus, brainstem nuclei, and even white matter. Copper deposition in the cornea leads to the characteristic Kayser-Fleischer ring of hyperpigmentation around the limbus; this physical finding is present in practically all patients with neurologic manifestations, but it may be subtle and only evident on slit-lamp examination in early cases.

Wilson disease is inherited in an autosomal recessive pattern. It is caused by mutations in the gene for ATP7B, an ATPase involved in the excretion of copper into the bile. Normal copper intake is approximately 1 mg per day, but the normal copper requirement is only about 0.75 mg per day. In healthy individuals, copper is absorbed in the upper intestine and transported to the liver, where it is taken up with high affinity. In hepatocytes, the ATP7B directs the incorporation of copper into a glycoprotein called apo-ceruloplasmin, which transports the copper into various enzymes and into the plasma. The ATP7B also helps direct the excess copper into a vesicular compartment near the canalicular membrane, and from here the copper is eliminated from the body by excretion into the bile. Mutations in the *ATP7B* gene are thought to interfere with the ability of ATP7B to direct the copper to the vesicular compartment, resulting in abnormal accumulation of copper in the hepatocyte. This eventually spills over into the blood and affects other organs, including the brain. The mechanism by which excess copper produces organ damage is not clear. Serum levels of ceruloplasmin are low in most patients with Wilson disease, and the reasons for this are also unclear. It may be that the *ATP7B* mutations result in reduced incorporation of copper into apoceruloplasmin, and without a full complement of bound copper the ceruloplasmin is subject to rapid intracellular and extracellular degradation.

A percutaneous liver biopsy to determine hepatic copper content is the single most reliable test for Wilson disease, but the diagnosis can usually be made in other ways. A slit-lamp examination will reveal Kayser-Fleischer rings in 98% of people with neurologic manifestations, but in only 50% of patients with exclusively hepatic manifestations. In neurologic Wilson disease, brain MRI scans typically show signal abnormalities in the basal ganglia, thalamus, or upper brainstem (or some combination of these locations). A 24-hour urine collection for copper is a good screening test because it is very sensitive if diligently collected: elevated levels of total excreted copper are almost universal in people with Wilson disease. This result is only specific when the level is extremely high, because other cholestatic disorders can also cause increased urine copper excretion. Total levels of serum copper are of little value, but elevated levels of free serum copper can be helpful. A serum ceruloplasmin level is often used as a screening test for Wilson disease, but ceruloplasmin levels are at the low end of the normal range in about 10% of individuals with the disease and low in about 10% of asymptomatic carriers. In situations where the diagnosis remains uncertain despite standard testing, genetic testing can be considered.

Without treatment, Wilson disease was once uniformly fatal. Patients are now treated with zinc, trientine, or penicillamine; neurologic symptoms may transiently worsen with the initiation of any of these medications, but especially penicillamine. Table 8.3 provides additional information regarding these medications. Therapy must be continued permanently. Orthotopic liver transplantation is currently reserved for patients with severe hepatic failure.

I. Tourette Syndrome

Tics are abrupt, transient, stereotyped, coordinated movements or vocalizations that are usually associated with a premonitory urge. Tourette syndrome is the most flagrant of a spectrum of tic disorders. It is a lifelong condition that begins in early childhood, usually between the ages of 3 and 8 years, and almost all patients manifest tics before adolescence. In addition to recurrent motor tics (such as blinking, eye rolling, or shoulder shrugging, often involving multiple muscle groups), there are frequent vocal tics such as grunting, barking, humming, or clearing of the throat. The most dramatic symptom is coprolalia, the involuntary utterance of obscenities, but this occurs in only a minority of patients. A patient may manifest different tics over the years, with certain tics predominating for months at a time, only to fade gradually and be replaced by other tics. Obsessive-compulsive disorder and attention deficit-hyperactivity disorder each occur in approximately 50% of patients; they can occur together or separately. These associated behavioral problems can be more disabling than the tics themselves.

Tourette syndrome has a strong hereditary component, and potential susceptibility genes have been identified, but the inheritance pattern is complex. Environmental triggers are also thought to play a role. The pathophysiology is unknown. The diagnosis is based on clinical features. Tics tend to become less severe over time. Most patients with mild tics require no treatment. When patients acknowledge their tics and are motivated to learn to suppress them, the first line of therapy is an approach called Cognitive Behavioral Intervention for Tics (CBIT), in which patients learn to initiate a voluntary behavior to manage the premonitory urge. When the decision is made to treat with medication for moderate or severe tics, the alpha$_2$-adrenergic agonists guanfacine and clonidine are considered the drugs of choice. Other medications that are sometimes used for Tourette syndrome are listed in Table 8.3. Deep brain stimulation (targeting either the centromedian/parafascicular nuclei of the thalamus or the internal segment of the globus pallidus) has been reported to reduce tics, depression, and obsessive-compulsive disorder, but this has not been conclusively established.

V. Supplementary Tables for Reference

Table 8.1 Medications Used for Parkinson Disease (PD)

Drug	Mode of Administration	Proprietary Name
A. Levodopa/carbidopa		
Immediate release	Oral	Sinemet
Sustained release	Oral	Sinemet CR
Extended release	Oral	Rytary
Rapid onset	Orally disintegrating	Parcopa
Immediate release	Oral, functionally scored	Dhivy
Continuous	Enteral suspension gel via percutaneous endoscopic gastrostomy/jejunal tube	Duopa
B. Levodopa	Inhaler	Inbrija
C. Dopamine agonists		
Pramipexole	Oral	Mirapex, Mirapex ER
Ropinirole	Oral	Requip, Requip XL
Rotigotine	Transdermal	Neupro
Apomorphine	Subcutaneous	Apokyn
	Sublingual	Kynmobi
D. COMT inhibitors		
Entacapone	Oral	Comtan
Tolcapone	Oral	Tasmar
Opicapone	Oral	Ongentsys

(Continued)

Table 8.1 Continued

Drug	Mode of Administration	Proprietary Name
E. Combination (levodopa, carbidopa, entacapone)	Oral	Stalevo
F. MAO-B inhibitors		
Selegiline	Oral Orally disintegrating	L-Deprenyl, Eldepryl Zelapar
Rasagiline	Oral	Azilect
Safinamide	Oral	Xadago
G. Anticholinergics		
Benztropine	Oral	Cogentin
Trihexyphenidyl	Oral	Artane
H. Adenosine A_{2A} receptor antagonist		
Istradefylline	Oral	Nourianz
I. Amantadine	Oral	Symmetrel, Gocovri, Osmolex ER

Table 8.2 Characteristic Protein Accumulations in Degenerative Dementing Illnesses and Movement Disorders

	Aβ-peptide (in Amyloid Plaques)	Tau	α-Synuclein
Alzheimer disease (AD)	+	+	
Frontotemporal dementia (FTD)—sometimes		+	
Dementia with Lewy bodies (DLB)			+
Parkinson disease (PD)			+
Multiple system atrophy (MSA)			+ (especially in glia)
Corticobasal degeneration (CBD)		+	
Progressive supranuclear palsy (PSP)		+	

Table 8.3 Medications Used for Less Common Movement Disorders

Disorder	Medications	Comments
Huntington disease		
Chorea	(1) Catecholamine-depleting agents (tetrabenazine, deutetrabenazine, valbenazine)	(1) Tetrabenazine and deutetrabenazine are FDA approved for chorea - Tetrabenazine can cause or exacerbate depression - Tetrabenazine thought to have more potential for side effects than deutetrabenazine and valbenazine
	(2) NMDA antagonists (amantadine, riluzole)	(2) NMDA antagonists less consistently effective
	(3) Phenothiazines	
	(4) Atypical antipsychotic agents	(4) Especially olanzapine
Behavior Disorder	(1) Phenothiazines	
	(2) Atypical antipsychotic agents	
	(3) Antidepressants, mood-stabilizing agents	
Friedreich ataxia	Omaveloxolone	
Tardive dyskinesia	(1) Catecholamine-depleting agents (tetrabenazine, deutetrabenazine, valbenazine)	(1) Deutetrabenazine and valbenazine are FDA approved for tardive dyskinesia - Tetrabenazine can cause or exacerbate depression - Tetrabenazine thought to have more potential for side effects than deutetrabenazine and valbenazine
	(2) Benzodiazepines, reserpine, clonidine, propranolol, vitamin E, donepezil, levetiracetam, gabapentin, valproic acid	(2) Only limited evidence for each of these agents

(Continued)

Table 8.3 Continued

Disorder	Medications	Comments
Dystonia	(1) Levodopa	(1) For DYT/PARK-*GCHI* dystonia and DYT/PARK-*TH* dystonia
	(2) Anticholinergic agents, baclofen, dopamine agonists, benzodiazepines, catecholamine-depleting agents	(2) For other dystonias, anticholinergic agents are the medications generally considered to be the most effective, but side effects are often limiting
Wilson disease	(1) Zinc	(1) Blocks intestinal absorption of copper; good choice for maintenance therapy but takes 4–8 months to achieve its effect
	(2) Trientene	(2) A chelating agent; promotes urinary excretion of copper
	(3) Penicillamine	(3) A chelating agent; formerly standard treatment, but it is no longer recommended because it is associated with a high incidence of adverse effects, including neurologic deterioration at the onset of treatment in 25–50% of patients
		- Trientine, like penicillamine, can result in neurologic deterioration initially, but it has fewer overall side effects
		- Temporarily supplementing zinc with trientine at the outset may help to achieve a more rapid clinical response

Table 8.3 Continued

Disorder	Medications	Comments
Tourette syndrome		
Tics	(1) Alpha$_2$-adrenergic agonists (guanfacine, clonidine)	(1) These are considered the drugs of choice
	(2) Selective serotonin reuptake inhibitors (SSRIs), serotonin-norepinephrine reuptake inhibitors (SNRIs), topiramate	(2) These are considered second-line agents
	(3) Antidopaminergic drugs (such as haloperidol, pimozide, or fluphenazine)	(3) These are the most effective medications for tics, but they are generally not used for initial treatment because of the potential for side effects (such as tardive dyskinesia) with long-term use
	(4) Atypical antipsychotics (olanzapine, quetiapine, aripiprazole, or risperidone)	(4) These may also be effective, with fewer side effects
	(5) Catecholamine-depleting agents (tetrabenazine, deutetrabenazine, and valbenazine)	(5) These have also been effective in some patients.
Obsessive-compulsive disorder	SSRIs	Cognitive-behavioral therapy is another option
Attention deficit hyperactivity disorder	(1) clonidine, guanfacine, or atmoxetine	(1) First-line treatment
	(2) Methylphenidate	(2) Controversial—may exacerbate tics
	(3) Bupropion, tricyclic antidepressants	(3) May also be helpful

VI. Discussion of Case Histories

Case 1: This woman has typical features of early Parkinson disease (PD). She may be frightened by this diagnosis, especially since PD was essentially untreatable when she was younger. It is important to make sure she understands that the disease is readily treatable but that it will require continuing attention. Because her symptoms have already caused her to limit her activities, it would be reasonable to initiate treatment with levodopa. Dose adjustments and decisions about adding other medications will depend on how her condition evolves over time.

She also relates symptoms that suggest she may be depressed. Her eating and sleeping habits, as well as her mood, need to be assessed. Depression is a common complication of PD, and it is often inadequately addressed because so many of the features resemble those of PD itself. A screening mental status examination should also be performed, and if it indicates any problems, formal evaluation of intellectual function and affect might provide a baseline to help assess any future decline.

Comment: This patient did very well on a low dose of levodopa, and the features of depression resolved once she had started on medication and received education and reassurance about her condition.

Case 2: Although this woman reports "generalized weakness," she actually has full strength on examination. Instead, the most prominent feature on her examination is parkinsonism. People with parkinsonian features commonly perceive or describe them as "weakness"—you must ask pointed questions about what they can and can't do to clarify what they mean. The neurologic examination is also critical. In this patient, the progression has been fairly rapid, and she already has bilateral parkinsonian findings on examination after only 3 months of symptoms. These atypical features suggest that she may not have idiopathic PD. In fact, this case illustrates the common phenomenon of drug-induced parkinsonism. The bradykinesia and tremor began almost immediately after starting metoclopramide (Reglan). All the usual symptoms of PD can be induced by even relatively brief exposure to this medication, and a careful history is the key to diagnosis. The first diagnostic maneuver is to stop the metoclopramide. Treating with anticholinergics or levodopa without stopping the metoclopramide would be inappropriate. Symptoms may take several weeks or more to subside, so follow-up evaluations will be necessary.

Regarding her report of foot numbness, the examination findings of hyporeflexia at the ankles and reduced vibration sense at the toes are consistent with peripheral polyneuropathy, a common complication of diabetes. Because her feet are not painful, the findings are mild, and there is a likely explanation, there is no need for further evaluation at this point. She has normal distal strength and joint position sense, so the polyneuropathy is probably not playing a major role in her gait disturbance.

Comment: This patient's motor symptoms disappeared within 3 weeks of stopping metoclopramide. She continued to have numbness in her feet, but this symptom did not bother her once it was explained to her.

Chapter 9

Sleep Disorders

I. Case Histories

Case 1. During one of his routine follow-up visits in the hypertension clinic, a 55-year-old man mentions that he was in an accident last week, but, luckily, nobody got hurt. He says he must have "fallen asleep at the wheel"—it happens to him every so often. He doesn't understand why he should be sleepy, because he goes to bed at 10 p.m. every night and sleeps through the night until he gets up at 7 a.m. the next morning. His wife confirms this but adds that she really couldn't say whether he is asleep that entire time because she sleeps in a different room to avoid his snoring.

The patient's general examination is notable for his hypertension, mild obesity, and a large neck circumference (48 centimeters, or 19 inches). His neurologic examination is normal.

Questions:

1. What diagnoses should be considered?
2. What investigations are necessary?
3. How should this patient be managed?

Case 2. A 45-year-old woman wonders if she is depressed because she has no energy, can't concentrate, and is tired all the time. She can never seem to fall asleep at night. In fact, she can hardly even lie in bed for any length of time, because of a constant unpleasant sensation in her legs, "like worms are crawling over them," causing an almost irresistible urge to move the legs. This feeling only goes away when she is moving her legs or walking. She prefers standing, anyway, because she often gets epigastric pain when she lies down. Her examination is normal.

Questions:

1. What diagnoses should be considered?
2. What investigations are necessary?
3. Should antidepressant medication be prescribed?
4. What other treatment options are available?

Case 3. A 4-year-old girl has been brought to the pediatric emergency room at 2 a.m. by her parents, who say that at 1 a.m. they were awakened by her frantic screaming. They rushed to her room and saw that she was agitated, sweating profusely, and breathing rapidly. They noted that her pulse was racing. They were unable to calm her, but over the next few minutes she gradually calmed down on her own and drifted back to sleep. In the emergency room, she seems to be normal, except that she is sleepy. She has no memory of the event. Two similar episodes occurred a month ago, but the family had just moved to a new city at the time and the girl's parents had attributed the episodes to the unfamiliar surroundings and the stress of adjusting to a new day care situation. The girl's examination is normal.

Questions:
1. What diagnoses should be considered?
2. What investigations are necessary?
3. What treatment should be given?

II. Approach to Sleep Disorders

In evaluating and managing patients with sleep disorders, three questions are fundamental:

1. Does the patient have trouble staying awake during the day?
2. Does the patient have trouble falling asleep or staying asleep at night?
3. Does the patient have abnormal sensations or behavior during sleep?

These symptoms often go together. For example, people who have trouble staying awake in the daytime may nap excessively during the day and then have trouble falling asleep at night. People who have trouble falling asleep at bedtime are insufficiently rested the following day, so they may have trouble staying awake. People who have abnormal behavior during sleep—and often their bed partners—may fail to get the required amount of normal sleep and have trouble staying awake the following day.

Despite the interconnections between these symptoms, it is helpful to consider them separately. Part IV of this chapter addresses Question 1, Part V addresses Question 2, and Part VI addresses Question 3. Part III presents some background information.

III. Background Information

A. Definitions

dyssomnia: a disorder resulting in insomnia or excessive daytime sleepiness (or both)

hypersomnia: excessive daytime somnolence

insomnia: the subjective impression of inadequate sleep

parasomnia: an abnormal movement or behavior that occurs during sleep or is brought on by sleep

sleep Definition #1 (conceptual): a reversible behavioral state of perceptual disengagement from and unresponsiveness to the environment

sleep Definition #2 (operational): a physiologic state defined by behavioral and physiologic criteria. The behavioral criteria include (1) minimal mobility, (2) closed eyes, (3) increased arousal threshold and reduced response to external stimulation, (4) increased reaction time, (5) reduced cognition, (6) characteristic sleeping posture, and (7) reversibility. The physiologic criteria are based on findings from electroencephalography (EEG), electromyography (EMG), and electrooculography (EOG).

B. Sleep Physiology

Sleep consists of a highly patterned sequence of cyclic activity in various regions of the brain; it is not simply a state of temporary unconsciousness. Although the brain is less responsive than normal during sleep, it is not totally unresponsive. In fact, during sleep the brain responds more readily to meaningful stimuli, such as a crying baby, than to other stimuli.

There are two principal states of sleep that alternate at about 90-minute intervals in the normal adult. *Rapid eye movement* (REM) sleep can be characterized as a period when the brain is active and the body is paralyzed, whereas in *nonrapid eye movement* (NREM) sleep the brain is less active but the body can move. Most elaborate dreams occur during REM sleep. REM sleep is characterized by EMG suppression, irregular low-voltage activity on EEG, and rapid eye movements. The eye movements sometimes correspond to dream content. The characteristic features of NREM sleep are normal resting EMG, progressive slowing of EEG activity, and the absence of rapid eye movements.

When healthy people fall asleep, they progress through three stages of NREM sleep (N1, N2, and N3) that are differentiated on the basis of EEG characteristics. The third stage (N3) is often called *slow-wave sleep* or *delta sleep* because it is characterized by high-amplitude, low-frequency waves (also called delta waves) on EEG. Delta sleep may last from a few minutes to an hour, depending on the subject's age, and the subject then reverts to stage N2 sleep. Shortly after this, the first REM sleep period begins. This lasts approximately 15–20 minutes and is followed by another NREM cycle. The REM and NREM phases continue to alternate, with a total of four to six cycles over the course of the night (Figure 9.1). The first two cycles are dominated by stage N3, but after the first third of the night this stage is less apparent, so NREM sleep later in the night consists primarily of N2 sleep, with brief periods of N1 sleep. Conversely, the periods of REM sleep grow longer as the night continues. Thus, the first third of the night is dominated by slow-wave sleep, and the final third is dominated by REM sleep. In healthy young adults, about 75% of total sleep time is spent in NREM sleep, and 25% in REM sleep. This cyclic activity is governed by several different neuronal systems.

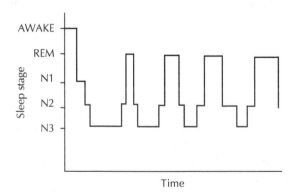

Fig. 9.1 Normal cycling of sleep stages; details explained in text. Note that delta sleep (stage N3) predominates early in the night, but as the night progresses, the amount of time spent in N3 sleep gradually shrinks while the amount of time spent in REM sleep grows.

In the awake state, ongoing thalamic input to the cortex results in stimulus-dependent—and thus, nonrhythmic—cortical activity. The EEG in normal wakefulness is therefore desynchronized and appears nearly random. The thalamus, in turn, receives excitatory input from a network of pathways originating in the brainstem, especially the midbrain. Stimulation of these pathways promotes wakefulness. The most potent and fast-acting wakefulness-promoting pathways employ glutamate or GABA as their neurotransmitter. More slowly acting pathways employing the monoaminergic neurotransmitters norepinephrine, serotonin, histamine, and dopamine are also involved in promoting wakefulness, possibly by modulating the activity of the glutamatergic pathways in response to the internal and external environment. Another set of wakefulness-promoting neurons utilize acetylcholine; these seem to be particularly important in maintaining the desynchronization of cortical activity in the awake state.

At the onset of NREM sleep, a group of GABA-ergic, "hypnogenic neurons" (located primarily in the ventrolateral preoptic nucleus of the anterior hypothalamus but also in the medulla) inhibit the wakefulness-promoting pathways. This suppresses thalamocortical activity. Progressive inhibition causes slower, more synchronized electrical activity in the cortex, eventually resulting in the typical appearance of slow-wave (delta wave) sleep. In this state, the cortex is effectively deafferented, or "closed off" from most sensory stimuli. At some point during slow-wave sleep, "REM-on cells" (a subpopulation of the wakefulness-promoting cells that are cholinergic and located primarily in the upper pons), begin to fire, stimulating the thalamus and basal forebrain. This results in renewed EEG desynchronization. During this stage (REM sleep), the EEG resembles that in awake subjects. In addition to activating the thalamus and basal forebrain, the REM-on cells have other brain and spinal cord projections that result in saccadic eye movements, suppression of other skeletal muscle activity, preserved respiratory and cardiovascular function, and (probably) increased activity in visual pathways. REM-on cells have a reciprocal inhibitory relationship with a population of neurons that are called REM-off cells, which are scattered across several locations in the brainstem and hypothalamus and contain serotonin, norepinephrine, and histamine. During REM sleep, the cholinergic REM-on cells are active and the REM-off cells are silent, but at some point during REM sleep, the REM-off cells become active, and the brain's activity returns to the pattern that characterizes non-REM sleep.

One component of the system regulating REM, NREM, and wakefulness is hypocretin (also called orexin), a peptide located in certain hypothalamic neurons near the fornix. These neurons have excitatory projections throughout the central nervous system, including projections to the REM-off cells and many of the nuclei that promote wakefulness. The hypocretin system appears to be critical for stabilizing the awake state. It inhibits REM sleep and stimulates feeding and motor activity. It also appears to be involved in the balance of motor excitation and inhibition during emotionally charged activities.

The alternation between wakefulness and sleep depends on the interplay of two processes. First, the brain contains a circadian rhythm generator, an "internal clock" in the paired suprachiasmatic nuclei (SCN) of the hypothalamus. The rhythm is generated by feedback loops of transcription and translation in several "clock" genes, which cycle at a very regular frequency. In patients who have been removed from environmental stimuli, the SCN cycles with a period of 24.2 hours, but it can be reset by external stimuli, primarily light. The SCN has reciprocal connections with the pineal gland, which releases melatonin at levels that fluctuate in a regular diurnal pattern. Both melatonin and light exposure can either advance or delay the circadian clock, depending on when they occur relative to an individual's natural sleep time.

The second process influencing the timing of sleep onset is the duration of prior wakefulness. The longer a person has been awake, the greater the tendency to sleep. Adenosine appears to be one of the major factors mediating this effect. Caffeine blocks adenosine receptors, which could explain the mechanism by which caffeine helps ward off sleepiness.

In summary, the sleep-wake cycle represents a complex interaction between many systems including glutamatergic, GABA-ergic, cholinergic, and monoaminergic (serotonergic, norepinephrine-containing, and histaminergic) cells in the brainstem that promote wakefulness, GABA-ergic neurons that initiate sleep, cholinergic REM-on cells, monoaminergic REM-off cells, and the hypocretin/orexin system. The timing of the cycle is a function of the circadian process of the SCN, in which melatonin is a factor, and the sleep debt process, in which adenosine is paramount.

C. Diagnostic Tests

Several diagnostic tests are available to supplement the clinical diagnosis of sleep disorders. A *polysomnogram* is an all-night recording of eye movements, EEG (frontal, central and occipital leads), electrocardiogram, EMG (chin and anterior tibialis surface leads), oximetry, airflow at the nose and mouth, and thoracic and abdominal wall motion. The testing sometimes includes video and additional EEG monitoring, or other physiologic assessments such as snoring sounds, position, esophageal pH, end-tidal pCO_2, or intrathoracic pressure. *Home sleep apnea tests* monitor fewer physiologic parameters—usually just airflow, respiratory effort, and oxygen saturation—but they are often sufficient for establishing the diagnosis in people who are thought to have a moderate or high risk of obstructive sleep apnea and who don't have complicating comorbidities. *Actigraphy* is a technique in which people wear an accelerometer on their wrist for days to weeks in their home environment to identify the periods in which they are awake and asleep and record their sleep-wake cycles. A *Multiple Sleep Latency Test* (MSLT) is a measure of daytime sleepiness. A subject is asked to take four or five brief naps at 2-hour intervals on the day after an adequate night's sleep (as confirmed by a polysomnogram). The EEG, EMG, and eye movements are monitored to determine the mean time the subject takes to fall asleep and to identify periods of REM sleep that occur during the naps. The *maintenance of wakefulness test*, in which subjects are asked to stay awake during four 40-minute test periods, is less commonly used because the results can be hard to interpret.

D. Classification of Sleep Disorders

The International Classification of Sleep Disorders published by the American Academy of Sleep Medicine designates six major divisions: (1) insomnia, (2) sleep-related breathing disorders, (3) central disorders of hypersomnolence, (4) circadian rhythm sleep-wake disorders, (5) parasomnias, and (6) sleep-related movement disorders. In this chapter, sleep disorders are grouped into three general categories, based on whether patients have trouble staying awake (Part IV), trouble sleeping (Part V), or abnormal behaviors during sleep (Part VI)—but as noted in Part II, these categories often overlap.

IV. Trouble Staying Awake

Excessive daytime somnolence (hypersomnia) can be obvious or subtle. At one extreme, people with chronic, severe hypersomnia can have "sleep attacks," in which they fall asleep even during activities where a nap is clearly inappropriate. The sleep attacks usually last about 15 minutes, at which point patients awaken feeling refreshed. They are not overwhelmed by sleepiness again for 1 or 2 hours. At the other extreme, some people may not even appreciate that they are sleepy. They may be more aware of the consequences of hypersomnia, including loss of energy, fatigue, headaches, lack of initiative, memory lapses, difficulty concentrating, and short temper. For these people, the barrier to diagnosis is a failure to recognize that there is a problem with sleep in the first place. Patients with symptoms that could be manifestations of hypersomnia should be asked directed questions to determine if they have an underlying sleep disturbance. Once hypersomnia has been identified, the most common causes—insufficient sleep, sleep apnea, and narcolepsy—are often easily recognized based on features of the history.

A. Insufficient Sleep

The demands of modern life (and the ready availability of artificial lighting) lead many people to allot themselves inadequate time for sleep at night. As a consequence, they suffer from unrecognized, self-imposed sleep deprivation. This problem is so common that many people consider it normal to be drowsy or even fall asleep during the day, especially in unstimulating situations or after a big lunch. This is not normal behavior for fully rested individuals, however. Be sure to ask patients what time they wake up on days when they don't set an alarm. If it is substantially later than their usual wake-up time, and they are less sleepy on those days, they probably are not allotting themselves sufficient time for sleep during the week. This problem is managed by educating the patient about healthy sleep habits ("sleep hygiene").

B. Sleep Apnea

Sleep apnea is a condition in which patients periodically stop breathing while asleep. Central sleep apnea results from abnormal central nervous system control of respiration, which can be caused by a variety of processes. Much more commonly, sleep apnea is caused by temporary obstruction of the upper airway. Obstructive sleep apnea is the most common medical cause of excessive daytime somnolence.

Even in healthy subjects, the pharyngeal muscles that maintain airway patency relax during sleep. There is normally enough residual volume in the airway to permit airflow, but in patients with obstructive sleep apnea, the muscle relaxation results in partial or complete occlusion of the airway. This leads to reduced inspiratory airflow and increased respiratory effort, vascular changes, hypoxemia, and hypercarbia, ultimately culminating in partial awakening, during which the airway re-opens and oxygen and carbon dioxide levels return to normal. Sleep cannot be fully restorative when it is disrupted repeatedly throughout the night by these episodes of partial arousal, and the result is excessive somnolence during the day.

The cornerstone of clinical diagnosis is a history of apneic episodes during sleep. Patients are often unaware of the episodes because they are brief and arousal is only partial, so the history usually must be obtained from bed partners. People with obstructive sleep apnea characteristically snore loudly, punctuated with bouts of interrupted breathing that often terminate with snorts or gasps. The diagnosis of obstructive sleep apnea is also supported by the presence of any conditions that can predispose to upper airway narrowing, including obesity (causing fat deposition around the upper airway), facial or mandibular configurations such as retrognathia (posterior positioning of the mandible), malignant infiltration of the soft tissue of the neck, laryngeal muscle weakness, and enlarged tonsils, adenoids, soft palate, uvula, or tongue. Polysomnography is used to confirm the diagnosis of sleep apnea and to quantify the severity in terms of the number of episodes of respiratory disturbance per hour, the degree of blood oxygen desaturation, and the presence of any significant cardiac arrhythmias. In people with a high likelihood of moderate-to-severe obstructive sleep apnea, a home sleep apnea test can substitute for an in-lab polysomnogram as long as certain contraindications are not present.

Sleep apnea can result in hypersomnia not only for patients but also for bed partners and others who suffer disrupted sleep because of the loud snoring. Chronic obstructive sleep apnea is associated with an increased risk of pulmonary hypertension, systemic hypertension, cardiac arrhythmias, sudden death, myocardial infarction, stroke, and motor vehicle accidents. Some evidence suggests that it may contribute to the metabolic syndrome and its components, such as diabetes and hyperlipidemia. Successful treatment of the sleep apnea can reduce the risk of at least some of those conditions. In children, sleep apnea is associated with hyperactivity and poor performance in school.

The standard treatment for obstructive sleep apnea is nasal positive airway pressure (PAP). This is most often administered continuously (continuous positive airway pressure, or CPAP), but other modalities include bilevel PAP (BiPAP), autoadjusting PAP (APAP), or expiratory PAP (EPAP). PAP raises the pressure in the oropharynx, and thus in the upper airway, reversing the pressure gradient across the wall of the airway and propping it open. This treatment is beneficial in 80–90% of patients; the main reasons for treatment failure are poor adherence (because the patient finds the nightly use of a mask over the nose uncomfortable or unappealing) and nasal obstruction. Other treatment options include weight loss for overweight patients (usually easier said than done), positional therapy for those whose apnea is much worse when sleeping on their backs, oral appliances that pull the lower jaw forward and widen the upper airway (primarily helpful for mild cases), uvulopalatopharyngoplasty (which is helpful in about one-half the patients, but it is difficult to predict which half), and surgical correction of other abnormalities that obstruct the airway (e.g., tonsillectomy or correction of facial and mandibular deformities). An implanted hypoglossal nerve stimulator can be effective in selected patients. An implanted phrenic nerve stimulator can be effective for some patients with central sleep apnea. Medications that have been proposed for obstructive sleep apnea include protriptyline (Vivactil), acetazolamide (Diamox), mirtazapine (Remeron), donepezil (Aricept), dronabinol, atomoxetine, and oxybutynin, but the evidence is inconclusive. In patients with residual sleepiness despite effective treatment of their upper airway obstruction, modafinil and armodafinil (initially developed for narcolepsy—see Section C) may be beneficial.

C. Narcolepsy

Narcolepsy is a syndrome consisting of excessive daytime somnolence and disordered regulation of REM sleep, resulting in intrusion of components of REM sleep into NREM sleep and the waking state. It usually begins in teenage years. The classic form, narcolepsy type 1, is caused by loss of hypocretin-producing neurons in the hypothalamus; in 90% of people with this condition, cerebrospinal fluid levels of hypocretin are undetectable or extremely low. Narcolepsy type 1 is characterized by four cardinal symptoms:

1. *Chronic excessive daytime somnolence.* Unlike somnolence from other causes, the sleepiness that occurs in narcolepsy cannot be relieved by any amount of sleep.
2. *Cataplexy* is a sudden loss of postural tone that occurs while the patient is awake but is otherwise identical to the atonia that occurs during REM sleep. The atonia may involve only a single muscle group, resulting in subtle manifestations such as slight buckling of the knees, drooping of the head or jaw, ptosis, or even just a subjective feeling of weakness, or it may be generalized and lead to complete bodily collapse and paralysis. Auditory function and consciousness are preserved before, during, and after the attack, although some patients pass directly from the attack into sleep. Attacks are precipitated by sudden, strong emotion, particularly laughter, and they typically last several minutes.

3. *Sleep paralysis,* like cataplexy, consists of atonia identical to that of REM sleep. It occurs at the onset of sleep or on awakening. The patient is conscious or half-awake but unable to move. This is often accompanied by intense fear and a sense of being unable to breathe.

4. *Hypnagogic* (or *hypnopompic*) *hallucinations* are vivid auditory or visual dream-like experiences that occur at *the onset of sleep* (or *on awakening*).

Excessive daytime somnolence is a universal feature, and it is required for the diagnosis. Almost everyone with narcolepsy type 1 has cataplexy. Cataplexy hardly ever occurs in people who don't have narcolepsy type 1. Between 53% and 69% of people with narcolepsy type 1 have sleep paralysis and 63–77% have hypnagogic/hypnopompic hallucinations, so these features are common but not universal. They also are non-specific. For example, about 10% of the general population experiences sleep paralysis at least occasionally. People with narcolepsy type 2 have typical features of narcolepsy, but no cataplexy. Again, excessive daytime somnolence is required for the diagnosis; sleep paralysis and hypnagogic/hypnopompic hallucinations each occur in 35–40% of patients. The cause of narcolepsy type 2 is not known.

The MSLT is used to support the diagnosis: people with either narcolepsy type 1 or type 2 characteristically have a mean sleep latency of 5 minutes or less, whereas rested individuals who don't have narcolepsy require an average of more than 10 minutes to fall asleep. The MSLT also provides a measure of the tendency to enter REM sleep prematurely, without the normal progression through stages 1–4 of NREM sleep. Any period of REM sleep that occurs in the first 15 minutes of sleep is noted and referred to as a sleep-onset REM period. Two or more sleep-onset REM periods, together with a mean sleep latency of 8 minutes or less, are considered diagnostic of narcolepsy.

Narcolepsy type 1 is closely associated with the HLA-DQB1-0602 and HLA-DR1501 alleles. This association is not sensitive or specific enough to be useful as a diagnostic test, but it suggests that an autoimmune process could be the underlying cause of narcolepsy type 1. Although an alternative interpretation is that the HLA locus simply lies near a susceptibility gene for narcolepsy, other observations also suggest that narcolepsy type 1 is an autoimmune condition. For example, there have been associations with H1N1 infections and other infections and with some H1N1 vaccines.

Excessive daytime sleepiness in people with narcolepsy is treated primarily with stimulant medications, especially modafinil (Provigil), armodafinil (Nuvigil), dextroamphetamine (Dexedrine), or methylphenidate (Ritalin).

Nighttime doses of sodium oxybate (the sodium salt of γ-hydroxybutyrate) also improve cataplexy and daytime somnolence. It is classified as a controlled substance because of concerns about its potential for abuse; it has achieved notoriety as a "date rape" drug. Solriamfetol (Sunosi) and pitolisant (Wakix) are more recently approved medications for sleepiness associated with narcolepsy. Sodium oxybate is currently the only medication with FDA approval for cataplexy, but some tricyclic antidepressants, selective serotonin-norepinephrine reuptake inhibitors (SNRIs), and selective serotonin reuptake inhibitors (SSRIs) are also effective. Pitolisant is also effective. Nonpharmacologic therapy of narcolepsy includes improved sleep hygiene and scheduled therapeutic naps.

D. Other Causes of Hypersomnolence

Excessive sleepiness may be caused by many medications, including sedative-hypnotics, antiseizure medications, antihypertensives, antidepressants, and antihistamines. Withdrawal from stimulants may also result in hypersomnolence. Many metabolic abnormalities can also cause sleepiness, or even obtundation or stupor. These include hepatic encephalopathy, uremic encephalopathy, hyperglycemia, hypoglycemia, hypercalcemia, and (severe) hypothyroidism. Other causes of hypersomnia include meningitis, encephalitis, chronic subdural hematoma, and post-concussion syndrome.

V. Trouble Sleeping

Many different physiologic and psychological factors can interfere with sleep, and many patients with insomnia have more than one of these factors. The goal is to identify the contributing factors and treat the ones for which therapy is available. There are three main patterns of insomnia: sleep-onset delay (trouble falling asleep), early morning awakening (trouble staying asleep), and sleep fragmentation (repeated awakenings).

A. Sleep-Onset Delay

1. Psychophysiologic insomnia
People who are trying to fall asleep sometimes focus on disruptive features such as pain, loud noises, other sensory stimuli, stressors, or emotions that they are currently experiencing or that they have experienced recently. This makes it difficult for them to relax and fall asleep, which, in turn, makes them anxious, making it even more difficult for them to initiate and maintain sleep. On subsequent nights, their anxiety about falling asleep

(and a heightened concern about the need for sleep) may be enough to provoke this cycle, even after the original disruptive features have resolved. Over time, patients may develop a conditioned association between their bed and unsuccessful sleep; they often find that they sleep better outside the bedroom. Psychophysiologic insomnia is the term used for this cycle of conditioned behavior, regardless of the original cause (and even when no specific cause can be identified).

In treating patients with insomnia, you should try to eliminate or at least minimize any ongoing disruptive features, such as depression, restless legs syndrome (see Part VI of this chapter), periodic limb movements or other parasomnias (see Part VI), dyspnea, orthopnea, pain, discomfort, and medications that might be interfering with sleep. You should treat any medical conditions that might be contributing to these features.

In addition to treating disruptive features and underlying conditions, the focus when treating psychophysiologic insomnia is behavioral intervention. Patients should be instructed to set a fixed time for retiring and awakening, eliminate daytime naps, refrain from caffeine after noon, avoid exercise or anxiety-provoking activities after dinner, and sleep in a dark, quiet, comfortable room. Patients should also be encouraged to associate the bed primarily with sleep; they should read, watch TV, and eat elsewhere. If they are lying in bed unable to fall asleep, they should leave the room and do something relaxing, returning to bed when they feel sleepy. In fact, it may be useful to restrict the total length of time they spend in bed (and prohibit any naps). This will make them sleepier, increasing the likelihood that when they do go to bed they will fall asleep readily and sleep continuously. Once this goal is achieved, the amount of time allowed for sleep can be gradually lengthened. For patients whose insomnia fails to respond to these simple interventions, a variety of structured techniques, known collectively as cognitive-behavioral therapy, are available.

In some situations, sedative-hypnotic medications are an appropriate adjunct to therapy, but there is some potential for drug dependence, especially with benzodiazepines. These agents are typically most helpful when applied for a limited number of nights. Benzodiazepines bind to the GABA receptor complex. Three nonbenzodiazepine drugs that bind to the GABA receptor complex—zaleplon (Sonata), zolpidem (Ambien), and eszopiclone (Lunesta)—and one melatonin agonist—ramelteon (Rozerem)—have been approved by the FDA for treatment of insomnia, and they are less likely than benzodiazepines to be associated with tolerance or withdrawal effects, although the benefits of cognitive-behavioral therapy are more enduring. Three hypocretin (orexin) receptor antagonists—suvorexant (Belsomra), lembrorexant (Dayvigo), and daridorexant (Quviviq)—have also been approved.

2. Delayed sleep-wake phase disorder

Some people are able to fall asleep readily and sleep for normal periods of time but do so at the "wrong times." These people have sleep-wake schedule disturbances. The most common example is delayed sleep-wake phase disorder. People with this condition do not feel sleepy at bedtime, so they stay up until 3 a.m. or later. They then sleep for a normal interval if allowed to do so, but if the demands of work or school require them to awaken at 8 a.m. or earlier they become chronically sleepy, especially in the mornings. These patients usually compensate by sleeping late on weekends. In some cases, they can adjust their work schedules to accommodate their sleep patterns, but this is not practical for most people. This disorder is sometimes familial, and in some families it is associated with mutations in circadian clock genes. Delayed sleep-wake phase disorder is treated with strategically timed melatonin, usually combined with timed exposure to light.

B. Early Morning Awakening

1. Psychiatric and psychological causes

Depression is the most common cause of early morning awakening in older patients. Depression is also associated with a shortened REM sleep latency, reduced slow-wave NREM sleep, and variable disturbance of sleep onset. Alcohol also disrupts sleep in the latter part of the night. This can result in a cycle whereby depressed individuals treat their own insomnia with alcohol (because it helps induce drowsiness); they then experience early morning awakening, resulting in more daytime sleepiness, so they take more alcohol on subsequent nights.

2. Psychophysiologic factors

Just as psychophysiologic factors can result in a cycle exacerbating sleep-onset delay, they can also increase the tendency to awaken early, producing greater daytime sleepiness, leading to more anxiety, resulting in even greater tendency to awaken early, and so forth. The behavioral interventions used to treat psychophysiologic insomnia are the same whether it manifests as sleep-onset delay or early morning awakening.

3. Advanced sleep-wake phase disorder

Advanced sleep-wake phase disorder is a sleep-wake schedule disturbance analogous to delayed sleep-wake phase disorder, except that these patients fall asleep and wake up too early. Mutations in genes for the circadian clock or a related protein have been identified in association with familial forms of this disorder. The cornerstone of treatment is exposure to bright light in the evening to delay circadian rhythms.

C. Sleep Fragmentation

Sleep that is frequently interrupted is not sufficiently restorative. Interruptions may result from sleep apnea (see Part IV of this chapter) or from other conditions such as nocturia, orthopnea, or gastroesophageal reflux. Cluster headaches and other parasomnias (see Part VI) may awaken patients and fragment their sleep. Sleep fragmentation may even result from the need to awaken to take prescribed medications. Endocrine disorders and medications (especially corticosteroids and dopaminergic agents) can also produce this problem.

Any of these conditions may initiate the same kind of psychophysiologic cycle that leads to delayed sleep onset or early morning awakening. The same behavioral interventions are indicated, together with treatment directed at the underlying conditions.

D. Sleep State Misperception

Occasional patients report unrelenting insomnia but are found to have no objective abnormalities on sleep studies. This uncommon condition is called paradoxical insomnia, or sleep state misperception. It may be caused by a failure to perceive sleep, or it may represent hypochondriasis or another psychiatric disturbance. Of course, it is always possible that existing techniques are simply not adequate to demonstrate the underlying abnormality.

VI. Abnormal Behavior During Sleep

Most of the undesirable movements or behaviors that occur during sleep are associated with NREM sleep, probably because the atonia of REM sleep prevents most movements and behaviors of any kind, desirable or undesirable. When parasomnias occur during REM sleep, they are usually associated with disruption of the normal atonia.

A. Nonrapid Eye Movement (NREM) Sleep Parasomnias

1. Night terrors

Night terrors (also called sleep terrors) occur primarily in children but occasionally in adults. The child suddenly arouses from slow-wave sleep, screams, and manifests intense anxiety and autonomic activation (e.g., dilated pupils, perspiration, tachycardia, tachypnea, and piloerection). The child cannot be awakened or consoled but calms down after several minutes and returns to sleep. There is usually amnesia for the event, although there may be a vague recollection of a frightful image or mood. In contrast to typical dreams or nightmares, there is no sense of a coherent theme or "plot." Reassurance is often the only treatment necessary, but intermediate- or long-acting benzodiazepines (typically clonazepam) can be used for particularly frequent and disruptive or dangerous events. Tricyclic antidepressants or selective serotonin reuptake inhibitors may also be effective.

2. Sleepwalking and sleep talking

In sleep talking, speech is often incoherent or elementary. Sleepwalking (somnambulism) involves complex behaviors that can include sitting up in bed, walking, dressing, eating, cooking, voiding, and even driving a car. Sleepwalkers have their eyes open and react partially to their environment; they can avoid objects, but their coordination is poor. Most episodes last a few seconds to a few minutes. Most children who exhibit sleepwalking outgrow it between ages 7 and 14 years.

In most cases of sleepwalking and sleep talking, no treatment is necessary except for reassurance. Safety restraints on doors, windows, and stairways may be required. When episodes are frequent, patients should be evaluated for sleep-related breathing disorders and managed accordingly. When no underlying disorder is identified, patients with frequent and disruptive episodes may be treated with clonazepam or a tricyclic antidepressant at bedtime.

3. Confusional arousals

Confusional arousals are characterized by confusion, slow responses, inappropriate behavior, and poor coordination, typically lasting a few minutes, following arousal from slow-wave sleep. Sudden, forced awakening can precipitate the episodes. They are very common in children less than 5 years of age, but most children outgrow them. They are present in about 4% of the adult population. A variety of medications, especially sedative-hypnotics, antihistamines, and antidepressants, can precipitate or exacerbate them. Conservative management is usually sufficient.

Sleep talking, sleepwalking, confusional arousals, and night terrors are all referred to as disorders of arousal. Many people have more than one of these disorders. Sleepwalking, confusional arousals, and night terrors arise in deep NREM sleep. Sleep talking can occur in any stage, but it usually occurs in light NREM sleep. There is a strong genetic predisposition to disorders of arousal. These disorders are sometimes associated with underlying sleep disorders such as sleep apnea. Although any of the disorders of arousal may be exacerbated by anxiety and psychosocial stress, they are usually not associated with severe psychopathology.

4. Enuresis

Enuresis (bedwetting) is involuntary micturition during sleep in an individual who has control of the bladder while awake. Enuresis is usually idiopathic, but it may be a symptom of underlying urogenital disease or another medical problem, or even sleep apnea. In many people, it probably represents delayed maturation; at age 5 years, about 15% of boys and 10% of girls have episodes of enuresis, which usually disappear by late childhood or adolescence. Psychological factors or family dynamics sometimes play a role. For frequent episodes, children may be treated with behavioral techniques (including enuresis alarms), deamino-8-d-arginine vasopressin (DDAVP, Desmopressin), or tricyclic antidepressants (typically imipramine) at low doses.

5. Periodic limb movements of sleep

Periodic limb movements of sleep usually involve the legs, typically resulting in dorsiflexion of the ankle and small toes, with flexion of the knee and hip, sometimes producing a "kicking" movement. These are the same muscles involved in the "triple flexion" response (see Chapter 2), but the movement is slower. These movements occur in "trains" during sleep. Similar movements may accompany arousals from sleep apnea, so it is important to exclude that diagnosis.

Some patients with periodic movements of sleep have restless legs syndrome when awake, but most do not. In contrast, 80–90% of all patients with restless legs syndrome also have periodic limb movements of sleep. Restless legs syndrome is characterized by an uncomfortable compulsion to move the legs, typically accompanied by deep paresthesias and crawling sensations in the calves and legs. The unpleasant sensations are relieved by stretching the legs or walking. These symptoms are more intense in the evening and at night than they are during the day, and they occur primarily when lying down or sitting. Restless legs syndrome can be associated with iron-deficiency anemia, and even patients with normal serum ferritin levels may have reduced ferritin levels in the CSF, suggesting that the condition may be related to impaired iron transport across the blood-brain barrier. When iron deficiency is present, iron replacement, is the first-line treatment. Restless legs syndrome commonly responds to L-dopa and dopamine agonists, although with long-term use these medications often cause augmentation: the restless legs symptoms start to appear earlier in the day, they grow increasingly intense, and they may spread to other regions of the body; meanwhile, the duration of medication effect gradually falls. Gabapentin, pregabalin, benzodiazepines, and opioids are also effective and less likely to cause augmentation.

6. Seizures

The synchronization that occurs during NREM sleep has the effect of promoting seizure propagation, whereas REM sleep inhibits epileptic discharges and seizures. Several epilepsy syndromes occur predominately or exclusively during sleep. Self-limited epilepsy with centrotemporal spikes (SeLECTS) is discussed in Chapter 5. Nocturnal frontal lobe epilepsy is characterized by episodes that occur in NREM sleep during which patients exhibit a variety of complex movements of the trunk and proximal extremities, including body rocking, kicking, boxing, pedaling, spitting, shouting, and swearing. Diagnosis may be difficult because many patients have a normal EEG even during the episodes. Other epilepsy syndromes are also associated with sleep.

7. Miscellaneous

About 60–70% of people have *hypnic jerks*—occasional isolated myoclonic jerks that occur at the onset of the first sleep interval of the night. Reassurance is the only treatment necessary. Some patients have conditions that produce more extensive myoclonus, which can sometimes disrupt their sleep or that of their bed partner. Most people grind their teeth at times, but in 5–15% of the population *bruxism* (tooth grinding) is severe or frequent enough to result in jaw discomfort or significant tooth wear. It may contribute to periodontal disease and temporomandibular joint dysfunction. *Sleep-related rhythmic movement disorder* is the label given to a group of uncommon parasomnias in which patients have stereotyped, repetitive movements such as banging of the head, side-to-side head movements, or rocking of the body, sometimes with rhythmic chanting or humming, just before sleep onset and continuing into light sleep. This typically occurs in normal infants or toddlers and usually resolves in the second or third year of life, but sometimes persists into older childhood or adulthood.

B. Rapid Eye Movement (REM) Sleep Parasomnias

1. REM sleep behavior disorder

REM sleep behavior disorder is a condition in which the atonia that normally accompanies REM sleep breaks down and patients "act out" parts of dreams. Motor activity is often vigorous enough to cause injury to patients or their bed partners. This disorder is associated with bilateral lesions in the upper pons (the region where the REM-on cells are located). Most patients are older than 50 years. The condition can be idiopathic, but most people with REM sleep behavior disorder eventually develop a disorder associated with α-synuclein accumulation, such as dementia with Lewy bodies (DLB), Parkinson disease (PD), or multiple system atrophy (MSA), as discussed in Chapters 7 and 8. The sleep disturbance sometimes precedes other neurologic manifestations of these diseases by a decade or more. It is sometimes difficult to distinguish REM sleep behavior disorder from nocturnal seizures on the basis of the history, and polysomnography can be helpful in this regard. Patients are usually treated successfully with clonazepam. Melatonin, L-dopa, dopamine agonists, donepezil, or sodium oxybate are second line agents that may also be helpful.

2. Nightmares

Nightmares are particularly vivid and disturbing dreams that often are associated with arousal from REM sleep. In contrast to night terrors, there is much less autonomic arousal, patients are readily awakened, and the patients can remember the dream, which usually has a story element. Chronic nightmares are often psychiatric in origin. Post-traumatic stress disorder is a common cause. Nightmares can be precipitated by some medications, such as L-dopa, beta-adrenergic blockers, and antidepressants, and also by abrupt withdrawal from some medications. Most patients need no treatment other than reassurance, but cognitive-behavioral therapy is sometimes necessary. A REM-suppressing agent, such as a tricyclic antidepressant or a selective serotonin reuptake inhibitor, is occasionally needed.

3. Miscellaneous

Cluster headaches typically occur during REM sleep and are sometimes included in discussions of parasomnias. Further details are presented in

Chapter 12. Penile erections are normal in REM sleep; very rarely they are painful enough to disrupt sleep. Catathrenia refers to expiratory groaning that typically begins 2–6 hours after sleep onset and occurs intermittently during the night; it is most common in REM sleep and the lighter stages of NREM sleep. It is not well understood, and no effective treatment is available.

VII. Discussion of Case Histories

Case 1. This person has hypersomnia. Falling asleep at the wheel outside the setting of sleep deprivation is never normal. This man allocates 9 hours for sleep each night, so he is not sleep deprived. One important consideration would be a medication effect, as antihypertensive agents can be associated with hypersomnia. The most likely diagnosis, however, is obstructive sleep apnea. The history of snoring, severe enough to prompt his wife to sleep in another room, strongly suggests the diagnosis. His obesity and big neck both could contribute to upper airway narrowing. Hypertension is present in about 40% of patients at the time of diagnosis of obstructive sleep apnea. You should ask the patient when he developed his hypersomnia, when he began snoring, and when he started gaining weight. He does not report any of the features that might suggest narcolepsy, although it would be important to inquire about them explicitly.

You should refer this man for polysomnography (especially because his wife cannot reliably say whether he is experiencing apneic episodes during sleep). If frequent episodes of apnea are documented, the study should be repeated with a trial of CPAP to see if the patient is likely to respond to this treatment. You should also encourage him to lose weight, and review his antihypertensive regimen to be sure it is not contributing to his problem. You should warn him not to drive alone until his hypersomnia has been adequately diagnosed and treated.

Case 2. This woman is correct that many of her symptoms can be features of depression, but they could also be manifestations of sleep disorders. Depression and sleep disorders have many common features, and it is often difficult to determine which problem is primary and which is secondary. In this case, the biggest clue that the delayed sleep onset might have a cause other than depression is the patient's report that she is unable to lie down for a prolonged period of time. The specific symptoms she describes are characteristic of restless legs syndrome. In addition, she notes epigastric discomfort when she is lying down, suggesting that she may also have gastroesophageal reflux. Both of these conditions can interfere with sleep onset, setting up a cycle of anxiety and insomnia as described in Part V.

The diagnosis of restless legs syndrome is based on the history. Patients should be evaluated for iron deficiency and uremia, both of which are associated with this disorder; iron replacement is indicated when the fasting serum ferritin level is 75 ng/mL or less. If restless legs symptoms persist, gabapentin or pregabalin should be prescribed. This patient should also receive appropriate treatment for gastroesophageal reflux; diagnostic studies are necessary only if her symptoms fail to respond.

This patient may also have established a pattern of psychophysiologic insomnia that will persist even after treatment of her reflux and restless legs syndrome. If so, she will need education about proper sleep hygiene, and she may require the kinds of behavioral interventions described in Part V. Only if depressive symptoms persist despite all these measures should treatment of depression be considered.

Case 3. The description of this girl's episode is classic for night terrors. The previous episodes may indeed have been exacerbated by the stress of a new home and day care environment, but the family should be informed that there is no evidence that this condition is caused by underlying psychiatric disease. If she has frequent recurrent episodes in the future, she will need to be evaluated for obstructive sleep apnea, but at this point, no additional investigations are necessary and no treatment is indicated other than good sleep hygiene and safety measures to prevent injury. The girl and her parents should be reassured that she does not have a serious disease, and she will probably outgrow these episodes, but they may recur during times of stress.

Chapter 10

Multifocal Central Nervous System Disorders

I. Case Histories

Case 1. A 29-year-old right-handed woman with a history of intravenous (IV) drug use has come to the emergency department because of the acute onset of inability to speak. Two days ago, she noticed weakness of the left arm after injecting heroin there and concluded that she must have "hit a nerve." She has been experiencing fevers, chills, and sweats for the past week, and feels tired all the time. Her general examination is notable for a temperature of 39°C and petechiae on both legs. Neurologic examination reveals almost no verbal output, nearly normal comprehension, left hemiparesis, and sensory loss to all modalities on her left side (face worse than arm worse than leg). Reflexes are increased throughout the left arm and leg, and a Babinski sign is present on the left.

Questions:

1. Where's the lesion?
2. What diagnoses should be considered?
3. What diagnostic tests would be helpful?
4. How should this patient be managed?

Case 2. A 35-year-old man has made an appointment with his family doctor because for the past 3 weeks, his left foot has had a tendency to drag after the third mile of his daily 5-mile run. Two years ago, he had a similar problem with the right foot, but he had twisted that ankle a week earlier, and when the symptoms resolved over the next month, he thought nothing more of them. He also had an episode of partial loss of vision in the left eye 8 months ago. It developed gradually over 5 days and resolved at almost the same rate; at the time, he attributed it to the stress of a divorce and a new job.

His general physical examination is normal. He has normal mental status. He has an afferent pupillary defect on the left, and his cranial nerves are otherwise normal. He has moderate weakness of left ankle dorsiflexion and walks with a mild foot drop on the left, but his motor examination is otherwise normal. Reflexes are increased at the left knee and ankle, and he has a Babinski sign on the left. Sensation is intact to all modalities.

Questions:

1. Where's the lesion?
2. What diagnoses should be considered?
3. What diagnostic tests would be helpful?
4. How should this patient be managed?

Case 3. A 67-year-old woman has come to the emergency department because of her second episode of Bell palsy within 6 months. The first episode resulted in only mild weakness of the right side of her face, so she was not treated. She has improved only minimally in the interim. The second episode began yesterday morning when she noted a tendency to drool out of the left side of her mouth, and she awoke this morning with complete inability to move the left side of her face. She has also noticed that her voice is hoarser than it used to be, and she thinks the hearing in her right ear is deteriorating. In addition, she reports that 2 weeks ago, she developed pain in her lower back on the right; for the last week, it has radiated into her right posterior thigh, leg, and little toe.

Her general physical examination is unremarkable. Neurologic examination confirms bilateral facial weakness (including forehead muscles), worse on the left, hearing loss in the right ear, reduced movement of the left side of the palate, and absent gag reflex on the left side. She has slight weakness of right ankle plantar flexion, but the motor examination is otherwise normal. She has no right ankle jerk, but all other reflexes are normal and symmetric. The sensory examination is normal.

Questions:

1. Where's the lesion?
2. What diagnoses should be considered?
3. What diagnostic tests would be helpful?
4. How should this patient be managed?

II. Approach to Multifocal Disorders

It is sometimes impossible to identify a single lesion site that explains all of a patient's symptoms and signs. Most systemic illnesses, neuromuscular diseases, dementing illnesses, movement disorders, and sleep disorders affect the nervous system diffusely. Still, even these diffuse conditions possess some pattern and symmetry. The particular pattern of involvement is generally the basis for making a diagnosis (see Figure 6.1 in Chapter 6 for a flowchart outlining an approach to diagnosing diffuse disorders of the peripheral nervous system).

This chapter addresses multifocal conditions. Unlike focal lesions and diffuse processes, multifocal conditions are characterized primarily by the lack of a consistent pattern. Fortunately, there are only a few conditions like this, so the diagnosis is often straightforward. In other words, the lack of pattern is itself a revealing pattern. The classic multifocal disease is multiple sclerosis (MS). Other inflammatory diseases and neoplastic processes can also produce multifocal manifestations. The time course and epidemiologic factors help to distinguish among these possibilities (see Chapter 3).

There are two broad categories of multifocal disorders. Some diseases propagate in random directions from a single focus. This is typical of infections and neoplastic diseases. Other processes are intrinsically multifocal. Most diseases in this category (including MS) are inflammatory but not infectious.

III. Focal Diseases with Multifocal Propagation

A. Neurologic Manifestations of Systemic Cancer

Central nervous system (CNS) metastases occur in 20–40% of patients with systemic cancer, and in more than two thirds of these patients, the metastases are symptomatic. The spinal cord may be involved by direct metastasis, or, more commonly, by epidural compression from a bony metastasis, as discussed in Chapter 15. Brain metastasis is particularly likely in patients with melanoma or testicular cancer, about half of whom have an intracranial tumor found at autopsy. Because lung cancer and breast cancer are common, they are the most likely sites of primary tumor in patients with brain metastases. Lung cancer accounts for 30–50% of all patients with brain metastases; breast cancer and melanoma each account for 10–20%.

The next most common primary tumors are gastrointestinal tumors and genitourinary tract tumors, each accounting for 5–10% of cases.

When patients with known cancer elsewhere in their body develop symptoms that localize to the brain and progress over a time course suggestive of a neoplasm (see Chapter 3), metastasis is the prime consideration. The preferred diagnostic test is an MRI scan of the brain. A metastasis typically appears on MRI or CT scans as a well-demarcated, contrast-enhancing, spherical lesion with surrounding edema, but this appearance is not specific, so a biopsy is sometimes necessary to establish the diagnosis even in patients with a known primary cancer. The MRI scan shows more than one lesion in up to 75% of patients with brain metastases, and the presence of multiple lesions with characteristic features (as opposed to a solitary lesion) increases the likelihood of metastases.

When the systemic cancer is controlled and only a single brain metastasis exists, it should be surgically resected, if possible. This is commonly followed by stereotactic radiosurgery, which uses multiple convergent beams of external irradiation to deliver a high single dose of radiation to a well-circumscribed region. Stereotactic radiosurgery is also an alternative to surgical resection when the metastasis is in a surgically inaccessible location or when the patient is not a surgical candidate.

Even when two or three metastatic lesions are present, resection may be appropriate if the lesions are surgically accessible, but stereotactic radiosurgery is often preferred. The more lesions there are, the less feasible surgical resection and stereotactic radiosurgery become. Patients who have widespread intracranial metastases and patients with a poor overall prognosis (based on their performance status, age, or the extent of systemic spread of their primary tumor) are generally treated with whole-brain radiation therapy. This can have palliative effects and prolong survival, but it is rarely curative. It is also associated with a high rate of delayed neurotoxicity. Chemotherapy may be effective in treating some brain metastases (such as metastases from testicular germ cell tumors), but the response is disappointing for most types of tumor. Targeted agents, such as tyrosine kinase inhibitors, are effective for some metastases from some types of primary tumor. Immune checkpoint inhibitors have beneficial effects for brain metastases from melanoma or non-small cell lung cancer.

Approximately 15% of patients with brain metastases have no known primary cancer and no other symptoms of malignancy at the time their CNS lesions are discovered. People with no known cancer who have brain lesions that look metastatic should be thoroughly evaluated for a primary neoplasm so that it can be treated appropriately. Furthermore, if the primary cancer can be found, and multiple brain lesions with typical characteristics of metastasis are present, there is no need for biopsy or surgical resection of the brain lesions. The evaluation should generally include CT scanning of the chest, abdomen, and pelvis. These patients also require thorough skin examinations and rectal examinations, and stool should be screened for occult blood. Male patients require careful testicular and prostate examinations, and female patients need careful breast examinations. If the diagnosis remains obscure, stereotactic brain biopsy (or surgical resection when there is only one lesion) is indicated.

Even before the diagnosis is established, many patients require treatment for the mass effect produced by the edema surrounding the metastases. Dexamethasone usually produces dramatic reduction in brain edema and clinical symptoms. The optimal dose is not known. A common practice is to give a loading dose of 10 mg, followed by a dose of 4 to 8 mg twice a day. When the mass effect is so great that there is a risk of cerebral herniation, higher initial doses may be used, and osmotic diuresis and hyperventilation may also be necessary (see Chapter 11). The dexamethasone dose is gradually tapered as clinically tolerated over subsequent days.

Seizures occur in approximately 25% of patients with brain metastases and are treated with antiseizure medications according to standard principles (see Chapter 5). For patients who have not yet seized, prophylactic antiseizure medications are usually not recommended, although some clinicians make an exception for metastatic melanoma, which has a high incidence of hemorrhage.

In 5–10% of people with systemic cancer, there is clinical evidence of spread to the meninges. This spread has been given a variety of labels, including leptomeningeal metastasis, carcinomatous meningitis, or meningeal carcinomatosis. It can occur with almost any cancer but is most commonly associated with breast cancer, leukemia, lymphoma, lung cancer, and melanoma. Leptomeningeal metastasis can present in several ways. It can cause meningeal irritation, producing a syndrome resembling meningitis. It may present with mental status changes and other symptoms of hydrocephalus when the cancer cells block CSF outflow. Tumor cells in the meningeal spaces may also compress nerve roots or cranial nerves as they leave the neuraxis, resulting in multiple cranial neuropathies or polyradiculopathies. The first step in diagnosis is an MRI scan of the brain and spinal cord, which typically shows linear or nodular enhancement of the meninges, particular in sulci or cisterns intracranially and along the surface of the spinal cord, cauda equina, or both. In some cases, the MRI findings are sufficient for establishing the diagnosis, but when the MRI findings are negative or nonspecific, a lumbar puncture should be performed. Cytologic identification of malignant cells in the CSF is the definitive diagnostic finding. Individual samples may be negative, so patients may require three or more lumbar punctures before the diagnosis is established. Additional CSF tests that may be helpful include flow cytometry (looking for a monoclonal population of B cells or T cells, especially in patients with hematologic malignancies) and assays for specific tumor markers. Meningeal enhancement on MRI scans can occur in normal subjects after a lumbar puncture, so it is best to obtain the MRI scan before performing any lumbar punctures. Intrathecal chemotherapy combined with radiation therapy helps to prolong life, and preliminary evidence suggests that tyrosine kinase inhibitors and systemic checkpoint inhibitors may be beneficial, but even with optimal treatment life expectancy for patients diagnosed with leptomeningeal metastasis is 6–12 months.

Cancers also can metastasize to the peripheral nervous system (PNS). Tumor cells can invade the brachial plexus and the lumbosacral plexus, and this is the first symptom of cancer in some patients. Individual peripheral nerves or muscles can also be sites of metastasis, but this is less common. Focal metastases in the peripheral nervous system are usually treated with radiation therapy.

Tumors can also cause remote effects without metastasizing; these manifestations are called *paraneoplastic syndromes* and are usually diffuse rather than multifocal. Examples include cerebellar degeneration, encephalitis, seizures, various forms of polyneuropathy (pure sensory neuropathy is the most specific), Lambert-Eaton myasthenic syndrome, and dermatomyositis. In many instances, the paraneoplastic syndrome becomes symptomatic before the patient has developed any other clinical manifestations of the underlying tumor. Paraneoplastic syndromes are thought to be the result of an autoimmune response to the tumor, but the precise pathogenic mechanisms are unknown. Table 10.1 lists some of the antibodies that are associated with these syndromes, but many others have also been identified. Serum and CSF paraneoplastic antibody panels are commercially available, but the abnormal antibodies may not be detectable early in the disease process. In some cases, the antibody panels are consistently negative; one reason is that there are probably additional paraneoplastic antibodies that have not yet been identified. Conversely, in some patients with positive antibodies, no primary tumor is ever found, suggesting that factors other than tumor sometimes trigger the autoimmune response. For example, autoimmune encephalitis can occur in association with antibodies to thyroglobulin or thyroid peroxidase or with antibodies to leucine-rich glioma-inactivated protein 1 (LGI1); these conditions often respond very well to high-dose steroid treatment. Patients with LGI1-associated encephalitis often have episodic, involuntary jerking movements of the arm and face on one side of the body, referred to as faciobrachial dystonic seizures; these can be a clue to the diagnosis.

When patients with no known tumor have symptoms and signs suggestive of a paraneoplastic syndrome, they should be evaluated for a primary cancer, typically with CT scanning of the chest, abdomen, and pelvis. Some antibodies have particular associations with specific tumors, as shown in Table 10.1, and this may be helpful in selecting additional diagnostic tests. If an underlying cancer is identified, it should be treated. Whether or not an underlying cancer is identified, patients are usually treated with some form of immune suppression—often high-dose intravenous steroids initially, sometimes followed by plasma exchange, intravenous immunoglobulin (IVIg), or steroid-sparing immunosuppressive medications. When the initial screening fails to identify a primary cancer, it should generally be repeated periodically for several years.

B. Central Nervous System Infections

Infectious agents can reach the CNS either by direct spread (from the sinuses or the inner ear, for example) or via the bloodstream. When infections reach the CNS, the resulting damage can be focal (e.g., an abscess or focal myelitis), multifocal (e.g., multiple abscesses), or diffuse (meningitis or encephalitis). This section concerns focal and multifocal infectious processes. Meningitis and encephalitis are discussed in Chapter 12, although encephalitis due to herpesviruses is also discussed later in this section.

1. Abscesses

An *abscess* is a localized area of suppuration and necrosis that forms when certain organisms reach a relatively hypoxic region of the body where host defenses are inadequate to eradicate the infection. Initially, the region of inflammation is poorly demarcated, but over the course of 2 or 3 weeks, a well-defined fibrous capsule forms. Anaerobic bacteria, aerobic bacteria, fungi, or parasites can cause CNS abscesses.

In many ways, CNS abscesses are analogous to metastatic tumors in the CNS. Both are mass lesions. The time course is characteristically subacute for abscesses and chronic for metastases, but this distinction is not always reliable. Abscesses and metastases are often indistinguishable radiographically—both characteristically appear as contrast-enhancing lesions with surrounding edema, and the area of enhancement often produces a ring around the lesion. The central core of an abscess is typically evident as a region of restricted diffusion on MRI scan. The likely diagnosis can sometimes be established by examining spinal fluid (cytopathology for metastases, cultures for abscesses), but the yield is often low, and brain herniation sometimes occurs when a lumbar puncture is performed on a patient in whom a focal mass lesion has produced a significant elevation of intracranial pressure. For both abscesses and metastases, definitive diagnosis usually requires direct tissue examination (i.e., biopsy or surgical resection), although this can sometimes be performed on lesions elsewhere in the body if they can be identified.

The optimal treatment of a solitary CNS abscess is either total excision or aspiration under stereotactic CT or MRI guidance, in conjunction with systemic antibiotic therapy. No controlled trials have compared excision to aspiration, but aspiration is more common. Excision is usually recommended for abscesses that are multiloculated, gas-containing, fungal, due to head trauma, or unresponsive to aspiration. Excision is most feasible when an abscess is solitary, superficial, and well-encapsulated. When multiple abscesses are present, systemic antibiotic therapy is the cornerstone of treatment, although the largest lesions may still be aspirated or (less often) excised. The choice of antibiotics depends on the underlying organism (or organisms), so even when neither excision nor aspiration is an option (e.g., when there are multiple small or deep abscesses), biopsy of one of the lesions may be desirable. When biopsy is not possible, patients are treated empirically, typically with a third-generation cephalosporin (cefotaxime or ceftriaxone) and metronidazole. Chloramphenicol also provides good coverage and CNS penetration but carries a greater risk of toxicity. When there are reasons to suspect a particular infectious agent, the antibiotic regimen should be tailored accordingly (e.g., antistaphylococcal agents such as vancomycin should be included when abscesses occur in the setting of recent head trauma or brain surgery).

2. Infective endocarditis

Infections in the heart are ideally situated for sending colonies in all directions. Cerebral embolism occurs in 20–40% of all patients with infective endocarditis. The emboli can be either sterile or infectious. Sterile emboli result in strokes that are indistinguishable from any other cardioembolic strokes. Infectious emboli can produce strokes by occluding arteries, or they may be deposited in the meninges or parenchyma, serving as foci for the development of meningitis or abscesses. In 2–4% of all patients with infective endocarditis, septic emboli infect the walls of the cerebral arteries themselves, leading to aneurysmal dilatation (*mycotic aneurysms*) that can rupture and cause subarachnoid, intraparenchymal, or intraventricular hemorrhage. Even if they don't rupture, mycotic aneurysms can be the source of emboli, resulting in downstream strokes. The mortality rate is 30% among patients with unruptured mycotic aneurysms and nearly 80% in patients with ruptured mycotic aneurysms.

Although anticoagulation is the standard treatment for most cardioembolic causes of stroke (see Chapter 4), it is generally avoided in patients with infective endocarditis because it does not prevent the growth of vegetations and may increase the risk of hemorrhagic transformation of a stroke or rupture of a mycotic aneurysm. The one exception is endocarditis on an artificial valve, in which the risk of recurrent embolization is so high that the benefits of anticoagulation probably outweigh the risks (but the exception to this exception is *S. aureus* endocarditis on an artificial valve, where the usual practice is to withhold all anticoagulation for at least the first 2 weeks of antibiotic therapy).

The presence of mycotic aneurysms does not affect therapy, except for aneurysms that have ruptured or increased in size, in which case coiling or clipping is often performed (although extending the antibiotic course is sometimes effective for unruptured aneurysms that have been enlarging). CT angiography (CTA) and MR angiography (MRA) are commonly used to evaluate for mycotic aneurysms, but because these aneurysms are often located distally in the arterial tree where CTA and MRA are less sensitive, intra-arterial catheter angiography is considered the gold-standard imaging modality for diagnosis.

One reasonable approach when patients have had one or more strokes (whether ischemic or hemorrhagic) in the setting of endocarditis is to perform a CTA or MRA as soon as it is safe and feasible. If this imaging shows a mycotic aneurysm, then it should be repeated at the conclusion of the antibiotic course. If the aneurysm is unchanged or larger, the patient will probably need coiling or surgical resection; if the aneurysm is present but smaller, a prolonged course of antibiotics would be reasonable. For patients whose initial CTA or MRA shows no mycotic aneurysm, the possibility remains that the imaging modality was not sufficiently sensitive, so those with intracerebral hemorrhage should have a catheter angiogram at the conclusion of the antibiotic course. Patients with purely ischemic stroke and no evidence of mycotic aneurysm on initial imaging may not need further testing for mycotic aneurysms unless long-term anticoagulation is being considered.

Stroke in the setting of endocarditis is not an indication for valve replacement surgery. When patients require acute valve replacement for other reasons (such as refractory congestive heart failure or perivalvular abscess), the surgery can result in further neurologic deterioration if performed within the first week or two of a stroke. For this reason, valve replacement surgery is usually delayed until at least a week after ischemic stroke and at least 3 weeks after a cerebral hemorrhage, if possible—but in some situations, the need for cardiac surgery is so urgent that it outweighs the neurologic risks.

3. Specific infectious agents

Certain infectious agents are particularly likely to produce multifocal nervous system disease. Most of these infections are relatively indolent, perhaps because more aggressive infections become symptomatic and are treated (or result in death) before they have a chance to form multiple disseminated colonies.

a. Human immunodeficiency virus (HIV)

Patients infected with HIV can develop dysfunction at any level of the nervous system. At least four factors predispose to neurologic involvement. First, these patients are at risk for many opportunistic infections and neoplasms that affect the nervous system. Second, HIV has a predilection for both the CNS and the PNS and may produce symptoms directly. Third, antigenic cross-reactivity between HIV and nervous system elements may occur, so that the inflammatory reaction provoked by HIV infection results in neurologic damage. Fourth, antiretroviral therapy (ART) and other medications used to treat HIV or its complications can have neurotoxic effects.

The most common PNS syndromes in people with HIV involve the muscles, nerves, plexuses, or nerve roots. Myositis most often occurs at the time of seroconversion, but it can develop at any stage of HIV infection. Four principal neuropathic syndromes are associated with HIV infection. The most common is a distal, symmetric peripheral polyneuropathy that tends to increase in incidence and severity with disease duration. This polyneuropathy is thought to be a direct effect of HIV infection, although other potential causes are often present (notably nutritional deficiencies and drug toxicity). Didanosine (ddI), zalcitabine (ddC), and stavudine (d4T) have been associated with neuropathy, and so have some of the drugs typically used to treat infectious manifestations of AIDS. The second type of neuropathic syndrome, inflammatory demyelinating poly-radiculoneuropathy, is much less common than axonal polyneuropathy. Acute inflammatory demyelinating polyradiculoneuropathy (AIDP) and chronic inflammatory demyelinating polyradiculoneuropathy (CIDP) may occur in HIV-positive patients who do not have AIDS. These conditions sometimes develop at the time of seroconversion, suggesting that they are caused by the inflammatory response to HIV and not by immunosup-pression or some other direct effect of HIV infection. Another, relatively rare, neuropathic syndrome is mononeuropathy multiplex, which can also occur early in the course of HIV infection. The fourth major variety of HIV-related neuropathic syndrome is progressive polyradiculopathy, typi-cally beginning with leg weakness and bladder or bowel problems, with progression to the arms over several weeks. This generally occurs with advanced immunodeficiency. Cytomegalovirus (CMV) appears to be the cause in many cases. Herpes varicella zoster reactivation is also common in HIV-infected patients, leading to a more localized radiculopathy. Cranial nerves may also be involved in patients with zoster, mononeuropathy mul-tiplex, AIDP, or CIDP.

In the CNS, the most common manifestation of HIV infection are referred to as HIV-associated neurocognitive disorders (HANDs), a term covering a spectrum that includes HIV associated dementia, minor neu-rocognitive disorder, and asymptomatic neurocognitive impairment (diag-nosed based on low neuropsychological test performance in people who have no symptoms or decline in function). Adequate ART reduces the like-lihood of developing HAND, especially the more severe forms, and ART is the main treatment for HAND. The non-nucleoside reverse transcriptase inhibitor efavirenz can cause psychiatric symptoms, so it should generally be avoided in people with HAND. People with HIV-associated dementia sometimes develop a myelopathy, with characteristic vacuolar changes noted in the spinal cord at autopsy; they often have incontinence, gait dis-turbance, and bilateral Babinski signs.

Focal lesions in the brain and spinal cord are common manifestations of HIV-associated secondary processes, especially toxoplasmosis, cryptococ-cus, and lymphoma. All of these can produce mass lesions (presenting with progressive, focal symptoms, usually with a subacute time course), but they can also be asymptomatic or produce diffuse symptoms. Cryptococcus, in particular, usually manifests with meningitis that can be fairly subtle—about 85% of patients experience headaches, but fever and neck stiffness each occur in only 35% of patients. Approximately 40% of patients with cryptococcal meningitis have altered mental status. Except for cranial neuropathies, focal findings are uncommon in cryptococcal meningitis. HIV also predisposes to progressive multifocal leukoencephalopathy (PML), a disease of white matter caused by the JC virus, an opportunistic papovavirus.

Because of the high incidence of mass lesions in the brain, an imaging study of the brain is usually the first test obtained in HIV-infected patients with headaches or mental status changes, even if there are no focal abnormalities on neurologic examination. When this study is normal, a lumbar puncture is usually performed to look for evidence of cryptococcal meningitis; cryptococcal antigen is present in the spinal fluid of 95% of patients with this infection. The CSF should also be evaluated for syphilis, tuberculosis, herpes simplex, and lymphoma.

When the brain imaging study is abnormal, differentiation between toxoplasmosis, lymphoma, PML, and less common conditions may be difficult. The condition that most readily responds to treatment is toxoplasmosis. Toxoplasmosis almost always represents reactivation of a latent infection in patients with CD4 counts below 200 cells/mm^3 (usually < 100 cells/mm^3), so toxoplasma IgG titers are consistently positive in patients with this manifestation, even early in the course. Thus, the standard approach in patients with HIV and CD4 counts below 200 cells/mm^3 who have multifocal mass lesions on a brain imaging study is to check serum toxoplasma IgG titers, and if they are positive, to treat empirically with the antibiotics sulfadiazine and pyrimethamine. The clinical and radiologic response is usually dramatic and rapid. If clinical and radiographic parameters fail to improve over the next 10 to 14 days, a biopsy should be performed. The main situation in which a trial of empiric antitoxoplasma medication is not recommended is when the brain MRI scan shows only a single lesion, because most patients with toxoplasmosis have multiple lesions visible on brain MRI. Even in this circumstance, empiric antitoxoplasma treatment is sometimes reasonable, particularly if CNS lymphoma is unlikely (for example, if the CD4 count is above 50 cells/mm^3). An urgent biopsy (rather than empiric toxoplasma treatment) is also indicated if the patient's clinical condition is deteriorating rapidly, or if the initial brain imaging study suggests a high risk of herniation. PML can sometimes be difficult to distinguish from toxoplasmosis and lymphoma on MRI scans, but it usually has a fairly distinctive appearance. When the scan looks typical of PML, empiric antitoxoplasma medicine is not necessary. Polymerase chain reaction (PCR) testing of CSF for JC virus DNA can be helpful in diagnosing PML, and positive Epstein-Barr virus PCR is evidence of CNS lymphoma. ART is the main treatment for PML in patients with HIV. Treatment of

CNS lymphoma in patients with HIV consists of ART combined with corticosteroids and high-dose methotrexate; recent results with rituximab and ibrutinib (a tyrosine kinase inhibitor) are promising. Cryptococcal meningitis usually responds readily to treatment with amphotericin and flucytosine for 2 weeks, followed by fluconazole consolidation therapy for 8 weeks. For both toxoplasmosis and cryptococcal meningitis, prolonged maintenance therapy is necessary to prevent relapses.

The *immune reconstitution inflammatory syndrome* (IRIS) is characterized by paradoxical clinical deterioration that usually occurs between 2 and 25 weeks after beginning ART. The main risk factor is a low CD4 count, especially in patients with a rapid rise in CD4 count and decline in HIV RNA viral load after ART is initiated. "Paradoxical" IRIS refers to worsening of a previously recognized opportunistic infection, whereas "unmasking" IRIS refers to the appearance of symptoms from a previously unrecognized opportunistic infection. PML and cryptococcal meningitis are the opportunistic infections most commonly associated with IRIS, so patients should be evaluated (and treated) for these conditions before starting ART. In patients who develop IRIS, ART should be continued and all opportunistic infections treated. Steroids are often administered, but they should be avoided in patients with cryptococcal meningitis.

Patients with AIDS have an increased incidence of syphilis, which may be hard to diagnose because some of the traditional serologic tests are less reliable in this setting. Patients who have AIDS may require more aggressive and sustained treatment for neurosyphilis than is necessary in immunocompetent individuals. Other conditions that may affect the nervous system in patients with AIDS include Kaposi sarcoma, atypical mycobacterial infections, nocardiosis, and fungal infections (e.g., candidiasis, aspergillosis, histoplasmosis, mucormycosis, and others). Patients with AIDS also have an increased incidence of strokes. In patients with AIDS, it is common for several different processes to affect the nervous system simultaneously.

b. Spirochetal infections

The initial clinical manifestation of syphilis (primary syphilis) is a skin lesion, or chancre, at the site of inoculation. In untreated patients, this heals spontaneously over 3–6 weeks; during this time, the spirochetes disseminate throughout the body, and in about 25–40% of infected patients, the nervous system is seeded. At this point, patients may develop the features of secondary syphilis (flu-like symptoms, rash, lymphadenopathy, and mucosal lesions). Neurologic symptoms are relatively rare; at most 5% of patients with secondary syphilis develop symptoms of aseptic meningitis (although asymptomatic lymphocytic meningitis is present in 25–40%). Some patients with disseminated organisms never manifest any symptoms of secondary syphilis. The symptoms (if any) of secondary syphilis resolve without treatment over a period of weeks to months, and patients enter a latent stage in which there are no clinical manifestations of infection for months to years. In 10–30% of untreated patients, the latent stage is followed by tertiary syphilis, which is characterized by skin, osseous, cardiovascular, or neurologic manifestations.

Neurosyphilis refers to nervous system involvement at any stage of syphilis. Most patients with neurosyphilis, regardless of the stage, are asymptomatic—only 4–6% of untreated patients with syphilis ultimately develop neurologic symptoms. These patients typically display one of several distinctive clinical syndromes. Aseptic meningitis can occur at any stage of the disease, from the first few weeks to many years later. It is characterized by headache and stiff neck, and it is often associated with cranial nerve involvement. Meningovascular syphilis can occur as early as 6 months after the primary infection, but it typically occurs 5–7 years after the primary infection. It is characterized by diffuse meningeal infiltrates and inflammation and fibrosis of arteries, causing brain and spinal cord lesions that may be focal, multifocal, or diffuse. The most delayed neurologic manifestations of syphilis are general paresis and tabes dorsalis, which usually occur 10–30 years after the initial infection. General paresis is a condition of diffuse cortical dysfunction, producing dementia, upper motor neuron findings, myoclonus, seizures, dysarthria, and pupillary abnormalities. Tabes dorsalis results from involvement of the posterior nerve roots as they enter the spinal cord. Typical symptoms are loss of proprioception, ataxia, lightning-like pains, and urinary incontinence. Deep tendon reflexes are usually absent in the lower extremities, though Babinski signs may be present when there is coexistent general paresis. The pupils are abnormal in more than 90% of patients; various abnormalities can occur, but the most characteristic finding is small, irregular, and unequal pupils that do not constrict in response to light but constrict when focusing on an approaching target.

Diagnosis of neurosyphilis is based on serologic studies from the blood and CSF, as well as other CSF features. Two types of serologic tests are currently available, nontreponemal and treponemal. Nontreponemal tests, such as the VDRL (Venereal Disease Research Laboratory test) or RPR (rapid plasma reagin), assay nonspecific antibodies made in response to a synthetic complex of cardiolipin, cholesterol, and lecithin. The sensitivity of these tests varies depending on the stage of disease. They are present in the blood of almost everyone with secondary syphilis and most people early in the latent stage of syphilis, but only about 70% of people with primary syphilis or late in the latent stage, and 50–60% of people with tertiary syphilis. A positive serum VDRL or RPR does not necessarily mean that a patient has neurosyphilis, but a positive result in the CSF is highly specific for neurosyphilis. Unfortunately, nontreponemal tests in the CSF have low sensitivity, so a negative CSF VDRL or RPR does not exclude the diagnosis of neurosyphilis. Serum treponemal tests, such as fluorescent treponemal antibody (FTA) or microhemagglutination–*Treponema pallidum* (MHA-TP), are highly sensitive at all but the earliest stages of the disease—and even in primary syphilis, they are positive in at least 75% of patients. These antibodies persist throughout life even when the infection itself is eradicated, so they are a reliable indicator of current or previous syphilitic infection but they do not indicate whether the infection is still active. CSF treponemal tests, like those in the serum, have high sensitivity but low specificity, in part because the treponemal antibodies may passively diffuse from blood into the CSF so they could be detectable even after the disease has been eradicated. Some studies suggest that CSF treponemal tests are more useful when higher cutoff values are used. Tests using PCR or monoclonal antibody reagents hold promise but are still experimental.

In a patient with aseptic meningitis, neurosyphilis can be diagnosed if either a nontreponemal or a treponemal test is positive. In a patient with clinical features suggestive of any other form of neurosyphilis, a negative serum treponemal test makes neurosyphilis very unlikely but a positive result simply means that the patient had an active syphilis infection at some point in their life. To determine if the infection is currently active in the CNS, a lumbar puncture should be performed, and the presence of any of the typical abnormalities (i.e., elevated white blood cell count, increased protein concentration, or positive VDRL) warrants treatment for neurosyphilis. Patients diagnosed with neurosyphilis should be treated with high doses of intravenous penicillin for 10–14 days.

In people with Lyme disease, the initial rash at the site of the tick bite is analogous to the initial chancre of syphilis—it can resolve without treatment, but meanwhile spirochetes disseminate throughout the body; 10–15% of patients will develop nervous system involvement. The most common neurologic manifestation is subacute or chronic meningitis that typically begins a few weeks to a few months after inoculation. The usual symptoms are headache and stiff neck, often with associated mood changes and difficulty concentrating. Cranial nerve palsies (almost always including one or both facial nerves) and radicular pain sometimes accompany the meningitis. Even in untreated patients, actual parenchymal infection of the brain or spinal cord is very rare, but when it occurs it can result in focal deficits or encephalitis. Patients with Lyme disease can also develop peripheral polyneuropathy.

Borrelia burgdorferi, the agent that causes Lyme disease, can almost never be cultured from the blood or spinal fluid, and even PCR has important limitations, so diagnosis is based on clinical characteristics and serologic antibody studies. Most laboratories use enzyme-linked immunosorbent assay (ELISA) techniques, which—like the treponemal tests for syphilis—indicate a history of exposure, but not necessarily active infection. A two-tier approach is recommended by the Centers for Disease Control and Prevention to support the diagnosis of Lyme disease: the first step is a sensitive ELISA. If this is negative, the patient is considered negative, and no further testing is performed. When the ELISA is positive, a Western blot assay is performed to identify the specific antigens to which the patient's antibodies react. Consensus criteria for what should be considered a positive result have been validated. Anti-Borrelia antibodies in the spinal fluid are specific for nervous system Lyme disease, but only if the titers are higher than in the serum, because otherwise they could just represent passive transfer across the blood-brain barrier. The sensitivity of CSF antibody testing is unknown; it is estimated to be 90% in acute disease and 50% in more chronic stages.

Patients with neurologic manifestations of Lyme disease should be treated with a 2- to 4-week course of IV ceftriaxone, IV cefotaxime, IV penicillin G, or oral doxycycline. The evidence for a "posttreatment Lyme disease syndrome" characterized by fatigue, chronic pain, paresthesia, and clouded thinking is unconvincing. A similar condition, "chronic Lyme disease," has been described in people with no history of typical symptoms of Lyme disease and only nonspecific laboratory abnormalities; the evidence for this entity is not compelling either.

c. Tuberculosis

Mycobacterium tuberculosis can spread to the nervous system via the bloodstream either during the initial infection or with subsequent caseation at the primary site or other sites. The resulting tuberculous foci (tubercles) can then remain dormant in the CNS for months or years before producing clinical symptoms. The most common neurologic manifestation is tuberculous meningitis, which occurs when a suitably located subpial tubercle grows or ruptures into the subarachnoid or intraventricular space. This meningitis is most marked at the base of the brain, ultimately forming a thick, gelatinous mass that engulfs the cranial nerves and blood vessels passing through it. Less often, tubercles located deep in the brain parenchyma may grow large enough to present as a mass lesion (a tuberculoma).

Tuberculous meningitis usually begins with a several-week prodrome of headache, malaise, personality change, and low-grade fever. The headache eventually becomes more severe and continuous, and patients develop nausea, vomiting, neck stiffness, confusion, papilledema, and cranial nerve abnormalities. Focal deficits (such as hemiparesis, paraparesis, and ataxia) can result from local pressure, venous congestion, or strokes that occur because blood vessels passing through the region of basilar meningitis become inflamed and thrombosed. Seizures may also occur. Patients subsequently progress to stupor and coma, with death typically occurring within 2 months of the onset of illness in untreated patients, but occasional patients follow a more indolent course over many months or even years. People with HIV have an increased risk of developing tuberculosis and progressing from latent to active disease, and tuberculosis can be associated with IRIS after initiating ART.

Tuberculous meningitis can be extremely difficult to diagnose, and antituberculous treatment often must be initiated even when the diagnosis is only presumptive. Positive tuberculin skin tests or blood interferon gamma release assays can provide evidence that a person has been sensitized to tuberculosis, but they don't help in determining whether there is active tuberculous infection in the nervous system. Even evidence of active tuberculous infection elsewhere in the body does not necessarily imply active infection in the nervous system. Conversely, the skin and serum tests have a high false-negative rate for tuberculous meningitis, and failure to find evidence of systemic tuberculous infection doesn't eliminate the possibility of tuberculous meningitis because the nervous system is sometimes the only site of active infection. CSF is usually the most important guide to diagnosis (see Table 12.1 in Chapter 12). Typical findings are elevated opening pressure, increased protein (usually 100–500 mg/dL), reduced glucose (<45 mg/dL in 80% of patients), and moderate pleocytosis (100–300 white blood cells per mm^3 in most patients). The cellular reaction is predominantly mononuclear, but polymorphonuclear cells may predominate in a significant minority of patients, especially early in the course. Acid-fast stains on CSF smears show mycobacteria in only 30–60% of cases. Mycobacterial cultures from the CSF require weeks to months for detectable growth, and even then the false-negative rate is at least 25%. The yield for both smears and cultures is increased by sending samples from several lumbar punctures (usually repeated on a daily basis); there is no need to delay treatment for this, because the yield from cultures remains good even after several days of therapy. The most useful diagnostic test in the short term is PCR on the spinal fluid. This test is extremely specific, but the sensitivity varies widely depending on the population under study and the particular assay used.

The optimal treatment regimen for tuberculous meningitis has not been established. Current recommendations are to treat for 2 months with isoniazid, rifampin, pyrazinamide, and a fourth drug selected from one of the following: streptomycin, ethambutol, levofloxacin, or ethionamide. After 2 months, the regimen can be simplified to isoniazid and rifampin, as long as the organism is fully sensitive to them. These drugs are continued for 7–10 more months. The specific agents used and the duration of therapy may be modified depending on the likelihood of drug resistance. Patients taking isoniazid should take pyridoxine (vitamin B6) concurrently to prevent neuropathy. Adjunctive corticosteroids are commonly included in the initial treatment regimen because they appear to help limit or even prevent the neurologic consequences of tuberculous meningitis, though this has never been convincingly demonstrated. They are tapered over 6 to 8 weeks. Tuberculomas can usually be adequately treated with medications, although the lesions are sometimes resected when the diagnosis is uncertain. Surgical procedures are sometimes required to treat increased intracranial pressure or hydrocephalus.

d. Herpesviruses

Herpesviruses have a tendency to lie dormant in the nervous system for years at a time, periodically reactivating and causing clinical symptoms. Several distinctive syndromes can result. The most serious is herpes simplex encephalitis (HSE), which can occur at any age. In neonates, HSE may be due to *Herpes simplex virus type 1* or *Herpes simplex virus type 2*; beyond the neonatal period it is almost always due to *Herpes simplex virus type 1*. HSE is the most frequent cause of fatal encephalitis, and it is the most common identified cause of acute, sporadic encephalitis. About two thirds of cases are due to reactivation, and a third are due to primary infection resulting from exposure to contaminated saliva or respiratory secretions. The clinical presentation is similar to that of any other form of encephalitis, with a prodromal phase characterized by malaise, fever, headache, and sometimes behavioral changes. The distinctive feature of HSE is a tendency to involve the frontotemporal lobes predominantly, resulting in focal signs and symptoms in at least 50% of patients. These can include hemiparesis, aphasia, visual field abnormalities, and cranial nerve deficits. Florid behavioral changes, amnesia, seizures, stupor, and coma are also common. The clinical course is extremely variable, with some patients progressing to coma within a few days but other patients stabilizing and demonstrating only a mild to moderate encephalopathy for several weeks.

Spinal fluid examination typically reveals a lymphocytic pleocytosis (50–500 cells per mm^3) with mild protein elevation and normal or moderately reduced glucose. In 25–40% of patients, red blood cells are present in the CSF. Regions of abnormal signal and microhemorrhage, especially in the temporal lobes, may be evident on MRI scans, and unilateral or bilateral lateralized periodic discharges in the frontotemporal regions are characteristic EEG findings. PCR testing for viral DNA in the spinal fluid is the gold standard diagnostic test, with an estimated sensitivity of 98% and a specificity of 99%, although false-negative results may be more common in the first 24–48 hours of illness. Whenever HSE is a realistic possibility, it is best to initiate empiric treatment with intravenous acyclovir (10 mg/kg every 8 hours for 14 to 21 days) while awaiting CSF PCR results. If the PCR result is negative but the clinical features are typical of HSE, the testing should be repeated (and empiric treatment continued), especially if the initial lumbar puncture was performed within 48 hours of symptom onset. The mortality rate in patients treated with acyclovir and supportive care is 20–30%, compared with 70–80% mortality in untreated patients. Some people who recover from HSE subsequently develop autoimmune encephalitis associated with antibodies to the N-methyl D-aspartate receptor (NMDAR); this primarily happens within 3 months of the acute illness.

Herpes varicella-zoster virus (VZV) remains latent in neurons of sensory ganglia after resolution of the primary infection (varicella, commonly called chickenpox). Zoster, or "shingles," occurs when the virus is reactivated years later. The lifetime risk of VZV reactivation is about 30%; older people and people with reduced immune function have the greatest risk of reactivation, but it may occur even in immunocompetent young people. Recombinant zoster vaccine reduces the risk of reactivation by more than 95%. The most common manifestation of VZV reactivation is sharp, burning pain in a dermatomal distribution, most often in a thoracic dermatome, followed 2–5 days later by a characteristic vesicular rash in the same distribution (though some patients never develop the rash). Another typical area of involvement is on the forehead in the territory of the ophthalmic division of the trigeminal nerve (*zoster ophthalmicus*). The most common neurologic complication is postherpetic neuralgia, which occurs in 10–15% of all patients with zoster, especially older patients (affecting 5% of patients younger than 60 years but 20% of patients older than 80 years). Recombinant zoster vaccine substantially reduces the risk of postherpetic neuralgia. Postherpetic neuralgia is characterized by steady, burning pain with superimposed lightning-like pains in the distribution of the preceding skin involvement, persisting for more than 4 weeks after the rash disappears. The area is often extremely sensitive to touch.

Acyclovir, famciclovir, and valacyclovir have all been shown to reduce the duration of the rash and the acute pain if they are initiated within 72 hours of the onset of the rash. Famciclovir and valacyclovir are generally preferred over acyclovir because they have also been shown to reduce the duration of postherpetic neuralgia. Acyclovir also requires more frequent dosing. Unfortunately, none of these agents has been definitively shown to reduce the incidence of postherpetic neuralgia. Other options for acute treatment of shingles include tricyclic antidepressants, antiseizure medications (especially gabapentin, pregabalin, and carbamazepine), opioids, and local anesthetics (including lidocaine patch and capsaicin cream). Although early studies suggested that the addition of glucocorticoids to the antiviral agent might be beneficial, subsequent meta-analyses have not confirmed this.

Other neurologic complications of zoster can occur when the virus spreads from the sensory nerve to involve other components of the nervous system. For example, spread to the anterior root can cause focal weakness, usually in the distribution of the nerve root that corresponds to the affected dermatome. Spread of the virus to the spinal cord may result in myelitis, and more diffuse spread may result in encephalitis or aseptic meningitis. About a third of patients with zoster ophthalmicus develop abnormalities of other cranial nerves, especially the third nerve. Other potential complications of zoster ophthalmicus include ocular involvement (in about 20% of patients) and, rarely, a thrombotic cerebral vasculopathy that results in delayed contralateral hemiparesis. Patients with these syndromes of more extensive nervous system involvement are usually treated with IV acyclovir, although its efficacy remains unknown. Ramsay Hunt syndrome (*zoster oticus, zoster auricularis,* or *zoster cephalicus*) is thought to represent spread of the virus from the geniculate ganglion of the facial nerve. It is characterized by vesicular eruption in the external auditory meatus accompanied by ipsilateral facial weakness, and often by hearing loss, tinnitus, or vertigo. Cranial nerves V, IX, and X are frequently involved, and there may be severe pain in the territories of these nerves.

e. Parasitic infections

Parasites are ideally adapted to colonize multiple sites in the nervous system and other organ systems without provoking overwhelming host responses. Many of these organisms are uncommon in the United States, but they account for significant worldwide morbidity and mortality. Parasitic infections that are particularly likely to involve the nervous system include malaria, toxoplasmosis, trypanosomiasis, amebic infections, strongyloidiasis, trichinosis, onchocerciasis, schistosomiasis, paragonimiasis, echinococcosis, and cysticercosis. Detailed descriptions of these parasites, their life cycles, and the diseases they cause are available in textbooks of infectious diseases.

f. COVID-19

Estimates of the frequency of neurologic symptoms in patients with COVID-19 vary widely, partly because of a lack of standardized definitions and ascertainment procedures and partly because of rapid epidemiologic changes. During the acute illness, at least a third of patients report nonspecific symptoms such as headache, cognitive changes, dizziness, fatigue, and myalgia. These are similar to the symptoms that occur with other systemic viral illnesses, and they may reflect an inflammatory response to systemic infection rather than direct infection of the nervous system. Anosmia is also common during acute COVID-19 infection. It is thought to be caused by viral invasion of the support cells of the nasal epithelium, resulting in inflammation that transiently obstructs olfactory clefts. Encephalopathy is common, especially in patients who are critically ill. It is typically multifactorial. Factors that may contribute to the encephalopathy include hypoxia, metabolic abnormalities, hypotension, and autoimmune phenomena. Older people, who have the greatest risk of becoming critically ill, are also the people most likely to have preexisting brain dysfunction (for example, from a degenerative dementia or previous strokes) that could predispose them to encephalopathy. SARS-CoV-2 can directly affect the central nervous system, but this appears to be rare. The main factor contributing to inflammation of the central nervous system is a cytokine-release syndrome. People with COVID-19 also have an increased risk of ischemic stroke and venous sinus thrombosis—and, and to a lesser extent, hemorrhagic stroke. COVID-19 may also be associated with an increased risk of Guillain-Barré syndrome, but the evidence is conflicting.

Many people who have had COVID-19 have chronic symptoms. In some cases, these represent persistence of symptoms that began during the acute illness; in other cases, the initial symptoms improved or resolved but new symptoms emerged weeks-to-months later. The terms used for this phenomenon include "long-COVID," "long-haul COVID," "post-COVID-19 syndrome," and "postacute sequelae of COVID-19 (PASC)." As already noted with respect to neurologic manifestations of the acute syndrome, the prevalence of this condition is unknown because of a lack of consistency in terminology and diagnostic criteria. The symptoms that have been reported include fatigue, cognitive dysfunction (often referred to as "brain fog"), headache, sleep disturbance, autonomic dysfunction, and persistent changes in the sense of smell or taste. The likelihood of developing these symptoms doesn't correlate with age or the severity of the initial symptoms—if anything, people who had a mild acute illness and never required hospitalization report more chronic symptoms than people who were hospitalized. The pathophysiology of these symptoms is unknown, and no specific treatment is available.

g. Potential agents of bioterrorism

In recent years, the risk of bioterrorism has required physicians to become aware of some pathogens that would otherwise be primarily of historical interest. Some of these agents can affect the nervous system.

Most cases of anthrax are of the cutaneous form. Spontaneous healing occurs in 80–90% of untreated patients with cutaneous anthrax. The rest develop bacteremia, which can lead to a fulminant and rapidly fatal hemorrhagic meningoencephalitis. Meningoencephalitis also occurs in up to 50% of cases of inhalational anthrax. This is the form of the disease most likely to be used as an agent of bioterrorism, although it accounts for only a minority of cases of naturally acquired anthrax. Patients typically present with fever, headache, vomiting, and delirium; they may also have seizures, myoclonus, increased tone, and focal abnormalities. The recommended treatment is a combination of IV ciprofloxacin, meropenem, and linezolid, together with an antitoxin, followed by oral ciprofloxacin or doxycycline for a total treatment course of 50 days.

Because of the successful global eradication of smallpox in 1980, immunization was discontinued. If bioterrorism results in the re-emergence of smallpox, historical experience suggests that neurologic complications will be uncommon, but some patients may develop encephalomyelitis 5–16 days after the onset of the typical rash. This can result in headaches, seizures, varying degrees of mental status change (up to and including coma), or a flaccid paralysis resembling poliomyelitis. Encephalomyelitis can also occur after vaccination, especially in children.

Meningitis can occur with any of the forms of plague (bubonic, septice-mic, and pneumonic), but it is uncommon. Plague is treated with either an aminoglycoside, a fluoroquinolone, or doxycycline; patients with menin-gitis are treated with intravenous chloramphenicol and a fluoroquinolone. Tularemia produces a variety of localized syndromes, but dissemination can also occur, associated with meningitis, encephalitis, or Guillain-Barré syndrome. Tularemia meningitis is treated with an aminoglycoside com-bined with either ciprofloxacin or doxycycline.

Botulism as a tool of bioterrorism would be disseminated via the toxin, not the actual infection. Botulinum toxin acts at presynaptic receptors to block release of acetylcholine and thereby prevent transmission at the neuromuscular junction, resulting in severe weakness (see Chapter 6). Diplopia, blurred vision, and ptosis are often the first symptoms, followed within 72 hours by dysarthria, dysphagia, and flaccid paralysis. Patients are treated with antitoxin and meticulous supportive care.

IV. Inherently Multifocal Diseases

A. Multiple Sclerosis (MS) and Related Disorders

Multiple sclerosis (MS) is the prototype of an inherently multifocal CNS disease. Most patients have discrete attacks of CNS dysfunction that arise over hours to days, typically last 2 to 6 weeks, and improve partially or completely over weeks or months. Early in the disease, the attacks occur at an average of once a year, but after the fifth year the frequency falls to an average of one attack every 2 years. The attacks can affect any pathway in the CNS, but the most common presenting symptoms involve the spinal cord (50%), optic nerve (25%), or posterior fossa structures (20%). Spinal cord lesions can produce numbness, paresthesias (e.g., tingling), dysesthe-sias (including Lhermitte phenomenon), pain, weakness, stiffness, clum-siness, urinary urgency, incontinence of bladder or bowels, constipation, or impotence. Lhermitte phenomenon is an electric sensation provoked by neck flexion, running into the limbs, down the back, or both. It can occur with any condition affecting the posterior columns of the cervical spinal cord, including vitamin B12 deficiency or extrinsic cord compres-sion. Optic nerve lesions can manifest with blurred vision, loss of vision, or eye pain. Brainstem or cerebellar involvement can result in diplopia, dys-arthria, dysphagia, clumsiness, vertigo, numbness, or weakness. The most common symptoms of MS are weakness in one or more limbs (40%), optic nerve symptoms (22%), paresthesias (21%), diplopia (12%), vertigo (5%), and urinary symptoms (5%). Tremor, fatigue, and cognitive impairment are common, especially in longstanding disease. Patients may also experience paroxysmal symptoms, including seizures, trigeminal neuralgia (see Chapter 12), other intermittent pains, episodic dysarthria or ataxia (usually lasting less than 20 seconds), and dystonic episodes (sometimes called "tonic seizures").

In an individual patient, it is extremely difficult to predict when the attacks will occur, what sites in the nervous system will be involved, the severity of the symptoms, and the degree of recovery. Four general patterns of clinical progression have been defined:

(1) *Relapsing-remitting:* clearly defined attacks (relapses), with no disease progression during the periods between the attacks. Patients typically recover from the attacks, but not always, and the recovery may be either partial or complete. If they have attacks from which they do not fully recover, their overall condition may deteriorate over time.

(2) *Primary-progressive:* continued disease progression from onset (though there may be occasional plateaus or temporary periods of minor improvement).

(3) *Secondary-progressive:* initial relapsing-remitting course, followed by continued progression (though there may be occasional plateaus, superimposed relapses, or temporary periods of minor improvement).

(4) *Progressive-relapsing:* continued progression from onset, but with clear superimposed relapses followed by partial or full recovery. There is continuing progression during the periods between relapses.

A minimum duration of 24 hours is arbitrarily required for symptoms to be classified as relapses. At onset, 85% of patients have a relapsing-remitting course, but by 10 years, 50% of the patients whose course was originally relapsing-remitting have evolved to a secondary-progressive pattern. About 10% of patients have a primary-progressive course, and about 5% have a progressive-relapsing course. MS affects females more than males (in a ratio of 3:1), and it preferentially affects young adults, with the age at onset typically between 10 and 59 years, although it can begin in early childhood or in later life. Primary-progressive MS tends to affect males and females equally, with a later age of onset.

Even in patients with relapsing-remitting disease, imaging studies show changes between relapses, suggesting that the disease is not truly "in remission." This has led some to question the distinction between relapsing and progressive courses, but the concept of a clinical relapse seems to have some clinical implications; for example, patients who have less frequent clinical relapses early in the disease tend to be less disabled later in the course. Patients who have minimal disability after 5 years of disease (i.e., patients who have recovered nearly completely from their relapses to date) also have a better prognosis.

The pathologic hallmark of MS is the demyelinating plaque. Macroscopically, plaques are well-demarcated areas of discoloration that can occur anywhere in the white matter; microscopically, they are perivascular collections of macrophages and lymphocytes, with numerous demyelinated axons demonstrated on myelin stains. Although the axons themselves are less prominently affected, they are reduced in number compared to normal brain, and axonal transection is common. Aggressive investigation has failed to identify a consistent infectious agent or other common factor responsible for inciting the inflammation, but environmental and genetic factors both play a role. For example, almost all people who develop MS have evidence of previous Epstein-Barr virus infection—but this can't be the only factor involved in pathogenesis, because most people with Epstein-Barr virus infection never develop MS. Likewise, someone who has an identical twin with MS has a risk of developing MS that is 200 times the risk in the general population, but the risk is not 100%; in fact, the majority of monozygotic twin pairs are discordant.

The diagnosis of MS is based on a history of "two or more CNS lesions separated in space and time," confirmed on physical examination. Many diseases can cause recurrent symptoms in a single location (e.g., seizures, TIAs, intervertebral disc herniation), and many monophasic illnesses are multifocal or diffuse (e.g., infections, metabolic disturbances), but very few conditions cause multiple, discrete episodes of transient dysfunction involving more than one area of the CNS. Of those that do, MS is by far the most common. Thus, when a patient's history and examination provide compelling evidence of two or more CNS lesions separated in space and time, it is usually reasonable to look for evidence of a systemic inflammatory disease, such as systemic lupus erythematosus, but if the results are negative, MS can be confidently diagnosed based purely on clinical grounds.

Several diagnostic tests can be used to supplement the history and examination, but no test is completely reliable. More than 90% of patients with a clear diagnosis of MS (based on history and examination) have typical abnormalities on MRI scans of the brain or spinal cord. MRI abnormalities can be helpful in establishing the diagnosis when the clinical evidence is strongly suggestive, but not diagnostic. Although the MRI signal changes that occur in MS have characteristic features, they are not specific—identical findings can result from other inflammatory conditions, ischemia, trauma, metabolic abnormalities, or even neoplasms (see Figures 10.1 and 10.2). The MRI scan can only be interpreted reliably in the context of the history and examination.

The second most useful test in patients whose diagnosis cannot be established from history and physical examination is CSF analysis. Patients with MS produce antibodies (especially IgG) within the CNS. Two tests are commonly used to look for evidence of CNS antibody production. One of

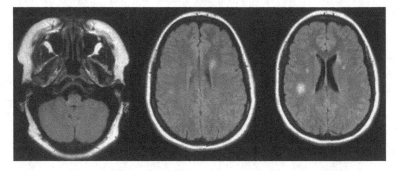

Fig. 10.1 MRI (FLAIR sequence, axial plane) images showing typical demyelinating lesions in a patient with relatively mild MS. (Source: Preston DC, Shapiro BE. Neuroimaging in neurology: an interactive CD. Elsevier, 2007).

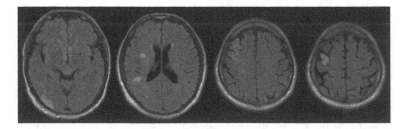

Fig. 10.2 MRI (FLAIR sequence, axial plane) images showing multiple small strokes in the distribution of multiple branches of the right middle cerebral artery (MCA). (*Source:* Preston DC, Shapiro BE. Neuroimaging in neurology: an interactive CD. Elsevier, 2007).

these tests looks for oligoclonal bands on electrophoretic analysis of CSF. Electrophoresis of CSF from healthy subjects usually produces a homogeneous blur of immunoglobulin. Patients with MS typically have a number of discrete bands distinct from the background, representing antibody produced by one or more clones of plasma cells. Bands that are present in the spinal fluid but not in the serum indicate active inflammation within the nervous system. The second CSF test for inflammation within the central nervous system is the IgG index, defined as:

$$\text{IgG index} = [\text{IgG(CSF)}/\text{albumin(CSF)}]/[\text{IgG(serum)}/\text{albumin(serum)}]$$

The ratio of IgG to albumin is used to be sure that an elevated IgG is not simply a manifestation of a generalized increase in protein. The normalization of this ratio in CSF with respect to the same ratio in serum is necessary to be sure that an elevated CSF IgG does not simply reflect passive migration of serum IgG across the blood-brain barrier in a patient with systemic inflammation. Neither an elevated IgG index nor the presence of oligoclonal bands is specific for MS as opposed to other causes of CNS inflammation, but in certain clinical settings this information can be very helpful.

A third group of tests sometimes used in diagnosing MS is evoked potentials. These are essentially measures of the speed with which sensory information reaches the brain (which is dependent on the function of myelinated pathways). EEG activity is recorded just before and just after a sensory stimulus. Because of the large amount of random activity in a routine EEG, the specific response to the stimulus cannot be distinguished from the background noise after a single stimulus. For this reason, the same stimulus is presented repetitively, and time-locked EEG activity is recorded. When these repetitive records are averaged, activity that is unrelated to the stimulus is likely to be randomly distributed across the recordings, sometimes positive and sometimes negative, and the sum is likely to be near zero. In contrast, brain activity that is a direct response to the stimulus will occur at the same delay after the stimulus on each recording, and that component of the EEG signal will be reinforced by summing across recordings. The resulting waveform can then be compared to normal controls, or even better, to the analogous waveform in the same subject stimulated on the opposite side. Abnormal function of the sensory pathway results in a prolonged latency of the signal (or, less reliably, reduced amplitude or complete absence of the signal). This may provide evidence of a clinical lesion not apparent on the neurologic examination. The standard evoked potential tests are visual, auditory, and somatosensory. The ones that most often provide useful information in diagnosing MS are the visual evoked potentials. Of course, abnormal evoked potential results do not in and of themselves provide information about the underlying cause of dysfunction or when it occurred, but taken in the context of the history and examination they can sometimes be very helpful. A fourth category of test used increasingly often in diagnosing MS is optical coherence tomography, a noninvasive imaging modality that provides cross-sectional images that yield quantitative measures of the retinal nerve fiber layer in the region adjacent to the optic nerve head.

In many cases, the history and physical exam provide compelling evidence of multiple CNS lesions separated in space and time. Other cases are less clear-cut. For example, at the time of presentation for one symptom, patients may report a history of a different symptom in the past, but the only abnormalities on neurologic examination correspond to the current symptom. A consensus panel has published a set of criteria for diagnosing MS (Table 10.2), including explicit discussion of situations like this. The diagnostic criteria summarized in Table 10.2 differ from previous criteria in several ways that facilitate diagnosing MS as early in the course as possible. This increased sensitivity comes at the expense of some reduced specificity. For example, the current criteria accept CSF oligoclonal bands as a substitute for evidence of dissemination in time, mainly because CSF oligoclonal bands have a high positive predictive value for MS—but CSF oligoclonal bands can be present in other inflammatory conditions, both infectious and autoimmune. The criteria specify that MS should be diagnosed only if there is no better explanation for the clinical presentation. In general, the criteria summarized in Table 10.2 are most reliable when applied to patients who present with a clinical syndrome that is characteristic of MS, and the criteria should be used cautiously when patients present with other symptoms.

The clinical presentations most characteristic of MS are optic neuritis, myelitis (i.e., a spinal cord lesion with CSF evidence of inflammation), and a brainstem or cerebellar syndrome. Patients who present with one of these *clinically isolated syndromes* and MRI scans showing multiple white matter lesions have a high probability of developing MS. Conversely, each of the clinically isolated syndromes can occur in patients who never proceed to manifest any subsequent neurologic symptoms, and this outcome is much more likely if the brain MRI scan is normal.

Another group of patients who do not have two discrete clinical episodes separated in time are those with primary-progressive MS. In these individuals, the diagnosis requires a consistent history and examination together with either MRI or CSF findings typical of MS (Table 10.3). Particular caution is required before making the diagnosis in these patients, so that a focal or multifocal structural process is not overlooked.

One condition that can be particularly difficult to distinguish from MS is *acute disseminated encephalomyelitis*, or *ADEM*. This is a multifocal condition that typically begins abruptly and progresses over hours, often with associated fever, headache, neck stiffness, and depressed level of consciousness. It is more common in children than adults, and there is typically a history of an antecedent infection (or, less often, vaccination). Some patients with ADEM subsequently develop MS, but not all.

Neuromyelitis optica spectrum disorders (NMOSDs) can also be difficult to distinguish from MS. The name of this group of disorders derives from the initial clinical description of patients who developed optic neuritis and myelitis, either separately or simultaneously, but no other MS lesions. Most of these patients were found to have serum antibodies to aquaporin-4, a water channel. Once this antibody was identified, it was found to be associated with several other clinical syndromes, which are now grouped together as NMOSDs. NMOSD, like MS, is an autoimmune disorder—but in NMOSD, the initial immune response involves astrocytes. Certain MRI features are also characteristic of NMOSD. For example, MRI scans of the spinal cord in patients with myelitis due to NMOSD usually show demyelinating lesions that extend over more spinal segments than a typical MS lesion, and the typical MRI appearance of optic nerve involvement (when it is present) differs in NMOSD and MS. The spinal fluid findings also tend to be different in MS and NMOSD: patients with NMOSD typically have a higher white blood cell count (30–50 cells/mm³), a neutrophilic predominance, and no oligoclonal bands. The core clinical syndromes of NMOSD are (1) optic neuritis; (2) acute myelitis; (3) unexplained hiccups or nausea and vomiting, attributed to a lesion in the chemoreceptor area in the area postrema of the medulla; (4) an acute brainstem syndrome; (5) symptomatic narcolepsy or acute diencephalic clinical syndrome with diencephalic lesions on MRI typical of NMOSD; and (6) a symptomatic cerebral syndrome with brain MRI lesions typical of NMOSD. A patient with any of these six syndromes and a positive aquaporin-4 antibody meets current diagnostic criteria for NMOSD. Patients without a positive aquaporin-4 antibody can also meet the diagnostic criteria if they have at least two of the core clinical syndromes and meet several other requirements. Some people with a clinical presentation suggestive of NMOSD have antibodies to myelin oligodendrocyte glycoprotein (MOG). Some clinical and imaging features differ between people who have antibodies to aquaporin-4 and those who have antibodies to MOG, but many features overlap; the degree to which NMOSD and MOG antibody disease (MOGAD) should be considered separate entities is debated. Other antibodies have occasionally been identified in patients with clinical syndromes resembling NMOSD, including antibodies to glial fibrillary acidic protein (GFAP).

Table 10.4 lists the medications that are currently approved as disease-modifying therapy for relapsing-remitting and secondary progressive MS with relapses. The primary endpoint for the randomized controlled trials that demonstrated the efficacy of each of these medications was a reduction in the relapse rate. The magnitude of the reduction is listed in the fourth column of Table 10.4. Many of the medications were also associated with improvement in secondary endpoints, such as degree of disability or MRI characteristics.

Patients who take any of the drugs listed in Table 10.4 are making a substantial commitment, and they must be thoroughly informed about what results they can expect. They must be advised that although the medications reduce the number of relapses and many of them slow disease progression, no medication has been shown to halt disease progression in all patients or to eliminate relapses in all patients. Some MS specialists advocate adjusting the therapeutic regimen until there is no evidence of disease activity, but it is unclear how often that goal can be achieved. One philosophy of MS treatment, the "early high-efficacy" or "intensive" approach, is to initiate treatment with one of the medications associated with a more dramatic reduction in relapse rate. An alternative philosophy, the "escalation" approach, is to start with one of the medications associated with a more moderate reduction in relapse rate, which tend to have fewer serious adverse effects. The medication is switched to one of the more aggressive medications if the patient has an inadequate response to the initial treatment (although there is no universally accepted definition of inadequate response).

Patients with relapsing-remitting MS should be encouraged to start a disease-modifying medication as early in the course as possible. Patients with a clinically isolated syndrome deserve special mention. As discussed previously, patients with a clinically isolated syndrome who have a normal MRI are unlikely to develop MS, but those who have multiple typical MRI lesions have a high risk of eventually developing MS. Controlled trials have demonstrated that initiation of disease-modifying therapy in this setting is beneficial, even if the patient doesn't meet criteria for the diagnosis of MS (for example, if all the MRI lesions appear to be the same age, and there are no CSF-specific oligoclonal bands; see Table 10.2). All of the medications listed in Table 10.4 except for cladribine, alemtuzumab, and mitoxantrone are approved for patients with clinically isolated syndrome. Glucocorticoids, such as prednisone and methylprednisolone, appear to accelerate the recovery from an acute MS relapse, but there is no consistent evidence for any long-term benefit. These agents should be considered for relapses that result in considerable discomfort or dysfunction, but they should not be used too frequently because of the high incidence of complications.

Symptomatic treatment is also important. Physical therapy, bladder and bowel regimens, drugs to reduce spasticity, and psychological support are essential components of patient management. Patients with fatigue should be evaluated for sleep disorders such as obstructive sleep apnea or restless legs syndrome and treated appropriately. Controlled trials have established that amantadine is effective in alleviating fatigue, but only some patients note a benefit, and the response is often incomplete. Modafinil, methylphenidate, and selective serotonin reuptake inhibitors may also be helpful. Dalfampridine, a sustained release form of 4-aminopyridine, is a potassium channel blocker that produces mild improvement in walking speed and lower extremity strength in patients with MS. Patients with trigeminal neuralgia are treated with carbamazepine, gabapentin, or the other standard agents used for this disorder. Lhermitte phenomenon often responds to carbamazepine and gabapentin, also. The paroxysmal dystonic episodes of MS usually respond dramatically to carbamazepine, phenytoin, or gabapentin. Tremors respond to the same treatments that are effective for tremor in non-MS patients.

The only medication that is currently approved for patients with primary-progressive MS is ocrelizumab. Many of the medications that have been shown to be effective for disease modification in MS are less effective for NMOSD, and they may even exacerbate it. The three medications that are FDA approved for treating NMOSD are eculizumab, inebilizumab, and satralizumab; rituximab is often used also.

B. Rheumatologic Diseases

Rheumatologic diseases characteristically involve widespread organ systems throughout the body, including the nervous system. Organ damage can be caused by immune complex deposition, vasculopathy, granuloma formation, or secondary damage due to musculoskeletal abnormalities. All levels of the nervous system can be affected. In some people, nervous system dysfunction is the initial or the predominant symptom of the disease.

Because these patients typically have multifocal neurologic deficits, they often resemble patients with MS. The main clues to the correct diagnosis are serologic tests and the eventual development of systemic symptoms.

Neurologic manifestations occur at some stage of the disease in 20–40% of people with *systemic lupus erythematosus* (SLE), and in some cases the initial manifestations are neurologic. The CNS symptoms associated with SLE include headache, cognitive impairment, psychosis, mood changes, and alteration of consciousness, although some of these associations may not be causative. About 1% of people with SLE develop a demyelinating syndrome, usually optic neuritis or myelitis; this is sometimes associated with aquaporin-4 antibodies, meeting criteria for NMOSD. Focal neurologic deficits in patients with SLE sometimes result from focal inflammation, but they are usually due to stroke (which, in turn, is most often related to a hypercoagulable state; see Section D). Seizures are also common, usually in an active phase of the disease. The most common PNS manifestation of SLE is a distal, symmetric polyneuropathy, but mononeuropathy multiplex and cranial neuropathies also occur.

The main CNS manifestations of *rheumatoid arthritis* result from compression of the spinal cord or brainstem due to arthritic changes in the spinal column. Rheumatoid nodules frequently form in the meninges, but they are usually asymptomatic. Aseptic meningitis can also occur, but it is uncommon. Symptomatic CNS vasculitis associated with rheumatoid arthritis is rare. In contrast, peripheral nerve involvement is relatively common, occurring in 10% of patients. It may take the form of mononeuropathy multiplex (due to either vasculitis or multiple sites of nerve entrapment) or a distal sensorimotor polyneuropathy.

People with *Sjögren syndrome* can develop a demyelinating syndrome in the brain, optic nerve, or spinal cord. Similar to SLE, many of these people have antibodies to aquaporin-4 and meet criteria for NMOSD. Some have suggested that these complications may be underreported. PNS manifestations are more common than CNS involvement. The most distinctive is a pure sensory neuronopathy, affecting the dorsal root ganglia and often resulting in sensory ataxia ("pseudoataxia") due to profound loss of proprioception. Other neuropathies that can occur in Sjögren syndrome include distal, symmetric, sensorimotor polyneuropathy, painful small-fiber sensory neuropathy (without ataxia), autonomic neuropathy, mononeuropathy multiplex, cranial neuropathies (especially trigeminal sensory neuropathy), and entrapment neuropathies (especially carpal tunnel syndrome). Patients may develop focal myositis. Patients with generalized myositis are usually considered to have secondary Sjögren syndrome (i.e., Sjögren syndrome that is associated with another rheumatologic disease). *Progressive systemic sclerosis* (*scleroderma*) only rarely affects the CNS, but focal CNS lesions have been reported on occasion. Trigeminal neuropathy is more common, and peripheral entrapment neuropathies, particularly carpal tunnel syndrome, may occur. There have been occasional reports of a sensorimotor polyneuropathy, with pathology suggesting a microangiopathy. Myopathies (mostly inflammatory) are common.

The neurologic features of *mixed connective tissue disease* (like the systemic features) overlap with those of SLE, rheumatoid arthritis, progressive systemic sclerosis, and polymyositis. The most common neurologic feature is aseptic meningitis. Trigeminal neuralgia and trigeminal sensory neuropathy are also common.

In most series of *Behçet disease*, less than 10% of patients have neurologic signs or symptoms. The most common neurologic manifestation is aseptic meningitis. There may be focal lesions at any level of the nervous system, with the brainstem and basal ganglia being the most commonly affected sites. Lesions often occur simultaneously at multiple locations, and clinical fluctuations are common, sometimes leading to an incorrect diagnosis of MS. Misdiagnosis is particularly likely in the 5% of patients who present with neurologic symptoms. Cerebral venous thrombosis may affect up to a third of patients with neurologic manifestations of Behçet disease. Peripheral nervous system manifestations are rare in Behçet disease.

Polyarteritis nodosa (PAN), also called periarteritis nodosa, is the prototypical vasculitic condition. It is a necrotizing vasculitis of small and medium-sized muscular arteries with preferential involvement of vessel branch points. Up to 80% of patients have neurologic manifestations, especially in the peripheral nervous system. PAN may produce an acute stroke syndrome with focal manifestations or a global syndrome characterized by headache and encephalopathy. The encephalopathy may present either acutely or chronically. Mononeuropathy multiplex is the classic peripheral nervous system manifestation, but distal, symmetric polyneuropathies, radiculopathies, and plexopathies also occur. Systemic vasculitides associated with antineutrophil cytoplasmic autoantibody (ANCA), including *granulomatosis with polyangiitis, eosinophilic granulomatosis with polyangiitis,* and *microscopic polyangiitis,* can all produce CNS and PNS manifestations similar to those that occur with PAN. In addition, the respiratory tract granulomas of granulomatosis with polyangiitis can extend to involve neighboring nervous system structures, especially the optic nerve in the orbit.

Primary angiitis of the CNS is a rare vasculitis restricted to small and medium-sized arteries of the CNS. The clinical manifestations resemble the CNS manifestations of PAN without the systemic symptoms. *Primary peripheral nervous system angiitis* is an analogous condition in the peripheral nervous system.

Patients with neurologic manifestations of rheumatologic diseases are treated in the same way as patients with manifestations in other organ systems, typically with immunosuppressive agents, including corticosteroids and cytotoxic agents.

C. Sarcoidosis

Sarcoidosis is a chronic, multisystem disorder of unknown cause characterized by noncaseating granulomas in several organs. It affects the nervous system in 5–10% of patients, and the nervous system is sometimes involved before other organ systems. The neurologic manifestations are similar in many ways to what occurs in tuberculosis. As with tuberculosis, there may be either parenchymal granulomas or meningeal involvement, particularly involving the meninges at the base of the brain and producing multiple cranial neuropathies. Unilateral or bilateral facial nerve palsy is particularly common. Cranial nerves II, V, VIII, IX, and X are also commonly involved, but any cranial nerve can be affected.

A common site of parenchymal involvement is the hypothalamus, leading to diabetes insipidus or other endocrine abnormalities. Granulomas can occur anywhere in the brain or spinal cord, resulting in focal dysfunction, obstructive hydrocephalus, or both. The most common pattern of peripheral nerve involvement is a chronic sensorimotor polyneuropathy, but mononeuropathy multiplex, pure sensory neuropathy, and plexopathy have also been described. Sarcoidosis commonly affects muscles. Typical granulomas are found on muscle biopsy in up to 50% of patients with sarcoidosis, but most of these are asymptomatic.

When clinical and radiologic findings suggest neurosarcoidosis, the most reliable way to establish the diagnosis is to demonstrate the typical pathologic findings in a tissue specimen. Because of the potential risk with a biopsy of CNS lesions, the usual approach is to search for a site of systemic involvement that is more accessible for biopsy. Although evidence of sarcoidosis outside the nervous system does not prove that the nervous system is involved, if the patient also has typical CSF findings (white blood cell count typically 10–100 cells/mm^3 with a mononuclear predominance, elevated protein, and low glucose) the diagnosis of neurosarcoidosis is very likely. Serum levels of angiotensin-converting enzyme (ACE) are typically elevated in patients with sarcoidosis, but this test is neither specific nor sensitive. In patients with neurologic manifestations of sarcoidosis, CSF ACE levels are more likely to be abnormal than serum ACE levels, but they are still normal in approximately 40% of patients with neurosarcoidosis, and they are sometimes abnormal in patients without neurologic involvement. Similarly, certain MRI findings can be helpful in supporting the diagnosis, but they aren't specific enough to permit a definitive diagnosis. Even the pathologic findings must be interpreted cautiously, because non-caseating granulomas can occur in a number of other diseases, including infections and malignancies.

Although controlled trials are lacking, patients with neurosarcoidosis usually improve when treated with corticosteroids, typically started at a dose of 0.5–1.0 mg/kg per day with a slow taper over many months or even years. Infliximab, a monoclonal antibody to tumor necrosis factor-alpha (TNF-α) is often used as a steroid-sparing agent when it seems that prolonged treatment will be required (or in refractory cases). Other options for maintenance treatment include cyclosporine, methotrexate, azathioprine, cyclophosphamide, chlorambucil, mycophenolate, etanercept, pentoxifylline, and thalidomide.

D. Coagulation Disorders

The physiologic pathways involved in maintaining hemostasis are complicated and can be compromised in many ways. Patients with hemophilia or other diseases predisposing to hemorrhage are usually diagnosed early in life because of uncontrolled bleeding after trivial injuries. Nervous system hemorrhages in these patients are treated as they would be in other patients. Hypercoagulability may occur because of a well-defined abnormality in the coagulation or fibrinolytic systems (primary hypercoagulable states) or in association with some other clinical condition in which the exact pathophysiology of thrombosis is unknown (secondary hypercoagulable states). The most common causes of primary hypercoagulability are resistance to activated protein C (most often due to a mutation in the gene for factor V Leiden), a mutation in the gene for prothrombin G20210, anti-thrombin III deficiency, protein C and protein S deficiency, and abnormalities of plasminogen or plasminogen activator. Most of these conditions are particularly associated with venous thromboembolism, and they are treated with anticoagulant medications. Causes of secondary hypercoagulable states include malignancy, pregnancy, congestive heart failure, extensive trauma, diabetes, nephrotic syndrome, vasculitis, and medications (including oral contraceptives and l-asparaginase). Many of these same conditions, but especially malignancies, can lead to nonbacterial thrombotic endocarditis, which results in an even higher incidence of nervous system involvement due to embolization. An increased risk of thrombosis and stroke is also associated with a heterogeneous family of antibodies known as antiphospholipid antibodies. Lupus anticoagulant and anticardiolipin antibody are two overlapping but not identical groups of antibodies included in this family. These antibodies occur not only in patients with SLE but also in association with other rheumatologic diseases, infections, neoplasms, and drugs, and they may be found in otherwise healthy individuals. People who have had a thrombotic event and are found to have a primary hypercoagulable state are typically started on lifelong anticoagulation. The optimal treatment for most secondary hypercoagulable states remains unknown. Thrombotic thrombocytopenic purpura (TTP), an extremely rare, life-threatening microcirculatory disorder, responds to plasma exchange; glucocorticoids are often added, and in specific circumstances rituximab or caplacizumab are used.

E. Functional Disorders

Some people have clinical symptoms that suggest dysfunction of the nervous system, but extensive evaluation reveals no evidence of any neurologic disease. These people have no objective abnormalities on neurologic examination, although they often have some of the anomalous or inconsistent exam findings described in Chapter 2, Part VI, Section D. Over the years, a variety of terms have been used for this type of clinical presentation, including "nonorganic symptoms," "conversion disorder," "somatoform disorder," "somatization," "psychogenic symptoms," "hysteria," and "functional disorder." Each of these terms is problematic. "Functional disorder" has been used with increasing frequency in recent years (after many years in which it had fallen out of favor); the *Diagnostic and Statistical Manual of Mental Disorders, Fifth Edition Text Revision* (*DSM-5-TR*) uses the diagnostic label "Functional Neurologic Symptom Disorder (Conversion Disorder)." The term "functional" is used to indicate that the underlying nervous system pathways are all *structurally intact*, but for some reason they aren't *functioning* normally. A commonly used analogy is that "the hardware is fine but there's a software problem." I find the term "functional" unfortunate, because of its potential ambiguity: in this context, it is being used to indicate a *lack of* function, whereas in many medical and rehabilitation settings, the word "functional" is used to indicate that despite impairment, the patient has *preserved* function. Additional ambiguity arises from the fact that the word "functional" is used to refer to certain types of neuro-imaging studies. This ambiguity could be avoided by using a term such as "utilization disorder" or "application disorder." In fact, the term "application disorder" would lend itself to the hardware/software analogy, because the condition could be likened to having downloaded a bad "app" on a smart phone—correcting the problem requires fixing or removing the app, not tinkering with the phone circuitry. Nonetheless, functional is the term currently in vogue.

Regardless of the terminology, almost any symptom can occur. Examples include weakness, tremor, other spontaneous movements, gait disturbance, decreased somatic sensation, altered vision, difficulty with language, speech, or swallowing, and psychogenic nonepileptic spells (PNES; see Chapter 5). It is generally accepted that the symptoms are involuntary, but the cause is not known. Abnormalities on functional neuroimaging studies have sometimes been reported in association with these symptoms, but they could be either the cause or the result of the clinical condition. Some of the terms that have been used for these conditions (such as psychogenic or conversion) reflect the theory that the underlying cause is some form of psychological distress that has been "converted" into a physical manifestation, but the evidence for this is not conclusive.

What seems clear is that psychological stress can exacerbate almost any clinical symptom, regardless of the cause. It stands to reason that if psychological stressors can be identified in people with functional symptoms, treatment of those stressors might help to alleviate the symptoms whether or not the stressors are the underlying cause. The rationale for treating psychological stressors is even stronger if there is any chance that they might be a causative factor. In some cases, explaining that the nervous system is intact and simply needs to be "reprogrammed" provides enough reassurance to alleviate symptoms. This explanation can sometimes be reinforced by demonstrating to the patient some of the anomalous exam findings. For example, it may be helpful to point out to patients that their tremor disappears when they are distracted, and to teach them techniques that allow them to take advantage of this—in essence, to learn ways to distract themselves. Cognitive behavioral therapy is a systematic program that is based on this type of approach.

The diagnosis of functional disorder should only be made when there is evidence to support it. Clinicians should avoid the trap of diagnosing functional disorder simply because they can't find any other diagnosis.

A corollary is that if functional disorder is a consideration, physicians should inform patients of that possibility up front, even if there are other things in the differential diagnosis that they want to evaluate with additional testing; otherwise, patients may draw the conclusion that, "The doctors couldn't figure it out, so now they're saying I'm crazy."

V. Supplementary Tables for Reference

Table 10.1 Common Associations between Paraneoplastic Syndromes, Antibodies, and Primary Tumors

Antibody	Most Commonly Associated Syndromes	Most Commonly Associated Primary Tumors
PCA-1 (Yo)	Cerebellar syndrome	Ovary, breast
ANNA-1 (Hu)	Sensory neuropathy/ neuronopathy, cerebellar syndrome, limbic encephalitis, myelitis	Small cell lung cancer
ANNA-2 (Ri)	Cerebellar syndrome, opsoclonus/myoclonus	Breast, lung
Ma1	Cerebellar syndrome, limbic or brainstem encephalitis	Lung, many others
Ma2	Brainstem or limbic encephalitis	Testicular
NMDAR	Limbic encephalitis	Ovarian teratoma, testicular
VGCC, P/Q type	LEMS, cerebellar syndrome	Small cell lung cancer
LGI1	Limbic encephalitis (including faciobrachial dystonic seizures)	Usually none; sometimes small cell lung cancer, prostate, or colon
thyroglobulin, TPO	Limbic encephalitis	Usually none

ANNA = antineuronal nuclear antibody; LEMS = Lambert Eaton myasthenic syndrome; LGI1 = leucine-rich glioma-inactivated protein 1; NMDAR = N-methyl D-aspartate receptor; PCA = Purkinje cell antibody; TPO = thyroid peroxidase; VGCC = voltage-gated calcium channels

Table 10.2 Diagnostic Criteria for Relapsing-Remitting MS

Number of Clinical Attacks (Separated in Space and Time)	Number of Lesions with Objective Clinical Evidence (Based on Physical Exam, Evoked Potentials, or Optical Coherence Tomography)	Additional Data Needed for a Diagnosis of MS
2 or more	2 or more	None
2 or more	1 (plus clear-cut historical evidence of a previous episode involving a lesion in a different CNS site)	None
2 or more	1	Dissemination in space [demonstrated by (a) an additional clinical episode implicating a different CNS site or (b) MRI[1]]
1	2 or more	Dissemination in time [demonstrated by (a) an additional clinical attack, or (b) MRI,[2] or (c) CSF-specific oligoclonal bands]
1	1	Dissemination in space [demonstrated by (a) an additional clinical episode implicating a different CNS site or (b) MRI[1]] AND dissemination in time [demonstrated by (a) an additional clinical attack, or (b) MRI,[2] or (c) CSF-specific oligoclonal bands]

Source: Thompson AJ, Banwell BL, Barkhof F, et al. Diagnosis of multiple sclerosis: 2017 revisions of the McDonald criteria. *Lancet Neurol* 2018;17:162–173.

[1] MRI evidence of dissemination in space requires at least one T2-hyperintense lesion characteristic of MS in two or more of the following CNS regions:
(a) periventricular
(b) cortical or juxtacortical
(c) infratentorial brain
(d) spinal cord

[2] MRI evidence of dissemination in time requires either (a) the simultaneous presence of gadolinium-enhancing and nonenhancing lesions or (b) a new T2-hyperintense or gadolinium-enhancing lesion on follow-up MRI with reference to a baseline MRI scan (obtained at any point in the past).

Table 10.3 Diagnostic Criteria for Progressive MS

---

1. At least 1 year of disability progression AND
2. At least two of the following:
   (a) one or more T2-hyperintense lesions characteristic of MS in one or more of the following locations:
       (i) periventricular
       (ii) cortical or juxtacortical
       (iii) infratentorial brain
   (b) two or more T2-hyperintense lesions in the spinal cord
   (c) CSF-specific oligoclonal bands

Source: Thompson AJ, Banwell BL, Barkhof F, et al. Diagnosis of multiple sclerosis: 2017 revisions of the McDonald criteria. *Lancet Neurol* 2018;17:162–173.

Table 10.4 Disease-Modifying Medications for MS

Drug [Brand Names in Brackets]	Side Effects	Monitoring Required	Annualized Relapse Rate Reduction (Relative to Placebo Unless Otherwise Noted)	Disability Reduction (Relative to Placebo Unless Otherwise Noted)
Injectable agents				
Interferon beta-1a (low dose) [Avonex]	Flu-like symptoms; depression; hematologic, thyroid, and liver abnormalities; injection site reactions	CBC, LFTs, TSH	18%	37%
Interferon beta-1a (high dose) [Rebif, Plegridy]	Same as low dose	CBC, LFTs, TSH	33%	30%

Table 10.4 Continued

Drug [Brand Names in Brackets]	Side Effects	Monitoring Required	Annualized Relapse Rate Reduction (Relative to Placebo Unless Otherwise Noted)	Disability Reduction (Relative to Placebo Unless Otherwise Noted)
Interferon beta-1b [Betaseron, Extavia]	Same as interferon beta-1a	CBC, LFTs, TSH	34%	No effect in RRMS; 20–40% in SPMS
Glatiramer acetate [Copaxone, Glatopa]	Postinjection flushing; injection site reactions	None	29%	28%
Ofatumumab [Kesimpta]	See ocrelizumab (below)	See ocrelizumab (below)	51–59% vs. teriflunomide	34% vs. teriflunomide
Oral agents				
Teriflunomide [Aubagio]	GI symptoms; alopecia; transaminitis; lymphopenia; TB reactivation; neuropathy; PREGNANCY CATEGORY X	LFTs, blood pressure, clinical monitoring for neuropathy	31–36%	30–31%
Dimethyl fumarate [Tecfidera]	Flushing; GI symptoms; transaminitis; leukopenia	CBC, LFTs	44–53%	21–38%
Diroximel fumarate[1] [Vumerity]				

(Continued)

Table 10.4 Continued

Drug [Brand Names in Brackets]	Side Effects	Monitoring Required	Annualized Relapse Rate Reduction (Relative to Placebo Unless Otherwise Noted)	Disability Reduction (Relative to Placebo Unless Otherwise Noted)
Monomethyl fumarate[1] [Bafiertam]				
Fingolimod [Gilenya, Tascenso]	Bradycardia/ heart block; macular edema; lymphopenia; transaminitis; infections; skin cancer. Pregnancy should be avoided.	Cardiac monitoring during first dose, CBC, LFTs, blood pressure, ophthalmology, dermatology	54% (52% vs. low-dose interferon beta-1a)	30%
Siponimod [Mayzent]	Same as fingolimod	EKG before first dose, CBC, LFTs, blood pressure, ophthalmology, dermatology	55%	21%
Ozanimod [Zeposia]	Same as siponimod; contraindicated in patients with severe untreated OSA or taking an MAO inhibitor	Same as siponimod	38–48% vs. low-dose interferon beta-1a	None
Ponesimod [Ponvory]	Same as siponimod	Same as siponimod	30.5% vs. teriflunomide	None

Table 10.4 Continued

Drug [Brand Names in Brackets]	Side Effects	Monitoring Required	Annualized Relapse Rate Reduction (Relative to Placebo Unless Otherwise Noted)	Disability Reduction (Relative to Placebo Unless Otherwise Noted)
Cladribine[2] [Mavenclad]	lymphopenia; headache; infections; malignancy. Contraindicated in pregnancy and breastfeeding; males taking cladribine should use contraception.	CBC, LFTs	58%	None
IV agents				
Mitoxantrone[3] [Novantrone]	Cardiac toxicity; leukemia; lymphoma; liver dysfunction; nausea/vomiting; alopecia; infections	CBC, LFTs, cardiac ejection fraction	68%	64%
Natalizumab [Tysabri]	PML; other infections; headaches; joint pain; infusion reactions	LFTs, JC virus antibody, MRI surveillance for PML if JC virus positive	68%	42%
Alemtuzumab[4] [Lemtrada]	Autoimmune conditions (ITP, glomerular nephropathy, thyroid); infusion reactions; malignancies	CBC, lymphocyte subsets, LFTs, TSH, creatinine, urinalysis	49–55% vs high-dose interferon beta-1a	42% in one study; none in another study vs. high-dose interferon beta-1a

(Continued)

Table 10.4 Continued

Drug [Brand Names in Brackets]	Side Effects	Monitoring Required	Annualized Relapse Rate Reduction (Relative to Placebo Unless Otherwise Noted)	Disability Reduction (Relative to Placebo Unless Otherwise Noted)
Ocrelizumab [Ocrevus]	Infusion reactions; infections (including skin); neutropenia; decreased serum immunoglobulin. Pregnancy should be avoided.	CBC, lymphocyte subsets, quantitative immunoglobulins, LFTs	47% vs. high-dose interferon beta-1a	40% vs. high-dose interferon beta-1a
Ublituximab [Briumvi]	See ocrelizumab	See ocrelizumab	41–49% vs. teriflunomide	None

Abbreviations: CBC = complete blood count (including differential and platelets); LFTs = liver function tests; MAO = monoamine oxidase; OSA = obstructive sleep apnea; PML = progressive multifocal leukoencephalopathy; TSH = thyroid-stimulating hormone (thyrotropin)

[1] Diroximel fumarate and monomethyl fumarate have the same active metabolite as dimethyl fumarate and were approved at doses yielding the same amount of that metabolite as the approved dose of dimethyl fumarate.

[2] Cladribine is only FDA approved for use in patients who have had a suboptimal response to at least one other disease-modifying medication.

[3] Mitoxantrone is FDA approved for use in patients with worsening relapsing-remitting MS, progressive-relapsing MS, or secondary progressive MS. Because of the risk of cardiotoxicity, a limit is placed on the cumulative lifetime dose.

[4] Alemtuzumab is only FDA approved for use in patients who have had a suboptimal response to at least two other disease-modifying medications.

VI. Discussion of Case Histories

Case 1. In a right-handed patient, aphasia is almost always due to a lesion in the left hemisphere. In this case, language output is nonfluent with relative sparing of comprehension, suggesting a left frontal lesion. This could not possibly account for the left-sided weakness, which is most likely due to a lesion in the right frontoparietal cortex, given the involvement of face, arm, and leg and the associated sensory loss. A single lesion large enough to produce both the aphasia and the left hemiparesis would involve such an extensive region of cortex bilaterally that impaired consciousness would be expected. Thus, the patient appears to have two separate lesions. The time course is acute, suggesting multifocal vascular disease. This has developed in the setting of an acute or subacute systemic illness. In someone who uses intravenous drugs, this clinical picture is suggestive of acute bacterial endocarditis. This patient is also in a risk group for AIDS, which is also associated with an increased risk of stroke, but it would be an unusual coincidence to develop fever, malaise, and cerebrovascular complications simultaneously as a result of HIV infection.

Cerebral emboli suggest left-sided valvular involvement, which is common in endocarditis whether or not the patient uses IV drugs (in contrast to right-sided involvement, which is much more common in people who use IV drugs than in any other group). Almost all patients with left-sided involvement have a heart murmur at some stage of the disease, but this may be absent on initial presentation.

The most important step in diagnosis is isolation of an organism from the blood. At least three separate venous blood cultures should be drawn. Echocardiography provides useful additional information, but a negative test does not rule out endocarditis. The sedimentation rate is almost always elevated in this condition, but it is nonspecific. An imaging study of the brain should also be performed, because even though the cerebral lesions are most likely ischemic, hemorrhages and even abscesses remain possible. An MRI/MRA provides good lesion visualization, and it is also the best noninvasive technique for detecting mycotic aneurysms. Finally, HIV testing should be offered to the patient, as the results will have an impact on her future medical condition even if unrelated to her current problem.

Even before culture results are available, empiric antibiotic treatment should be initiated. This should cover *Staphylococcus aureus*, streptococci, and enterococci. Vancomycin is a reasonable choice. Anticoagulation is avoided in this setting.

Case 2. The examination corroborates this man's report of left lower extremity weakness. The hyperreflexia there indicates an upper motor neuron lesion (i.e., a left-sided lesion in the spinal cord or low medulla, or a right-sided lesion above the medulla). The left afferent pupillary defect indicates a lesion anterior to the optic chiasm on the left. A single lesion could not produce both deficits without impairing consciousness. Thus, this patient has a multifocal condition. Based on his history, the two lesions appeared 8 months apart, and the left eye symptoms actually resolved in the interim. Accordingly, there is evidence of multiple CNS lesions separated in space and time, and this patient meets criteria for the diagnosis of MS. Although some rheumatologic diseases can mimic MS, these would be unlikely in a patient who has had no other systemic symptoms even after 2 years of neurologic symptoms.

Given the convincing examination findings, no additional diagnostic tests are necessary. Most practitioners would obtain an MRI scan of the brain in this setting, as it is the single test most likely to lend support to the diagnosis, but a normal scan would not rule out MS. It would also be reasonable to order serologic testing for SLE and other rheumatologic diseases.

Because the current exacerbation began 3 weeks ago, has not progressed, and is still producing only mild dysfunction, many clinicians would elect not to treat it acutely. Others would recommend a brief course of high-dose corticosteroids. With three exacerbations in a 2-year period, this patient should be strongly encouraged to begin disease-modifying therapy.

One of the most important aspects of management at this stage of the disease is patient education. Misconceptions about MS are widespread, and many people assume that the disease is rapidly disabling or even fatal. Although people with MS need to be aware that they could eventually become severely disabled, it is equally important that they realize that there is also potential for a relatively benign course. Unfortunately, there are no reliable prognostic indicators, and patients must understand that the course is unpredictable. People with MS who have minimal disability after 5 years of disease (i.e., people who have recovered nearly completely from their relapses to date) have a better prognosis than other people with MS.

Case 3. In this woman, multiple cranial nerves are impaired. A mass lesion in the pons and medulla could conceivably cause this, but with such extensive bilateral impairment in the brainstem, long-tract signs in the limbs (such as weakness, spasticity, hyperreflexia, ataxia, or sensory loss) would be expected, and alteration of consciousness would also be likely. Involvement of the cranial nerves as they exit the brainstem is therefore more plausible. In addition, she has signs and symptoms consistent with a right S1 radiculopathy. This suggests a meningeal process producing multifocal involvement of nerve roots and cranial nerves as they leave the neuraxis. The chronic time course suggests a neoplastic process, such as leptomeningeal metastasis or lymphomatous meningitis, but chronic inflammatory conditions such as tuberculous meningitis, Lyme disease, rheumatologic diseases, and neurosarcoidosis should also be considered. Diagnosis depends on CSF examination and a search for other systemic manifestations of these conditions.

In this case, CSF cytopathology revealed lymphomatous cells, and there was no evidence for any other systemic involvement. The diagnosis of primary leptomeningeal lymphoma was made. This is an extremely rare condition. The patient was treated with craniospinal radiation and intrathecal methotrexate, but symptoms continued to progress and she died 6 months after diagnosis.

III

Common Symptoms

Chapter 11

Acute Mental Status Changes

I. Case Histories

Case 1. You are called to evaluate a 72-year-old woman with diabetes because of an acute alteration in mental status. She had been admitted to the hospital yesterday for evaluation of exertional chest pain and had undergone cardiac catheterization earlier today. When you arrive, the patient is awake but agitated and unable to follow commands. She makes occasional attempts at speech, but everything she says is unintelligible. She seems to be able to move her limbs symmetrically and withdraws to noxious stimulation in the arms and legs. With difficulty, you examine her further and find no focal abnormality.

Case 2. A 19-year-old college student was brought to the emergency department by friends after they found him unconscious in his dorm room. He had been to a fraternity party the night before and reportedly looked well at 1 a.m., just before heading to his room. His friends report that he is "not a party animal"; he rarely, if ever, drinks alcohol and never uses drugs. On examination, his pulse is 110 and his blood pressure is 120/70. Temperature is slightly elevated at 38.3°C. Respirations are 24 per minute. Neurologic examination reveals no response to voice and only brief eye opening to noxious stimulation. Pupils are equal and react normally to light. His eyes don't move in response to the doll's eyes maneuver. Reflexes are depressed but present and symmetric throughout, and the plantar responses are normal.

Questions:

1. What initial approach should be taken with both of these patients?
2. How does each clinical setting affect your diagnostic considerations and the workup?
3. How will you manage each of these cases?

Case 3. A 38-year-old weekend softball player was brought to the emergency department after being hit on the left side of the head with a bat. When first hit he stumbled but quickly got back on his feet. He told his teammates that he could play despite the pain in his head, but they insisted on bringing him to the hospital. On arrival in the emergency department, he was able to speak to the triage nurse without difficulty and signed all his admission papers. When you first examine him 20 minutes later, he requires constant stimulation to stay alert. The left pupil is slightly larger than the right, but both react to light. The rest of his examination is normal.

Case 4. You are asked to evaluate a 20-year-old woman who was thrown from a horse and hit her head on the ground. There was no loss of consciousness at the time of the fall. She has a severe headache but otherwise feels all right. On examination, she is alert and her mental status is normal. She has no focal abnormalities on neurologic examination. She has a large occipital laceration.

Questions:

1. What is the proper approach to these two patients?
2. What determines whether a patient who has sustained a head injury needs a head CT scan? When do you need the assistance of a neurosurgeon?
3. Which patients can be sent home after a head injury, and what advice do you give them?
4. What problems can follow head injury?

II. Background Information

A. Definitions

coma: a state in which subjects lie with eyes closed and demonstrate no conscious responses to external stimuli, even after vigorous attempts to rouse them

consciousness: awareness of self and the environment, with the ability to react to internal and external stimuli

delirium: an acute, transient, fluctuating confusional state characterized by impairment in maintaining and intentionally shifting attention, often associated with agitation, disorientation, fear, irritability, illusions (misperceptions of sensory stimuli), or hallucinations (imagined perceptions with no basis in the external world)

encephalopathy: any state of altered level of consciousness or clouded sensorium

minimally conscious state: a condition of severely altered consciousness in which there is minimal but definite behavioral evidence of awareness of self or environment

obtundation: a condition of mild to moderate reduction of consciousness in which subjects appear to be drowsy or asleep, with reduced interest in the environment; they respond sluggishly to verbal or slightly painful stimuli, but when the stimulation stops they slip back into their previous state of reduced alertness and environmental interaction

stupor: a state of unresponsiveness resembling deep sleep, from which subjects can be roused only by vigorous and repeated stimulation, and even then they tend to have reduced alertness

vegetative state: a condition characterized by the complete absence of behavioral evidence for awareness of self or of the environment, but with preserved capacity for spontaneous or stimulus-induced arousal, including a sleep-wake cycle

B. Focal Mental Status Changes vs. Altered Level of Consciousness

Acute mental status changes can be either focal (such as aphasia, neglect, or visual hallucinations) or diffuse (such as delirium or stupor). Acute, focal mental status changes, like other acute, focal symptoms, are usually due to TIAs, strokes, or seizures (or—less often—migraines). These conditions are covered in other chapters. Transient global amnesia is another example of an acute, focal change in mental status. It is a distinctive syndrome in which a person loses the ability to lay down new memories and has variable degrees of retrograde amnesia (inability to remember previously stored memories) but has normal cognition and behavior otherwise. Characteristically, people with this disorder keep repeating the same questions over and over. The condition is self-limited and usually resolves completely within 2–12 hours; the cause is unknown, and no treatment is indicated. In contrast to these focal syndromes, this chapter focuses on acute, *diffuse* mental status changes, and specifically, acute changes in level of consciousness.

C. Physiology of Normal and Altered Consciousness

Consciousness can be thought of as consisting of three components: arousal, awareness, and cognition. As discussed in Chapter 9, a variety of wakefulness-promoting projections from the brainstem to the thalamus mediate *arousal*. Unlike sleep, in which the activity in these projections is modulated in a precise, cyclical pattern, stupor and coma are characterized by nonspecific suppression of activity in the wakefulness-promoting pathways. *Awareness* is poorly understood, and not even well-defined, but it seems to be closely related to the ability to direct and maintain attention. Thus, this aspect of consciousness may be mediated by the prefrontal cortex and its connections, especially with the thalamus. *Cognition* is a function of widespread cortical networks.

It follows that altered consciousness can result from damage to the thalamus or the brainstem, and also from widespread cortical damage. Many metabolic abnormalities, including hyponatremia, hypernatremia, hypoglycemia, hyperglycemia, hypomagnesemia, uremia, hepatic dysfunction, hypothyroidism, hypoxia, acidosis, alkalosis, and a host of toxins, can cause such damage. A structural lesion can only affect consciousness if (1) it directly involves the wakefulness-promoting systems in the brainstem or thalamus, (2) it is located elsewhere, but it is so large that it exerts pressure on the wakefulness-promoting projections, or (3) it is so extensive that it produces diffuse, bilateral cortical damage.

Delirium can be considered the mildest form of altered level of consciousness. It is characterized by inattentiveness and confusion. People with delirium may be agitated or withdrawn, combative or cooperative, but the consistent feature is that they can't engage in a sustained conversation or anything else that requires sustained, lucid thought processes. Obtundation, stupor, and coma are more severe alterations of consciousness. Individuals in these states are not only unable to maintain attention, they are unable to maintain arousal. People who are obtunded can be aroused by stimuli of varying intensity, such as shouting or shaking. In stupor, patients can be aroused only with extremely vigorous stimuli, and as soon as the stimulation ceases, they become unresponsive again. In the most extreme form of altered consciousness, coma, patients are unarousable no matter how vigorously they are stimulated.

These levels of altered consciousness form a continuum, rather than a set of discrete steps. In recent years, functional imaging techniques (such as PET and functional MRI) have provided evidence that some people with minimal behavioral response nonetheless have patterns of brain activity that suggest residual cognitive function; this has been referred to as cognitive motor dissociation or covert consciousness. Traditional approaches to classification may require modification in the future.

III. Approach to Acute Changes in Level of Consciousness

The potential causes of coma, stupor, and delirium are the same. When you evaluate a patient with any of these conditions, you should address the potential causes systematically from most urgent to least urgent. For the less urgent causes, you have time to be analytical and individualize the management plan, but for the most urgent conditions, diagnosis and therapy should proceed rapidly and systematically. The initial management of these patients should be almost automatic. Conceptually, the evaluation should proceed in the following order:

A. ABCs (airway, breathing, circulation)
B. oxygen, glucose, naloxone
C. pupils, doll's eyes, motor asymmetry
D. other electrolytes, renal, hepatic, temperature
E. everything else

In practice, it is often convenient to take some steps out of order. For example, the blood necessary for the tests in Step D can be drawn and sent to the laboratory along with the glucose in Step B. In fact, as with any other medical emergency, there are bound to be many things happening at once, producing a sense of controlled anarchy. The evaluation may simultaneously reveal several potential causes of altered mental status, which makes it even more important to have a clear idea of which problems must be addressed most urgently.

A. ABCs: Airway, Breathing, Circulation

As in most other clinical emergencies, the most important initial management goal is to ensure the adequacy of cardiopulmonary function by evaluating the patient's ABCs (airway, breathing, circulation). All other evaluations should be deferred until it is clear that blood pressure and ventilation are adequate. Even if ventilation is adequate, it should be monitored closely, as patients with a depressed level of consciousness are at risk for both hypoventilation and aspiration. If there is any hint that ventilation is failing, elective intubation should be considered.

B. Oxygen, Glucose, Naloxone

Once it is clear that cardiopulmonary function is adequate, you must explicitly address the possibilities of hypoxia and hypoglycemia. Both conditions can be fatal or result in irreversible damage if left untreated for even a short period, but both can be corrected rapidly once recognized. A clear airway and normal breathing pattern are no guarantee that oxygenation is adequate. A pulmonary embolus, interstitial pneumonitis, or anything else that produces a significant ventilation-perfusion mismatch may cause hypoxia without significantly altering breathing. If a reliable measure of arterial oxygen saturation can't be obtained immediately, 100% oxygen by face mask should be started empirically. Analogously, if a reliable serum glucose measurement is not immediately available, a 50 mL IV bolus of a 50% dextrose solution (one amp of D50) should be given empirically (immediately after collecting a venous sample to send to the lab). If there is any possibility that the patient might have thiamine deficiency (because of alcohol use or malnutrition), 100 mg of IV thiamine should be given with the dextrose to avoid precipitating or exacerbating Wernicke encephalopathy. The potential harm that could result from these interventions (e.g., the risk that the patient has chronic CO_2 retention and depends on hypoxia for respiratory drive, or the risk that the patient is already hyperglycemic and the glucose bolus will render them more so) is mostly theoretical and far outweighed by the potential harm that could result from withholding oxygen from someone who is hypoxic or glucose from someone who is hypoglycemic.

Unless the cause of coma is obvious, empiric treatment with naloxone (Narcan), 0.4–0.8 mg IV, for possible opiate/opioid overdose should be administered at the same time. This measure is not as urgent as oxygen or glucose administration because patients often recover fully from opiate/opioid overdose even when it is prolonged. Like oxygen and glucose, however, naloxone is a generally benign treatment that can produce dramatic reversal of mental status changes in the appropriate situations. This rapid improvement may be sufficient to establish the diagnosis and save the patient from more invasive and expensive diagnostic testing. When the clinical setting makes benzodiazepine toxicity particularly likely, you should also give flumazenil.

While treating for drug overdose, you should also consider the possibility of drug withdrawal. In particular, alcohol withdrawal can produce a delirious state (*delirium tremens*) characterized by agitation, confusion, hallucinations, and autonomic overactivity, including fever, tachycardia, and profuse sweating. This condition typically occurs 3 or 4 days after the last drink; common settings are alcohol detoxification programs or several days after a patient is incarcerated or admitted to a hospital. You should always consider this diagnosis in the setting of delirium, even if the person has no known history of alcohol use. The main goals of treatment are to address the autonomic overactivity, maintain hydration and electrolyte balance, and prevent self-injury. To this end, large doses of benzodiazepines may be required to control agitation. Less severe alcohol withdrawal produces tremulousness and agitation; a similar picture can occur with benzodiazepine or barbiturate withdrawal.

C. Pupils, Doll's Eyes, Motor Asymmetry

After addressing the most urgent conditions that can affect mental status—systemic derangements like hypotension and hypoglycemia—the possibility of structural brain damage must be considered. Not until this point in the evaluation does the neurologic examination become critical. The most urgent structural problem is transtentorial herniation, in which a mass lesion located above the tentorium expands downward and puts pressure on the brainstem, resulting in a depressed level of consciousness. The most useful elements of the examination for assessing transtentorial herniation are the pupillary light reflex and the vestibulo-ocular reflex (assessed by examining the response to the doll's eyes maneuver or ice water caloric testing; see Chapter 2).

The clinical features of herniation differ depending on whether the downward expansion originates on one side or in the midline. A mass lesion located laterally in one cerebral hemisphere typically exerts pressure on the ipsilateral temporal lobe, causing the medial aspect of the temporal lobe, the uncus, to herniate over the free tentorial edge (*uncal herniation*). This puts pressure not only on the midbrain, but also on the third nerve, which exits the midbrain at this level, so the first sign of uncal herniation is usually an ipsilateral third nerve palsy. Because of the impaired level of consciousness, the abnormal eye movements may be difficult for the examiner to appreciate, so the most prominent feature is usually a large, unreactive pupil—often referred to as a blown pupil—on the same side as the mass lesion (although occasionally the herniating temporal lobe pushes the midbrain to the other side and compresses the contralateral third nerve, resulting in a large, unreactive pupil contralateral to the mass lesion). In contrast, when the downward expansion occurs in the midline (*central transtentorial herniation*), it exerts pressure first on the thalamus, and then on the midbrain, where it disrupts both the parasympathetic and the sympathetic circuitry mediating pupillary constriction and dilation. As a result, both pupils are unreactive to light and they are fixed at an intermediate size.

If the herniation progresses beyond the level of the midbrain and reaches the pons, it can disrupt the circuitry that mediates the vestibulo-ocular reflex, because the afferent limb of this reflex is in the vestibular nerve (cranial nerve VIII), which enters the brainstem at the pontomedullary junction, and the efferent limb originates in the abducens (cranial nerve VI) nucleus. Because the circuitry mediating the vestibulo-ocular reflex is below the circuitry mediating the pupillary reflex, a supratentorial mass that is exerting pressure downward and causing transtentorial herniation—whether central or uncal—will disrupt pupillary function before it disrupts the vestibulo-ocular reflex. This leads to a useful rule: *In a comatose patient, if the pupils are normal but the doll's eyes response is not, the coma is not due to transtentorial herniation.*

To rephrase, when a comatose patient has an abnormal response to the doll's eyes maneuver but the pupils respond normally to light, a systemic metabolic abnormality is more likely than a structural lesion. This situation is surprisingly common, primarily because the response to the doll's eyes maneuver is relatively fragile and can be disrupted by even mild metabolic abnormalities, especially from exogenous toxins (notably benzodiazepines and barbiturates). In contrast, the pupillary reflex is resistant to such disturbances and is often preserved when altered mental status is due to metabolic causes. This is not always true, of course—in particular, a variety of drugs can affect pupillary size (see Table 11.1)—so when the

Table 11.1 Drugs That Commonly Affect Pupil Size

Large Pupils	Small Pupils
Anticholinergics	Cholinergics (e.g., glaucoma eye drops)
Sympathomimetics (e.g., bronchodilator inadvertently splashed in eye; cocaine; amphetamine)	Cholinesterase inhibitors
	Opiates/opioids

pupillary responses and doll's eyes responses are *both* abnormal, the cause of coma could be *either* structural or metabolic. Nonetheless, patients with abnormal responses to the doll's eyes maneuver but intact pupillary responses are common enough that the rule is well worth remembering. Also note that unless drugs are applied directly to just one eye, they affect both pupils equally. When the pupillary responses are markedly asymmetric in a patient with reduced level of consciousness, you should suspect a structural lesion.

Even when there is no evidence of transtentorial herniation, a patient with an unexplained alteration of consciousness must be evaluated for a structural lesion. The main feature to look for is asymmetry—of reflexes, sensory function, or motor responses. Even though many components of the standard neurologic examination must be modified or eliminated when impaired cognitive function prevents full patient cooperation (see Chapter 2, Part VI, Section C), deep tendon reflexes and resistance to passive manipulation can still be assessed, and the response to painful stimulation of the limbs often provides important information. An asymmetric withdrawal response to pain can signify hemiparesis or hemisensory loss. When evaluating responses to painful stimuli, you should distinguish purposeful withdrawal from local reflex responses and also from central reflexes (decorticate or decerebrate posturing). A useful technique to avoid confusion is to pinch the inner aspect of the arm or leg. Abduction of the stimulated limb is purposeful withdrawal, whereas adduction is most likely a local reflex. Flexion of the hip, knee, or ankle may simply be a local reflex, flexion of the elbow may indicate decorticate posturing, and extension of the leg could represent decerebrate or decorticate posturing.

When the examination suggests an expanding structural lesion, you should immediately obtain a brain imaging study (usually non-contrast CT scan), while contacting neurosurgeons to alert them that their help might soon be necessary. If the physical examination strongly suggests increased intracranial pressure (ICP), you may need to initiate the treatment measures described in Part IV, Section B even before the CT scan is done.

When the physical examination indicates that the altered mental status is most likely due to a metabolic cause, you can defer a brain imaging study and proceed with the next steps in the evaluation. If the diagnosis remains obscure after that, a brain imaging study may still be necessary eventually, but it is a lower priority than in patients whose examination suggests a structural lesion.

D. Other Electrolytes, Renal, Hepatic, Temperature Abnormalities

At this point in the diagnostic process, all of the most urgent conditions have already been considered, and you can spare a little time for deliberation. Many of the remaining causes of altered mental status are serious conditions requiring prompt treatment, but they can only be corrected gradually. Rapid treatment is impossible for some of these conditions and potentially dangerous for others.

Hyponatremia, hypernatremia, hypocalcemia, hypomagnesemia, hepatic disease, and uremia can all produce a wide spectrum of mental status changes, from irritability to coma, and there is nothing specific about the clinical picture associated with any one of them (except that the presence of tetany suggests hypocalcemia or hypomagnesemia). Laboratory testing is required for diagnosis. As noted earlier, the necessary laboratory tests should generally be requested at the same time that blood samples are sent for glucose and blood gas determinations, so the results will be available by the time this step in the evaluation process is reached. Treatment for each of these conditions is discussed in textbooks of internal medicine.

Body temperatures below approximately 34°C or above 39–40°C can produce mental status changes ranging from agitation or lethargy to stupor or coma. They can also produce many systemic abnormalities, including many of the metabolic derangements listed in the previous paragraph. These metabolic disturbances are often resistant to treatment until the underlying thermal disorder has been corrected. Treatment of hyperthermia and hypothermia is discussed in textbooks of intensive care medicine and emergency medicine.

E. Everything Else

The first four steps in the evaluation process address problems that are common, and patients often have more than one of these problems. For example, someone with hyperglycemia will often be dehydrated, resulting in both hypotension and hyponatremia. Opiate/opioid overdose may be associated with hypothermia and hypotension. Thus, it is usually appropriate to proceed through all of the first four steps even if one of the initial steps has already revealed an abnormality. In most cases, those four steps will uncover the likely cause (or causes) of acutely altered mental status. It is only necessary to search further when the first four steps have been unrevealing or when something specific in the patient's history or examination suggests another potential cause (e.g., a febrile patient should be evaluated for infection, even if hypotension and hypoglycemia have already been discovered).

Opioids, opiates, and benzodiazepines are not the only drugs that can produce altered mental status. Drugs with anticholinergic activity (including atropine, scopolamine, and tricyclic antidepressants), amphetamines, cocaine, LSD, and phencyclidine are other potential culprits. A urine toxin screen should generally be sent, and you should explicitly ask the patient's friends and relatives about drug use. A state's prescription drug monitoring program is also a useful resource, but only for agents that were prescribed.

Patients may be agitated or stuporous in the postictal period after a seizure (see Chapter 5). The diagnosis is often straightforward because of witnessed rhythmic movements or a known history of epilepsy but these clues may be absent. Patients discovered in bed in the morning with altered consciousness may have had a seizure in their sleep. Make every effort to find witnesses and ask them about abnormal movements or behavior preceding the alteration in mental status and about any history of similar events. Even witnessed seizures may be difficult to recognize, especially when they have no motor component. Clinicians should always be alert to the possibility of subclinical seizure activity, and obtain an EEG whenever the cause of an acute mental status change remains unclear. Unexplained fluctuations in mental status also increase the likelihood of subclinical seizures. Prolonged EEG monitoring is sometimes required to establish this diagnosis.

Patients with acute, severe hypertension, patients on immunosuppressive medication, and patients with eclampsia sometimes develop a syndrome known as *posterior reversible encephalopathy syndrome (PRES)* or *reversible posterior leukoencephalopathy syndrome (RPLS)*, characterized by mental status changes, visual symptoms (often blindness), other focal symptoms, and sometimes seizures, with brain imaging studies (especially MRI) showing edema in the white matter of the posterior cerebral hemispheres. The mechanism is unknown, but it is commonly thought to be a breakdown of cerebrovascular autoregulation. As the name implies, both the clinical and the radiologic abnormalities usually resolve when the underlying problem is successfully addressed.

Bacterial, viral, and fungal meningitis and encephalitis can all cause alterations in mental status. Fever, stiff neck, and headache are all clues to the diagnosis. Subarachnoid hemorrhage can mimic meningitis. The approach to these disorders is discussed in Chapter 12. Mental status changes also occur with sepsis and even with apparently localized infections such as pneumonia or urinary tract infections (especially in the elderly or people with dementia), presumably because of clinically undetectable spread of the organism to the nervous system or because of metabolic effects of the infection. If the first four steps of the evaluation are unrevealing, patients should generally be evaluated with chest x-ray and cultures of blood, sputum, urine, and spinal fluid, even if they are afebrile and have normal white blood cell counts.

Other inflammatory conditions, such as lupus and primary angiitis of the CNS, may also produce acute mental status changes. Hyperthyroidism, hypothyroidism ("myxedema coma"), addisonian crisis, and Cushing's syndrome (either iatrogenic or endogenous) are other potential causes. Unless there are specific features pointing to these diagnoses, they should only be considered when more common conditions have been excluded.

IV. Special Circumstances

A. Head Trauma

Altered mental status is no surprise when someone has sustained trauma to the head. Even so, the initial evaluation should proceed through the same steps as for anyone else with altered mental status because there could be additional factors contributing to the encephalopathy. These other factors might even have precipitated the head trauma (e.g., a motor vehicle accident could have resulted from depressed consciousness caused by hypoglycemia).

Management should be aimed at determining whether the head trauma caused any structural damage to the nervous system and whether that damage will require neurosurgical intervention. You should carefully inspect and palpate the head and scalp for evidence of laceration, fracture, or hematoma. If you detect any scalp lacerations, probe them with a sterilely gloved finger to look for a fracture or foreign body. You should inspect the periorbital and temporal regions for evidence of ecchymoses, which could indicate basilar skull fracture, and examine the nares and external auditory canals for evidence of a cerebrospinal fluid leak or hemotympanum. Progressive focal abnormalities on neurologic examination or changes in the patient's level of alertness could indicate progressive brain damage. Some people lose consciousness at the time of the head trauma, quickly return to normal for minutes to hours, and then have progressive decline in level of consciousness. The temporary normalization is called a "lucid interval." It is classically associated with epidural hematoma but it is neither specific nor sensitive—it can occur with any expanding intracranial mass, and it occurs in fewer than a third of people with epidural hematoma. To monitor for a decline in consciousness, patients should be observed every 30 minutes during the first 2 hours after the head trauma, every hour for the next 4 hours, and every 2 hours until at least 12 hours after the injury.

The Glasgow Coma Scale (GCS—see Table 11.2) is a quick, reproducible method for assessing level of alertness. Possible scores range from 3 to 15. Patients with a score of 8 or less are classified as severe head injury, those with scores of 9–12 are classified as moderate, and those with scores of 13–15 are classified as mild. In patients who are intubated, in whom assessment of best verbal response is impossible, the score is annotated by adding a "t" and the potential scores range from 3t to 11t. The GCS score is useful for making a rough estimate of prognosis, and it is often used as

Table 11.2 Glasgow Coma Scale*

I. Best motor response	
Obeys	6
Localizes to pain	5
Withdraws to pain	4
Abnormal flexion (decorticate)	3
Extension (decerebrate)	2
No response	1
II. Verbal response	
Oriented	5
Confused but converses	4
Inappropriate words	3
Incomprehensible sounds	2
No response	1
III. Eye opening	
Spontaneous	4
To speech	3
To pain	2
None	1

* Coma score = score I + II + III.
© Glasgow University

a basis for acute management decisions, such as whether to do a head CT scan, whether to intubate, whether to monitor intracranial pressure, and so forth. For example, a GCS score less than 15 is an indication for obtaining a head CT scan according to the two most commonly used decision rules, the "New Orleans criteria" and the "Canadian CT head rule." The other indications for obtaining a head CT scan according to the New Orleans criteria are (1) headache, (2) vomiting, (3) age > 60 years, (4) drug or alcohol intoxication, (5) persistent anterograde amnesia, (6) visible trauma above the clavicles, and (7) seizure. According to the Canadian CT head rule, the additional indications for obtaining a head CT scan are (1) suspected open or depressed skull fracture, (2) any sign of basilar skull fracture, (3) two or more episodes of vomiting, (4) age ≥ 65 years, with "medium risk" indications, (5) retrograde amnesia to the event ≥ 30 minutes, and (6) "dangerous" mechanism of head trauma.

Head injuries are often accompanied by injury to the cervical spine. Before removing a cervical collar, a helical cervical CT scan should be obtained, except when the mechanism of injury was not high risk and the patient is fully alert and asymptomatic, with a normal neurologic examination (and no intoxication or painful distracting injury that could confound the examination), free range of cervical motion, and no midline cervical tenderness. Traumatic events that result in head injury can also cause intra-abdominal or intrathoracic injury, and these possibilities should not be ignored.

When thorough evaluation reveals no evidence of a process that might require surgical intervention, many people with uncomplicated head injuries can be allowed to return home under close supervision by friends or family members. Patients' families should be instructed to awaken the patient every two hours during the first twelve hours after the injury and to return to the emergency department if the patient has reduced responsiveness, severe headache, or nausea and vomiting.

Concussions, especially those due to sports-related injuries, have received increasing attention in recent years. A concussion is a clinical syndrome of altered brain function, typically affecting memory and orientation, resulting from head trauma. It may result in loss of consciousness, but it may not. Patients may also have abnormal speech or coordination. Concussion is thought to be due to abnormal intracellular processes triggered by shear injury to axons. The optimal treatment is not known, but there is general consensus that patients should avoid physical and mental exertion until the symptoms have resolved.

In the days and weeks after a head injury, patients can develop a condition known as post-concussion syndrome, or post-traumatic syndrome, characterized by any combination of a diverse set of symptoms that include headaches, diffuse pain, abnormal sensation, weakness, dizziness, difficulty with thinking and memory, depression, hypersomnolence, behavioral changes, and seizures. The mechanism underlying this syndrome is not understood, and there is ongoing debate about the role played by secondary gain and compensation issues. Treatment is symptomatic. Fortunately, the symptoms usually resolve spontaneously over a period of months, although they may last several years in some patients.

B. Increased Intracranial Pressure

The only definitive treatment for increased ICP is elimination of the underlying cause. In many cases, this requires a neurosurgical procedure. Several measures can reduce ICP transiently, limiting neurologic deterioration while awaiting definitive treatment. Unfortunately, every available strategy has potential risks. One simple and safe intervention, once you have established that the patient has a stable cervical spine, is to remove the cervical collar and anything else that might interfere with venous drainage from the head. For similar reasons, many clinicians elevate the head of the bed to 30°, although this is more controversial because it can also reduce arterial blood flow to the head. Ventilator pressures should be minimized, to improve the pressure gradient for venous return from the head.

Hyperosmolar agents that do not readily cross the blood-brain barrier produce an osmotic gradient that pulls fluid out of the brain parenchyma and into the blood vessels. An osmotic diuresis also occurs because these agents are not reabsorbed from the renal tubule. It is not clear which of these effects is most significant in lowering ICP. Some maintain that the main effect of hyperosmolar agents is improved perfusion due to the decreased viscosity of blood that results from the increased intravascular water content. In any event, the effect is transient, presumably because the agents eventually do permeate tissue barriers, eliminating (and eventually reversing) the osmotic gradient. The most commonly used osmotic agents are hypertonic saline or mannitol.

Another way to reduce ICP is to remove CSF using an external ventricular drain, which can also be used to monitor ICP. The potential risks are hemorrhage and infection.

Hyperventilation results in decreased arterial pCO_2, which induces cerebral vasoconstriction and hence a reduction in intracranial blood volume.

This technique lowers ICP within 2 to 30 minutes, but the effect is transient. Furthermore, this treatment requires intubation and mechanical ventilation and carries the risk of ischemia if the vasoconstriction is excessive. For this reason, levels of pCO_2 below 25 mm Hg should be avoided; some authors recommend a target of 35 mm Hg.

Paralytic agents and sedatives, such as pentobarbital, can reduce the toxic by-products of brain metabolism that occur with brain injury. Unfortunately, they can also cause hypotension, leading to reduced cerebral perfusion, and they can make it difficult to evaluate the neurologic examination. Consequently, this approach is generally considered a second-line therapy. Induced hypothermia is another second-line therapy with no proven benefit.

For tumors and abscesses, increased ICP is usually a result of edema formation around the lesion. In this setting, glucocorticoids often produce dramatic improvement. In fact, improvement may be so dramatic that the underlying lesion is no longer evident on imaging studies, complicating subsequent attempts to establish a specific diagnosis and management plan. Thus, when a brain biopsy of a mass lesion may be necessary, glucocorticoids should generally be deferred until immediately before the procedure as long as the patient's medical condition and neurologic status are stable. A typical glucocorticoid regimen is 10 mg of IV dexamethasone (Decadron), followed by maintenance doses of 4 to 8 mg twice a day, but the optimal dosing regimen is unknown. There is no evidence that steroids are effective in treating edema related to ischemic or hemorrhagic stroke or in treating edema related to metabolic or hypoxic injury.

These measures are at best temporizing maneuvers that can help limit deterioration while awaiting definitive treatment. Neurosurgical consultation should be requested as soon as possible whenever operative intervention is a consideration.

C. Brain Death

With mechanical ventilators and other means of artificial support, it is possible to maintain some bodily functions indefinitely. As a result, philosophical questions regarding the definition of death have immediate practical relevance, especially in the context of organ transplantation. Is it ethical to remove life-sustaining organs from a donor whose heart is still beating?

The United States and almost every industrialized nation in the world formally recognize the principle that conscious and unconscious brain functions are fundamental to human life, so a person who has permanent loss of all brain function is dead. Explicit rules governing the determination of brain death have been established, although some of the details and even the underlying philosophical principles and legal applications remain the subject of debate. In essence, declaration of brain death requires that the cause of coma is known, it is irreversible, and there is no evidence of cortical or brainstem function. The patient does not respond to visual or auditory stimuli. All brainstem reflexes are absent, including the pupillary reflex, corneal reflex, gag reflex, the respiratory reflex in response to hypercarbia, and the vestibulo-ocular reflex—assessed with both the oculocephalic (doll's eyes) maneuver and the ice water caloric procedure. Noxious stimuli provoke no response other than possibly triggering reflexes mediated at the level of the spinal cord.

The most common reason to assess for brain death is to decide if a patient is eligible to be an organ donor. Most decisions about withdrawal of medical support do not involve brain death. Many comatose patients who still have some brainstem function have a poor prognosis. In such cases, even though the patient is clearly not brain dead, it is appropriate to withdraw support if family members agree that this is what the patient would have wanted. Most of the clinical features and diagnostic test results traditionally used for determining prognosis are imperfect, so in most situations it is prudent to wait for at least 72 hours from the onset of coma before concluding that the neurologic prognosis is bleak.

V. Discussion of Case Histories

Case 1. The initial approach to this patient should be the evaluation discussed in the body of this chapter: (1) ABCs; (2) oxygen, glucose, naloxone; (3) pupils, doll's eyes, motor asymmetry; and (4) other electrolytes, renal, hepatic, temperature. Particular concerns in this setting would be the possibilities of hypoglycemia (if she was given her usual doses of insulin or oral hypoglycemic agents despite being NPO for the procedure), drug toxicity (from opiates or sedatives given for the catheterization), or multiple cerebral emboli dislodged from the heart or aorta because of the catheterization (less likely given the nonfocal examination).

Comment: In this case, none of the initial steps provided an explanation for the patient's altered mental status. Careful review of her medication chart revealed that she had received several sedative-hypnotic drugs before and after the catheterization. With frequent reassurance, verbal orientation, and removal of unnecessary stimuli, she became less agitated. Her physicians ordered a sitter to stay by her bedside and she gradually returned to normal. She had little recall of her agitated state. Follow-up examinations were normal.

Case 2. The initial management of this patient is the same as that in Case 1. Starting to get the picture? This is the initial approach that should be followed in *all* cases of diffuse altered mental status. The normal pupillary response in a patient with no eye movements in response to the doll's eyes maneuver is strong evidence that the cause of this patient's coma is toxic/metabolic.

Comment: Despite the history given by his friends, this patient had opiates and benzodiazepines on a urine toxin screen, and drug ingestion was the ultimate diagnosis. A lumbar puncture was performed because of the patient's fever, and the results were normal. His remaining blood tests, including complete blood cell count and electrolytes, were normal. He awoke quickly after receiving naloxone and went home a day later.

Case 3. This patient has progressively worsening mental status, and his asymmetric pupils suggest a structural lesion of the brain. A CT scan should be obtained as soon as possible while consulting a neurosurgeon.

Comment: He had suffered a fractured skull with laceration of the middle meningeal artery and epidural hemorrhage (consistent with his lucid interval). Prompt evacuation of the hematoma saved his life, and he went home after a 2-week hospital stay.

Case 4. Because the patient has a normal mental status and normal neurologic examination, she can be allowed to go home (after the laceration is stitched) if friends and family members agree to observe her closely.

Comment: Aside from mild residual headache, she felt well at a follow-up visit 4 weeks later.

Chapter 12

Headache

I. Case Histories

Case 1. A 28-year-old man has come to the emergency department because he is experiencing the worst headache of his life. He first started having headaches when he was 16 years old, but they used to occur only two or three times a year. In the last 2 years they have been more frequent, up to twice a week. They always start on one side of the head—usually the right, but sometimes the left—and progress to involve the entire head. They are associated with photophobia and nausea. They usually go away if he takes two aspirin and lies down in a dark room. His current headache started 12 hours ago, and it is qualitatively similar to his previous headaches, but more severe. The pain is continuing to get worse, even though he has taken eight aspirin.

Questions:

1. What diagnoses should be considered?

2. What tests are necessary?

3. What treatment would you give?

Case 2. A 54-year-old woman with a history of chronic obstructive pulmonary disease and hypertension has come to your office for her routine quarterly checkup. She mentions in passing that she has been having daily headaches for the past 3 or 4 months. They are always on the right side of her head. The pain is not severe, just a nagging ache that usually gets better when she takes two aspirin and goes away completely when she takes two more aspirin 4 hours later. She can live with the pain at this level, but she thought she should mention it because she never used to have headaches at all. On examination, she has her baseline level of wheezing and a chronic cough. You find a mild left hemiparesis, and when you point it out she says she never noticed it before, but it's probably just because she is strongly right-handed and hardly uses her left side. You also find mild but definite hyperreflexia on the left, and she tends to extinguish left-sided stimuli on double simultaneous stimulation.

Questions:

1. What diagnoses should be considered?
2. What tests are necessary?
3. What treatment would you give?

II. Approach to Headache

Four questions must be addressed in evaluating and managing a patient with headaches:

1. Is the situation an emergency?
2. Are the headaches primary or secondary?
3. If the headaches are secondary, what is the underlying cause?
4. If the headaches are primary, which of the established headache syndromes do they most resemble?

Question 1 is addressed in Part IV. Question 2 is addressed in Parts V and VI. Question 3 is addressed in Parts IV and V, and Question 4 in Part VI. Part III presents some background information.

III. Background Information

A. Primary vs. Secondary Headaches

Headaches can occur independently of any other disease processes (*primary headache disorders*) or they can be associated with a wide variety of underlying neurologic and systemic conditions (*secondary headache disorders*). The pathophysiologic mechanisms are incompletely understood. Most research has focused on migraine headaches; other headache syndromes, both primary and secondary, presumably have similar mechanisms.

B. Pathophysiology of Migraine

The brain itself is not sensitive to pain. Pain signals from other structures within and around the skull—including the first few centimeters of the major arterial branches supplying the brain; the dura and its arterial supply;

the dural venous sinuses; the skin, muscles, fascia, blood vessels, and bones of the scalp, face, and neck; the sinus mucosa; and the teeth—are conveyed via the trigeminal nerve and cervical nerve roots to second-order neurons in the brainstem and cervical spinal cord (the "trigeminocervical complex").

Although we typically think of pain perception as an afferent, ascending process, it also includes efferent components. One of these components is "neurogenic inflammation." A sensory nerve is analogous to a riverbed, with numerous tiny tributaries joining to form the main channel. When a peripheral branch of the nerve is stimulated, an electric impulse travels up the axon toward the cell body. Along the way, the impulse passes numerous branch points marking the sites where other peripheral "tributaries" join the main channel. At each branch point, the electrical impulse splits into two signals that propagate in opposite directions. One impulse keeps traveling along the main channel toward the nerve cell body, while the other turns to travel along the tributary, away from the cell body to the tributary's peripheral terminal, where it stimulates release of neuropeptides that provoke an inflammatory response. This inflammation activates other nearby branches of the nerve, sending additional electrical impulses toward the cell body, which also bifurcate at branch points and propagate both toward and away from the nerve cell body. Again, the impulses traveling away from the cell body stimulate release of neuropeptides at the tributary terminals, establishing a positive feedback loop that results in an ever-growing pain signal. Two prominent molecular mediators of neurogenic inflammation are serotonin and calcitonin gene-related peptide (CGRP).

Another efferent component of pain perception involves descending, inhibitory pathways that modulate the activity in the ascending pain pathways, ultimately influencing the intensity of perceived pain. Serotonin is one of the principal neurotransmitters released by the neurons in one of these descending pathways.

Several lines of evidence suggest that auras (the neurologic symptoms that are often prominent before, during, or after the headache in people with migraine) are a manifestation of cortical spreading depression. This is a phenomenon characterized by dramatic ionic shifts and changes in electrical excitability and blood flow that march across large regions of the cortex unrelated to arterial territories. In experimental animals, a variety of stimuli can trigger this phenomenon.

Even between attacks, the cerebral cortex of people with migraine appears to be hyperexcitable. One theory is that a migraine occurs when a person with this hyperexcitability experiences something in the external or internal environment that triggers a wave of cortical spreading depression.

The spreading depression activates the trigeminocervical complex and initiates a cycle of neurogenic inflammation, and at the same time interferes with the normal modulating function of the descending inhibitory pathways. An alternative theory is that because of their cortical hyperexcitability, people with migraine sometimes experience increased activity in the trigeminocervical complex, either spontaneously or because of an environmental trigger. This trigeminocervical activation—or the resulting neurogenic inflammation—can cause cortical spreading depression. These theories are not mutually exclusive. It could be that the process flows in one direction on some occasions and the opposite direction at other times. Regardless, CGRP plays a key role in activating the trigeminocervical complex, as well as neurogenic inflammation. Serotonin is an important mediator of neurogenic inflammation and modulation of the pain pathway. Adenylate cyclase-activating polypeptide is another neurotransmitter that activates the trigeminocervical complex.

Just as it is not clear which process is primary, cortical spreading depression or trigeminocervical complex activation, it is not clear what terminates these processes—but something does. Migraines are self-limited, so they do not represent a medical emergency, even though they can be extremely unpleasant and disabling. Other primary headache syndromes do not constitute emergencies, either. In contrast, secondary headaches reflect the urgency of the underlying cause.

IV. Headache Emergencies: Subarachnoid Hemorrhage and Bacterial Meningitis

The two causes of headache that require urgent management are subarachnoid hemorrhage (SAH) and bacterial meningitis. For both of these conditions, early intervention has the potential to be life-saving and to reduce the likelihood of residual deficits. People with SAH must be evaluated for an aneurysm so that it can be repaired before it bleeds again and causes further damage. Bacterial meningitis is an extremely aggressive condition that has a high mortality rate; antibiotics must be started as early as possible in the course. The principal situations in which to consider the diagnoses of bacterial meningitis and SAH are:

1. a severe headache that is *qualitatively* different from any headache the patient has ever experienced before, and/or
2. a headache that is accompanied by fever, stiff neck, or a focal neurologic abnormality not documented with the patient's previous headaches.

Either of these situations represents an emergency—the patient must be assumed to have either a subarachnoid hemorrhage or bacterial meningitis until proven otherwise. This is a little more nuanced than the common adage that someone reporting the "worst headache of my life" should be presumed to have a life-threatening illness until proven otherwise. Anyone with chronic headaches who happens to develop a particularly severe headache could be experiencing "the worst headache of my life." In fact, people who go to the trouble of coming to an emergency department will probably use this or a similar phrase to make the staff appreciate the severity of the pain. The important thing to determine is whether this headache is *qualitatively* different from other headaches the person has experienced in the past. If the difference is only quantitative—that is, if the patient has a long history (>1–2 years) of similar headaches, and the current one is simply lasting longer or hurting more than usual—no diagnostic studies are required, and the patient can be treated with medications appropriate for their chronic headache syndrome. On the other hand, if the current headache is different in character from anything the patient has ever experienced before, *this is an emergency!*

Meningitis and SAH can't be reliably differentiated based on clinical characteristics. The onset of pain is typically more abrupt in SAH, and fever is more common (and usually more pronounced) in meningitis, but there are exceptions to these generalizations. Patients should be evaluated for both conditions simultaneously, and empiric intravenous antibiotics for bacterial meningitis should be administered immediately (2 g of either cefotaxime or ceftriaxone, plus 1 g of vancomycin for resistant pneumococcal strains; in patients older than 50 years, ampicillin should be added to cover *Listeria monocytogenes*, and in patients with impaired cellular immunity the recommended regimen is vancomycin, ampicillin, and either cefepime or meropenem). Antibiotics should only be deferred if the clinical suspicion of meningitis is low and the patient is afebrile with completely normal cardiovascular, respiratory, and mental status. Dexamethasone should be given with or just before the first dose of antibiotics (although the benefits of this practice have been demonstrated most clearly for children with meningitis resulting from *Haemophilus influenzae* and adults with meningitis resulting from *Streptococcus pneumoniae*).

The diagnostic test for meningitis is a lumbar puncture (spinal tap). Once antibiotics have been given, CSF must be obtained promptly, or cultures may be falsely negative. Because SAH can also be diagnosed by examining the CSF, one reasonable approach would be to perform a lumbar puncture immediately in any patient with a severe, unprecedented headache.

This is an invasive test, however, with the potential to provoke herniation in patients who have a cerebral mass lesion. In 95% of people with SAH scanned within 48 hours of symptom onset, the SAH can be visualized on a noncontrast CT scan, and the sensitivity is closer to 99% within the first 6 hours, so if a CT scan can be obtained immediately, it should be done before doing a lumbar puncture. Unless the clinical suspicion of meningitis is very low, empiric antibiotics should be started before doing the CT scan—and if there is any possibility that the CT scan will introduce a delay of an hour or more, the CT scan should be omitted and a lumbar puncture performed immediately, unless the examination strongly suggests that the patient has a mass lesion.

If the CT scan can be obtained immediately and it clearly establishes the cause of the headache (either SAH or a mass lesion), a lumbar puncture is unnecessary. If the CT scan is normal, the next step is to perform a lumbar puncture—both to evaluate further for subarachnoid hemorrhage and to diagnose meningitis. If there are no white blood cells in the CSF, no further antibiotics are necessary, but if there are more than five white blood cells per mm^3, bacterial meningitis remains a possibility. A CSF white blood cell count less than 100 per mm^3, a lymphocytic predominance, and a normal CSF glucose increase the likelihood that the meningitis is viral rather than bacterial (see Table 12.1), but there are exceptions to all of these rules. A multiplex PCR panel for the most common bacterial and viral pathogens responsible for meningitis has high specificity but false negatives can occur, and it does not include all potential bacteria and viruses that can cause meningitis. As a general rule, patients with a clinical presentation consistent with bacterial meningitis who have more than five white blood cells per mm^3 in their CSF and negative PCR testing should be maintained on IV antibiotics until cultures have been negative for 48 hours.

The hallmark of SAH is the presence of red blood cells in the CSF. This must be distinguished from a traumatic tap, in which local blood vessels are punctured during the procedure and blood enters the CSF at the puncture site. For this reason, whenever SAH is a consideration, it is imperative to use a centrifuge to spin down the CSF immediately. Blood cells that have been present for 12 hours or more will already have started to break down, producing xanthochromia (a yellow tinge to the supernatant). If all the blood present in the CSF was introduced at the time of the lumbar puncture, the cells will not yet have started to break down. They will aggregate at the bottom of the tube and the supernatant will be completely colorless.

If the CT or lumbar puncture suggests SAH, neurosurgical consultation should be obtained immediately. A CT angiogram (CTA) is often obtained

Table 12.1 Typical CSF Patterns in Meningitis

	Healthy Adult	Bacterial Meningitis	Viral Meningitis	Fungal Meningitis	TB Meningitis
CSF pressure	<200 mm H_2O	200–500 mm H_2O	Normal	Mildly elevated	Elevated
White blood cells	0–5 cells/mm³	>1000 cells/mm³	10–200 cells/mm³	50–800 cells/mm³	100–300 cells/mm³
Predominant cell type	Lymphocytes	Neutrophils	Lymphocytes	Lymphocytes	Lymphocytes
Protein	15–45 mg/dL	>100 mg/dL	15–100 mg/dL	40–500 mg/dL	100–500 mg/dL
Glucose	>50% of serum glucose	<40% of serum glucose	Normal	10–40 mg/dL	<45 mg/dL
Gram stain	Negative	Positive	Negative	Positive	Negative
Cultures	Negative	Positive	Negative	Positive	Positive (eventually)

in conjunction with the CT scan and it is often sufficient for identifying an aneurysm, but if it is negative a digital subtraction angiogram should be done. If an aneurysm is present, the patient should be admitted to a closely monitored bed in a dark, quiet room. The goal is to avoid clinical deterioration and to occlude the aneurysm by coiling (when technically feasible) or clipping within 3 days of the initial hemorrhage (see Chapter 4), before the period when vasospasm is most likely. Severe hypertension should be treated, but hypotension should be avoided—it is usually best to use short-acting agents that can be stopped quickly if necessary. Oral nimodipine should be started, because a regimen of 60 mg every 4 hours has been shown to improve outcomes, although the mechanism of benefit is not clear.

One condition that can be mistaken for SAH is the reversible cerebral vasoconstriction syndrome (RCVS), characterized by the sudden onset of an explosive headache, often referred to as a "thunderclap" headache. This condition is discussed later in this chapter (Part V, Section I).

V. Other Secondary Headaches

In patients who do not have subarachnoid hemorrhage or bacterial meningitis, the next step is to consider other systemic or neurologic causes of secondary headache. Although these are not emergencies in the same sense as SAH or bacterial meningitis, many of them require prompt treatment. These conditions are often apparent from the patient's medical history or examination. Features that increase the likelihood that headaches are secondary include systemic symptoms such as fever or weight loss, abnormal exam findings such as hepatomegaly or asymmetric reflexes, abrupt onset, a consistent correlation between body position and headache severity, age of onset greater than 50 years, known diagnosis of an illness that commonly causes headache, and current or recent pregnancy. You should be sure to ask whether the patient developed any other symptoms at about the same time the headaches began, and whether the patient started or stopped any medications at about that time.

A. Viral Meningitis or Encephalitis

Viral meningitis is not really an emergency, because there is no specific treatment, so delayed diagnosis does not affect outcome. The clinical presentation is essentially indistinguishable from that of bacterial meningitis, however, so these patients need a lumbar puncture urgently. As explained in Part IV, a non-contrast CT scan should be done first if it can be done expeditiously, because SAH is also in the differential diagnosis, and antibiotics should be administered empirically unless bacterial meningitis seems truly implausible. Both the clinical features and the spinal fluid findings tend to be less dramatic in viral meningitis than in bacterial meningitis (see Table 12.1), but there is sufficient overlap that unless PCR testing identifies a viral pathogen it is usually safest to continue treating empirically with antibiotics until bacterial cultures have been negative for 48 hours.

The clinical features of viral meningitis and viral encephalitis overlap considerably, but as a rule, fever, headache, and stiff neck are more prominent than mental status changes in people with meningitis and the converse is true in people with encephalitis. Seizures may occur with either, but they are more common in encephalitis. About 10% of people with encephalitis due to West Nile virus develop flaccid paralysis because of involvement of motor neurons in the anterior horns of the spinal cord. Most cases of viral meningitis are due to enteroviruses that enter the bloodstream from the intestines. This is also the source of some cases of viral encephalitis, but most cases of viral encephalitis are caused by arboviruses injected directly into the bloodstream by an insect vector, usually a mosquito or a tick. Diagnosis is usually based on serologic testing of the blood or spinal fluid. As is the case with viral meningitis, there is no specific treatment available for most types of viral encephalitis. People who have viral encephalitis often develop associated problems that require hospitalization, and the prognosis is generally much worse for encephalitis than for meningitis. The one type of viral encephalitis for which treatment is available is Herpes simplex encephalitis (HSE). As discussed in Chapter 10, clinicians should remain mindful of this diagnosis, and they should start acyclovir empirically whenever HSE is a realistic possibility.

B. Fungal or Tuberculous Meningitis

The clinical presentation of tuberculous meningitis is discussed in Chapter 10; the clinical features of fungal meningitis are similar. In general, both tend to be more indolent than viral meningitis, and they can occasionally smolder for months or even years. Cryptococcal meningitis, the most common cause of fungal meningitis, occurs nearly as often as bacterial meningitis in the United States. It is most common in individuals who are immunocompromised, but can also occur in people who are immunocompetent. CSF findings for both fungal and tuberculous meningitis are generally intermediate between those of viral meningitis and those of bacterial meningitis (see Table 12.1). CSF cryptococcal antigen is a sensitive and specific test for cryptococcal meningitis, which is the most common cause of fungal meningitis. The treatment of tuberculous meningitis is discussed in Chapter 10. Fungal meningitis is treated with amphotericin or other antifungal agents.

C. Mass Lesions

The vast majority of people with headaches have primary headaches, not secondary headaches. Even among the secondary causes of headache, mass lesions are rare. People whose headaches are due to structural abnormalities in the brain, such as tumor, abscess, stroke, parenchymal hemorrhage, subdural or epidural hematoma, or hydrocephalus, typically have papilledema or focal neurologic abnormalities. The main exceptions to this rule are lesions that developed so recently that they have not yet produced any focal findings or papilledema. My general rule is that I obtain a brain MRI when the headaches began less than a year ago or the examination reveals optic disc swelling or a focal abnormality. When someone with a headache has had qualitatively similar headaches for a year or more—even if they have recently become more frequent or more severe—and their examination is normal, I reassure them and do not order an imaging study. If an MRI is done and it shows a mass lesion, subsequent evaluation and management depend on the appearance of the lesion and the patient's risk factors.

D. Giant Cell (Temporal) Arteritis

Giant cell arteritis, also known as temporal arteritis, is a generalized disorder of medium and large arteries that occurs almost exclusively in patients over 50 years of age; some evidence suggests that it may be triggered by herpes varicella-zoster. Giant cell arteritis can result in a variety of focal neurologic deficits, or it may present with generalized mental status changes, but it usually presents with head pain that is dull and superficial, with superimposed lancinating pains. The pain may be unilateral or bilateral, and although it is often temporal, it may occur in any location. Patients frequently report temporal artery tenderness and jaw claudication (mandibular pain or fatigue provoked by chewing and relieved by stopping). About 40–50% of patients also have polymyalgia rheumatica, manifested by pain and stiffness of the limbs. The most concerning manifestation of giant cell arteritis is vision loss, which is usually due to ischemia of the anterior optic nerve, but giant cell arteritis can also cause central or branch retinal artery occlusion or posterior optic nerve ischemia. Permanent bilateral blindness occurs in up to 50% of untreated patients, so even though the clinical course is self-limited and lasts only 1–3 years, prompt treatment is essential.

A sedimentation rate should be checked in all patients older than age 50 with headaches of recent onset. The sedimentation rate is a useful screening test because it is elevated in 95% of patients (and > 100 mm/hour in 60%). Sensitivity can be improved by simultaneously checking the C-reactive protein. The sedimentation rate and C-reactive protein are not specific, so the diagnosis must be confirmed with a temporal artery biopsy. The combination of sedimentation rate and C-reactive protein is not 100% sensitive, so when the clinical suspicion is high enough, a temporal artery biopsy should be performed even if both the sedimentation rate and C-reactive protein are normal. Temporal artery biopsies are specific, but their sensitivity is less than 100%, partly because the pathologic process is often patchy. If the biopsy result is negative and the clinical suspicion is high, a repeat biopsy is often performed on the contralateral temporal artery (or occasionally a facial or occipital artery). A color Doppler ultrasound may be an alternative confirmatory test when performed by experienced operators.

Because of the risk of vision loss, people who are thought to have giant cell arteritis should be treated empirically with 60–80 mg per day of prednisone even before the diagnosis is confirmed with a temporal artery biopsy. An initial brief course of intravenous methylprednisolone (1–2 grams per day) is recommended if vision loss is already present. The biopsy should be obtained as soon as possible to minimize the duration of high-dose steroid treatment if it is not necessary. If the diagnosis is confirmed, patients should remain on this dose of prednisone for at least 4–6 weeks, with a subsequent slow taper guided by clinical symptoms and sedimentation rate. When tocilizumab is added to the prednisone, less cumulative prednisone is necessary.

E. Idiopathic Intracranial Hypertension (IIH)

As the name implies, idiopathic intracranial hypertension (IIH) is a condition in which intracranial pressure is elevated for no known reason. It has an overwhelming female predominance and typically presents during the reproductive years. It has a strong association with obesity. The headache is typically diffuse, with no distinctive characteristics. Other commonly reported symptoms include transient visual obscuration, diplopia, pulsatile tinnitus, and back or neck pain. Almost everyone with IIH has papilledema; some have unilateral or bilateral sixth nerve palsies. These clinical features can occur with elevated intracranial pressure from any cause, including brain tumors (which is why IIH was previously called pseudotumor cerebri), so patients with presumed IIH need a brain imaging study to exclude a mass lesion, followed by a lumbar puncture to document elevated intracranial pressure (and to exclude inflammatory disease as the cause). Other potential causes of increased intracranial pressure, such as venous sinus thrombosis, hypoadrenalism, or exposure to certain medications (including vitamin A, retinoids, tetracycline, and sulfa drugs) should also be excluded. The most recent diagnostic criteria require the documentation of elevated opening pressure on a lumbar puncture together with either papilledema or a sixth nerve palsy. Certain imaging features—such as flattening of the posterior globe—are characteristic of IIH, but they are neither sensitive nor specific. IIH is generally a self-limited condition, but it may lead to permanent vision loss. Weight loss has been shown to reduce intracranial pressure and improve symptoms, and it can induce remission. Unfortunately, maintaining weight loss is difficult. The most commonly used medication is acetazolamide (Diamox), a carbonic anhydrase inhibitor. Topiramate (Topamax) also inhibits carbonic anhydrase, and its potential side effect of weight loss is often desirable in people with IIH. Patients who do not respond to medication are sometimes treated with ventriculoperitoneal shunting, lumboperitoneal shunting, or fenestration of the optic nerve sheath. When headaches persist despite these treatments, patients are usually treated with the same medications used for migraine.

F. Spontaneous Intracranial Hypotension

Spontaneous intracranial hypotension is characterized by a postural headache, precipitated or aggravated by sitting up or standing, and relieved by lying down. It is similar to the headache that can occur after a lumbar puncture, but it has no apparent precipitant. Patients may also experience blurred vision, visual field defects, diplopia (especially from sixth nerve palsy), dizziness, nausea, vomiting, hypoacusis, tinnitus, personality changes, or mental status changes—some even have a presentation that resembles frontotemporal dementia. MRI scans typically show diffuse dural enhancement and features suggesting a "sagging brain." In some of these patients, but not all, evaluation reveals a spinal fluid leak. The condition often resolves spontaneously after several weeks, but when it doesn't, it may respond to treatment with hydration, caffeine, theophylline or aminophylline, corticosteroids, intrathecal or epidural saline infusion, or epidural blood patch. When these measures fail, an aggressive search for a CSF leak should be conducted, and if one is found, it should be repaired surgically.

G. Cerebral Venous Thrombosis

Most people with cerebral venous thrombosis experience headaches. Many, but not all, also have some combination of seizures, focal neurologic deficits, and confusion. Cerebral venous thrombosis primarily occurs in people who have a coagulation disorder or who are severely dehydrated, so such patients probably should have an MRI/MRV (magnetic resonance imaging with magnetic resonance venography) even if their headaches appear to be innocuous. Recent COVID-19 infection or COVID-19 vaccination may also predispose to cerebral venous thrombosis. Cerebral venous thrombosis is typically treated with low-molecular-weight heparin, with subsequent conversion to oral anticoagulation; the evidence for endovascular therapy is weak (see Chapter 4, Part V, Section A).

H. Arterial Dissection

Arterial dissection is usually suspected when patients present with TIAs or strokes, especially in the setting of recent head trauma or cervical manipulation, but these patients often say that they have had a fairly non-specific headache or neck pain dating from around the time of the trauma. This suggests that arterial dissection may occur much more often than appreciated. The optimal management strategy is not known, but these patients are usually treated with an antiplatelet agent or anticoagulation (see Chapter 4, Part VI, Section G).

I. Reversible Cerebral Vasoconstriction Syndrome (RCVS)

Reversible cerebral vasoconstriction syndrome (RCVS) is characterized by recurrent episodes of severe headache that come on suddenly and reach peak intensity within a minute, "like a thunderclap." The headache is often accompanied by mild confusion and sometimes focal neurologic abnormalities. Imaging studies show regions of constriction and dilation of large and medium-size cerebral arteries. Reversible cerebral edema may also be present, and ischemic or hemorrhagic strokes sometimes occur. RCVS is thought to be related to cerebrovascular dysregulation, similar to posterior reversible encephalopathy syndrome (PRES; see Chapter 11, Part III, Section E), and the two conditions sometimes coexist. RCVS is associated with pregnancy (especially in the setting of eclampsia) and with a variety of drugs (including sympathomimetic medications, selective serotonin reuptake inhibitors, serotonin-norepinephrine reuptake inhibitors, triptans, cocaine, marijuana, and oral contraceptives). No specific treatment has been proven beneficial, and symptoms typically resolve spontaneously over several weeks, but calcium channel blockers are often administered.

J. Systemic Conditions

Headaches can occur with a wide variety of systemic infections, autoimmune diseases, neoplasms, endocrine disorders, and metabolic disturbances. Almost every class of medication can provoke headaches in some patients. A thorough discussion of all the substances and conditions that can cause secondary headaches would, in effect, be a textbook of medicine (and pharmacology). In most cases, the characteristics of the headache are nonspecific, and the underlying condition is diagnosed based on other features of the illness (or, in the case of medications, based on a focused history and sometimes a trial off medication).

K. Secondary Headache Syndromes with Diagnostic Ambiguity

1. Sinus disease

People with acute sinusitis often experience headaches that are typically exacerbated by changes in head position. The diagnosis is usually apparent because of additional symptoms, such as nasal discharge, congestion, conjunctival injection, cough, and sinus tenderness. Sphenoid sinusitis may be difficult to detect because the sphenoid sinus does not communicate directly with the nasal passages, so patients may experience headaches without any of the other associated symptoms that are typical of sinusitis. Patients with sphenoid sinusitis are at substantial risk for developing meningitis and require a prolonged course of antibiotic therapy, often intravenously.

The role of *chronic* sinusitis in producing headaches is less clear. Many people with chronic headaches have some opacification in one or more sinuses on imaging studies, but many people without headaches have similar findings. There is no compelling evidence that these patients respond to antihistamines, antibiotics, or sinus surgery, so they should be treated with the same medications used for tension and migraine headaches.

2. Temporomandibular disorders

People who have structural malalignment of the temporomandibular joint often experience pain that can be local, referred, or both. It is unclear how much of the pain is due to abnormal jaw biomechanics and how much is due to other factors, such as a reduced pain threshold, sustained contraction of muscles around the head and neck, or a primary headache disorder. Still, if a patient reports a correlation between chewing and headaches, and if the temporomandibular joint is easily dislocated on examination, a temporomandibular disorder should be considered. No high-quality evidence is available to guide management. Patients should be educated regarding optimal head posture and avoidance of triggering behaviors such as pen chewing or nail biting. A soft diet, bite splints, and jaw exercises are often recommended. Local injections and surgery are occasionally used for severe cases.

3. Post-concussion (or post-traumatic) syndrome

As discussed in Chapter 11, Part IV, Section A, it is common for people who have had head trauma to develop headaches as a component of the concussion syndrome. This is usually a self-limited condition, but in some patients the symptoms persist. The headache pain is often continuous, but waxes and wanes in severity. These individuals often report memory difficulties, sleep disturbance, mood swings, depression, neck and back pain, dizziness, and diffuse sensory symptoms. Imaging studies are usually normal (but should be obtained once, to exclude chronic subdural hematomas and to exclude structural problems in the spine if the patient has symptoms there). Superimposed legal and disability issues often complicate this syndrome, and because all features are subjective, there is no way to rate the severity of this condition or even to be sure it is present. In most cases, the symptoms resolve spontaneously—usually within a year—but they sometimes last as long as 3 years. In approximately 10% of patients, symptoms persist beyond that point. While waiting for resolution, only symptomatic treatment is available. The headaches should be treated in the same way as migraine and tension headaches; antidepressants are often used because the patients also have symptoms of depression.

VI. Primary Headaches

As explained in Parts IV and V, certain characteristics should prompt you to evaluate for secondary headaches that might require expeditious or even urgent treatment: (1) headache onset (or clear change in character, not just severity or frequency) within the past year, (2) fever and stiff neck, (3) focal abnormalities on neurologic examination, (4) optic disc swelling, (5) acute or subacute mental status changes, (6) strong correlation between headache and body position, (7) prominent systemic symptoms or exam abnormalities, (8) known diagnosis of an illness that commonly causes headache, (9) current or recent pregnancy, and (10) age of onset more than 50 years. Most people with headaches have none of these characteristics—they have a long history of similar episodes, a normal neurologic examination, no fever or neck stiffness, and no other features to suggest a secondary headache disorder. These patients have a primary headache disorder, and the next step is to classify their headaches as carefully as possible so that the appropriate treatment can be given. This classification is based purely on the history.

A. Migraine and Tension Headaches

Most people with headaches have symptoms that fall somewhere on a spectrum that includes the symptoms of migraine and tension headaches. These have traditionally been viewed as two completely separate conditions with distinct etiologies, but many investigators believe that they may simply be varying manifestations of a single underlying pathophysiologic process. Certainly, many people say that their headaches are not all identical—they describe some with symptoms that suggest migraine and others with features that sound like tension headaches. It is also common for individual headaches to have some attributes of migraine and other characteristics that suggest tension headache. The same medications are effective for treating both classes of headache. For this reason, I often use the term *migraine/tension spectrum* to refer to both categories together.

Even though the distinction between migraine and tension headache doesn't influence management, it is useful to characterize patients' headaches as precisely as possible. This helps in monitoring patients over time and assessing their response to therapy. Furthermore, it's possible that differentiating between migraine and tension headache will ultimately be shown to have therapeutic implications, so it is worth knowing the traditional distinctions.

Migraine headaches are typically unilateral (although the side of the headache may vary from one episode to the next). The pain is usually throbbing or pulsing. Nausea, vomiting, photophobia, and phonophobia are common accompaniments. Some patients develop focal neurologic symptoms or signs. The most common are visual (scintillations and scotomata), but focal numbness, weakness, aphasia, dysarthria, dizziness, and even syncope may occur. Patients who experience focal neurologic symptoms during, after, or immediately before a migraine are said to have migraine with aura, and patients with no neurologic symptoms are classified as having migraine without aura.

Migraines may last from hours to days. Many people note that specific triggers can precipitate their headaches. These can include alcohol (especially red wine), chocolate, cheese, pickled items, processed meats, monosodium glutamate, menstrual periods, weather conditions, irregular eating or sleep habits, and stress. Compared to headache-free individuals, people with migraine are more likely to have a history of motion sickness and more likely to have other family members with headaches.

Tension headaches are typically bilateral, often involving either the forehead or the back of the head and neck, and sometimes the entire head. The pain is described as pressure, tightness, or a squeezing sensation. Nausea may occur, but most of the other features that can accompany migraine are absent. The only common precipitating factor is stress.

Some people with migraine or tension headaches can achieve adequate control simply by identifying and eliminating triggers. Even something as straightforward as taking care to eat and sleep on a regular schedule may have a big impact on headache frequency. It is worth considering whether use of hormonal contraceptives might be one of a patient's triggers. Even when there does not seem to be a clear correlation between the onset of a patient's headaches and initiation of the contraceptive, an empiric trial off the contraceptive sometimes produces significant improvement in headaches. A separate concern with hormonal contraceptive use is the risk of thromboembolic events, including stroke. Migraine (especially migraine with aura) and use of hormonal contraceptives (especially those with high estrogen doses) are both associated with an increased risk of stroke. Although the evidence is imperfect, it suggests that people with both of these risk factors have a substantially higher incidence of stroke than people with either risk factor alone. Even so, stroke is so uncommon in young females that even when both risk factors are present the magnitude of the increased incidence remains low. Patients should be informed of these issues so that they can make informed choices. People with migraine—especially migraine with aura—who use hormonal contraceptives should consider using formulations with a low estrogen dose. They should minimize other stroke risk factors, such as cigarette smoking. In fact, I usually advise patients who have migraine with aura that if they continue to smoke they shouldn't use hormonal contraceptives, and if they use hormonal contraceptives, they should stop smoking. Of course, there are many additional reasons to recommend stopping smoking.

Elimination of trigger factors can reduce the frequency of headaches, but it usually doesn't abolish them. Nonpharmacologic treatments such as neck stretching exercises, mindfulness meditation, physical therapy, yoga, acupuncture, and biofeedback may be helpful, but most people also require medications. Pharmacologic treatment is centered on two kinds of medications: abortive and prophylactic (preventive). An abortive agent is taken as soon as possible when a headache begins, with the goal of stopping the headache. A prophylactic agent is taken on a regular basis, even when the patient does not have a headache, to prevent headaches or reduce their frequency. The most commonly used abortive and prophylactic agents are listed in Tables 12.2, 12.3 and 12.4.

People who have infrequent migraine/tension headaches do not require prophylactic medications if they can find an abortive agent that consistently and rapidly relieves their symptoms. The key factor in deciding whether to start a prophylactic agent is the degree to which patients' headaches disrupt their lives. Even people who have found an effective abortive regimen often experience a substantial period of discomfort before the drug takes effect, and this can be severe enough to interfere with normal activities. If this happens frequently, work productivity and quality of life can be affected. Furthermore, most abortive agents seem to be less effective if used too frequently. In fact, people who take abortive agents on a daily basis often have particularly intractable headaches, leading to the concept of "medication overuse headache" or "rebound headache." This term is used differently by different people. At one level, it can be interpreted to mean that individuals who take abortive medication frequently will be uncomfortable if they miss one or more doses of the medication. Few people would dispute this. At another level, "medication overuse headache" can be interpreted to mean that frequent use of abortive medication *causes* headaches to be more frequent or more severe than they would have been otherwise. This statement is far less intuitive, and the evidence for it is not compelling. Regardless of whether this version of the "medication overuse headache" concept is valid, someone who uses abortive medication frequently would generally benefit from prophylactic medication. In general, people with more than one severe headache a week should consider starting a prophylactic medication, but this is only a rough guideline that must be modified based on each individual patient's circumstances and preferences. For example, some people with only one headache a month may require a prophylactic agent if the headaches last several days and are disabling despite abortive treatment. Others may choose to experience several headaches a week rather than take a medication regularly, especially if their headaches are mild or they get prompt relief from an abortive agent.

The choice of which abortive or prophylactic agent to use is typically based on side-effect profiles, dosing characteristics, patient preferences, and concurrent medical problems (which might contraindicate some medications, whereas other medications might have the potential to "kill two birds with one stone"). Efficacy is usually less of a consideration. It is impossible to know which treatments will work best for which individuals. It is also impossible to predict what dose will be required; standard practice is to start at a low dose, building gradually to higher doses if necessary (and switching to a different medication if intolerable side effects occur). The medications for which the evidence of efficacy is strongest are indicated with an asterisk in Tables 12.2, 12.3 and 12.4, but this is somewhat misleading. Controlled trials demonstrating efficacy were required for FDA approval of medications that were recently developed for headache, whereas medications that were approved for other indications and subsequently found to be effective for headache may not have been studied as rigorously, despite a large reservoir of anecdotal clinical evidence supporting their use.

Side-effect profiles are a particular concern in pregnant patients. No medication is considered absolutely safe during pregnancy (or breastfeeding). Headaches often subside during pregnancy, but they may persist or get worse; in some cases, headaches begin during pregnancy or soon after delivery. If a patient requires medication, it is best to try to control the headaches with abortive agents alone. Acetaminophen and metoclopramide are generally thought to be the safest abortive agents. Other dopamine-blocking antiemetic medications are commonly used also. Triptans may also be used; they have traditionally been avoided during pregnancy, but a systematic review found no evidence of adverse outcomes. Codeine and other opioids/opiates are relatively safe, but discouraged because of the risk of dependence, and frequent use has been associated with various congenital malformations. If a prophylactic agent is necessary, magnesium, riboflavin, and coenzyme Q10 are the safest choices. Cyproheptadine may be the safest prescription medication, but it is not always effective. Nonsteroidal anti-inflammatory drugs (NSAIDs) can cause premature ductus closure and consequent pulmonary hypertension; they may also increase bilirubin and impair renal function. They are generally considered relatively safe in the first two trimesters. Metoprolol (Lopressor) is considered fairly safe. Propranolol (Inderal) has an oxytocic effect and may cause growth retardation, respiratory depression, and hypoglycemia. It carries more risk than metoprolol but may be more effective for some patients. Calcium channel blockers may be relatively safe in pregnancy, but there is a theoretical risk of reduced uterine blood flow due to hypotension. Fetal limb reduction abnormalities, other bone deformities, and hand swelling have been reported with tricyclic antidepressants. Antiseizure medications should be avoided in the first trimester because of teratogenic potential, and valproic acid should generally be avoided in anyone who could potentially become pregnant.

Four noninvasive neuromodulation devices are FDA approved for acute migraine treatment: external trigeminal nerve stimulation (eTNS, also known as transcutaneous supraorbital nerve stimulation), single-pulse transcranial magnetic stimulation (sTMS), noninvasive vagus nerve stimulation (nVNS), and remote electrical neuromodulation (also known as distal transcutaneous electrical stimulation, or distal TENS). The studies demonstrating that these devices are effective are complicated by the fact that is difficult to ensure that patients are blinded to their treatment arm. Side effects are usually mild, but the devices can be costly and they are not usually covered by insurance. Some evidence, mostly from open-label studies, indicates that eTNS and sTMS may also be effective for headache prophylaxis. These approaches might be particularly attractive to people who have difficulty tolerating pharmacologic treatment or are opposed to taking systemic medications; they might also be an option to consider during pregnancy or breastfeeding.

B. Trigeminal Neuralgia

Trigeminal neuralgia (tic douloureux) is characterized by a paroxysmal, "electric shock-like" pain that lasts about a second, usually in the V2 distribution (along the maxilla) or V3 distribution (along the mandible), but in some patients it affects the V1 distribution (the forehead). It tends to occur in trains lasting 5–30 seconds. In most patients, the pain can be triggered by lightly touching a particular spot on the face, called a trigger zone. The location of the trigger zone differs among patients.

Cold wind, brushing teeth, or chewing may also trigger the pain. It usually does not wake patients from sleep. There is often a superimposed dull, continuous ache, especially when the condition has been present a long time.

Trigeminal neuralgia is usually a benign condition, either idiopathic or associated with compression of the trigeminal sensory root by blood vessels, but it can also be associated with other structural lesions of the fifth nerve, and it occurs fairly frequently in people who have multiple sclerosis. Symptoms usually begin after age 50 but may occur as early as the teen years. The younger the age of onset, the greater the likelihood that the trigeminal neuralgia is secondary to some other condition, especially multiple sclerosis. An MRI scan of the brain, with special attention to the posterior fossa, should be done if the symptoms begin before age 50, if there are focal abnormalities on examination, or if symptoms began or changed in character within the past 2 years. Some people develop trigeminal neuralgia (or symptoms that mimic it) as a result of dental problems, including microabscesses, so all patients should be carefully evaluated for dental disease.

Table 12.5 lists medications used to treat trigeminal neuralgia; carbamazepine is usually prescribed first unless the patient has contraindications. At least several of these agents should be tried before considering surgical treatment. When the pain can't be controlled even after advancing to doses as high as the patient can tolerate and imaging studies identify a blood vessel compressing the nerve, microvascular decompression of the trigeminal nerve is generally the preferred surgical option. Some clinicians advocate this procedure even when imaging fails to show a compressive vessel, but most clinicians recommend one of the neuro-ablative procedures listed in Table 12.5 in that circumstance. These neuroablative procedures are also favored in people who are poor candidates for craniotomy. Unfortunately, a few patients develop "anesthesia dolorosa" after the neuroablative procedures. This is a condition of numbness and extremely painful paresthesias over part of the face, notoriously refractory to treatment.

C. Glossopharyngeal Neuralgia

The pain characteristics and clinical features of glossopharyngeal neuralgia are similar to those of trigeminal neuralgia, except that the pain typically starts in the oropharynx and extends upward and backward toward the ear (sometimes in the reverse direction). Swallowing (especially sour or spicy foods), yawning, sneezing, coughing, cold liquids in the mouth, or touching the ear can be triggers. Unlike trigeminal neuralgia, the pain frequently awakens patients from sleep. The pain is sometimes associated with bradycardia, hypotension, or syncope. Medical treatment is the same as for trigeminal neuralgia, and surgical treatment is analogous. Glossopharyngeal neuralgia is very rare (trigeminal neuralgia is 75 times more common).

D. Cluster Headaches

Cluster headaches have several distinctive features:

(1) temporal clustering—The patient may go for months or years without headaches but then experiences a cluster of daily headaches. Clusters usually last 4–8 weeks and occur once or twice a year, but this is quite variable. Within a cluster there may be one or more headaches a day, but at least one of the headaches typically occurs at the same hour every day, often during the first REM period after falling asleep.

(2) excruciating pain/agitation—The headaches typically last 30 minutes to 2 hours (an average of 45 minutes), and the onset is explosive. Patients prefer to be upright. They often cannot sit or stand still, and many will even hit their head against a wall. This is a marked contrast with migraine, in which patients usually try to be as motionless as possible.

(3) unilaterality—Whereas people with migraine typically have left-sided headaches on some occasions and right-sided headaches on other occasions (and many of them have bilateral headaches), most people with cluster headaches experience every headache on the same side.

(4) autonomic symptoms—People with cluster headaches commonly have lacrimation, redness of the eye, nasal congestion, and rhinorrhea on the same side as the head pain. An ipsilateral partial Horner syndrome is sometimes present during the attack, and it may persist between attacks. All of these features may also occur with migraine, but they are more common and more severe with cluster.

In some people with cluster headaches, the remissions between clusters gradually disappear; this is referred to as chronic cluster headache. Occasionally, the chronic cluster time course is present from the onset.

Management is two pronged (see Table 12.6). One prong focuses on aborting the individual headaches (with treatments that must act rapidly, given the short duration of the headaches). The other prong focuses on shortening the cluster. For patients who have only short time intervals between clusters, or those with chronic cluster headaches, a third management prong focuses on long-term preventive ("maintenance") therapy, but most of the evidence for this type of maintenance treatment comes from open-label trials.

E. Other Trigeminal Autonomic Cephalalgias (TACs)

Cluster headache is by far the most common of a group of disorders known as trigeminal autonomic cephalalgias, or TACs, all of which cause intense unilateral pain and autonomic symptoms in the distribution of the ipsilateral trigeminal nerve, usually the V1 division. Paroxysmal hemicrania is a rare condition characterized by attacks in which the pain and accompanying autonomic symptoms are similar to cluster headache, but the temporal profile is different: the headaches are short (usually 2–30 minutes, an average of 13 minutes) and recur frequently throughout the day (4–38 attacks a day, an average of 14). No nocturnal predominance is apparent. Most people with paroxysmal hemicrania have the chronic subtype—their headaches occur daily throughout the year, with no remissions. About 20% of people with paroxysmal hemicrania have the episodic subtype, with remissions of at least 3 months each year. This contrasts with cluster headache, where the episodic subtype is much more common than the chronic subtype. Unlike people with cluster headache, people with paroxysmal hemicrania tend to stay quietly in one place. Paroxysmal hemicrania responds reliably and dramatically to indomethacin (Indocin), though dose requirements may vary.

Hemicrania continua is another TAC, similar to paroxysmal hemicrania except that the pain is constant, with exacerbations at times. This condition is also exquisitely responsive to indomethacin.

Another subgroup of TACs, short-lasting unilateral neuralgiform headache attacks (SUNHAs), can be thought of as resembling trigeminal neuralgia in the V1 distribution together with ipsilateral autonomic symptoms similar to those that occur in paroxysmal hemicrania and cluster headaches. SUNHA is subdivided into SUNCT (short-lasting unilateral neuralgiform headache with conjunctival injection and tearing), in which both conjunctival injection and tearing are prominent, and SUNA (short-lasting unilateral neuralgiform headache attacks with cranial autonomic symptoms), in which one or both are absent. SUNHA is characterized by paroxysms of pain that last 1–600 seconds, but typically 15–30 seconds, averaging 28 attacks per day (with a range of 1–77). As with the other TACs, both episodic and chronic forms of SUNHA are defined based on whether remissions occur. Many people with SUNHAs have cutaneous triggers, similar to those of trigeminal neuralgia. Despite the resemblance to paroxysmal hemicrania, SUNHA does not respond to indomethacin. It is usually treated with the same medications (and in refractory cases, surgical interventions) as trigeminal neuralgia. The best available evidence is for lamotrigine.

Migraine, paroxysmal hemicrania, hemicrania continua, and SUNA have a female predominance, whereas cluster headache and SUNCT have a male predominance, but the ratio is not overwhelming for any of these conditions.

F. Primary Stabbing Headache

Very brief paroxysms of stabbing pain, lasting at most a few seconds (usually less than a second) without autonomic symptoms, are common in people who are subject to migraine, but they can also occur in people with no prior headache history. This condition has been called "ice-pick headache" but it is currently referred to as "primary stabbing headache." It typically responds to indomethacin.

G. Persistent Idiopathic Facial Pain

People with headaches that do not fit cleanly into any well-defined category are classified as having persistent idiopathic facial pain (previously referred to as atypical facial pain). They often have some features of migraine, but other features suggestive of a neuralgia or a TAC, and they may have some features that are not typical of any defined headache syndrome. This diagnosis obviously has no consistent pathophysiologic correlate, and treatment is usually a matter of trial and error with medications used for one of the more well-defined conditions. As with other headache syndromes, diagnostic testing is only necessary if the neurologic examination shows focal abnormalities or if there has been recent onset or change in the character of the patient's symptoms.

VII. Supplementary Tables for Reference

Table 12.2 Abortive Agents for Headaches in the Migraine/Tension Spectrum

Drug Category	Specific Agents (Routes of Administration; Brand Names)
Nonsteroidal anti-inflammatory drugs (NSAIDs)	Aspirin* (PO), diclofenac* (PO; Cataflam), ibuprofen* (PO; Advil, Motrin), indomethacin (PO, PR; Indocin), ketorolac (PO, IM, IV; Toradol), naproxen* (PO; Naprosyn, Aleve)
Other nonopioid analgesics	Acetaminophen* (PO; Tylenol), lidocaine (NAS), tramadol (PO; Ultram)
Combination analgesics	Acetaminophen/aspirin/caffeine* (PO; Excedrin, Excedrin Migraine)
Combination analgesic/barbiturates [**AVOID PRESCRIBING** due to risk of barbiturate dependence]	Acetaminophen/butalbital/caffeine (PO; Fioricet, Esgic), aspirin/butalbital/caffeine (PO; Fiorinal), acetaminophen/codeine combinations
Dopamine-blocking antiemetics	Chlorpromazine (PO, IM, IV; Thorazine), droperidol (IV, IM; Inapsine), metoclopramide (PO, IM, IV; Reglan); prochlorperazine (PO, PR, IM, IV; Compazine)
Triptans (serotonin-$_{1B/D}$ agonists)	Almotriptan* (PO; Axert), eletriptan* (PO; Relpax), frovatriptan* (PO; Frova), naratriptan* (PO; Amerge), rizatriptan* (PO, ODT; Maxalt, Maxalt-MLT), sumatriptan* (PO, NAS, SQ; Imitrex), zolmitriptan* (PO, ODT; Zomig)
Ergots	Dihydroergotamine (NAS*, IV, IM, SQ; Migranal, DHE 45, Trudhesa)
Gepants (CGRP antagonists)	Rimegepant* (ODT; Nurtec), ubrogepant* (PO; Ubrelvy), zavegepant* (NAS; Zavzpret)
Ditans (serotonin-$_{1F}$ agonists)	Lasmiditan* (PO; Reyvow)

CGRP = calcitonin gene-related peptide; IM = intramuscular; IV = intravenous; NAS = intranasal; ODT = orally dissolving tablet; PO = oral; PR = rectal; SQ = subcutaneous

* = Strong evidence of efficacy

Table 12.3 Options for Aborting Headaches in the Emergency Department

IV hydration (1–2 liters of normal saline)

Any of the medications listed in Table 12.2, if not already tried (commonly used: dopamine-blocking antiemetics, IV; ketorolac, IV or IM; triptans—especially sumatriptan, SQ, 6 mg; dihydroergotamine, IV, 1 mg)

Magnesium (IV, 2 grams)

Valproic acid (IV; Depacon, 5–10 mg/kg)—after ensuring that patient is not pregnant

Diphenhydramine (PO; Benadryl, 25–50 mg)

Baclofen (PO; Lioresal, 10 mg)

Oxygen, 100% by Non-rebreather mask at 12 L/min for 15–30 minutes

Corticosteroid—dexamethasone (IV; Decadron, 10 mg), hydrocortisone (IV; 100–250 mg), or methylprednisolone (IV; Solumedrol, 1 gram)

Lidocaine, 4% drops without epinephrine, 2 mL per nostril

Opioids/opiates—AVOID IF POSSIBLE (strongest evidence of efficacy is for butorphanol [NAS; Stadol, 1 mg in one nostril])

IM = intramuscular; IV = intravenous; NAS = intranasal; PO = oral; SQ = subcutaneous

Table 12.4 Prophylactic Agents for Headaches in the Migraine/Tension Spectrum

Drug Category	Specific Agents (Routes of Administration; Brand Names)
Nonsteroidal anti-inflammatory drugs (NSAIDs)	Aspirin (PO), indomethacin (PO, PR; Indocin), naproxen (PO; Naprosyn, Aleve)
Herbal and nutritional supplements	Coenzyme Q10 (PO), feverfew (PO), magnesium (PO), riboflavin (PO; vitamin B2)
Beta-blockers	Atenolol (PO; Tenormin), metoprolol* (PO; Lopressor, Toprol), nadolol (PO; Corgard), propranolol* (PO; Inderal), timolol* (PO; Blocadren)
Calcium channel blockers	Flunarizine (PO), verapamil (PO; Calan, Verelan)
Angiotensin-converting enzyme inhibitors	Lisinopril (PO; Prinivil, Zestril)
Angiotensin receptor blockers	Candesartan (PO; Atacand)
Tricyclic antidepressants	Amitriptyline (PO), nortriptyline (PO)

Table 12.4 Continued

Drug Category	Specific Agents (Routes of Administration; Brand Names)
Serotonin-norepinephrine reuptake inhibitors (SNRIs)	Duloxetine (PO; Cymbalta); venlafaxine (PO; Effexor)
Antiseizure medications	Gabapentin (PO; Neurontin), levetiracetam (PO; Keppra), topiramate* (PO; Topamax), valproate* (PO; Depakote), zonisamide (Zonegran)
CGRP monoclonal antibodies	Eptinezumab* (IV; Vyepti), erenumab* (SQ; Aimovig), fremanezumab* (SQ; Ajovy), galcanezumab* (SQ; Emgality)
CGRP antagonists	Atogepant* (PO; Qulipta), rimegepant* (PO; Nurtec)
Neurotoxins	Botulinum toxin* (IM; Botox)
Antihistamines	Cyproheptadine (PO; Periactin)
N-Methyl-d-aspartate (NMDA) antagonists	Memantine (PO; Namenda)
Ergots	Methylergonovine (PO; Methergine)

CGRP = calcitonin gene-related peptide; IM = intramuscular; IV = intravenous; PO = oral; PR = rectal; SQ = subcutaneous
* = Strong evidence of efficacy

Table 12.5 Medical and Surgical Treatments for Trigeminal Neuralgia

Medical Treatments	Surgical Treatments
Carbamazepine* (Tegretol)	Microvascular decompression of the trigeminal nerve (posterior fossa surgery)
Oxcarbazepine* (Trileptal)	Percutaneous lesion of the trigeminal ganglion or exiting branches (by radiofrequency thermocoagulation, glycerol injection, or balloon compression
Gabapentin (Neurontin)	Stereotactic radiosurgery of the trigeminal nerve root
Baclofen (Lioresal)	Partial rhizotomy of the sensory root of the trigeminal nerve
Lamotrigine (Lamictal)	
Botulinum toxin	
Eslicarbazepine (Aptiom)	
Topiramate (Topamax)	

(continued)

Table 12.5 Continued

Medical Treatments	Surgical Treatments
Valproate (Depakote)	
Phenytoin (Dilantin)	
Levetiracetam (Keppra)	
Amitriptyline or nortriptyline	
Acute treatment during a severe attack: fosphenytoin (IV), lidocaine (IV), or sumatriptan (NAS or SQ)	

IV = intravenous; NAS = intranasal; SQ = subcutaneous
* = Strong evidence of efficacy

Table 12.6 Cluster Headache Treatment

Treatments for Aborting an Individual Headache	Treatments for Shortening a Cluster	Preventive Treatments for Patients with Frequent Clusters or Chronic Cluster
SQ: octreotide, sumatriptan*	Oral corticosteroids* (prednisone, dexamethasone)	Verapamil
NAS: capsaicin, dihydroergotamine, lidocaine (4%), sumatriptan,* zolmitriptan*	Verapamil*	Lithium
IV/IM: dihydroergotamine	Galcanezumab*	Occipital nerve stimulation
PO: zolmitriptan	Suboccipital steroid injections*	Noninvasive vagus nerve stimulation (nVNS)
Oxygen* (100% by non-rebreather mask at 7–12 L/min)	Melatonin	
Noninvasive vagus nerve stimulation (nVNS)—three consecutive 2-minute stimulations	Noninvasive vagus nerve stimulation (nVNS)	
Sphenopalatine ganglion stimulation		

IM = intramuscular; IV = intravenous; PO = oral; SQ = subcutaneous
* = Strong evidence of efficacy

VIII. Discussion of Case Histories

Case 1. Even though this man is experiencing the worst headache of his life, it is not qualitatively different from the headaches he has been having for 12 years. If his examination is normal—in particular, if he is afebrile, with a supple neck, and no focal neurologic abnormalities—no imaging study is necessary. He is too young to have giant cell arteritis, so a sedimentation rate is not necessary. The description of his headache is consistent with the migraine/tension spectrum. He should be given an abortive agent. Nonsteroidal medications should be avoided because he has already taken eight aspirin tablets; subcutaneous sumatriptan (Imitrex) or intravenous DHE would provide the most rapid relief. Since he is now having up to two headaches per week, he should be sent out of the emergency department with a prescription for a prophylactic agent; naproxen (Naprosyn) or propranolol (Inderal) would each be reasonable choices, but many options are available. If naproxen is prescribed, he should also be given a prescription for some abortive agent other than aspirin.

Case 2. Although this woman's headache is not severe, it has two features that increase the likelihood of an underlying systemic or neurologic process: It has only been present 3 months, and there are focal abnormalities on examination (localizing to the right frontal and parietal lobes). She seems to have some anosognosia (unawareness of her own deficits), a common accompaniment of nondominant parietal lobe lesions. Given a focal lesion and a chronic time course, a neoplasm is a prime concern (see Chapter 3). This patient needs an imaging study of the brain as soon as possible, and treatment will depend on what it shows. At the same time, she could be given symptomatic treatment for her headaches, using the same approach that would be followed in a patient with migraine or tension headaches.

Comment: A CT scan revealed a ring-enhancing lesion in the right frontal and parietal lobes, with substantial edema surrounding it. A chest x-ray showed an apical lesion in the right lung that had not been present on previous studies, the most recent of which had been obtained 9 months earlier. A non-small cell lung cancer was found at bronchoscopy. The cerebral mass was presumed to be a metastasis, and the patient was started on dexamethasone to treat the cerebral edema. This eliminated the headaches, also. She was referred to an oncologist for management of her primary cancer, and the cerebral metastasis was treated with resection followed by stereotactic radiosurgery.

Chapter 13

Visual Symptoms

I. Case Histories

Case 1. A 22-year-old woman has been experiencing discomfort and blurring of vision in her left eye for several days. She has never had similar symptoms before and has otherwise been healthy. She has 20/20 vision in her right eye, measured with a near vision card while her left eye is covered. With the right eye covered, she is unable to read newsprint and her acuity is 20/300. Her pupils are equal, but she has a left afferent pupillary defect. The left optic disc appears slightly pale; the right appears normal. She reports discomfort in the left eye during testing of visual pursuit. The remainder of her examination is normal.

Case 2. A 75-year-old man noticed blurred vision in his left eye several days ago and it has slowly been getting worse. He has no eye pain, but when he tries to chew meat he experiences pain in his jaw. Even with his glasses, he is barely able to count fingers with the left eye, but right eye visual acuity is normal. He has a left afferent pupillary defect and a swollen left optic disc. The remainder of his examination is normal.

Case 3. A 60-year-old woman reports episodes of loss of vision in the left eye. Each spell begins suddenly and gradually worsens over 15–30 seconds. She can't provide any details, except that at the height of the episode "everything is dark in that eye." The vision loss lasts for several minutes before resolving completely. She has no pain or other symptoms with these spells. The first episode occurred 2 months ago, and she has had four more episodes since. Her examination is normal.

Questions:

1. How is the approach to these patients the same?
2. How does their evaluation differ?
3. What steps must be taken urgently?

II. Background Information

A. Definitions

diplopia: double vision

homonymous: affecting the same side of the visual field in both eyes

heteronymous: affecting different sides of the visual field in each eye

B. Overview of the Visual System

Information from each eye travels separately to the optic chiasm, where fiber pathways cross and sort themselves so that fibers carrying information from analogous portions of the visual fields of the two eyes travel together to the primary visual cortex in the occipital lobe. The visual information is subsequently forwarded to many other specialized regions of cortex where features such as form, color, depth, and motion are analyzed. Most of the individual cells in these different regions of visual cortex receive input from both eyes. For these cells to function properly, the two eyes must be exquisitely aligned. This is accomplished by the ocular motor system, which directs the output of cranial nerves III, IV, and VI in such a way that both eyes are always fixated on the same point.

When the ocular motor system malfunctions so that the two eyes fixate on slightly different points, the brain receives two visual images of the world that are a little displaced from each other. The result is diplopia. In contrast, lesions of the visual pathways produce a degraded image in the affected visual field regions, but the visual fields of the two eyes remain aligned, so patients experience loss of vision, rather than diplopia.

III. Approach to Visual Symptoms

The key to diagnosing visual symptoms is an accurate description. Does the patient have diplopia or loss of vision? If the problem is vision loss, does it involve one eye or both, and does it involve the entire visual field of the affected eyes or only a portion of the field? Are the symptoms transient, static, or progressive? If the symptoms are transient, are there any precipitating factors? Are the episodes stereotyped, and, if so, what is the temporal progression of the symptoms?

People who have static or progressive deficits can be examined while symptoms are present. When the symptoms are transient, however, the patient is often completely free of symptoms during the examination and may have trouble providing a detailed description of the episodes. In these cases, it is helpful to instruct patients that if they have more episodes in the future they should cover each eye in turn during the episodes and pay careful attention to how this affects their symptoms.

IV. Monocular Vision Loss

Vision loss confined to a single eye usually implies a lesion anterior to the optic chiasm because this is the only portion of the visual pathway (with minor exceptions) that does not receive input from both eyes. The cause of monocular vision loss can usually be deduced from the age of the patient and the time course of symptoms.

Examination findings are helpful in distinguishing diseases of the optic nerve from other ocular causes of loss of vision. A careful ocular examination (including measurement of intraocular pressure) will usually reveal disease situated in the non-neural tissue of the eye. Unless the vision loss is mild, the "swinging flashlight test" (see Chapter 2) almost always reveals an afferent pupillary defect when the problem is in the optic nerve. Regardless of the cause of monocular vision loss, the most straightforward way to determine severity and follow the clinical course is to measure visual acuity in each eye separately. In a few conditions, especially glaucoma and increased intracranial pressure, visual acuity is relatively spared, so disease progression must be assessed in other ways.

A. Acute or Subacute Monocular Vision Loss in Young People

In young patients, the acute onset of monocular vision loss usually signifies *optic neuritis* (much less common causes include sinus mucocele, vasculitis, and optic nerve infiltration by carcinomatous or granulomatous processes). The vision loss of optic neuritis may progress over 7–10 days. Eye pain, which is usually exacerbated by eye movement, may precede or accompany the loss of vision. Optic neuritis may occur in isolation or as a manifestation of multiple sclerosis (MS) or another demyelinating disease. Patients should be asked explicitly about any previous neurologic symptoms that might suggest MS. Those with no prior history of neurologic symptoms have a 30% risk of developing MS within 5 years, a 40% risk within 10 years, and a 50% risk within 15 years. Patients with multiple white matter lesions on MRI scan of the brain have a higher (72% at 15 years) likelihood of developing MS, whereas only 25% of those with completely normal MRI scans develop MS over the next 15 years. People with optic neuritis who receive a 3-day course of high-dose IV methyl-prednisolone (followed by oral prednisone for 11 days) recover slightly more quickly than those who receive placebo, but there is no difference in visual function between the two groups 6 months later.

Acute vision loss can also result from traumatic injury to the eye, but this is usually obvious from the history and examination. In young people with diabetes, vitreous hemorrhage should be considered. Acute iritis typically presents with blurred vision, pain, and redness, sometimes in one eye only. Iritis can be a symptom of systemic autoimmune disease, so people who have iritis should be asked about problems of the skin, joints, or visceral organs.

B. Acute, Subacute, or Chronic Monocular Vision Loss in Older People

In older patients, monocular loss of vision may be due to acute glaucoma, retinal detachment, macular degeneration, cataract, retinal artery occlusion, or acute ischemic optic neuropathy. Glaucoma is usually a chronic condition causing gradually progressive field loss, but one type of glaucoma, angle-closure glaucoma, is characterized by acute obstruction of aqueous outflow causing sudden vision loss accompanied by severe eye and face pain, nausea, vomiting, and dilation of the pupil. Retinal detachment is commonly associated with myopia, diabetes, intra-ocular inflammation, or cataract surgery; it can also occur after trauma (even minor trauma, such as jogging). Central retinal artery occlusion and branch retinal artery occlusion both present with sudden, severe visual loss without associated pain. Most people with branch retinal artery occlusion recover, but most people with central retinal artery occlusion do not. A variety of interventions are available, but their efficacy has not been established. Most cases of retinal artery occlusion are thought to represent embolic events, so evaluation for a carotid or cardiac source and secondary stroke prevention are indicated (see Chapter 4, Part VI).

Retinal artery occlusion can also result from *giant cell arteritis (temporal arteritis)*, which is discussed in more detail in Chapter 12 (Part V, Section D). A more common manifestation of giant cell arteritis causing loss of vision is *acute ischemic optic neuropathy*. Most cases of acute ischemic optic neuropathy are nonarteritic. The mechanism of nonarteritic ischemic optic neuropathy is not known, but it may be due to small vessel disease. It is usually not due to embolism, so the carotid artery and heart are generally not evaluated.

Cataracts and macular degeneration (and most cases of glaucoma) produce gradual vision loss progressing over years and are usually evident on examination.

V. Transient Vision Loss (Monocular or Binocular)

Transient visual obscuration in one or both eyes may be caused by ischemia, migraine, or increased intracranial pressure. The visual phenomena associated with migraine are typically distinctive, often described as flashing lights or jagged lines on the edge of a scotoma in which vision is obscured or totally absent. The abnormal region often expands gradually or moves off toward one side of the visual field. When a typical headache develops before, during, or after these characteristic visual symptoms, the diagnosis is usually straightforward. Diagnosis can be more difficult in people who have the visual symptoms without any headache or symptoms that are atypical in some way; it is usually prudent to evaluate these people for vascular disease or structural abnormalities before concluding that their symptoms are due to migraine.

Transient vision loss in one eye can represent a transient ischemic attack (TIA) due to atherosclerotic disease in the ipsilateral carotid artery (or, less likely, caused by cardioembolism). The vision loss typically progresses over a matter of minutes and resolves completely within an hour—usually within minutes. Patients' descriptions of the symptoms and the time course vary greatly, and many people just can't remember the details of how the symptoms evolved. The possibility of TIAs should always be considered when people at risk for atherosclerotic disease experience transient monocular vision loss.

People can also experience transient vision loss as a result of TIAs affecting the cerebral cortex, but in this case the symptoms involve only one half of the visual field, and both eyes are affected. It may be difficult to appreciate the hemi-field character of the deficit from the history, either because the patient didn't notice it or because both sides became ischemic simultaneously, resulting in visual deficits in both right and left fields of both eyes (so-called lone bilateral blindness). Another reason the history of hemi-field loss may be obscured is that patients sometimes mistakenly interpret the field cut (which is binocular) as an inability to see out of one eye. You should be sure to ask patients explicitly whether they checked their vision in each eye separately.

People who have increased intracranial pressure sometimes experience transient visual symptoms triggered by even minor changes in intracranial pressure. For example, they may note visual disturbance in one or both eyes whenever they sit up from a lying position, when they stand from a lying or sitting position, or when they bend forward. The characteristic physical finding is bilateral optic disc edema in the presence of normal optic nerve function. Increased pressure can result from obstruction of cerebrospinal fluid outflow. An appropriately placed mass lesion can cause this (see Chapter 11), or it may occur without any obvious structural cause; this is called *idiopathic intracranial hypertension,* or *pseudotumor cerebri* (see Chapter 12).

VI. Persistent Binocular Vision Loss

Soon after the visual pathways leave the optic chiasm, the input from the two eyes is aligned so closely that any lesion posterior to the chiasm produces a homonymous visual field defect. Lesions in the chiasm itself typically affect the fibers that are in the process of crossing from right to left or vice versa; these are the fibers from the nasal half of each retina, corresponding to the temporal half of each eye's visual field. The result is a heteronymous (bitemporal) hemianopia. As noted in Chapter 2, this lesion may go undetected by the patient, because the "bad" field in each eye corresponds to the "good" field in the other eye. The deficit is only evident when each eye is tested separately. The differential diagnosis of lesions affecting the chiasm includes pituitary adenomas, suprasellar meningiomas, craniopharyngiomas, gliomas, and internal carotid artery aneurysms.

For lesions affecting the visual pathway posterior to the optic chiasm, the differential diagnosis is based on demographic considerations and the time course of symptoms, as described in Chapter 3, and management is predicated on the underlying disease process.

VII. Diplopia

A. Localization

Lesions in the ocular motor pathway proximal to the brainstem nuclei of cranial nerves III, IV, and VI result in a gaze palsy (see Chapter 2): the patient has difficulty moving the eyes in a certain direction, but the impairment affects both eyes equally, so the eyes remain aligned with each other and the patient does not experience diplopia. The brainstem horizontal gaze center is in the nucleus for cranial nerve VI, so lesions of that nucleus also cause a gaze palsy. More distal lesions in the ocular motor system cause the eyes to be misaligned, resulting in binocular diplopia. Thus, binocular diplopia suggests a problem in cranial nerves III, IV, and VI, the muscles they innervate, the medial longitudinal fasciculus (MLF), or the nuclei of cranial nerves III or IV. Generalized diseases of muscle or the neuromuscular junction can also interfere with the ability to keep the eyes aligned, and so can anything affecting the mechanical properties of the eyeballs themselves (e.g., a soft tissue mass in the orbit restricting movement of the eyeball).

The first issue to address in someone with diplopia is whether all of the findings could be caused by dysfunction of a single cranial nerve. There are three specific patterns to recognize:

1. *Sixth nerve lesion:* limitation of abduction (lateral movement) of one eye only; all other movements intact.
2. *Fourth nerve lesion:* impaired ability of one eye to look down and in (i.e., toward the nostril); people with this deficit often compensate by tilting the entire head in the direction the affected eye cannot move (i.e., away from the affected eye).
3. *Third nerve lesion:* limitation of adduction (medial movement), supraduction (upward movement), and infraduction (downward movement) of one eye only, sometimes associated with ipsilateral ptosis and dilated pupil.

If one of these patterns is found, then the correct localization is almost always at the level of the cranial nerve or its nucleus. The same is true even if some components of the pattern are missing (e.g., a patient with a third nerve lesion may have all the eye movement abnormalities without a dilated pupil or ptosis). A disease of muscle or neuromuscular junction can sometimes produce a pattern that resembles an isolated lesion of the third, fourth, or sixth cranial nerve, but this is less common because there is no particular reason for a generalized disease process to affect only the muscles innervated by a single cranial nerve. Another pattern to remember is internuclear ophthalmoplegia (INO), caused by a lesion in the MLF; this results in impaired adduction of the ipsilateral eye and nystagmus of the contralateral eye when it abducts (see Chapter 2, Part V, Section B).

If the patient's eye movement problems do not all fit into the syndrome expected with a lesion of a single cranial nerve or the MLF, the next question is whether the findings could all be explained by combined lesions of two cranial nerves, especially two that are neighbors at some point in their course (such as both sixth nerves, or the left third and left fourth nerves). If so, this is the likely localization.

Whenever the cause of the eye movement abnormality appears to be malfunction of one or more cranial nerves, the next issue to address is whether the lesion is intra-axial (within the substance of the brainstem itself) or extra-axial (affecting cranial nerves after they have exited the brainstem). This requires a search for involvement of fiber tracts passing through the brainstem but not entering or exiting at that level, so that a purely extra-axial process could not possibly affect them. Thus, patients should be examined closely for limb weakness, sensory changes, ataxia, and hyperreflexia.

When a lesion of just one or two cranial nerves cannot explain the pattern of eye muscle abnormality and there are no sensory deficits or findings to suggest an intra-axial brainstem lesion, a primary muscle or neuromuscular junction problem should be considered, especially when muscles of both eyes are involved. Meningeal inflammation or cancer can also affect multiple cranial nerves (see Chapter 10), and mechanical limitation of eye movement from structural problems in the orbit (including soft tissue swelling) should not be ignored.

B. Differential Diagnosis and Management

Diseases primarily affecting the neuromuscular junction or muscle are discussed in Chapter 6. Initial symptoms are often restricted to extraocular muscles, and sometimes these are the only muscles involved throughout the entire course of the illness. The principles of diagnosis and management are the same as for patients with these diseases who have more widespread muscle involvement.

When the disease appears to be affecting one or more cranial nerves, the differential diagnosis depends on whether the process is intra-axial or extra-axial and on how many cranial nerves are affected. An intra-axial lesion can be analyzed according to the approach presented in Chapter 3, using the time course and epidemiologic factors to guide diagnosis and management. An extra-axial process affecting multiple cranial nerves is almost always caused by meningeal infiltration, either from inflammatory disease (including infection) or from neoplastic disease. Evaluation should include cerebrospinal fluid examination and a search for systemic evidence of a neoplasm or inflammatory disease. On rare occasions, meningeal biopsy may be diagnostic when less invasive studies are not.

Extra-axial involvement of a single cranial nerve is usually caused by either compression or focal ischemia. People with diabetes are particularly likely to develop isolated third, fourth, or sixth nerve palsies, and these are generally attributed to small-vessel ischemia. As with small vessel disease elsewhere in the nervous system, no specific treatment is available; fortunately, spontaneous recovery gradually occurs in approximately 50% of cases. Compressive lesions, in contrast, often signal the need for urgent treatment, because an expanding mass at this level may go on to produce brainstem compression and death. Because early treatment of a compressive lesion can potentially prevent devastating consequences, people with extra-axial involvement of a single cranial nerve should be considered to have a compressive lesion until proved otherwise. An MRI of the brain with attention to the brainstem should be obtained as soon as possible. This is particularly true when there is isolated impairment of third nerve function. As discussed in Chapter 11, a mass lesion situated laterally in one cerebral hemisphere can exert medially directed pressure on the ipsilateral temporal lobe (*uncal herniation*), compressing the third nerve. Third nerve compression may also result from an expanding arterial aneurysm, which is almost as urgent a problem as herniation, because of the high morbidity and mortality associated with aneurysmal rupture (see Chapters 4 and 12). If the aneurysm can be found and repaired before it ruptures, the patient may be spared these dire outcomes. Treatment of a compressive lesion usually involves surgical intervention and the techniques for treating increased intracranial pressure discussed in Chapter 11.

VIII. Discussion of Case Histories

Case 1. The monocular visual symptoms indicate a lesion in the visual pathway anterior to the optic chiasm, and the left afferent pupillary defect implies that the lesion is in the left optic nerve. In this age group, the most common cause of acute optic nerve dysfunction is optic neuritis. Her examination is typical of that condition.

Comment: An MRI scan of the brain showed eight white matter lesions that were 5–10 mm in diameter, and one of them enhanced with contrast. Her physician explained to her that this MRI finding in the setting of optic neuritis indicates a high likelihood of developing MS, and that disease-modifying therapies have been proven to improve outcomes in this situation (see Chapter 10). She was given a brief course of IV methylprednisolone to shorten the duration of her acute episode, and after learning about the available treatment options, she decided to begin treatment with dimethyl fumarate.

Case 2. This patient also has monocular visual symptoms and a left afferent pupillary defect, again suggesting a lesion in the left optic nerve. Of the various potential causes of monocular vision loss in this age group, the time course is most consistent with acute ischemic optic neuropathy. The jaw pain when chewing (jaw claudication) suggests that his acute ischemic optic neuropathy is due to giant cell (temporal) arteritis.

Comment: His sedimentation rate was greater than 100 mm/hour, and temporal artery biopsy showed arteritis. He was treated with prednisone for just over 6 months, and all of his symptoms resolved. The prednisone was very gradually tapered off over the subsequent 6 months.

Case 3. This patient has been experiencing TIAs involving the retinal artery. Evaluation and management of TIAs are discussed in Chapter 4.

Both Case 2 and Case 3 represent urgent problems, because the symptoms described by each of the two patients may be associated with underlying conditions (giant cell arteritis and TIAs) for which prompt treatment can prevent serious and irreversible consequences (blindness in Case 2 and stroke in Case 3).

Chapter 14

Dizziness and Disequilibrium

I. Case Histories

Case 1. A 40-year-old school bus driver is terrified that she is going to lose her job. For the past 6 weeks, she has been experiencing severe nausea and a spinning sensation every time she looks up and to the right to check her rearview mirror. She has stopped driving, because even though the symptoms always resolve within 30 seconds, she reasons that this is plenty of time for an accident to happen. A routine physical examination is entirely normal.

Questions:

1. Where's the lesion?
2. What additional examination techniques would be useful in this case?
3. What is the likely diagnosis?
4. What additional diagnostic and treatment measures should be taken?
5. What is the prognosis?

Case 2. A 45-year-old right-handed man is "having problems walking straight." For the past 6 months, he has needed to hold on to walls or furniture for support when he walks, because it feels as if the ground slants to the left. He thinks the problem is getting worse, because 3 days ago he actually fell down for the first time. He has also noticed that the right side of his face "feels funny," but he thinks he may be imagining it. His handwriting is getting sloppier, but it has always been poor. He also mentions that he has had tinnitus and hearing loss in his right ear for the past 2 or 3 years, but attributes it to "all those rock concerts in college."

His examination is notable for reduced sensation on the entire right side of his face, with an absent corneal reflex on the right. He has left-beating nystagmus with a slight rotatory component, most prominent when looking to the left. He has reduced hearing in his right ear, and his right arm and leg movements are ataxic.

Questions:

1. Where's the lesion?
2. What is the likely diagnosis?
3. What additional diagnostic and treatment measures should be taken?
4. What is the prognosis?

Case 3. A 60-year-old woman has an unsteady gait that has been getting progressively worse over the past 6 months. She sometimes stumbles so much that others worry for her safety. She has had increasing trouble climbing ladders because of stiffness in her legs. She has a long history of mild neck discomfort. She has had several episodes of urinary incontinence. On examination, her mental status and cranial nerves are normal. Her gait is stiff and unsteady, and she tends to fall if not supported. The intrinsic muscles of her hands are atrophic, and she has spasticity and weakness in her lower extremities. Her reflexes are brisk at the knees and ankles, normal in the arms, and symmetric throughout. Both of her plantar responses are extensor (i.e., she has bilateral Babinski signs).

Questions:

1. Where's the lesion?
2. What is the likely diagnosis?
3. What additional diagnostic and treatment measures should be taken?

Case 4. A 78-year-old man is no longer able to walk. He first noticed some problems with his balance about a year ago, but he was still able to complete his daily 3-mile walks. He slipped on some ice 4 months ago and fractured the neck of his left femur. This was treated with open reduction and internal fixation, and he had no surgical or postoperative complications. He was started on gabapentin and opioids for pain after his fall, and these were continued for postoperative pain, but he was able to taper off the opioids over the next 2 months. He has been unable to walk since the surgery. He also has a history of primary hypertension, type 2 diabetes, osteoarthritis of the hips and knees, and cataracts. He takes metformin, lisinopril, atorvastatin, and gabapentin. On examination, his blood pressure is 105/65. He has mild bilateral corneal opacities and visual acuity of 20/50 in both eyes. His reflexes are mildly reduced throughout the upper extremities, knee reflexes can only be elicited with reinforcement (Jendrassik) maneuvers, and ankle reflexes are absent. Vibration and position sensation are absent at the toes, moderately reduced at the ankles, and slightly reduced at the knees. He initially says that he is too weak to walk, but with encouragement he is able to walk while holding the examiner's arms, moving slowly and cautiously with normal base and stride length, no swaying or swerving, and no tendency for either leg to give way. He exerts very little downward force on the examiner's arms and maintains his balance when the examiner briefly pulls away so that he is standing unsupported.

Questions:

1. Where's the lesion?
2. What is the likely diagnosis?
3. What additional diagnostic and treatment measures should be taken?

II. Approach to Dizziness

People use the word "dizzy" in many different ways. It can be helpful to ask your patients to describe their symptoms using other words, mainly to be sure that they aren't using dizziness to refer to some other type of symptom, such as confusion or difficulty with coordination. More precise delineation is of limited benefit. An unequivocal report of vertigo—defined as a false sense of movement—suggests dysfunction of the vestibular system, whereas a vague feeling of lightheadedness is more suggestive of global cerebral hypoperfusion, but people often have difficulty characterizing their symptoms precisely. When they are offered terms and asked to select the ones that describe their symptoms, the terms they choose show a poor correlation with the ultimate diagnosis. Furthermore, their responses change even after an interval of only 6 minutes. Instead of focusing on the quality of the dizziness, it is more informative to ask whether the dizziness is constant or intermittent, whether there are consistent triggers, what makes the dizziness better or worse, and whether there are any associated symptoms.

III. Localization

The processes that affect the peripheral vestibular system are distinct from those that affect the central portions of the vestibular pathway. Several features help to distinguish central from peripheral lesions. Because the vestibular end-organ (the labyrinth) is connected to the auditory end-organ (the cochlea), and the vestibular and cochlear nerves remain next to each other all the way to the brainstem, hearing loss and tinnitus frequently accompany peripheral vertigo. In contrast, because the auditory pathways proceed bilaterally as soon as they enter the brainstem, a unilateral central lesion generally does not produce significant hearing loss, so it is unusual for central vertigo to be associated with prominent auditory symptoms. Instead, the typical abnormalities accompanying central vertigo include dysarthria, dysphagia, diplopia, limb numbness, limb weakness, or ataxia, reflecting the fact that this portion of the vestibular pathway is located in the brainstem and cerebellum.

Both central and peripheral vertigo are commonly associated with nystagmus. The specific characteristics of the nystagmus can provide clues to the cause. When vertigo is due to displaced otoliths in the semicircular canals, the nystagmus is only present in certain head positions. When vertigo is due to a fixed structural lesion in the peripheral portion of the vestibular system (the semicircular canals or vestibular nerves), the nystagmus is almost always unidirectional (with the direction of the fast beat away from the side of the lesion) and it usually has both linear and rotatory components. The nystagmus becomes more intense when looking in the direction of the fast beat. When vertigo is due to a CNS lesion, the nystagmus may be either unidirectional or multidirectional (i.e., the direction of the fast beat of the nystagmus changes depending on the direction of gaze), and it may be purely horizontal, purely vertical, purely rotatory, or any combination. Multidirectional gaze-evoked nystagmus almost always indicates a CNS lesion. All these rules have exceptions, but they are usually reliable.

When these clinical features are not sufficient to determine whether the lesion is central or peripheral, specialized testing in a vestibular laboratory may be helpful. An audiogram can also be useful in demonstrating unilateral hearing loss that would make a peripheral disorder more likely. In theory, brainstem auditory evoked potentials (see Chapter 10) could help localize defects in the auditory pathway, but they are generally not reliable enough to be very useful. When localization remains uncertain, imaging studies of the brain (especially the posterior fossa) and skull (especially the auditory canal) may be necessary.

IV. Differential Diagnosis

The differential diagnosis of vertigo depends primarily on two factors: (1) whether the lesion is central (in the CNS portion of the vestibular system) or peripheral (in the vestibular end organs or vestibular nerves) and (2) the time course of symptoms.

A. Central Vertigo

Central vertigo that is getting progressively worse is usually due to a mass lesion, such as a neoplasm, vascular malformation, or abscess (see Chapter 3). Central vertigo of acute onset usually signifies a vascular process (or trauma, in the appropriate setting). Recurrent, transient spells can represent transient ischemic attacks, migraines, seizures, or paroxysmal manifestations of multiple sclerosis; the time course and associated symptoms usually distinguish these possibilities (see Chapters 4, 5, 10, and 12). In particular, many people with recurrent episodes of vertigo have a personal or family history of migraine, and anecdotal reports (but no controlled trials) suggest that their episodes of vertigo become less frequent or less severe (or both) when they take prophylactic migraine medications. The term vestibular migraine refers to individuals who have a current or past history of migraine, at least five episodes of vertigo, and at least 50% of their episodes accompanied by headache, sensitivity to light and sound, visual aura, or some combination. It remains unclear whether migraine can also be responsible for episodic dizziness without accompanying headache, visual aura, or sensitivity to light and sound, and whether it can result in continuous dizziness.

B. Peripheral Vertigo

Peripheral vertigo that is getting progressively worse suggests inflammatory or neoplastic disease. The most common tumors in the cerebellopontine angle are meningiomas and vestibular nerve schwannomas. Vestibular schwannomas usually arise from the vestibular division of the eighth nerve, but the initial symptoms are usually auditory; disequilibrium, ipsilateral facial numbness and weakness, and ipsilateral ataxia often develop later in the course. A few specific toxins cause progressive, bilateral eighth nerve dysfunction, notably aminoglycosides and cisplatin.

Most often, peripheral vertigo begins acutely and does not progress (though it may persist for days, weeks, or even months). In this situation, the diagnoses to consider depend on whether similar episodes of vertigo have occurred in the past.

a. Recurrent episodes

The distinction between peripheral and central vertigo may be especially difficult when the symptoms are episodic and the patient is asymptomatic at the time of examination, so even when a patient with recurrent episodes of vertigo has symptoms that sound peripheral, central disorders such as migraine, vertebrobasilar TIA, seizure, and multiple sclerosis must be considered. Nonetheless, episodic vertigo is usually due to a disorder of the peripheral portion of the vestibular system.

(a) Benign paroxysmal positional vertigo (BPPV) is the most common cause of recurrent vertigo. People with BPPV experience brief episodes of vertigo whenever the head is in certain positions, and they have no vertigo in other head positions, although they may have a prolonged or constant sense of unsteadiness at other times. They typically report that the vertigo occurs when they extend their head to look up, or when they turn over in bed. The vertigo usually begins about 5–10 seconds after the head assumes the symptomatic position. It usually lasts less than 30 seconds and almost always less than a minute. The vertigo generally becomes less severe if the head is placed in the symptomatic position several times in a row. These features can often be demonstrated by performing the *Dix-Hallpike test* (Figure 14.1): Start by having the patient sit near one end of the examination table, with the body facing the far end of the table and the head turned 45° to one side. Next, help the patient recline to a supine position with the head hanging over the edge of the table and the neck extended 20–30°, still turned to the same side. Keep the patient in this position for at least 20 seconds and ask the patient to report any symptoms of vertigo, while you observe the patient's eyes for nystagmus. Then return the patient to the seated position, and repeat the maneuver with the head rotated 45° to the other side. To establish the diagnosis of BPPV, one of these positions should trigger a burst of upbeat and torsional nystagmus that lasts about 10–30 seconds.

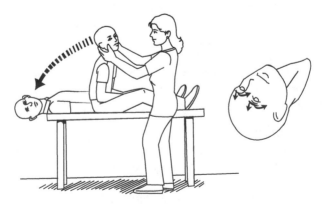

Fig. 14.1 Dix-Hallpike test for diagnosing benign paroxysmal positional vertigo (BPPV); details explained in text.

BPPV is caused by calcium carbonate particles (otoliths) that have become dislodged from the otolith membrane and migrated to one of the semicircular canals, where they typically float free in the endolymph though occasionally they can adhere to the cupula. The condition may follow head trauma or labyrinthitis, but usually no obvious precipitant is apparent. The most common form of BPPV is posterior canal BPPV, which is readily treatable with particle repositioning maneuvers (either the *Epley maneuver*, shown in Figure 14.2, or the *Semont-plus maneuver*) designed

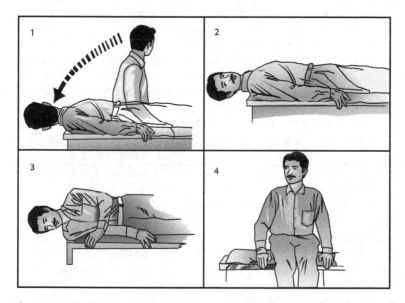

Fig. 14.2 Epley maneuver for treating posterior semicircular canal BPPV. The first steps (1) are the same as in the Dix-Hallpike test (note that this patient's displaced particles are in the left ear, whereas Figure 14.1 shows a patient whose problem is in the right ear). Keep the patient in the initial position (in this case, head extended 20–30° over the end of the table and turned all the way to the left) for at least a minute, then (2) rapidly turn the head all the way to the other side (still keeping the head extended 20–30° over the end of the table). Keep the head in this position for at least a minute, then (3) roll the patient's body in the direction the head is already turned, maintaining the rotated position of the head relative to the body so that the patient's face is now pointed toward the floor. Keep the patient in this position for at least a minute, then (4) have the patient sit up, maintaining the rotated position of the head relative to the body.

to move the particles from the canal back into the central chamber of the inner ear, the vestibule.

Less common forms of BPPV involve the horizontal or anterior canals. In horizontal canal BPPV, the nystagmus is in the horizontal plane and is best triggered by having the patient lie supine and then turn the head to either side. Patients exhibit nystagmus in one direction when the head is turned to the right, and in the opposite direction when the head is turned to the left. (Note that this does not contradict the rule that peripheral lesions cause unidirectional nystagmus, because that rule applies only to fixed structural lesions; BPPV is caused by moving particles. Similarly, the rule that multidirectional nystagmus indicates a central lesion refers to direction-changing, *gaze-evoked* nystagmus, whereas BPPV results in direction-changing *positionally induced* nystagmus.) Horizontal canal BPPV does not generally respond to the Epley maneuver; other particle repositioning maneuvers are available for this variant, but it also tends to resolve spontaneously within days. In anterior canal BPPV, the Dix-Hallpike test triggers a burst of downbeat, torsional nystagmus. This condition usually responds to the Epley maneuver (thereby providing evidence that the patient does not have positional downbeat nystagmus due to a central lesion, which would require neuroimaging).

(b) *Ménière disease* is characterized by episodic vertigo and tinnitus superimposed on a condition of hearing loss. The hearing loss is fluctuating and completely reversible early in the disease, but it eventually becomes progressive. The episodes of vertigo typically begin with a sensation of fullness and pressure in one ear, accompanied by tinnitus and reduced hearing in that ear. The vertigo reaches maximum intensity within minutes and slowly subsides over the next few hours, but the patient usually continues to feel vaguely unsteady and dizzy for the next few days. Nausea, vomiting, and ataxia may accompany the episodes. These attacks occur irregularly, at intervals of weeks, months, or years.

Ménière disease is associated with increased endolymph volume throughout the labyrinth, but it is not clear whether this "endolymphatic hydrops" is involved in pathogenesis, because it is also observed in people with no symptoms of Ménière disease. Ménière disease can occur after labyrinthitis but is usually idiopathic. It is typically treated with salt restriction and diuretics, although the evidence supporting their efficacy is anecdotal. Dopamine-blocking antiemetics or low-dose benzodiazepines are sometimes used at the onset of attacks. As the disease progresses, some people experience sudden drop attacks without loss of consciousness, as if an external force pushed them to the ground; this is generally considered an indication for ablative therapy. The rationale for ablative therapy is that the brain can eventually habituate to the complete loss of vestibular function on one side better than it can adjust to fluctuating vestibular function. The least complicated ablative procedure is intratympanic gentamicin injection, although this does not always control the vertigo and there is a 25% risk of hearing loss in that ear. Labyrinthectomy is more consistently effective, but also results in hearing loss. These procedures are most appropriate when patients have already lost functional hearing on the affected side. A vestibular nerve section is the procedure most likely to preserve hearing, but it is more complicated and less reliable.

(c) *Perilymphatic fistula* is characterized by episodes of vertigo that are often precipitated by sneezing, coughing, loud noises (*Tullio phenomenon*, which may also occur in Ménière disease and superior canal dehiscence), exertion, or airplane flights. The fistula consists of a small tear in the oval window or the round window, but the mechanism by which this produces symptoms is unclear. Most people recover spontaneously, so treatment is usually conservative: bed rest, head elevation, and measures to reduce straining. Surgical correction is possible when conservative measures are ineffective.

(d) *Dehiscence of the superior semicircular canal* is a rare condition in which the part of the temporal bone that overlies the superior semicircular canal is thin or absent. The symptoms are similar to those of perilymph fistula (including Tullio phenomenon), together with mild low-frequency hearing loss and hypersensitivity to bone-conducted sounds (sometimes including the movement of the eyeballs in their sockets). Patients may be particularly bothered by autophony—hearing their own voice unusually loudly in the affected ear. Surgical repair can be attempted if the symptoms are debilitating, but many people do well with conservative management.

(e) *Vestibular paroxysmia* is a rare condition that is thought to result from vascular compression or another irritant of the vestibular pathway (either centrally or peripherally), analogous to some cases of trigeminal neuralgia (see Chapter 12). Patients experience very brief episodes (lasting seconds or at most a few minutes) of vertigo, sometimes accompanied by hearing loss, hyperacusis, or tinnitus. Like trigeminal neuralgia, this syndrome can respond to carbamazepine or oxcarbazepine.

2. Single episode

(a) Acute labyrinthitis is characterized by the sudden or subacute onset of severe vertigo, nausea, vomiting, and imbalance, associated with hearing loss, tinnitus, or both. Symptoms are usually severe for hours to days, with residual symptoms gradually resolving over days to months. This condition is generally thought to be due to a virus, and it may occur in association with a systemic viral illness. Less often, it is associated with a documented bacterial infection of the middle ear or an autoimmune process. When a clear bacterial cause can be found, appropriate antibiotics should be given.

(b) Acute idiopathic unilateral peripheral vestibulopathy (also called *acute peripheral vestibulopathy, acute unilateral vestibulopathy,* or *acute vestibular syndrome*) is an analogous and much more common condition. The symptoms usually develop over several hours, but sometimes in a matter of seconds or minutes. Patients experience intense vertigo that is worst when they move their head, but present even at rest, and most patients have nausea and vomiting. Unlike people with acute labyrinthitis, those with acute vestibular syndrome have normal hearing. This condition is widely presumed to be viral or postviral (specifically, reactivation of herpes simplex virus type 1) based on some epidemiologic and pathologic evidence, but the etiology has not been convincingly demonstrated. This condition is often referred to as vestibular neuritis.

People with either acute idiopathic unilateral peripheral vestibulopathy or acute labyrinthitis have unidirectional horizontal and rotatory nystagmus with the fast component away from the affected ear. The nystagmus is most intense when they are looking away from the affected ear (in the direction of the fast phase). With the head impulse test, or head thrust maneuver (see Chapter 2), they maintain fixation on the target when you turn their head away from the affected ear, but when you turn the head toward the affected ear, their eyes move off the target (in the direction of the head movement), so that at the conclusion of the head movement they have to make one or more corrective saccades (in the direction opposite to the way in which the head was just moving). When the head thrust maneuver does not show this abnormality, a lesion in the cerebellum or brainstem becomes a serious consideration.

Corticosteroids may hasten recovery from acute peripheral vestibulopathy, but they have not been shown to improve clinical outcome. The only other available treatments are symptomatic and may include bed rest, antiemetics, antihistamines, and vestibular rehabilitation programs.

All of the conditions in the differential diagnosis of recurrent peripheral vertigo must also be considered in a patient with a single episode—after all, there must be a first episode even for recurrent symptoms. For example, if the patient has no spontaneous or gaze-evoked nystagmus, the Dix-Hallpike test should be performed. Ischemic disease merits special mention. The traditional teaching that ischemia never causes isolated vertigo without ataxia or brainstem dysfunction is false. Some people with small cerebellar strokes have a syndrome virtually indistinguishable from acute idiopathic unilateral peripheral vestibulopathy. Nonetheless, such patients are uncommon. The main situations in which someone presenting with the acute vestibular syndrome may need an MRI scan to look for ischemia are when (1) the symptoms or examination are not typical of vestibular neuritis (for example, they don't have the typical pattern of nystagmus, or they have a normal response to head thrust maneuver in both directions); (2) the patient has signs suggesting a lesion in the cerebellum or brainstem (such as limb ataxia, dysarthria, asymmetric deep tendon reflexes, or skew, a vertical misalignment of the eyes); or (3) the patient has strong risk factors for stroke (such as a recent neck injury that might have caused a vertebral artery dissection, or multiple atherosclerotic risk factors).

V. Disequilibrium

To maintain balance, the brain must receive detailed, accurate information about the position of the body relative to the environment and generate an appropriate, coordinated motor response. Any condition that disturbs either the sensory input or the motor output can produce disequilibrium. The visual, proprioceptive, and vestibular pathways are the most important sensory systems for determining body position. The auditory pathway also contributes, but to a lesser degree. The history and examination should be directed at detecting dysfunction in any of these pathways. The Romberg test is a useful screen. Normal individuals can maintain balance with their eyes closed, because even after visual information has been removed the remaining sensory modalities are sufficient to provide a sense of body position. In contrast, people with dysfunction of the proprioceptive or vestibular system rely heavily on visual input, and although they may be able to maintain equilibrium with their eyes open, they lose their balance when they close their eyes.

People whose disequilibrium is due to an inadequate motor response usually have difficulty maintaining their balance even with their eyes open, so the Romberg test does not apply. An inadequate motor response can result from a purely mechanical problem (such as a hip fracture), weakness, stiffness (either because of spasticity or due to extrapyramidal disease), ataxia, or cognitive deficits. All of these possibilities should be evaluated in the course of the history and the physical examination.

If any sensory or motor abnormalities that could contribute to disequilibrium are found, they should be evaluated and treated according to principles presented elsewhere in this book. For example, vestibular diseases are discussed in Parts III and IV of this chapter, neuromuscular causes of proprioceptive disturbance are discussed in Chapter 6, parkinsonism is discussed in Chapter 8, and so forth. Disequilibrium is often multifactorial; individuals may have several minor abnormalities combining to produce considerable impairment of balance even though each of the abnormalities in isolation would be unlikely to cause serious problems. Psychological factors can also contribute—even one or two falls can result in escalating levels of anxiety that can exacerbate whatever problems were originally responsible for the disequilibrium.

Treatment of gait difficulty should include an assessment of the patient's home environment. People with gait disturbances who have difficulty climbing stairs can be helped by a stair-lift or by moving to a ground-floor apartment or bedroom. Loose rugs are a hazard and should be removed whenever possible. Strategically placed handrails can help to make the home safer. Wall-to-wall carpeting is more easily negotiated in smooth-soled shoes than sneakers, whereas sneakers are better for walking on the sidewalk or street.

VI. Discussion of Case Histories

Case 1. The consistent relationship of this patient's symptoms to a specific head position, the brevity of the symptoms, and the intensity of the vertigo all suggest a peripheral lesion, and specifically, BPPV. Positional vertigo can occasionally occur with central lesions, however. The Dix-Hallpike test should be performed.

Comment: The Dix-Hallpike test precipitated vertigo and a burst of upbeat and torsional nystagmus when the patient's head was turned to her right, establishing the diagnosis of right posterior canal BPPV. The physician immediately proceeded to perform a particle repositioning procedure, with prompt and complete resolution of the patient's symptoms. She returned to her job, and she has had no recurrence of symptoms.

Case 2. The fact that this patient's vertigo is associated with tinnitus and hearing loss in only one ear makes a peripheral lesion almost certain. The unidirectional nystagmus with both horizontal and rotatory components also makes a peripheral lesion more likely than a central lesion. The fast component of the nystagmus is toward the left, suggesting a right-sided lesion (the fact that the nystagmus is most prominent when looking to the left adds no localizing information, because with unilateral peripheral vestibular lesions the nystagmus is always most prominent when the patient is looking in the direction of the fast component). With a right-sided vestibular lesion, the left vestibular apparatus is relatively unopposed, accounting for the patient's subjective impression of the ground slanting to the left. All of the examination findings are consistent with a focal lesion located at the right cerebellopontine angle (see Chapter 1). In this case, the symptoms were progressive, with a time course of several years, suggesting neoplastic disease.

The history is typical of a vestibular nerve schwannoma, but other inflammatory and neoplastic diseases are certainly possible. This patient needs an MRI scan. If it is consistent with a vestibular nerve schwannoma, and if it is relatively large, the treatment of choice is surgical excision using microsurgical techniques, with intraoperative electrophysiologic monitoring of the facial nerve. For small vestibular schwannomas, conservative management with serial imaging to monitor tumor growth may be the preferred approach; radiosurgery is also an option. The prognosis is good.

Case 3. This patient has disequilibrium, not vertigo. She has upper motor neuron signs in the lower extremities and lower motor neuron signs in the intrinsic hand muscles. Although a combination of upper and lower motor neuron signs can indicate motor neuron disease, this patient's lower motor neuron findings are confined to the distribution of the C8 and T1 nerve roots. A lesion compressing the nerve roots and spinal cord at this level would produce lower motor neuron findings locally and upper motor neuron signs in the lower extremities, while sparing structures higher up, explaining the normal arm reflexes (mediated by roots C5–C7), cranial nerves, and mental status. The symptoms have been progressive, with a chronic time course. A chronic, focal lesion is generally a neoplasm. She needs an imaging study of the cervical spine.

Comment: In this case, an MRI scan of the cervical spine showed degenerative spine changes and compression of the spinal cord. A multilevel decompressive laminectomy was performed with slight benefit.

Case 4. This patient, like the patient in Case 3, has disequilibrium rather than vertigo. His examination is notable for findings consistent with his known history of cataracts, as well as findings suggestive of polyneuropathy (reduced sensation and reflexes with a distal-to-proximal gradient). His gait is cautious, but stable, with no evidence of weakness, ataxia, or parkinsonism. The impaired vision due to cataracts and reduced proprioception due to peripheral polyneuropathy (which is most likely due to diabetes) could easily explain the mild balance problems he began to notice about a year ago. The fact that his gait got so much worse after the surgery, without any examination findings to suggest a new neurologic problem, is most likely due to a combination of factors. First, he probably developed mild atrophy of some of his lower extremity muscles due to disuse. Second, his blood pressure is low—perhaps his lisinopril requirement is lower given his reduced activity—which could be causing some light-headedness. Third, he now takes gabapentin, which can cause dizziness. Fourth, the osteoarthritis at the hips and knees could be affecting the mechanics of his gait. Fifth, and probably most important, he seems to be very anxious when he walks, a common and understandable reaction after a severe fall, especially one that resulted in surgery. Of course, the initial factors responsible for balance problems—impaired vision and proprioception—are still present also.

Comment: The lisinopril dose was reduced, and the gabapentin was tapered off. The patient was referred for physical therapy, where he was taught techniques to stabilize his gait and exercises to strengthen his lower extremity and trunk muscles. The physical therapists and physicians reassured him that they expected his gait to improve slowly but surely, and that is what happened. He will be having cataract surgery soon.

Chapter 15

Back Pain and Neck Pain

I. Case Histories

Case 1. While lifting a heavy box yesterday, a 55-year-old patient suddenly developed a sharp pain that started in their low back and shot into the right buttock, posterior thigh, and posterior leg. The pain has been present ever since. They have smoked a pack of cigarettes a day for 40 years, and they had resection of a left upper lobe non-small cell lung cancer 1 year ago. On examination, you note a positive straight leg raising sign on the right, slight weakness of right ankle plantar flexion, and a reduced right ankle reflex.

Case 2. A 50-year-old man has come to the emergency department "to get some relief." Over the years, his back would "go out" on him now and then, but he would stay in bed for a day, apply heat, and wear a corset for the next 2 weeks and he would be "as good as new." Six weeks ago his back went out on him again, but it did not resolve as it had previously. If anything, it seems to be getting worse. It keeps him awake at night, and he is having trouble concentrating at work. He has no pain in his legs, and no difficulty with bladder or bowel function. He has hypertension, diabetes, and obesity, and he takes lisinopril, metformin, and atorvastatin. His examination is notable only for tight muscles and mild tenderness on both sides of the midline throughout his lower back, with no tenderness along the spine. His motor examination, reflexes, and sensory examination are all normal.

Questions:

1. What diagnoses should be considered?
2. What tests should be ordered?
3. What treatment should be prescribed?

II. Approach to Back or Neck Pain

There are two principal questions to address in evaluating someone with back or neck pain:

A. Do they have a condition that might require urgent treatment?
B. Even if it isn't urgent, will surgery be necessary?

A. Emergency Situations

Anyone with known cancer who develops back or neck pain requires an MRI scan (or in rare circumstances, a myelogram) to look for a spinal metastasis. The entire spine should be imaged, not just the painful region, because of the possibility of additional, asymptomatic metastases. Only when the likelihood of metastatic disease is extremely low (specifically, when the pain is characterized as a dull ache confined to the paraspinal area, there have been no recent constitutional symptoms such as fever or weight loss, the neurologic examination is completely normal, and plain x-rays of the symptomatic region of the spine are benign) is it safe to treat the patient symptomatically without further testing.

People without a history of cancer who develop back or neck pain don't need urgent imaging unless they have symptoms or signs suggesting rapidly progressive damage to the spinal cord or multiple nerve roots, in which case they should have an urgent MRI scan (or, occasionally, a myelogram) of the involved area of the spinal canal. If a soft tissue mass is compressing the spinal cord or multiple nerve roots, it could be a metastasis, an epidural abscess, a primary tumor, a hematoma, or an acute disc herniation. If the imaging characteristics are ambiguous, especially in a person with no known cancer, a surgical procedure will generally be necessary, both to establish a diagnosis and to decompress the spinal cord (and sometimes to stabilize the spine).

People who have spinal cord compression due to a metastatic lesion should be started immediately on high-dose dexamethasone (Decadron). The details of subsequent definitive treatment depend on the mechanical stability of the spine and radiosensitivity of the tumor. For example, in the absence of spinal instability, previously untreated radiosensitive tumors can generally be treated with conventional external beam radiation alone, whereas people with spinal instability should have spine stabilization surgery followed by radiation therapy.

If imaging studies do not reveal a compressive lesion, individuals with focal signs or symptoms should be evaluated for noncompressive causes of the neurologic abnormalities. For example, patients with myelopathy should be evaluated for transverse myelitis, vitamin B12 deficiency, and other inflammatory and metabolic conditions.

B. Non-Urgent Indications for Surgery

Even when people do not require urgent decompression, their back or neck pain could still be caused by a structural lesion that might eventually require surgical intervention. The main indications for surgery are the following:

1. Spinal cord compression,
2. Compression of one or more nerve roots causing persistent motor deficits or abnormal control of bladder or bowels,
3. Lumbar spinal stenosis, or
4. A mass lesion of unknown etiology.

Surgery is also performed on occasion when patients have pain that is refractory to all nonsurgical treatment, if the pain is in a distribution that clearly corresponds to the structural lesion.

Thus, people who have symptoms or signs that suggest lumbar spinal stenosis or damage to the spinal cord or to one or more nerve roots should have an MRI scan (or myelogram) of the appropriate region of the spinal canal. The imaging study can be scheduled electively to be done within the next few weeks as long as the patient has no known cancer, no erosive bone lesions on plain films of the spine, and no clinical evidence of rapid progression.

III. Specific Conditions Causing Back or Neck Pain

A. Musculoskeletal Pain

In the vast majority of people who have back or neck pain, the pain is diffuse, with no specific signs or symptoms to suggest damage to individual nerve roots. This is a very common situation, but it is not well understood. It is generally thought to be a musculoskeletal problem related to frequent excessive stress on the bones, muscles, and connective tissue elements that support the back. The pain generally improves over time even in untreated patients. If the neurologic examination is normal, further diagnostic testing is unnecessary. In the past, people with low back pain were routinely instructed to stay at strict bed rest for 2 weeks or more, but the evidence indicates that patients who are instructed to continue with their ordinary activities have better outcomes than patients assigned to bed rest.

Many treatment modalities are used for chronic low back pain, but the evidence that any of these treatments can change the long-term course of the condition is weak. In fact, even short-term beneficial effects have not been demonstrated for many of the treatment approaches. The modalities for which a short-term benefit has been most convincingly demonstrated are cognitive behavioral therapy, physical therapy, yoga, chiropractic manipulation, acupuncture, nonsteroidal anti-inflammatory drugs, and serotonin-norepinephrine reuptake inhibitors (SNRIs). There is no convincing evidence of efficacy for other commonly used treatments, including tricyclic antidepressants, heat, ultrasound, skeletal muscle relaxants, antiepileptic drugs (notably gabapentin), soft tissue injections (with anesthetic agents, steroids, or botulinum toxin), or spinal cord stimulation. A reasonable approach is to prescribe a nonsteroidal anti-inflammatory drug and to instruct the patient to continue a moderate level of activity, but to focus on correct postures and avoid major back strain or lifting. Recovery occurs within 4 weeks in most patients. Physical therapy should be considered in those who fail to improve. Patients may require trials of several physical therapy regimens or medications.

The approach to musculoskeletal pain in the neck is similar to that in the low back. Anecdotal evidence suggests that chiropractic manipulation of the neck can cause arterial dissection, but the evidence is inconclusive.

B. Disc Herniation

A herniated intervertebral disc can exert pressure on a nerve root and produce pain. This is far less common than musculoskeletal pain. The classic history for a lumbosacral disc herniation is a sudden pain in the low back during heavy lifting, later radiating into one lower extremity in a band conforming to the distribution of the L5 or S1 nerve root. Pain in this distribution is often referred to as *sciatica*, because it is in the territory supplied by the sciatic nerve, but this term should be avoided because it has been used in so many different ways that it is ambiguous. The pain of a herniated disc is worst when sitting and it is exacerbated by coughing, sneezing, or straining at bowel movements. These classic features are not always present, however. For example, many patients have no precipitating event, some have only lower extremity pain with no back pain, and others have the opposite.

A straight leg raising sign is characterized by extreme pain when the hip is passively flexed while holding the knee extended. This pain is exacerbated by dorsiflexion of the ankle and relieved by flexion of the knee. This sign is sensitive but not specific. Some people with a herniated disc will have weakness in the distribution of the involved nerve root, and some may have reduction of the relevant tendon reflex. When the nerve root irritation is severe, abnormalities may be detected on EMG and motor nerve conduction studies.

For cervical disc herniation, the antecedent injury—when there is one—often involves rapid head turning. Pain or numbness extends from the neck into one arm or the medial scapula, conforming to the territory of a single cervical nerve root (or two adjacent nerve roots). Patients may also have weakness, atrophy, and hyporeflexia in the distribution of the affected nerve root.

For both cervical and lumbar discs, the risk of neurologic impairment is greatest when the herniation is in the midline, rather than lateral. In the case of a cervical disc, this can put pressure on the spinal cord, which can affect function of the lower extremities, bladder, or bowels. People who have cervical disc herniation may have little or no neck pain, presenting instead with gradually progressive gait disturbance. Many of these people are found to have completely normal strength in the lower extremities; their gait problems are primarily a result of spasticity. When a lumbar disc herniates centrally, it can compress the cauda equina, resulting in diffuse lower extremity weakness and numbness, as well as loss of bladder and bowel control.

Disc herniation, like musculoskeletal pain, is incompletely understood. Although the symptoms suggest nerve root irritation, and imaging studies show impingement on the nerve root by the disc, those imaging findings often persist even after the symptoms have spontaneously resolved. Disc herniation is often present as an incidental finding on imaging studies of people who have no history of any pain or neurologic symptoms. The degree of inflammatory reaction around the nerve root may be an important factor in determining whether a herniated disc produces symptoms.

The symptoms of disc herniation, like those of musculoskeletal pain, often resolve even without specific therapy. The same treatment modalities are used, with the same lack of clear evidence that they improve the already favorable natural course of the disease. Controlled trials are scarce, and the results are inconsistent. Randomized trials have shown no significant difference in long-term outcome between patients treated surgically and patients treated conservatively, although the rate of perceived recovery is faster for patients in the surgical group. Studies comparing open surgery to minimally invasive procedures (such as microdiscectomy or percutaneous discectomy) have not demonstrated any consistent differences in outcome.

Surgery is usually reserved for people who have failed to respond to conservative treatments (especially analgesics and physical therapy), people with substantial motor deficits (especially when they are progressive), or people with involvement of bladder or bowels. Patients who do not fall into one of these categories should be treated in the same way as patients with musculoskeletal pain, and imaging studies may not even be necessary.

C. Spinal Stenosis

Over time, there may be growth of bony elements in the spinal canal, resulting in significant narrowing of the canal (especially when superimposed on a congenitally narrow canal). In the cervical spine, this produces the same symptoms as those of a herniated disc, and the management is analogous. In the lumbar canal, spinal stenosis often produces a syndrome known as neurogenic claudication—pain in the low back or legs provoked by standing and relieved by bending over or sitting down. Unlike vascular claudication, the pain is related to position and not to exertion (walking is no worse than standing, and riding a bike may produce no pain at all). First-line treatment is physical therapy, activity modification, and the same medications used for musculoskeletal pain; if symptoms persist despite these conservative treatments, surgical decompression is associated with improved short-term outcomes, but no long-term benefit has been demonstrated.

IV. Discussion of Case Histories

Case 1. This patient has characteristic features of an acute S1 radiculopathy and most likely has a disc herniation at L5–S1. Even so, with the history of recent cancer, you must be sure they do not have a metastatic lesion at this level. You should order an urgent MRI (or if it is not possible, a myelogram) of the lumbosacral spine. If metastatic disease is present, start dexamethasone (Decadron) and arrange radiation therapy; if it is not, prescribe a nonsteroidal anti-inflammatory drug, activity modification, and a gentle stretching program.

Case 2. This is an example of musculoskeletal pain. There is no radiation of the pain along a nerve root, and there are no focal findings on examination. The normal neurologic examination despite a long history of similar problems makes it very unlikely that the patient has a new structural lesion, and no imaging studies are necessary. This kind of pain may be just as severe as the pain from a herniated disc or metastatic cancer.

The patient has already discovered for himself several of the conservative measures that are often used to treat this problem. Because his symptoms persist despite these measures, he should be given a prescription for a nonsteroidal anti-inflammatory drug and possibly a tricyclic antidepressant (which may be synergistic), while embarking on a physical therapy program designed to teach him gentle stretching exercises and educate him about correct posture. Ultimately, weight loss would help to relieve the mechanical stress on his spine and might reduce the risk of future exacerbations.

Chapter 16

Incontinence

I. Case Histories

Case 1. A 55-year-old woman has been experiencing "accidents" with her bladder whenever she sneezes or coughs. Otherwise, she is able to void normally and has no bowel or sexual dysfunction. She has no other symptoms. She has a history of hypertension, controlled by diet and exercise, and hypothyroidism. She is gravida 4 para 4, and all of the births were spontaneous vaginal deliveries without complications. She went through menopause at age 45. Her only daily medication is levothyroxine. Her neurologic examination is normal.

Case 2. A 40-year-old man with limb-girdle muscular dystrophy has had episodes of bowel and bladder incontinence for the past several months. He has no difficulty sensing when he "needs to go." He has started using a bedside commode, and this has solved his problem with nocturnal incontinence, but he still has difficulty when he is away from his home. He has started scouting out the restrooms whenever he goes somewhere unfamiliar, because he can avoid accidents as long as he reaches the restroom quickly enough. He has also noticed progressive difficulty with walking over the past year. He has no sensory symptoms. His sexual function has been normal. His examination is notable for profound proximal weakness of the legs and arms, and a slow, waddling gait. Perianal sensation and rectal tone are normal. Deep tendon reflexes are normal and plantar responses are flexor.

Case 3. A 60-year-old woman with chronic back pain due to degenerative lumbar spine disease has developed urinary incontinence characterized by frequent dribbling of small amounts of urine without any sensation of a need to void. She has also noted mild lower extremity weakness and an increase in her baseline lower extremity numbness. Examination is notable for weakness of ankle dorsiflexion, absent ankle reflexes, and numbness on the lateral borders of the feet and in the perianal region. Rectal tone is decreased.

Questions:

1. What is the likely explanation for each patient's incontinence?

2. Which of these is an urgent problem?

II. Background Information

The normal bladder stores a large volume of urine at low pressure. Continence is maintained (generally unconsciously) by contraction of muscle fibers in the bladder neck (internal sphincter) and proximal urethra (external sphincter). A micturition reflex is triggered when a sufficient volume of urine collects in the bladder. Except at extremely high bladder volumes, a healthy individual is able to inhibit this reflex until a socially convenient time. The reflex produces a coordinated event in which the internal and external sphincters open and the detrusor muscle in the bladder wall contracts, while the junctions between the bladder and the ureters are compressed to prevent reflux toward the kidney. The coordination between bladder and sphincter contraction is largely mediated by a micturition center in the pons.

The majority of detrusor motor innervation is cholinergic from the pelvic parasympathetic plexus, which derives from the S2–S4 nerve roots. Sympathetic adrenergic fibers originating at the T10–L2 levels provide the major motor innervation of the distal ureters, trigone, and bladder neck. Voluntary sphincter control is mediated by the pudendal nerve, which is derived from the S2–S4 nerve roots.

III. Approach to Incontinence

Incontinence is a particularly distressing symptom for patients and their families, and this would be reason enough to evaluate it promptly. In addition, although incontinence is not an emergency in and of itself, it sometimes indicates the presence of an underlying neurologic condition that must be addressed urgently. This chapter focuses on urinary incontinence, but the same principles apply when evaluating neurologic causes of fecal incontinence. Neurologic conditions more often produce urinary incontinence than fecal incontinence, and when both occur, urinary incontinence generally appears first.

Two questions must be addressed in evaluating someone with urinary incontinence:

A. Is the problem related to nervous system control of bladder function?
B. If so, what level of the nervous system is involved?

A. Non-neurologic Causes of Incontinence

The most common cause of incontinence is weakness of the mechanical structures supporting the urethral sphincters. This produces *stress incontinence,* characterized by leakage of small amounts of urine during any activity that results in increased intra-abdominal pressure, such as coughing or sneezing. Ordinarily, increased abdominal pressure is transmitted equally to the bladder and proximal urethra, so that the pressure across the sphincter remains constant. Stress incontinence occurs when there is relaxation of pelvic floor musculature and partial herniation of the proximal urethra through the pelvic floor, so that increases in abdominal pressure result in an increased pressure gradient across the sphincter. This problem is unusual in males unless their urinary sphincters have been damaged during prior surgery, but it is common in females, especially those who have had vaginal deliveries. The prevalence and severity increase with age; obesity is also a risk factor. There are generally no associated abnormalities on neurologic examination. Treatment consists of pelvic floor exercises, sometimes supplemented with biofeedback, pessaries (instruments placed in the vagina to support the uterus), or a midurethral sling procedure.

The term *functional incontinence* applies to any condition that results in difficulty reaching a toilet quickly in someone whose bladder, its associated sphincters, and their nerve supply all function normally. The most self-evident example is a person in mechanical restraints. Limb pain or weakness may be less obvious, but no less an obstacle to mobility. Confused individuals may manifest functional incontinence simply because they can't find the bathroom. Making the diagnosis of functional incontinence can sometimes be tricky, especially when the condition limiting mobility is a neurologic problem that could also be affecting bladder function directly. The main question is whether the problem would persist even if the person could get to the bathroom quickly. Some patients can answer this question directly. If they have trouble answering this question, they should be asked whether they can recognize when their bladder is full and whether they can inhibit urination for a brief time. Functional incontinence is managed by maximizing mobility, providing adult diapers, and placing commodes in strategic locations in the home.

A damaged urinary sphincter may be inadequate to maintain a tight seal, resulting in leakage of urine from the bladder. This may be the result of prior surgery or trauma. A midurethral sling is the standard surgical procedure for this condition also. In males, an artificial urinary sphincter can be inserted; these have greater long-term efficacy than perineal slings. Other non-neurologic causes of incontinence include medication side effects (e.g., diuretics and alpha-adrenergic antagonists), volume overload, diabetes mellitus, diabetes insipidus, urinary tract infection, and reduced bladder compliance.

B. Central vs. Peripheral Nervous System Causes of Incontinence

Lesions at any level of the nervous system can cause incontinence. The main localizing distinction is between a *spastic bladder* and a *flaccid bladder*. People with a spastic bladder experience *urge incontinence*—a sudden, uncontrollable urge to void, with complete emptying of the bladder contents. In contrast, with a flaccid bladder the muscle in the bladder wall does not contract either voluntarily or reflexively; people with this problem tend to retain urine, and the bladder expands passively until its capacity has been surpassed, at which point urine may leak out. This is called *overflow incontinence*. Unlike stress incontinence, this can occur even without any elevation of intra-abdominal pressure. The volume leaked may be small or large. Overflow incontinence may be associated with urinary hesitancy or slow flow. Overflow incontinence can also be due to urinary outlet obstruction (e.g., from prostatic hypertrophy); patients with this problem often need to strain in order to pass their urine.

A spastic bladder indicates an upper motor neuron problem and can result from lesions in the brain or spinal cord. Associated symptoms and examination findings may permit a more precise localization. For example, limb hyperreflexia and a sensory level on the trunk suggest myelopathy. Mental status testing is important, because dementing illnesses may result in dysfunction of the cortical pathways involved in sphincter control.

A flaccid bladder corresponds to a lower motor neuron lesion. It can result from any condition that disturbs the nerves that supply the bladder after they have exited the spinal cord. For example, overflow incontinence is the typical pattern that occurs in people with diabetic polyneuropathy. Associated symptoms and signs again provide clues to the site of pathology; someone with sacral numbness, leg weakness, and hyporeflexia at the ankles and knees, for example, may have a lesion of the cauda equina. Overflow incontinence can also occur in individuals who have an upper motor neuron lesion that is below the level of the pontine micturition center. Such lesions produce not only a spastic bladder but also *detrusor-external sphincter dyssynergia*, in which the timing of bladder and sphincter contraction is poorly coordinated so that the bladder contracts against a closed sphincter. This condition often leads to ureteral reflux.

When historical information and examination findings are insufficient to discriminate between a flaccid bladder and a spastic bladder, useful information may be obtained from urodynamic studies, in which the bladder pressure is measured at different volumes. The point at which the subject feels an urge to void and the point at which the urge to void cannot be overcome are recorded, as is any residual volume in the bladder after voiding. This study is called a cystometrogram. Even if a complete urodynamic study is not feasible, the post-void residual can be measured by catheterizing the bladder or performing an ultrasound immediately after the patient voids spontaneously.

Neurogenic incontinence is treated by addressing the underlying neurologic problem to the extent possible. When there is a structural lesion affecting the spinal cord or the cauda equina, urgent decompressive surgery may be necessary. For patients with a spastic bladder, pelvic floor exercises may be helpful. Symptomatic improvement can often be achieved using anticholinergic (in particular, antimuscarinic) medications or beta-3 adrenergic agonists to inhibit bladder wall contraction (Table 16.1). Timed voiding may help prevent the bladder from filling to the point where reflex emptying occurs. Patients are often counseled to limit their evening fluid intake to minimize nocturia, but the effectiveness of this approach has not been proven. Electrical stimulation of the S3 nerve root, the pudendal nerve, or the tibial nerve has been advocated for selected patients. Another option is botulinum toxin injection into the detrusor muscle, although this can cause urinary retention. In some patients, catheterization is necessary, especially when detrusor-external sphincter dyssynergia is present.

IV. Supplementary Table for Reference

Table 16.1 Medications Used for Spastic Bladder

Antimuscarinic Agents

Darifenacin (Enablex)

Fesoterodine (Toviaz)

Oxybutynin (Ditropan)

Solifenacin (Vesicare)

Tolterodine (Detrol)

Trospium (Sanctura)

Beta-3 Adrenergic Agonists

Mirabegron (Myrbetriq)

Vibegron (Gemtesa)

V. Discussion of Case Histories

Case 1. This patient is describing typical stress incontinence. In the absence of other symptoms or examination abnormalities, no tests are indicated. This is not an urgent problem. Treatment is described in Part III, Section A.

Case 2. This patient has functional incontinence that is the result of deteriorating ability to walk because of his progressive muscle disease. The diagnosis is based on the history and examination; no tests are indicated. This is a serious but not urgent problem. Treatment of the incontinence is described in Part III, Section A. Unfortunately, no treatment is available for his underlying muscular dystrophy.

Case 3. This patient's incontinence is an important clue to an urgent neurologic problem. The lower extremity weakness and decreased reflexes suggest a lower motor neuron problem, and this is consistent with the flaccid character of her urinary symptoms. Many of the abnormalities on her neurologic examination are distal and symmetric, suggesting a peripheral polyneuropathy, but this would not explain the reduced sensation in the perianal region or the reduced rectal tone. These additional findings suggest a more proximal problem, involving the lower sacral nerve roots. The ankle dorsiflexion weakness could be explained by bilateral L5 radiculopathies, and the absent ankle reflexes and reduced sensation along the lateral borders of the feet could be explained by bilateral S1 radiculopathies. The most likely lesion localization would be the cauda equina. The time course is difficult to determine. Her urinary symptoms are subacute, but she has had chronic back pain and lower extremity numbness. This suggests a chronic process that has recently accelerated. A chronic, focal lesion is most likely a tumor. This patient needs an imaging study urgently, and she may need emergency surgery for diagnosis and decompression.

Comment: An MRI scan of the lumbosacral spine showed a prominent disc herniation with compression of multiple sacral nerve roots. This is yet another example of how the rules of Chapter 3 are approximations, lumping many different "new growths" into the category of neoplasm. Even so, cancer was a realistic possibility, and use of the rules resulted in the appropriate diagnostic test with the correct level of urgency. This patient was taken for decompressive surgery immediately, because a delay could have resulted in permanent loss of bladder and bowel function.

IV

Bookends

Chapter 17

Pediatric Neurology

I. Case Histories

The five questions below apply to all the case histories that follow:

1. What additional historical information would be most useful?
2. Which parts of the neurologic examination would most likely provide helpful data?
3. What diagnoses should be considered?
4. How should this individual be evaluated?
5. How should this individual be managed?

Cases 1 and 2: Spells

Case 1. A 7-year-old girl was well until about a month ago, when she started having spells in which she awakens shortly after going to sleep and walks out to the living room, where her parents are usually reading. She says nothing, or at most a few words, and her parents notice that one side of her mouth twitches and she drools. She appears to be able to understand what they say to her during the episodes. She has had four episodes in all, each lasting 1–5 minutes.

Case 2. An 8-year-old boy has been exhibiting unusual repetitive movements for the past 3 months. For the first 2 months, he repeatedly blinked his eyes and jerked his head. These symptoms resolved spontaneously, but they were followed 2 weeks later by intermittent episodes of repetitive hand clapping and throat clearing.

Cases 3 and 4: Ataxia

Case 3. Ten days after recovering from a viral illness, a 5-year-old girl suddenly developed severe unsteadiness. She was able to sit up, but she was unable to walk. She was mentally alert, and when she was lying down she had normal strength in all four limbs.

Case 4. A 4-year-old boy has been experiencing occasional headaches for the past several months. He has also had some vague stomach problems and vomiting over the same period. For the past week, his gait has been increasingly unsteady, and he has fallen a few times.

Cases 5 and 6: Toe Walking

Case 5. A 3-year-old girl walks on her toes, and her parents are concerned. She has walked this way ever since she began walking. Her parents were initially told that it would probably resolve, but it hasn't. The patient and her twin sister were born at gestational age 30 weeks. The patient has made steady developmental progress, but all motor milestones have been delayed relative to her twin.

Case 6. A 6-year-old boy has recently developed a tendency to walk on his toes. He was born at term, and his initial development was considered normal, although he lagged a little behind his twin sister in all aspects of development. He walked at age 18 months. He has always had trouble running or climbing stairs, but recently he has been stumbling and falling more frequently.

Cases 7, 8, and 9: School Problems

Case 7. A 7-year-old girl has been referred for unusual behavior and problems at school for the past 3 months. She was a model student last year, but lately her school performance has been inconsistent. The girl's teacher has observed that she often appears to be daydreaming, and she sometimes fails to complete tasks. The family has noted similar behavior at home but didn't think much of it until the teacher drew their attention to it.

Case 8. A 9-year-old boy has just transferred to a new school, and an initial evaluation indicates that he is 18 months behind in his reading skills. He was previously diagnosed with dyslexia and attention deficit hyperactivity disorder (ADHD), for which he is being treated with dextroamphetamine-amphetamine. The boy's parents and pediatrician all think that his attention and behavior have improved markedly with this treatment. The boy's family is also concerned because he has not learned how to ride a bicycle, and he is less coordinated than his peers.

Case 9. A 10-year-old boy is being evaluated for a decline in school performance over the past 6–9 months. He had always been an "A" student before but is now failing in all subjects. He is apathetic and insolent to his teacher, who says that he "seems like a different boy." His parents divorced about a year ago, and the boy's difficulties were initially attributed to psychosocial stress. He has had no headaches, seizures, or loss of motor skills.

II. Developmental Considerations

Children are immature. This is hardly a revelation, yet it expresses a fundamental principle of human biology. Although the human brain has an enormous capacity for complex processing, most of its potential is unrealized at birth. In other species, a newborn is able to walk, swim, or fly almost immediately, with full adult function acquired within a few years at most. In humans, the process takes more than a decade (and, of course, "some kids never grow up"). This confers great flexibility, allowing children to develop functions that are directly adapted to their particular environment. In essence, the process results in "custom-made" brains, rather than assembly line products. The most obvious example is language. Different cultures, different regions, and above all, different eras have vastly different vocabulary needs, and the rate at which evolution proceeds is far too slow to accommodate them. Instead, heredity provides a general program for linguistic processing, but environmental exposure determines the specific language elements that an individual acquires. The same principle of developmental plasticity applies to most aspects of perception, motor function, and cognition. Without plasticity, there would be no learning.

Developmental plasticity is the main feature distinguishing pediatric neurology from adult neurology. The diagnostic principles presented in the first three chapters of this book still apply, but many of the nervous system functions typically assessed in adults are not fully operational until months or years after birth. Obvious examples are walking, talking, and control of bladder and bowel function. Incontinence in an adult patient is clearly abnormal and suggests a set of specific lesion sites (see Chapter 16). Incontinence in a pediatric patient may be significant or not, depending on the patient's age. The same is true of the inability to walk or talk. Conversely, some reflexes normally present in infancy disappear as children age. Thus, a child's developmental stage determines how the examination is interpreted and how it is performed.

The effects of disease also vary depending on an individual's developmental stage. The developing nervous system is extremely vulnerable to some injuries that have little effect on the mature nervous system, whereas developmental plasticity permits more complete recovery from some injuries in children than in adults.

This chapter is not meant to be a comprehensive survey of the vast array of diseases that affect the developing nervous system. Rather, the goal is to present a general approach to some of the more common clinical situations that occur primarily in the pediatric population.

III. Hypotonic Infants

Newborn infants have very limited behavioral repertoires. The most common manifestation of neurologic disease at this age is abnormal motor activity. In particular, parents report a "floppy baby," and physicians observe hypotonia. There are several ways to assess an infant's tone. One way is to pull the baby by the hands from a supine to a seated position. A healthy full-term baby will flex the neck to lift the head from the surface along with the body; a hypotonic infant's head will fall back (Figure 17.1A). Another way to assess tone is to suspend the baby with the abdomen lying on your outstretched hand—infants with normal tone will straighten their back, flex their limbs, and hold their head straight or extended. A hypotonic infant held in this way will be limp, with head and limbs drooping down over your hand (Figure 17.1B). Infants who have normal tone can be held vertically by supporting the axillae, whereas a hypotonic infant tends to "slip through" the examiner's hands (Figure 17.1C). The assessment of tone requires a fair amount of experience with the expected range of variation among healthy infants and knowledge of how the expectation changes with gestational age. When examining infants, it can be difficult to differentiate muscle tone (resistance to *passive* manipulation) from strength (maximum *voluntary* resistance to a movement). To assess an infant's strength, the examiner usually observes spontaneous movement or applies a noxious stimulus; often, the only conclusion that can be reliably drawn is whether or not the infant can overcome gravity.

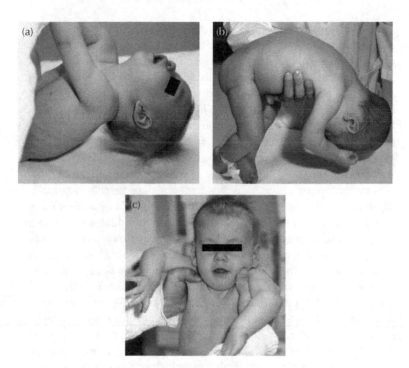

Fig. 17.1 Physical examination features of hypotonia. A) "pull-to-sit", B) ventral suspension, C) shoulder suspension. (Modified, with permission, from Bodensteiner JB. The evaluation of the hypotonic infant. Semin Pediatr Neurol 2008;15:10–20.)

Unlike adults, in whom hypotonia implies a lesion in the LMN (and increased tone implies an UMN lesion), infants manifest hypotonia with lesions anywhere in the motor pathway. Consequently, features other than tone must be used to distinguish between central and peripheral lesions. Infants with peripheral hypotonia (caused by lesions at the level of anterior horn cell, nerve root, peripheral nerve, neuromuscular junction, or muscle) typically have severe weakness, with reduced or absent tendon reflexes. When hypotonia is due to lesions at the level of the spinal cord or higher, the hypotonia is usually more profound than the weakness, and tendon reflexes are normal or brisk. When the lesion is in the cerebral hemispheres, there are often additional manifestations of cerebral malfunction (such as seizures or reduced alertness).

Central hypotonia may be idiopathic, or it may result from intrauterine or perinatal hypoxic-ischemic events, intracranial hemorrhage, ischemic strokes, genetic abnormalities (such as chromosomal abnormalities, inborn errors of metabolism, and leukodystrophies), congenital malformations, infections, and a variety of metabolic derangements including hypoglycemia, hyperbilirubinemia, hypothyroidism, and drug intoxication. Many of these conditions can be identified by taking a careful history (especially family history and history of intrauterine and postnatal drug exposure), obtaining an imaging study of the brain, checking serum electrolytes and glucose, or doing genetic or metabolic testing.

Some of the peripheral causes of hypotonia are hereditary (especially myotonic dystrophy, some metabolic myopathies, and some neuropathies), so the diagnosis can sometimes be made by taking a careful family history or examining family members, but genetic testing is usually key. It is important to diagnose spinal muscular atrophy (SMA) as early as possible to maximize the benefit of genetic therapy (see Chapter 6, Part IV, Section A). Approximately 15% of infants born to mothers with myasthenia gravis have hypotonia and weakness, traditionally attributed to passive transfer of maternal antibodies. The average duration of symptoms is 18 days. Hereditary neuromuscular junction disorders exist, but they are very rare. Infant botulism is caused by ingestion of food (most often honey) or soil containing the bacterium, which colonizes the gut and produces toxin (in contrast to adults, who have defenses against the bacterium and only acquire the disease by ingesting already-manufactured toxin). Detailed questions about what the child has recently eaten or where they have been playing sometimes provide a clue to the diagnosis. A history of constipation is typical. Other historical information may provide clues to other metabolic or toxic conditions. For some peripheral causes of hypotonia, specific biochemical assays, nerve conduction studies, EMG, and muscle biopsy may help clarify the diagnosis.

IV. Developmental Delay and Developmental Regression

The process of development varies considerably from one child to the next, but it proceeds in the same general sequence and in a similar time frame in all children. When children reach developmental milestones at a slow rate that is clearly outside the usual range, it is called *developmental delay*. Because the process of development is so variable, and the stigma associated with developmental delay is so great, this label should only be applied when a child is unequivocally failing to achieve developmental milestones within the expected age range.

When children lose some of the skills they have already acquired, it is called *developmental regression*. This determination does not require comparison to standard developmental milestone expectations, because it is based purely on a child's own previous development. Nonetheless, caution must be exercised in diagnosing developmental regression, because many children intermittently regress slightly.

An isolated, time-limited insult to the nervous system, such as an infection or head trauma, can result in developmental delay. Although the event itself may be transient, the damage it produces may severely limit or even abolish the nervous system's capacity to develop further. In contrast, regression usually implies an ongoing disease process.

Developmental delay can affect various domains of function—motor, language, cognitive, and social—either in isolation or in combination, and the differential diagnosis depends on which functions are affected. Global developmental delay (affecting motor function, language, overall cognition, and social interaction) can result from genetic abnormalities, in utero or perinatal processes (including infections, toxins, or hypoxic-ischemic injury), or the same kinds of ongoing disease processes that typically produce developmental regression (see the final paragraph of Part IV). The most common inherited cause of global developmental delay is *fragile X syndrome*, caused by an expanded triplet repeat in an uncoded region of a gene on the X chromosome that codes for a protein involved in learning-dependent synaptic changes, called the fragile X messenger ribonucleoprotein (FMRP). Children who have fragile X syndrome have little or no FMRP. They have problems with cognition, behavior, and motor function, together with characteristic craniofacial features and joint abnormalities. Because the gene is on the X chromosome, the disease affects males more severely and more frequently than females. As discussed in Chapter 8 (Part IV, Section D), carriers with triplet expansions of 55–200 repeats may develop fragile X–associated tremor ataxia syndrome (FXTAS), usually presenting after age 55 years. This condition is not due to an absence of FMRP; instead, the triplet expansion is thought to exert a neurotoxic effect by sequestering and perturbing the function of nuclear proteins.

The list of potential causes of delayed motor development includes most of the conditions that can cause central hypotonia in infants, although as children mature and their nervous systems myelinate, the hypotonia is typically replaced by spasticity. Nonprogressive limitation of motor control due to prenatal or perinatal CNS dysfunction has traditionally been referred to as *cerebral palsy*. It can involve a single limb, one side of the body, both lower extremities, or all four limbs. The usual motor manifestation is spasticity, but some children have dystonia, ataxia, or hypotonia. In children who were born preterm, the most common manifestation of motor delay is spasticity, typically affecting the legs more than the arms. This is because the most common cause of both motor and cognitive delay in children born before 32 weeks' gestation is neonatal white matter injury, also known as periventricular leukomalacia. This condition preferentially affects the white matter tracts adjacent to the lateral ventricles, especially the medial motor fibers of the corticospinal tract that control the lower extremities (with relative sparing of the lateral fibers that control the upper extremities). Preterm white matter in these regions is particularly vulnerable to hypoxic-ischemic insults and other factors. The white matter dysfunction is usually not clinically evident in infancy but becomes more apparent as the child develops.

The most common cause of an isolated delay in language development is reduced hearing. Children with language delay should be promptly referred for formal audiologic testing; language skills often improve dramatically when children are able to hear more clearly. Other developmental causes of isolated language difficulty include hereditary factors and perinatal injury. In older children who have difficulty with reading and writing despite normal initial language development, dyslexia is an important consideration.

Some children have widespread cognitive delay, affecting other intellectual functions in addition to language, without any motor delay. These children should still have their hearing tested, because reduced hearing could be a potentially treatable factor underlying their cognitive delay, but it is unlikely to be the only factor. The differential diagnosis for widespread cognitive delay without motor involvement is similar to that for global developmental delay. *Attention deficit hyperactivity disorder (ADHD)* is another potential cause of delayed learning. It has received a great deal of publicity in recent years, with a wide range of prevalence estimates that probably reflects the lack of a biological marker. ADHD is characterized by symptoms of inattention, impulsivity, distractibility, and hyperactivity that affect function and occur in more than one setting. The recommended treatment for ADHD is behavioral therapy in preschool children and stimulant medication (often in conjunction with behavioral therapy) in school-age children. The use of stimulant medication in children who do not meet specific diagnostic criteria for ADHD remains a subject of intense controversy. Psychological factors can also impede school performance; a useful clue is that the child's problems are often restricted to particular activities, with relative sparing of language skills, self-care ability, and performance in recreational activities.

The most common cause of delayed social development is *autism spectrum disorder*, characterized by impairment in social communication, restricted interests, and repetitive behaviors. This is generally considered to be a heterogeneous set of conditions with no single cause. About a third of people with autism spectrum disorder have intellectual disability. Gastrointestinal difficulties and sleep disturbances are more prevalent among people with autism spectrum disorder, and 12% have epilepsy.

A vast array of disease processes can cause intellectual and motor *regression*. These include infections, tumors, toxic exposure, vascular conditions, metabolic conditions, some generalized epilepsy syndromes, inflammatory/autoimmune diseases, and endocrine disorders. Many of these conditions involve components of the nervous system and other organ systems in specific patterns that provide clues to the diagnosis. The age of onset is also helpful in narrowing the diagnosis. Even when the family history is negative, genetic testing is often revealing. More detailed algorithms and tables are available in standard textbooks of pediatric neurology.

V. Paroxysmal Symptoms

As noted in Chapter 3, the most common causes of paroxysmal focal neurologic symptoms in adults are transient ischemic attacks, seizures, and migraines. Of these, the most common in children are seizures and migraines. Cerebrovascular disease certainly occurs in children, but it is primarily due to diseases other than atherosclerosis, so it is usually not associated with transient ischemic attacks. Other paroxysmal conditions that can occur in childhood include breath-holding spells, night terrors, other NREM parasomnias, narcolepsy/cataplexy, tics, other paroxysmal movement disorders, syncope, psychogenic spells, and benign paroxysmal vertigo. Most of these conditions are discussed in previous chapters, but several merit additional comment.

A. Migraine

Headaches are common in childhood. The same principles of evaluation and treatment that apply to adults (see Chapter 12) also hold for children. Most of the abortive and prophylactic medications that are prescribed to adults are also effective in children, but the specific drugs used may differ because of different concerns about side effects. Cyclic vomiting (characterized by recurrent episodes of nausea and vomiting) and periodic abdominal pain are two variants of migraine that arise almost exclusively in childhood. These two syndromes frequently overlap. There is often no accompanying headache, but approximately 75% of these children develop typical migraine later in life; in many cases, the cyclical vomiting responds to typical migraine medications. Much less commonly, recurrent episodes of vomiting or abdominal pain may represent seizures, with associated EEG changes.

B. Seizures

Seizures in children are classified, evaluated, and managed according to the same principles that apply in adults (see Chapter 5). It is sometimes more difficult to recognize seizures in children than in adults, however. In neonates especially, the immaturity of the nervous system interferes with propagation of epileptic discharges, so classic tonic-clonic convulsions are rare. More common are brief episodes of hypertonia, atonia, or localized clonic movements. Neonatal seizures may also manifest with rhythmic or sustained eye movements, chewing, or unusual limb movements. Most neonatal seizures are not clinically evident and can only be diagnosed with EEG; conversely, many neonatal behaviors that look like seizures are not. Another unique feature of pediatric epilepsy is that certain seizure types arise only at particular ages. Infantile spasms, for example, usually present between the ages of 3 and 11 months and almost always before 2 years of age. Absence seizures almost always begin in childhood, typically between the ages of 5 and 9 years. Self-limited epilepsy with centrotemporal spikes (SeLECTS) presents between the ages of 18 months and 13 years, usually between the ages of 5 and 10 years, and is typically outgrown by puberty. Juvenile myoclonic epilepsy (JME) generally presents around the time of puberty. For more details regarding these conditions, see Chapter 5.

The same underlying processes that produce seizures in adults can cause seizures in children. Congenital brain defects and antenatal or perinatal injuries (especially hypoxic-ischemic and infectious) are common causes. Febrile seizures represent a separate category (see Chapter 5).

C. Breath-Holding Spells

Breath-holding spells are common in infants and children ages 6 months to 6 years, with the first attacks usually occurring before age 18 months. The episodes become less frequent with advancing age, and disappear by the age of 5 or 6 years. There are two types of breath-holding spells. The cyanotic variety occurs when children get upset or angry about something, cry briefly, and then hold their breath in forced expiration, quickly becoming cyanotic. This may be followed by going limp and losing consciousness. The pallid variety of breath-holding spell is less common. It is caused by bradycardia or brief asystole due to vagal hypersensitivity. The spells are typically precipitated by a minor fall or a blow to the head or upper body. After a brief delay (30 seconds or less), the child loses consciousness, stops breathing, and becomes pale, diaphoretic, and limp. This may be followed by increased tone in the trunk and extremities, incontinence, and sometimes low-amplitude clonus. The family should be reassured that these spells are benign, and they usually disappear by the age of 5–6 years; almost all children stop having spells by the age of 8 years, with no sequelae. Iron-deficiency anemia is more prevalent in children with either type of breath-holding spells than in the general population, so blood counts and iron studies are warranted. Iron supplementation reduces the frequency of spells in iron-deficient children, and even children who are not iron-deficient may respond to iron supplementation, perhaps due to improvement in the blood's capacity to carry oxygen.

D. Benign Paroxysmal Vertigo

Benign paroxysmal vertigo of childhood is characterized by recurrent episodes of vertigo, vomiting, nystagmus, and diffuse pallor. The attacks usually last a few minutes or less. Children may fall during the attack, but they do not lose consciousness. Onset is usually between the ages of 1 and 4 years. The episodes eventually become less frequent and either disappear or are replaced by symptoms that are characteristic of migraine.

VI. Gait Disturbance

In both children and adults, abnormal gait can be a result of either focal lesions or diffuse processes. When the history and examination implicate a focal lesion, evaluation and treatment proceed in the same manner in children as in adults. When the symptoms are symmetric, the three most likely problems in all age groups are spasticity, weakness, and ataxia. The diagnostic considerations for each of these problems differ in children and adults.

A. Spasticity

As discussed in Part IV, conditions that produce central hypotonia in infants—notably intrauterine or perinatal damage, especially from hypoxic-ischemic events, hemorrhage, and infections—commonly result in spasticity later in childhood. Spasticity that affects the legs more than the arms is typical of neonatal white matter injury (periventricular leukomalacia) in children who were born preterm. When evaluating children with spastic gait, you should ask about birth history, intrauterine or perinatal complications, and delayed motor or intellectual milestones. Structural lesions in the spinal cord or metabolic diseases (such as leukodystrophies) can also produce lower extremity spasticity, but the symptoms are usually progressive, resulting in loss of previously acquired function.

B. Weakness

The most important consideration in evaluating a diffusely weak child is whether the weakness is central or peripheral. Associated hyperreflexia and spasticity suggest a central process. As discussed in the previous paragraph, intrauterine or perinatal damage commonly results in spasticity that remains static over time, and spinal cord damage or metabolic disease typically causes progressive spasticity. Hypotonia, hyporeflexia, and muscle atrophy suggest disease at the level of the anterior horn cell, nerve root, peripheral nerve, neuromuscular junction, or muscle. The evaluation of neuromuscular disease is discussed in Chapter 6. The same principles apply in children and adults, but the particular diseases differ in the two groups. Muscular dystrophies and hereditary neuropathies are more likely to be important diagnostic considerations in children than in adults, for example, whereas conditions like inclusion body myositis (IBM) or diabetic polyneuropathy are common in adults but not in children.

C. Ataxia

In children, acute ataxia most commonly occurs in the setting of an infection or nonspecific febrile illness. A wide variety of infectious agents have been implicated; varicella virus is the classic example. Postinfectious ataxia may occur at any age, but it is most common between the ages of 1 and 5 years. It is characterized by the sudden onset of truncal ataxia, resulting in rapid deterioration of gait. Nystagmus is present in about half of the patients, and there may be prominent tremors of limbs, head, or trunk. The symptoms resolve completely in most children, usually within several months, but some children have permanent residua. The acute ataxia syndrome can also occur after children receive the varicella vaccine—which contains live, attenuated virus—but the incidence is much lower.

Another cause of acute ataxia is toxic exposure, primarily to antiseizure medications, alcohol, antihistamines, heavy metals, and mercury. Neuroblastomas are associated with a paraneoplastic syndrome consisting of ataxia, myoclonus, and opsoclonus (irregular, multidirectional involuntary eye movements). This syndrome is often the initial clinical manifestation of the tumor. The same syndrome sometimes occurs in children or adults who have no associated tumor, and no explanation is found. Intermittent episodes of acute ataxia may occur with some metabolic diseases, such as disorders of amino acid metabolism, and also with ion channel diseases.

Posterior fossa tumors can also cause acute ataxia, but they are much more likely to produce gradually progressive, chronic symptoms. Other causes of chronically progressive ataxia include Friedreich ataxia and ataxia telangiectasia, both of which are discussed in Chapter 8, Part IV, Section D. A number of metabolic conditions can also cause chronic, progressive ataxia.

VII. Functional Disorders

Some children, especially adolescents, have clinical symptoms that suggest dysfunction of the nervous system, but extensive evaluation reveals no evidence of any neurologic disease. All the principles that apply to "functional disorders" of adults (see Chapter 10, Part IV, Section E)—including the fact that the term "functional" is problematic—apply equally to children.

VIII. Discussion of Case Histories

Case 1. This patient has paroxysmal symptoms, and they sound most like seizures. They could conceivably be tics, but tics usually occur more randomly, rather than in discrete episodes lasting up to 5 minutes. Given the onset shortly after going to sleep, NREM parasomnias such as sleepwalking must be considered, but the mouth twitching and drooling would be atypical. Migraine is unlikely, as the symptoms are not typical of migraine and she has no associated headache. None of the symptoms suggest any of the other paroxysmal conditions of childhood. Given the focal nature of the symptoms and the apparent preservation of consciousness, these would be classified as focal seizures. In particular, they are typical of the seizures that occur in the syndrome of self-limited epilepsy with centro-temporal spikes (SeLECTS) (see Chapter 5, Part V, Section B).

The history and examination should be directed at confirming this diagnostic impression and excluding any other type of seizures that might signal the need for more extensive evaluation. Thus, questions about family history are important. The patient and family should be asked about any symptoms that might suggest other kinds of seizures and about any progressive neurologic deficits. Children with SeLECTS typically have a normal neurologic examination, so any focal abnormality on examination should prompt further evaluation. If the history and examination do not suggest progression, focality, or multiple seizure types, the diagnosis of SeLECTS can be confirmed by finding characteristic abnormalities on EEG (epileptiform activity in the region of the Sylvian fissure). If the EEG does not show these abnormalities, an MRI would be indicated. Patients with SeLECTS often require no treatment other than reassurance. Antiseizure medications may be used to reduce the frequency of seizures in some cases. This condition resolves near the time of puberty, so life-long treatment is not necessary.

Case 2. This patient also has paroxysmal symptoms. They could conceivably be seizures, but the change in clinical characteristics after 2 months would be atypical. This would be more suggestive of a tic disorder. None of the other paroxysmal conditions of childhood are considerations in this case.

Further historical information that would be useful could be obtained by asking whether there is any impairment of awareness associated with the spells (which would be consistent with seizures). People with tics usually experience a sense of urgency just before the tic is expressed; they can temporarily suppress the tic, but this results in the urgency becoming even more difficult to resist. They feel a sense of relief when they stop resisting and "release" the tic. The boy and his family should be asked about these features. The parents should also be asked whether he has exhibited any other potential vocal tics in addition to his repetitive clearing of the throat. They should be asked about weight loss, exercise tolerance, and behavioral changes to evaluate the possibility of hyperthyroidism, which can precipitate tics. A family history would also be pertinent. On examination, direct observation of the involuntary movements would be particularly helpful. Because tics can often be transiently suppressed, they may be difficult to observe in the doctor's office even when they are reported to be very frequent at home or at school. Families should be encouraged to take videos and bring them to appointments. Close observation of the patient (and family members) during the medical visit sometimes reveals subtle involuntary movements that the family may never even have noticed.

If the information gathered from the history and examination confirms that the movements are most likely tics, no further diagnostic testing is necessary. Symptoms often resolve spontaneously, so treatment is usually reserved for symptoms that have persisted and are significantly disruptive to the child (see Chapter 8, Part IV, Section I and Table 8.3).

Case 3. This history is very suggestive of postinfectious ataxia. Varicella is the infectious agent that is classically associated with this disorder, but it can occur with a wide variety of infectious agents, and the proportion of cases associated with varicella has declined as a result of widespread vaccination programs. If the history and examination confirm that the patient has ataxia with no weakness, reflex changes, or other abnormalities, there is no evidence of pre-existing neurologic dysfunction, and there are no other potential causes of ataxia (especially toxic exposure), then additional tests may be unnecessary. It is sometimes appropriate to obtain an MRI scan of the brain (looking for hydrocephalus or a mass lesion in the posterior fossa) and a lumbar puncture (to exclude ongoing infection). If these tests are normal (or at most show a mild lymphocytic pleocytosis in the cerebrospinal fluid), only supportive therapy is required.

Case 4. This patient is also ataxic, but the several-month history of associated symptoms suggests a more chronic condition. If his ataxia were intermittent, migraine would be a consideration, but this boy's gait has been growing progressively worse over the past week. The headaches and vomiting suggest increased intracranial pressure, making a posterior fossa mass lesion or hydrocephalus the two leading considerations. The history and examination should focus on any focal abnormalities that might help localize a mass lesion. In addition, increased intracranial pressure often causes papilledema, so a funduscopic exam is very important. The examiner should look carefully for eye movement abnormalities that can result from pressure on cranial nerves III, IV, or VI. In younger children, it would also be important to measure head circumference, because subacute decompensation of long-standing hydrocephalus may produce increased intracranial pressure.

If the examination confirms elevated intracranial pressure, an imaging study should be obtained urgently, because even children who look healthy may deteriorate rapidly. Either a CT scan or an MRI scan would be adequate to diagnose hydrocephalus, but an MRI scan is the optimal imaging technique in this setting because it provides much better resolution in the posterior fossa. Immediate neurosurgical evaluation is indicated if either hydrocephalus or a mass lesion is found. Temporizing treatment of increased intracranial pressure with dexamethasone, mannitol, or hyperventilation may also be necessary (see Chapter 11).

Case 5. This history suggests developmental delay rather than regression. Additional historical information about intellectual and motor milestones should be elicited to confirm or refute this impression. Given the clear history of prematurity, developmental delay is not surprising. An MRI scan would probably show evidence of neonatal white matter injury (periventricular leukomalacia); if it doesn't, further testing might be indicated. The cornerstone of management is physical therapy. Additional interventions for spasticity, such as tendon release procedures or botulinum toxin injections, are sometimes necessary.

Case 6. Like the patient in Case 5, this patient had delayed motor development, but in this case the history also indicates motor regression, suggesting an ongoing disease process. The main goal in the history and examination is to determine whether the prominent abnormality is ataxia, weakness, or spasticity. If there were no history of regression, and the patient had a normal neurologic examination and serum creatine kinase (CK) level (making muscular dystrophy unlikely), it would be reasonable simply to observe the child over time, because some children who toe walk have no specific neurologic deficits. In this case, however, the history of recent deterioration requires prompt evaluation.

Comment: This patient's examination was notable for prominent calf muscles and proximal weakness in all four limbs. He exhibited the "Gowers sign": he marched up his legs with his hands in order to stand up from the floor. These findings suggest a primary muscle disorder, and in particular, the prominent calf muscles are typical of Duchenne muscular dystrophy. Elevated CK and genetic testing confirmed this diagnosis. The patient was referred to a muscular dystrophy clinic, where he was enrolled in an ongoing physical therapy program and started on prednisone and gene therapy.

Case 7. Although the prominent feature of this case is intellectual regression, the frequent daydreaming (both in school and at home) also suggests paroxysmal symptoms. Daydreaming is often the only symptom reported for children with absence seizures, and physicians (and teachers) must be alert to this possibility. Some forms of focal seizures may also manifest as daydreaming spells. Daydreaming may not raise any concerns until it leads to problems at school. Further historical information about the daydreaming spells would be helpful: Can the patient respond during the spells? Are there any associated eye or face movements? Does she have any unusual feelings before, during, or after the spells? The examiner should search for focal neurologic abnormalities (which would support the diagnosis of focal seizures) and should also instruct the child to hyperventilate while observing her for absence seizures. An EEG should be performed.

Comment: This girl's neurologic examination was normal, and hyperventilation provoked a typical absence attack. Her EEG showed 3-Hz generalized spike-and-wave activity, and ethosuximide was started. Her daydreaming spells and school problems resolved promptly.

Case 8. In contrast to the previous case, nothing suggests that this boy has a paroxysmal condition. There has been no regression noted, and if further questioning reveals no evidence of epilepsy or developmental deterioration, the clear response to dextroamphetamine-amphetamine would suggest that the diagnosis of ADHD is correct. A family history of this condition would also support the diagnosis. The main goal of the examination is to exclude a structural lesion. It would not be unusual if this patient's examination revealed some "soft neurologic signs"—subtle abnormalities that do not clearly correlate with discrete, focal lesions, and that might be considered normal in a younger child. These are present in many patients with ADHD and other learning disorders, and they have uncertain significance.

If the history reveals no evidence of a paroxysmal or progressive disorder and the examination shows no significant focal abnormalities, then no diagnostic studies are indicated. The dextroamphetamine-amphetamine treatment should continue.

Case 9. Like the girl in Case 7, this boy has experienced intellectual regression, but in this case, nothing suggests paroxysmal symptoms, so the likelihood of progressive neurologic disease is greater. On the other hand, the problems began at a time of significant psychological stress, and it was reasonable for his teachers and physicians to wonder about a connection. Historical information should be elicited regarding his behavior outside of school. If he continues to perform well at extracurricular activities he enjoys and he still gets along with his friends, an underlying neurologic disease is unlikely. Historical evidence for a focal lesion (such as language disturbance or hemiparesis) and focal examination deficits should also be sought. A family history of neurologic disease would help considerably in narrowing the differential diagnosis.

If these considerations fail to reveal a specific diagnosis, an MRI scan of the brain should be done, looking for either a focal abnormality or a diffuse process such as leukodystrophy or hydrocephalus. Depending on the age of onset, time course, family history, associated physical examination findings, and MRI findings, more specific tests for particular metabolic, genetic, infectious, and neoplastic diseases may be indicated.

Comment: This boy's behavior problems extended to the playground, where he had been getting in more and more fights. Even though he had not lost any motor skills, his examination revealed lower extremity spasticity. This prompted an MRI scan of the brain, which showed symmetric abnormalities in the cortical periventricular white matter bilaterally. This suggested the diagnosis of adrenoleukodystrophy. The diagnosis was confirmed by measuring very long chain fatty acids in serum. Unfortunately, the boy's clinical and MRI manifestations were sufficiently advanced that he was unlikely to respond to hematopoietic stem cell transplant. Because of the potential for adrenal insufficiency he was referred to an endocrinologist.

Chapter 18

Geriatric Neurology

I. Case Histories

Case 1. An 82-year-old man who was diagnosed with Alzheimer disease a year ago has had four episodes of urinary incontinence in the past 3 weeks. His family members understand that people with Alzheimer disease are often incontinent, and they want advice on how they should deal with the problem. The patient is unable to describe the episodes of incontinence in any detail. He cannot remember whether he felt any urge to void before any of the episodes, and he is embarrassed to talk about them at all. Despite his dementia, he still converses normally, has no difficulty showering or dressing, does simple chores like dishwashing and yard work, and plays golf twice a week.

His general physical examination is unremarkable. He is alert, attentive, and jovial. He talks fluently, but he has some word-finding problems. He can follow one- and two-step commands but typically makes slight errors when he tries to follow three-step commands. He has a normal digit span. He can only remember one of three items after a 5-minute delay, even with prompting. He cannot name the current president and cannot remember the ages or birth order of his children. He has eight grandchildren but cannot name any of them. He is able to perform one-digit addition and subtraction in his head, but no calculations more complicated than that.

His cranial nerve examination is normal. He walks stiffly, with no obvious asymmetry. He has marked spasticity in both lower extremities, but his strength is normal throughout all four limbs, and individual limb coordination is intact. He has diminished biceps and brachioradialis reflexes, but triceps reflexes are brisk bilaterally, and he has unsustained clonus at the knees and ankles, with bilateral Babinski signs. His mental status makes a detailed sensory examination difficult, but he seems to react much more strongly to pinprick in the upper extremities, neck, and face than in the trunk and lower extremities.

Questions:

1. Is this man's incontinence likely to be due to Alzheimer disease?
2. Are any other investigations necessary?
3. What interventions are indicated?

Case 2. A 78-year-old woman tells her family physician that she has chronic pain in her elbows, hips, and knees, and it is worse at the end of the day. The woman's history, examination, and x-rays are all consistent with degenerative joint disease, but she is noted to have absent ankle reflexes and markedly diminished vibration sense in her toes.

Questions:

1. Is this woman's pain likely to be caused by peripheral polyneuropathy?
2. What additional diagnostic tests are necessary?

Case 3. A 70-year-old man has had an unsteady gait since an open reduction and internal fixation procedure for a hip fracture 2 months ago. He received physical therapy after discharge, and it helped, but he continues to feel like "any puff of air would blow me over." He has fallen on two occasions when he got up in the middle of the night. He is afraid that he may sustain another fracture if he falls again.

His history is notable for type 2 diabetes, for which he takes metformin. His general physical examination is normal. He has normal mental status, although he is clearly anxious. His cranial nerves are notable only for decreased visual acuity and reduced hearing bilaterally. When the examiner points this out, the patient says that he had been scheduled for cataract surgery, but it was canceled because he fractured his hip 4 days before the operation date. His wife has been urging him to get his hearing checked, but he has been too busy. His gait is tentative, and he limps favoring the side of the surgery, but he needs no support and has no tendency to sway to either side. He has normal coordination and strength throughout all four limbs. His upper extremity reflexes are normal, his knee reflexes are brisk, and ankle reflexes cannot be elicited. His plantar responses are flexor. Vibration sense is absent at the toes, moderately reduced at the ankles, and mildly reduced at the knees. Position sense is reduced at the toes, but normal elsewhere. He can distinguish sharp from dull throughout his body but says a pin feels less sharp in his feet and lower calves than elsewhere.

Questions:

1. What might be responsible for this man's gait disturbance?
2. What diagnostic tests should be done?
3. What interventions are necessary?

II. Geriatric Issues

Three facts distinguish the neurologic assessment of older individuals. First, and most important, people accumulate more diseases the longer they live. Second, some diseases occur primarily in the elderly. Third, even in the absence of any apparent disease, some components of the aging nervous system gradually deteriorate.

One consequence of the first fact is that older people often have numerous symptoms referable to more than one organ system. The standard approach of trying to localize all symptoms to a single lesion is untenable in many cases. Instead, the question is whether the patient has a degenerative disease affecting sites distributed diffusely throughout the nervous system or a combination of unrelated diseases. The neurologic examination provides useful information for answering this question, but accurate interpretation of the examination requires knowledge of the changes that occur during healthy aging.

III. Effects of Aging on the Neurologic Examination

It is harder than one might expect to characterize the changes that normally occur with aging. There is a wide range of variation even among subjects with no known diseases, so a population study is required. The simplest kind of population study to conduct is a cross-sectional study, in which specific features are systematically observed in a random group of healthy people of one age and compared to the same features in a random group of healthy people of a different age. Cross-sectional studies can be misleading, however, because it is difficult to ensure that the groups being compared differ only in age and are identical in all other respects. For example, the elderly group might have a higher proportion of subjects with mild hypertension, cervical stenosis, or subclinical strokes than the younger group. An intended comparison of two "healthy" groups then becomes a comparison of two groups with different (and often unrecognized) disease profiles.

Longitudinal studies are more reliable in this regard, but they are much more difficult to conduct. In a longitudinal study, a single group of randomly selected healthy people is observed serially over many years. Even with this kind of study it is impossible to control for the fact that some members of the group might develop diseases during the period of observation. This would result in overestimation of the changes that occur with normal aging. Conversely, the changes could be underestimated if individuals with changes proved to be more difficult to follow over time. For example, suppose that even in the absence of any disease, 50% of healthy individuals become so absent-minded as they age that they are unable to keep their appointments, whereas memory function remains completely intact in the other half of the population. A study based only on the people who were able to return for regularly scheduled memory testing would conclude that no memory problems occur in normal aging.

Even when a healthy elderly subject demonstrates an abnormality on neurologic examination, its meaning may be ambiguous. It is often difficult to unravel the role played by intrinsic processes in the nervous system and the contribution of other, non-neurologic factors. For example, changes in gait can be related to fractures, sprains, and peripheral vascular disease as well as neurologic problems. Moreover, even within the nervous system there is interaction between different components. Gait changes may relate to abnormalities of sensation, strength, or coordination. Apparent changes in mental status may simply be due to primary sensory problems, especially hearing loss. Older people may seem to forget things just because they never heard them in the first place, and this can also cause them to ask the same question repeatedly. Speed of response is often important in interpreting the mental status examination, and this can be influenced by motor system problems. One example is parkinsonism, which sometimes causes patients to respond so slowly that examiners assume they don't know the answer and move on to another item.

Despite these limitations, some age-related changes in the "normal" neurologic examination have been consistently identified. All these changes are of relatively low magnitude—the variability between individuals of a given age is much greater than the change that occurs in any individual with aging. Even so, an awareness of these age-related changes is important when interpreting the neurologic examination in older people.

A. Mental Status

The interpretation of age-related changes in the mental status examination is confounded by the deterioration that occurs in other processes (such as hearing loss and motor slowing), as discussed in the preceding paragraphs. Nonetheless, careful testing strategies that minimize these confounding factors permit the following general observations. First, older individuals have difficulty thinking of words but relative sparing of vocabulary (i.e., they are still able to recognize and define words). Second, a generalized slowing of central processing occurs with aging. Third, recent memory and ability to learn new information decline, with relative sparing of remote memory. Note that the boundary between normal aging and mild cognitive impairment (see Chapter 7) is not sharply defined.

B. Cranial Nerves

The most common age-related changes noted in the cranial nerve examination relate to changes in sensory end-organs rather than intrinsic nervous system deterioration. The lens grows less clear and less elastic, the pupil becomes smaller and less elastic, rods and cones decrease in number, and the receptive fields of retinal ganglion cells change. As a result, older subjects have decreased light perception, reduced light/dark adaptation, impaired near vision (presbyopia), and changes in contrast sensitivity and color vision. Similarly, pure tone hearing declines with aging (presbycusis), especially for high-frequency tones, and speech discrimination is diminished. As discussed in Chapter 7 (Part II, Section B), hearing loss is associated with an increased risk of dementia. Taste and smell discrimination often deteriorate slightly with aging also.

As they grow older, people often develop impairment of upward gaze. This is a supranuclear problem, so the vestibulo-ocular reflex elicits full upward excursion even though the subject cannot achieve this voluntarily. The smooth pursuit mechanisms also become less robust with aging, so "jerky" or "saccadic" intrusions during pursuit eye movements are fairly common. Aging is the most common cause of ptosis; it is generally attributed to stretching of the skin and muscles of the eyelids over time, resulting in reduced elasticity.

C. Motor System

The single greatest change in station and gait that occurs with aging is a reduced ability to stand on one leg with the eyes closed. Older subjects have increased postural sway and reduced postural reflexes. They walk with a widened base, a stooped posture, shortened steps, and reduced arm swing, similar to someone with mild Parkinson disease.

Older subjects are less coordinated when manipulating small objects. They are mildly uncoordinated without frank dysmetria when performing finger-to-nose and heel-knee-shin testing. Their movements are slowed compared to younger subjects. Postural and kinetic tremors are increasingly common with advancing age.

Muscle bulk declines with age, especially in the intrinsic muscles of the hands and feet. Power is also reduced. The EMG reveals changes consistent with partial denervation and reinnervation. Paratonia is common in the elderly.

D. Reflexes

Deep tendon reflexes become less brisk as people age, with a distal-to-proximal gradient, although at least 80% of truly healthy elderly subjects still have detectable ankle reflexes. Babinski signs are rare in healthy people, regardless of age. All the so-called primitive reflexes (grasp, snout, root, suck, and palmomental) increase in prevalence with age, but except for the grasp reflex, all of them are sometimes present in younger healthy subjects, also.

E. Sensation

Ability to sense vibration declines with age, again with a distal-to-proximal gradient. Healthy subjects who are more than 70 years of age are often unable to detect vibration at the toes. Position, light touch, and pain sensation also deteriorate, but to a lesser degree.

IV. Common Neurologic Symptoms in the Elderly

A. Dizziness

As discussed in Chapter 14, it is difficult and often futile to try to characterize what people mean when they say they are dizzy. These difficulties are magnified in older people, who frequently have several coexisting problems. Arrhythmia, congestive heart failure, and orthostatic hypotension can all contribute to cerebral hypoperfusion, and they are all common in the geriatric population. Many of the medications that are prescribed to older patients can cause either hypotension or vertigo. The likelihood of ischemic disease in the posterior circulation increases with advancing age. Many age-related changes in sensory function, including visual, auditory, and proprioceptive deterioration, can result in disequilibrium. When an elderly individual reports dizziness or disequilibrium, it is usually wise to consider all of these potential underlying conditions simultaneously. In many instances, dizziness is determined to be a result of many different abnormalities, each of which, in isolation, would be too mild to produce appreciable symptoms.

B. Gait Disturbance

The most common factors in older individuals with gait difficulty are cervical stenosis, polyneuropathy, and mechanical problems such as fractures. All the causes of dizziness and disequilibrium discussed in the preceding paragraph can also interfere with walking. Other potential causes of gait disturbance that must be considered in elderly patients include parkinsonism, strokes (causing focal weakness, spasticity, or ataxia), cerebellar deterioration (often from chronic alcohol use), and subdural hematomas (acute or chronic). Normal pressure hydrocephalus is uncommon but is worth considering because of the potential for improvement with treatment. As with dizziness, extensive evaluation of elderly patients with gait problems often reveals multiple potential causes, each of which by itself would produce only minimal symptoms but when combined cause serious impairment.

C. Incontinence

Elderly people who are incontinent should be evaluated according to the principles presented in Chapter 16. The evaluation can be particularly difficult in people with dementia, who often have difficulty providing the historical information necessary to distinguish a spastic from a flaccid bladder. In these individuals, diagnosis may depend on associated symptoms, physical examination findings, and results of urodynamic studies. Dementia can result in incontinence because of impairment of the normal cortical inhibition of the micturition reflex, but other causes of incontinence must also be considered. Incontinence may be the only symptom of prostatic hypertrophy or a urinary tract infection in someone with dementia. Medications frequently contribute to the problem, also. Because gait impairment is so common in the elderly, many older people have functional incontinence caused by an inability to reach the bathroom in time. Again, the problem often proves to be a combination of many slight abnormalities, none of them severe enough in isolation to cause notable symptoms. The most important practical objective is to determine whether any of the factors contributing to the incontinence are treatable.

D. Dementia

The most common dementing illnesses occur primarily in the elderly population, so the points made in Chapter 7 do not need modification here.

E. Pain

The principles of evaluation and management of painful conditions are the same in the elderly as in younger people, except that older individuals are more likely to have more than one painful condition simultaneously. Many chronic painful conditions are incurable, and over time these may combine with accumulated injuries and mechanical stress on the musculoskeletal system to the point where some older people experience constant or debilitating pain. Depression may intensify pain and complicate management. Depression is common in the elderly, and chronic pain may itself lead to depression. In addition, older people have heightened sensitivity to the side effects of drugs, and patients with several chronic conditions are often taking multiple medications. As a result, they can develop confusion or depression, further complicating pain management.

A few painful conditions occur exclusively or more commonly in older patients. Polymyalgia rheumatica (with or without giant cell arteritis), postherpetic neuralgia, and trigeminal neuralgia are examples.

V. Discussion of Case Histories

Case 1. Although it is true that people with Alzheimer disease may be incontinent, other potential causes, especially prostate hypertrophy and urinary tract infections, should always be considered. This is particularly true in someone whose cognitive deficits are as mild as this man's. In this case, the examination strongly suggests a spinal cord lesion. There are unambiguous upper motor neuron findings in the lower extremities, indicating a lesion above the lumbar region of the spinal cord. The brisk triceps reflexes further localize the lesion to above the C7 level, whereas the diminished brachioradialis and biceps reflexes indicate that the lesion is not above C5. In short, the reflexes alone localize the lesion to the C5 or C6 level of the spinal cord. The sensory examination cannot be performed in enough detail in this patient to provide precise localizing information, but the suggestion of a sensory level is at least consistent with a spinal cord lesion. Since the patient and his family don't even seem concerned about his gait disturbance, it probably developed gradually, but his urinary symptoms are new, indicating that the spinal cord lesion is getting worse. He needs an MRI scan of the cervical spine as soon as possible. The most likely cause of cervical myelopathy in this age group is compression from herniated discs or osteophytes. Despite his age and dementia, surgery is a realistic option. He appears to be active, productive, and happy; if he were paraplegic, his quality of life would deteriorate markedly and the cost of his medical and nonmedical care would rise dramatically.

If the MRI scan shows a mass lesion unrelated to degenerative disease, the imaging characteristics will determine subsequent evaluation and management (including a search for a primary cancer if the mass looks like metastatic disease, and possible steroid treatment and radiation therapy). If no mass lesion is found, nonstructural causes of myelopathy should be considered. These include vitamin B12 deficiency, thyroid disease, and neurosyphilis. Motor neuron disease is another consideration, but it would be more likely if there were evidence of lower motor neuron dysfunction at a level below C6. The suggestion of a sensory level also reduces the likelihood of motor neuron disease. The triad of incontinence, gait disturbance, and dementia invokes the possibility of normal pressure hydrocephalus, but this diagnosis is unlikely in someone with evidence for myelopathy on examination. Similarly, vascular cognitive impairment is a consideration in someone with focal neurologic signs and dementia, but vascular cognitive impairment would not explain the reflex gradient or the possible sensory level.

Case 2. This woman's pain is located in her joints, not in her distal extremities, so the cause is much more likely to be joint disease than peripheral polyneuropathy. The examination findings of absent ankle reflexes and decreased distal vibratory sensation are not uncommon in the elderly. Without any other examination findings or symptoms suggestive of peripheral polyneuropathy, there is no need to evaluate for it. The focus should be on evaluating and managing her joint disease.

Case 3. This man has many problems that could potentially contribute to disequilibrium. He has impaired vision, presumably caused by cataracts. He also has hearing impairment that is probably caused by end-organ degeneration, suggesting that his vestibular end-organ might be similarly affected. Note that he did not think to mention his cataracts or hearing loss when asked about his medical history—most patients don't. You should get in the habit of asking elderly patients about cataracts, glaucoma, and hearing loss explicitly, not just with open-ended questions. This man also has reduced position sense in the lower extremities, probably due to peripheral polyneuropathy in view of the other findings on his examination. All of these sensory deficits can interfere with his ability to determine the position of his body relative to the environment, so they could all be contributing to his gait disturbance.

In addition, this man now has an impaired motor response because of the mechanical limitations imposed by his hip fracture (which may have resulted from a fall caused by his unsteady gait—further questioning would be necessary to determine the cause). A hint of an upper motor neuron lesion exists as well, because his knee reflexes are brisk despite evidence for a peripheral polyneuropathy. The most likely cause would be cervical myelopathy from degenerative disease. Finally, psychological factors now seem to be playing a significant role in limiting his gait. He appears to be nervous about walking even though he is not particularly unsteady.

It may prove impossible to identify which of these problems is primarily responsible for the patient's gait impairment. Indeed, each of the problems seems to be fairly mild and in isolation would be unlikely to produce significant disability. All of the problems should be addressed and treated to the extent possible. You should urge him to follow through with the cataract surgery and also to be evaluated for hearing aids. Although the polyneuropathy is probably due to his diabetes, other potential causes should be explored, especially thyroid disease and vitamin B12 deficiency, because these two treatable conditions can cause both polyneuropathy and myelopathy. With no evidence of myelopathy other than the brisk knee reflexes, no surgery would be indicated even if he had significant degenerative disease of the cervical spine, but an MRI scan would still be reasonable to be sure he doesn't have spinal metastases. Finally, he should receive additional physical therapy to increase his confidence while walking and to prevent deconditioning. If the evaluation reveals no evidence of severe ongoing disease, you should make a point of reassuring him. Anxiety about another fall can cause some people to restrict their walking so much that they ultimately develop disuse atrophy that is a more serious limitation than any of their original problems.

Chapter 19

Practice Cases

I. Case Histories

For each of the following cases, answer the following questions:

1. Is the lesion focal, multifocal, or diffuse?
2. What is the temporal profile?
3. What diagnostic category is most likely?
4. What is the most likely diagnosis?

Case 1. A 55-year-old woman came to the emergency room because of trouble speaking. She had some pain behind her left ear yesterday, but was otherwise fine until this morning, when she noted that water was leaking out of the left side of her mouth as she was brushing her teeth. Several hours later, while on the phone, she realized that her words were slurred. She looked in the mirror and saw that the left side of her face was drooping. She came immediately to the emergency department. On examination, she has weakness of eye closure, smile, and forehead wrinkling on the left side of her face. She has mild, flaccid dysarthria. The rest of her examination is normal.

Case 2. A 72-year-old right-handed man came to see his primary care physician because of trouble speaking. He is not sure exactly when it began, but he thinks it was less than 4 months ago, because at that time he delivered an important speech and neither he nor anyone else noted any problems. Over the past 2 months or so, his speech has grown progressively more slurred, to the point where he has stopped speaking on the telephone. In the past few weeks, he has also choked while drinking water on several occasions. On examination, he has marked dysarthria, with both spastic and flaccid components. His tongue is atrophic, with prominent fasciculations. He also has some fasciculations in his quadriceps and deltoid muscles bilaterally. He has diffuse hyperreflexia and bilateral Babinski signs.

Case 3. A 3-year-old boy was brought to the pediatrician because of trouble speaking. He attempts only single-word utterances, and his speech is loud, harsh, and imprecise. His other developmental milestones are also very delayed compared to his older sister. He has no other siblings. On examination, he has a long face, with prominent ears. He avoids eye contact, and says only a few, poorly articulated words. He does not follow directions. There are no focal abnormalities on his examination.

Case 4. A 56-year-old woman came to her physician because of trouble speaking. She first noticed the problem about 2 years ago, but when she mentioned it to her husband he told her she was just being neurotic. The problem has progressed slowly but steadily, to the point where her husband now acknowledges it. Her examination is notable for marked dysnomia, labored speech, and frequent paraphasic errors. Her mental status is otherwise normal, and so is the rest of her examination.

Case 5. A 58-year-old person who identifies as nonbinary has come to the physician because of lower extremity pain. They initially noted tingling in their toes about 8 months ago, but this gradually spread to involve both feet, and over the past month it has spread above the ankles about a third of the way to the knees. The pain has a burning quality, and they have a very hard time falling asleep. They have not noticed any weakness. Their examination is notable for obesity, slight weakness of ankle dorsiflexion bilaterally, reduced knee reflexes, absent ankle reflexes, and reduced sensation to all modalities from the mid-calf down, worse distally.

Case 6. A 72-year-old woman has come to the physician because of lower extremity pain. She has no problems when she is sitting or lying down, but within a minute of standing she develops severe pain in her thighs and calves bilaterally. This problem has been getting gradually worse over the past 9 months. She has found that bending over a shopping cart relieves the pain to some degree. She continues to swim half a mile each day, and this does not cause her any pain. Her examination is normal.

Case 7. A 29-year-old man has come to the physician because of involuntary movements. The problem began about a year ago and has been getting gradually worse. His neck feels as if it is being pulled to the right.

He can overcome the pulling if he tries hard enough, but he finds it very painful. Superimposed on the chronic deviation to the right, he has intermittent jerking movements of the head in that direction. His examination is normal except for his head position.

Case 8. A 69-year-old woman has come to the physician because of involuntary movements. They never happen during the day, but sometimes in the middle of the night while she's sleeping she suddenly begins thrashing wildly with her arms. She has fallen out of bed on a few occasions. During one of these episodes, her husband shook her awake, and she told him that she had been dreaming that burglars had broken into the house and were trying to tie her up. She has had this problem for at least 15 years, but it has been getting worse, and has now reached the point where her husband will no longer sleep in the same bed. Her husband is also concerned about her memory. Her examination is notable for mild dementia, cogwheel rigidity at both wrists, a stooped posture, short steps, and slow turning.

Case 9. A 27-year-old man has come to the physician because of visual symptoms. The problem began 4 months ago, but resolved by the next morning, and since that time he has had about five episodes in all, each lasting 2 days or less. The episodes consist of double vision, which resolves if he closes either eye. He has also noticed that the two images tend to be much farther apart later in the day. His examination is notable for ptosis of the left eyelid and trouble maintaining upward gaze for more than 30 seconds.

Case 10. A 33-year-old woman has come to the physician because of visual symptoms. Her vision starts to "tunnel down" to the point where everything is momentarily black, and returns to normal within 15 seconds. These episodes can occur at any time, but she has noticed that they are particularly likely to happen when she first stands up from a chair. She has had this problem for 5 months, and during that time she has also had a dull, constant headache. Her examination is notable for obesity and bilateral optic disc swelling.

Case 11. A 52-year-old man has come to the emergency department because of trouble using his left hand. He has had intermittent tingling in the fourth and fifth fingers of his left hand for more than a year, and for the past month the tingling has been continuous. His left hand has been getting gradually weaker over the past month, and over the past 2 weeks he has noticed that the hand is shrinking. He has no neck pain. His examination is notable for atrophy and weakness of the intrinsic muscles of his left hand, with reduced sensation to all modalities in the fourth and fifth digits of that hand. Percussion at the left elbow exacerbates the tingling in his fourth and fifth fingers (Tinel sign).

Case 12. A 22-year-old woman has come to the emergency department because of trouble using her left hand. She had experienced some neck pain for the past few weeks, but it had responded to chiropractic manipulation, and she was otherwise fine until about 10 a.m. today, when she suddenly dropped her coffee cup. When she tried to clean up the mess, she discovered that she could not control her left hand. She came immediately to the emergency department, where her examination reveals marked ataxia of the left upper extremity and mild ataxia of the left lower extremity. Her strength, reflexes, and sensation are normal, as are her mental status and cranial nerves. She has no history of previous medical problems, takes no medications (including contraceptive medications), and does not smoke.

II. Answers

Case 1.

1. focal (left facial nerve)
2. acute
3. vascular
4. Bell palsy

Comment: This is a situation in which the principles of Chapter 3 lead to the wrong diagnostic category—Bell palsy is thought to be an inflammatory condition, not a vascular one. The principles lead to the correct diagnostic approach, however, because vascular disease must always be considered in a patient with acute facial weakness. Patients must be examined carefully for additional neurologic findings (especially weakness or numbness of the ipsilateral arm and leg) before diagnosing Bell palsy. This patient had a completely normal examination except for her left facial weakness. She received a prescription for a 10-day course of prednisolone and instructions for eye care to prevent corneal injury. Her face continued to get weaker for a day, then reached a plateau. It started to improve 3 weeks later and returned to baseline over the subsequent 4 weeks.

Case 2.

1. diffuse (upper motor neurons and lower motor neurons)
2. chronic
3. degenerative
4. ALS

Comment: This patient was started on riluzole and BiPAP, but developed aspiration pneumonia about a month after his disease was diagnosed. In accordance with his advance directives, he was treated with antibiotics but not intubated, and when his respiratory function continued to deteriorate he was given opiates to minimize his discomfort. He died shortly thereafter.

Case 3.

1. diffuse (supratentorial)
2. chronic
3. congenital-developmental
4. fragile X syndrome

Comment: Although the craniofacial abnormalities suggested fragile X syndrome, this boy had careful testing for hearing impairment and other potentially treatable causes of developmental delay. Genetic testing eventually confirmed the presumptive diagnosis of fragile X syndrome, and he was enrolled in a therapy program directed at speech, language, and behavioral problems. His parents were also provided with extensive counseling, including genetic counseling.

Case 4.

1. focal (left frontal lobe)
2. chronic
3. neoplasm
4. frontotemporal dementia

Comment: This is another situation in which the principles of Chapter 3 lead to the wrong diagnostic category, but the correct diagnostic approach, because neoplasm must be considered in any patient with a progressive focal lesion. In this patient, an MRI scan was normal except for mild left frontal atrophy. The syndrome of nonfluent/agrammatic progressive aphasia can occur in patients with PSP, CBD, or, less commonly, FTD. A PET scan showed prominent abnormalities in the left frontal and temporal lobes, and the patient had no eye movement abnormalities, parkinsonian features, or other motor abnormalities, so she was diagnosed with FTD. This patient and her husband were counseled regarding the diagnosis, prognosis, and techniques for facilitating her communication.

Case 5.

1. diffuse (sensory and motor peripheral nerves)
2. chronic
3. toxic-metabolic
4. polyneuropathy

Comment: This patient had a normal fasting glucose, but an abnormal 2-hour glucose tolerance test. The results of all other tests for common causes of polyneuropathy were normal. They were diagnosed as having impaired glucose tolerance and counseled regarding exercise and diet. Studies have shown that patients with impaired glucose tolerance who adhere to dietary modification and a regular exercise program are less likely to progress to overt diabetes during the follow-up period; these measures also produce a short-term improvement in small-fiber nerve function and a more sustained benefit with respect to pain.

Case 6.

1. focal (cauda equina/lumbosacral nerve roots)
2. chronic
3. neoplasm
4. lumbar spinal stenosis

Comment: As discussed in Chapter 3, structural disease of the spine is another situation in which the diagnostic principles lead to the wrong diagnosis but the right approach. This patient's lumbar MRI scan showed no neoplasm, but significant lumbar spinal stenosis. She responded well to surgery.

Case 7.

1. focal (though specific site unknown – left basal ganglia?)
2. chronic
3. neoplasm
4. cervical dystonia (spasmodic torticollis)

Comment: The failure to reach the correct diagnostic category in this case is hardly an indictment of the principles of Chapter 3, because the etiology of dystonia remains unknown. This patient had an excellent response to botulinum toxin injections, and said that only after he started "to feel normal again" did he appreciate how much his symptoms had been limiting his activity.

Case 8.

1. diffuse (basal ganglia and cerebral cortex bilaterally)

2. chronic

3. degenerative

4. REM sleep behavior disorder as a component of DLB (dementia with Lewy bodies)

Comment: Her history was classic for REM sleep behavior disorder, and a polysomnogram confirmed the diagnosis. This syndrome often pre-cedes other manifestations of degenerative disease by years or decades, as it did in this case. Her sleep disorder responded to a low dose of clonazepam at bedtime. Her examination also revealed dementia and parkinsonism, consistent with DLB. This can be difficult to distinguish from Parkinson disease (PD), but when people with PD develop demen-tia it is usually later in the course, whereas this woman's parkinsonism is mild, to the point where she and her husband don't even seem to be aware of it. She was given a prescription for donepezil; she and her husband thought that it made her thinking a little sharper, but the effect was not dramatic.

Case 9.

1. multifocal (neuromuscular junction)

2. intermittent

3. inflammatory

4. myasthenia gravis

Comment: Because this patient's symptoms are intermittent, the prin-ciples summarized in Table 3.1 do not apply. The purely motor manifes-tations, the predilection for ocular muscles, the intermittent time course, and the worsening at the end of the day all suggest myasthenia gravis. His symptoms responded to pyridostigmine. A thymectomy was recom-mended, but deferred.

Case 10.

1. focal (increased intracranial pressure)

2. chronic

3. neoplasm

4. idiopathic intracranial hypertension (IIH, pseudotumor cerebri)

Comment: It may seem strange to think of this case as focal, because the symptoms and signs were symmetric, but it is probably best to consider increased intracranial pressure focal until proven otherwise, with the assumption that a focal lesion has interrupted the flow of CSF or the brain's venous outflow. In fact, that is the basis for the previous name, pseudotumor—this condition mimics a tumor. An MRI scan was normal, and a lumbar puncture revealed an opening pressure of 300 mm of water (normal opening pressure is 180 mm or less). This patient's symptoms responded to acetazolamide. She managed to lose 55 pounds over the next 2 years, at which point the medication was successfully tapered.

Case 11.

1. focal (left ulnar nerve)

2. chronic

3. neoplasm

4. compression neuropathy of ulnar nerve at the elbow (cubital tunnel syndrome)

Comment: This patient's sensory and motor symptoms could be consistent with a lesion either of the ulnar nerve or of the C8 nerve root, but the fact that the symptoms could be reproduced by percussion at the elbow is strong evidence for an ulnar nerve lesion, because the elbow is the most common site of ulnar nerve compression. This is another situation in which "neoplasm" must be understood in its most general sense ("new growth"). Although cancer is certainly in the differential, connective tissue is responsible for the compression in most cases. Conservative therapy with protective elbow padding is usually adequate, but the rapid progression of weakness in this patient prompted his physician to recommend surgical decompression. His sensory symptoms resolved soon after the surgery, and his strength gradually returned to baseline.

Case 12.

1. focal (left cerebellar hemisphere)

2. acute

3. vascular (ischemic)

4. stroke, likely due to vertebral artery dissection

Comment: A stroke in a young person with no cardiovascular risk factors raises the possibility of less common causes. In this case, the recent chiropractic manipulation suggested the possibility of arterial dissection, which was confirmed with MRI/MRA scanning. Fortunately, her symptoms improved considerably over the next 48 hours, and they completely resolved over the following week. She was treated with aspirin.

Index

For the benefit of digital users, indexed terms that span two pages (e.g., 52–53) may, on occasion, appear on only one of those pages.

Tables and figures are indicated by *t* and *f* following the page number

AADC (aromatic L-amino acid decarboxylase), 281
ABCs (airway, breathing, circulation), 381–82
Abdominal pain, periodic, 475–76
Abdominal reflexes, 60
Abducens nerve (cranial nerve VI), 384
  assessment of, in altered level of consciousness, 96–98
  lesions of, 430–32, 433
Aβ-peptide (beta amyloid)
  accumulations in AD, 249–51, 250*f*, 253–54, 255, 298*t*
  accumulations in IBM, 229
  accumulations in movement disorders, 283, 298*t*
Abscess(es)
  case histories, 117–18
  CNS, 333–35
  definition of, 333
  dementia and, 244
  increased ICP and, 392
Absence seizures, 476
  case histories, 165, 198, 468, 483
  childhood absence epilepsy, 180
  clinical characteristics of, 170
  EEG pattern, 173, 483
  management of, 189–90, 194*t*, 197*t*
Abstraction, 52
Abulia, 62
Acalculia, 62, 74
  case histories, 108–9, 118, 239

ACA (anterior cerebral artery) occlusion, 129*f*, 130*t*, 132
Accessory nerve (cranial nerve XI), 83
ACE inhibitors. *See* Angiotensin converting enzyme inhibitors
Acetaminophen (Tylenol), 413–14, 419*t*
Acetaminophen/aspirin/caffeine (Excedrin, Excedrin Migraine), 419*t*
Acetaminophen/butalbital/caffeine (Fioricet, Esgic), 419*t*
Acetaminophen/codeine, 419*t*
Acetazolamide (Diamox), 289, 313–14, 405–6, 502
Acetylcholine receptor antibodies, 224, 235
Acetylcholinesterase inhibitors, 225–26, 254. *See also* Cholinesterase inhibitors
Achilles (ankle) reflexes, 59, 91
Actigraphy, 310–11
Action tremor, 273, 276
Activated protein C, 361–62
Acupuncture, 452
Acute ataxia, 478–79
Acute disseminated encephalomyelitis (ADEM), 355
Acute idiopathic unilateral peripheral vestibulopathy, 444–45
Acute inflammatory demyelinating polyradiculoneuropathy (AIDP), 220–22
  common features of, 232*t*
  emergency measures for, 230
  in HIV-positive patients, 336–37

Acute ischemic optic neuropathy, 428
Acute labyrinthitis, 444
Acute mental status changes, 377–94
    approach to, 381–88
    case histories, 109, 377–78, 393–94
    definitions, 378–79
    with headache, 410
    special circumstances, 388–93
Acute monocular vision loss
    in older people, 428–29
    in young people, 427–28
Acute motor axonal neuropathy
    (AMAN), 232t
Acute motor-sensory axonal neuropathy
    (AMSAN), 232t
Acute myelitis, 355–56
Acute myocardial infarction, 144–45
Acute peripheral vestibulopathy, 444–45
Acute sinusitis, 408
Acute stroke
    management of, 134–39
    neurologic complications of, 136–38
    rehabilitation for, 138–39
    restoration of blood flow in, 134–36
    systemic factors, 138
Acute symptoms, 111, 115t
    case histories, 116, 118–19
    in toxic and metabolic
        diseases, 113–14
    in vascular diseases, 113
Acute traumatic disorders, 114
Acute vestibular syndrome, 444–45
Acyclovir
    for Bell palsy, 217–18
    for HSE, 345, 403
    for meningitis or encephalitis, 116–17
    for VZV, 346
    for zoster ophthalmicus, 346
Addisonian crisis, 388
ADEM (acute disseminated
    encephalomyelitis), 355
Adenosine, 310
Adenosine A$_{2A}$ receptor antagonists,
    281–82, 297t
ADHD. See Attention deficit-
    hyperactivity disorder
Adrenergic agonists, 286–87
Adrenoleukodystrophy, 467, 483–84
Aducanumab, 255
Advance directives, 230, 256–57, 499
Advanced sleep-wake phase disorder,
    319
Advil (ibuprofen), 419t

AEDs (antiepileptic drugs). See
    Antiseizure medications (ASMs)
Afferent pupillary defects, 76–78, 79f,
    371–72, 427
    case histories, 425, 433–34
Aging, normal, 487–90
Agitation
    in AD, 252, 256
    after seizure, 387
    case histories, 237–38, 377, 393–94
Agnosia, 62
Agraphia, 63, 74
Agrin, 222
AIDP. See Acute inflammatory
    demyelinating
    polyradiculoneuropathy
AIDS, 336–37, 339
Aimovig (erenumab), 420t
Airway, breathing, circulation
    (ABCs), 381–82
Airway protection, 138
Ajovy (fremanezumab), 420t
Akinesia, 273
Alcohol
    and ataxia, 479
    chronic use, 491
    and early morning awakening, 318
    and myopathy, 227
    polyneuropathy associated with, 220
    and seizures, 179
    and stroke, 156–57
Alcohol intoxication, 389–90
Alcohol withdrawal, 182, 383
Alemtuzumab (Lemtrada), 356–57, 366t
Alertness. See Consciousness
Aleve (naproxen), 419t, 420t
Alexia, 63, 74
    in stroke, 130t, 132
Alien limb phenomenon, 285
Allodynia, 204–5
Almotriptan (Axert), 419t
Alpha-adrenergic agonists, 286–87,
    299t, 460
α-secretase, 249–50, 250f
Alpha tocopherol (vitamin E), 254–55
ALS. See Amyotrophic lateral sclerosis
Alteplase, 134
Altered level of consciousness
    bihemispheric disease, 116–17
    case histories, 116–17
    in DLB, 257
    examination of, 94–98
    vs focal mental status changes, 379

lesion localization, 42–43
physiology of, 380–81
temporary loss of consciousness, 177–78
Altered mental status. *See* Mental status
changes
Alternating movements, rapid, 57
Alzheimer disease (AD), 75, 112, 248–57
case histories, 118, 237–38, 269–70,
485–86, 492–93
characteristic protein
accumulations, 298*t*
characteristic protein aggregates, 267*t*
clinical features of, 251–52, 267*t*
course of, 252
diagnostic tests for, 252–54
differential diagnosis of, 257–58
epidemiology of, 248–51
etiology of, 248–51
mutations when familial, 267*t*
pathology of, 248–51
prevalence of, 248
treatment of, xxi, 254–57, 258
AMAN (acute motor axonal
neuropathy), 232*t*
Amantadine (Symmetrel, Gocovri,
Osmolex), 281–82, 297*t*, 299*t*, 357
Amaurosis fugax, 128
Ambien (zolpidem), 317–18
Amerge (naratriptan), 419*t*
Aminoglycosides, 225, 349
Aminophylline, 179, 406–7
Amiodarone, 276, 279–80
Amitriptyline, 420*t*, 421*t*
Amnesia, 63, 344–45, 389–90
Amphetamine-dextroamphetamine,
468–69, 483
Amphetamines, 384*t*, 387
Amphotericin, 338–39
Ampicillin, 399
AMSAN (acute motor-sensory axonal
neuropathy), 232*t*
Amyloid angiopathy, cerebral, 126
Amyloid cascade hypothesis, 251, 255
Amyloid plaques, 249–50, 283
Amyloid precursor protein (APP), 249–
50, 250*f*
Amyloid-related imaging abnormalities
(ARIA), 255
Amyotrophic lateral sclerosis (ALS),
209–12, 235
dementia and, 258–59
flowchart for identifying, 207*f*
Analgesics, 179, 419*t*

Anatomic definitions, 272–73
ANCA (antineutrophil cytoplasmic
autoantibody), 359
Anemia, iron-deficiency, 476–77
Anesthesia, 204–5
Anesthesia dolorosa, 415
Anesthetics, 346, 452
Aneurysms
case histories, 118
clipping, 151–52, 335, 400–2
coiling into, 151–52, 335, 400–2
mycotic, 335
saccular or berry, 126
thrombosis of, 151–52
Angiitis, 360
Angiography
computed tomography (*see* Computed
tomography angiography [CTA])
digital subtraction, 400–2
intra-arterial, 134, 150–51
magnetic resonance (*see* Magnetic
resonance angiography [MRA])
Angiomas, 126
Angioplasty, carotid, 147, 156
Angiotensin converting enzyme
(ACE), 360–61
Angiotensin converting enzyme (ACE)
inhibitors, 140*t*, 152–53, 162–
63, 420*t*
Angiotensin receptor blockers (ARBs),
140*t*, 152–53, 420*t*
Anisocoria (asymmetric pupils), 75–76,
77*f*, 105
Ankle dorsiflexion
nerve roots and peripheral nerves
corresponding to, 85, 87*f*, 105
testing, 58
weakness, 33–34, 45, 327–28, 457–
58, 462–63
Ankle plantar flexion, 58
nerve roots and peripheral nerves
corresponding to, 85, 87*f*
weakness, 328, 449
Ankle (Achilles) reflexes, 59, 91
ANNA-1 (antineuronal nuclear antibody-
1), 270, 364*t*
ANNA-2 (antineuronal nuclear antibody-
2), 364*t*
Anomia, 30*f*, 30–33, 63
Anosognosia, 63, 74–75, 423
Anterior cerebral artery (ACA) occlusion,
129*f*, 130*t*, 132
Anterior circulation, 125

Anterior horn cells, 205
Anthrax, 348
Anti-arrhythmics, 225
Antibiotics, 334, 335, 371, 399–400
Antibody assays, 209, 234–35, 332–33
Anticardiolipin antibody, 361–62
Anticholinergics
  for dystonia, 299*t*
  for incontinence, 461
  for PD, 281–83, 297*t*
  side effects of, 269, 384*t*, 387
Anticoagulation therapy. *See also*
    Warfarin
  for arterial dissection, 407
  avoid use, 371
  for cerebral venous thrombosis, 407
  for stroke prevention, 136, 144, 145,
    148–49, 151, 154–55, 161
Antidepressants
  for behavior disorder, 299*t*
  for post-concussion syndrome, 409
  side effects of, 179, 316, 320–21, 323
  tricyclic (*see* Tricyclic antidepressants)
Antidopaminergic drugs, 299*t*
Antiemetics
  for headache, 413–14, 419*t*, 420*t*
  for movement disorders, 279–80
  for vertigo, 442–43, 444–45
Antiepileptic drugs (AEDs). *See*
    Antiseizure medications (ASMs)
Antihistamines
  for acute peripheral
    vestibulopathy, 444–45
  for headache, 420*t*
  side effects of, 269, 316, 320–21, 479
Antihypertensives
  for hypertension, 152–53
  side effects of, 269, 316, 324
Antimuscarinics, 281–82, 461, 462*t*
Antineuronal nuclear antibody-1
    (ANNA-1), 270, 364*t*
Antineuronal nuclear antibody-2
    (ANNA-2), 364*t*
Antineutrophil cytoplasmic autoantibody
    (ANCA), 359
Antiphospholipid antibodies, 149, 361–62
Antiplatelet therapy
  for arterial dissection, 407
  for stroke prevention, 136, 140*t*, 142,
    144, 148–49, 154
Antipsychotics
  for agitation in AD, 256
  for Huntington disease, 299*t*

sensitivity to, 257, 258
side effects of, 179, 279–80, 283
for tics, 299*t*
Antiretroviral therapy (ART), 336–
    37, 338–39
Antiseizure medications (ASMs), 182–85
  broad-spectrum, 183
  drug interactions, 191–92
  for dysesthesia, 230
  for headache, 413–14, 420*t*
  for musculoskeletal pain, 452
  for neuropathic pain, 230
  rationale for not starting, 188
  risks and benefits, 188
  for seizures, 137, 179, 182–85, 192*t*,
    194*t*, 331
  for shingles, 346
  side effects of, 316
  for status epilepticus, 182, 189–
    90, 197*t*
  teratogenic effects of, 199–200, 413–14
  toxicity, 479
Antisynthetase syndrome, 227–28, 233*t*,
    234–35
Antithrombotic therapy, 154–55
Antitoxin administration, 225–26
Anxiety, 446, 494
Aortic arch disease, 149
Aortic stenosis, 177
APAP (autoadjusting positive airway
    pressure), 313–14
Apathy, 469
Aphasia, 63
  Broca, 30*f*, 30–33, 63
  case histories, 107, 116, 327, 370–71
  classification of, 30*f*, 30–33
  conduction, 30*f*, 30–33, 63
  expressive, 64
  fluent, 63
  global, 30*f*, 30–33
  in herpes simplex encephalitis, 344–45
  lesion localization, 42
  mixed transcortical, 30*f*, 30–33, 74
  nonfluent, 64
  primary progressive (PPA), 246–47,
    258–59, 266*t*
  receptive, 64
  in stroke, 129–32, 130*t*, 143
  terminology for, 65–66
  transcortical, 64, 74
  transcortical motor, 30*f*, 30–33, 74
  transcortical sensory, 30*f*, 30–33, 74
  Wernicke, 30*f*, 30–33, 64, 74

Aphemia, 63
Apixaban, 140*t*, 144, 161–62
Apnea. *See* Sleep apnea
Apokyn (apomorphine), 297*t*
Apolipoprotein E (ApoE), 248, 253–54
Apomorphine (Apokyn, Kynmobi), 297*t*
Apoptosis, 127
APP (amyloid precursor protein), 249–50, 250*f*
Apraxia, 63, 74
    oculomotor, 288
    progressive, of speech, 247
Aptiom (eslicarbazepine), 192*t*, 421*t*
Aquaporin-4 antibody, 355–56, 358–59
Arboviruses, 403
ARBs (angiotensin receptor blockers), 152–53, 420*t*
ARIA (amyloid-related imaging abnormalities), 255
Aricept (donepezil), 254, 313–14
Aripiprazole, 299*t*
Armodafinil (Nuvigil), 313–14, 315–16
Arm weakness
    case histories, 107–8, 117, 123–24
    lesion localization, 45
    in stroke, 123–24, 129–32, 130*t*
    weakness, 327
Aromatic L-amino acid decarboxylase (AADC), 281
Arousal
    confusional, 320–21
    mediation of, 380
Arrhythmias, 177, 226–27, 230
ART (antiretroviral therapy), 336–37, 338–39
Artane (trihexyphenidyl), 297*t*
Arterial dissection, 148–49, 407
    case histories, 498, 503
Arteriolosclerosis, 125, 126
Arteriovenous malformations (AVMs), 126
Artificial urinary sphincter, 460
Artificial valves, 334–35
ASCVD. *See* Atherosclerotic cardiovascular disease
Aseptic meningitis, 340–41, 358, 359
ASMs. *See* Antiseizure medications
Aspiration pneumonia, 236
Aspirin
    for headache, 395–96, 419*t*, 420*t*, 423
    for stroke, 123, 136, 140*t*, 142, 144–45, 148, 156–57, 161–63, 503

Aspirin/acetaminophen/caffeine (Excedrin, Excedrin Migraine), 419*t*
Aspirin/butalbital/caffeine (Fiorinal), 419*t*
Atacand (candesartan), 420*t*
Ataxia
    case histories, 109, 118–19, 435–36, 468, 481–82, 498, 503
    in children, 468, 478–79, 481–82
    definition of, 273
    episodic, 289
    fragile X-associated tremor/ataxia syndrome (FXTAS), 289–90, 473
    Friedreich, 287, 299*t*, 479
    hereditary, 287–90
    medications for, 299*t*
    in MS, 349–50
    in MSA, 286
    postinfectious, 468, 478–79, 481
    spinocerebellar, 288–89
    in stroke, 130*t*, 132
    in syphilis, 340
    in tuberculous meningitis, 343
Ataxia telangiectasia, 288, 479
Ataxia telangiectasia mutated *(ATM)* gene, 288
Ataxic movement disorders, 274–75
Atenolol (Tenormin), 420*t*
Atherosclerotic cardiovascular disease (ASCVD)
    case histories, 162–63
    lipid management, 175
    risk calculators, 153–54
    risk factors, 143
Athetosis, 57–58
    choreoathetosis, 288, 294
    definition of, 273
    pseudoathetosis, 205
ATM (ataxia telangiectasia mutated) gene, 288
Atogepant (Qulipta), 420*t*
Atomoxetine, 299*t*, 313–14
Atonia
    in cataplexy, 314
    of REM sleep, 319
    in sleep paralysis, 315
Atonic seizures, 170, 194*t*
Atorvastatin, 140*t*, 161–63
ATP7B, 295
Atrial fibrillation
    case histories, 118–19, 161–62
    stroke prevention in, 139–40, 140*t*, 144, 154–55

Atrophy, 84
  disuse, 494
  multiple system (MSA), 286–87,
    298t, 323
  muscular (see Muscle atrophy)
  posterior cortical, 246, 251, 267t
  spinal muscular (SMA), 472
  testicular, 226–27
Atropine, 387
Attention, 51
Attention deficit disorder, 198
Attention deficit-hyperactivity disorder
    (ADHD), 296, 299t, 474–75
  case histories, 468–69, 483
Attention deficits, 130t
Aubagio (teriflunomide), 366t
Audiography, 438
Auditory pathway, 19, 437–38
Augmentation, 321–22
Auras, 169, 397, 411–12
Autism spectrum disorder, 475
Autoadjusting positive airway pressure
    (APAP), 313–14
Autoimmune diseases, 113
  conditions associated with large-
    fiber sensory neuropathy or
    neuronopathy, 231t
  conditions associated with small-fiber
    sensory neuropathy, 231t
  encephalitis, 332–33
  encephalopathies, 265
  neuropathies, 221–22
  plexopathies, 215
Automatisms, 169
Autonomic dysfunction, 257, 278, 347–48
Autonomic instability, 203
Autonomic insufficiency
  emergency measures for, 230
  in MSA, 286
Autonomic nervous system, 204
Autonomic nervous system lesions, 204–5
AVMs (arteriovenous malformations), 126
Avonex (interferon beta-1a), 366t
Awareness, 380
Axert (almotriptan), 419t
Axonal neuropathies, 220
Azathioprine, 225, 361
Azilect (rasagiline), 297t

Babinski sign, 84. See also Extensor
    plantar response
  age-related changes in, 490
  bilateral, 108, 337, 436, 485–86, 495–
    96, 499

case histories, 107, 108, 116–17, 202,
    327–28, 485–86, 495–96, 499
  in Friedreich ataxia, 287
  in HIV-associated neurocognitive
    disorder, 337
  reflex examination, 59
  significance of, 72
  in syphilis, 340
Back pain, 449–55
  approach to, 450–51
  case histories, 109, 449, 454–55
  emergencies, 450–51
  musculoskeletal, 451–52
  non-urgent indications for
    surgery, 451
  in radiculopathy, 205–6
  specific conditions causing, 451–54
Baclofen (Lioresal), 299t, 420t, 421t
Bacterial endocarditis, 144–45. See also
    Infective endocarditis
Bacterial meningitis, 398–402, 401t
Bafiertam (monomethyl fumarate), 366t
Balance impairment, 203, 436–37, 448
Balint syndrome, 246
Ballism, 273
Ballismus, 57–58
Balloon compression, 421t
Banzel (rufinamide), 192t
Barbiturates, 384–85, 419t
Barbiturate withdrawal, 179, 383
Basal ganglia, 272, 274–75
Basilar artery, 148
Basilar meningitis, 343
Basis pontis, 8–10
Becker muscular dystrophy, 226
BECTS (benign epilepsy with
    centrotemporal spikes), 180
Bed rest, 444–45, 451
Bedside evaluation of swallowing, 138
Bedwetting, 321
Behavioral abnormalities
  in AD, 251
  case histories, 198
  in CBD, 285
  in CJD, 262–63
  in FTD, 258–59
  in PSP, 284–85
  during sleep, 178, 319–24
Behavioral changes
  in HSE, 344–45
  in Huntington disease, 290
Behavioral therapy, 321
  Cognitive Behavioral Intervention for
    Tics (CBIT), 296–97

cognitive behavioral therapy, 299*t*, 317–18, 323, 363, 452
Behavior disorders, 299*t*
Behavior problems
 in AD, 270
 case histories, 468–69, 483–84
 school problems, 468–69, 483–84
 in Tourette syndrome, 296
Behçet disease, 359
Bell palsy, 217–18. *See also* Facial nerve palsy
 case histories, 328, 495, 498
Bell phenomenon, 100*t*
Belsomra (suvorexant), 317–18
Benadryl (diphenhydramine), 420*t*
Benign epilepsy with centrotemporal spikes (BECTS), 180
Benign paroxysmal positional vertigo (BPPV), 440–42
 case histories, 435, 446–47
 Dix-Hallpike test for, 440*f*, 440, 442
 Epley maneuver for, 441*f*, 441–42
Benign paroxysmal vertigo of childhood, 477
Benign rolandic epilepsy, 180
Benzodiazepines, 384–85
 for dystonia, 299*t*
 for insomnia, 317–18
 for night terrors, 320
 for restless legs syndrome, 321–22
 side effects of, 269
 for status epilepticus, 190
 for tardive dyskinesias, 299*t*
 for tremor, 276–77
 for vertigo, 442–43
Benzodiazepine toxicity, 382
Benzodiazepine withdrawal, 179, 383
 case histories, 377, 394
Benztropine (Cogentin), 297*t*
Berry aneurysm, 126
Beta-adrenergic agonists, 276, 461, 462*t*
Beta-adrenergic antagonists (beta blockers), 269
 for headache, 420*t*
 side effects of, 323
 for tremor, 276–77
Beta amyloid (Aβ-peptide)
 accumulations in AD, 249–51, 250*f*, 253–54, 255, 298*t*
 accumulations in IBM, 229
 accumulations in movement disorders, 283, 298*t*
Beta amyloid precursor protein (APP), 249–50, 250*f*
Beta interferon, xxiv–xxv

Betaseron (interferon beta-1b), 366*t*
β-secretase, 249–50, 250*f*
Biceps reflex, depressed, 34
Biceps reflex pathway, 22, 26*f*
Biceps reflex testing, 59, 91
Bihemispheric disease, 116–17
Bilateral blindness, lone, 429
Bilateral cortical lesions, 82
Bilateral optic disc edema, 429–30
Bilateral prefrontal cortex disease, 75
Bilateral sensory and motor deficits, 40–41
Bilateral tremors, 271–72, 302–3
Bilevel positive airway pressure (BiPAP), 212, 236, 313–14, 499
Binocular diplopia, 42
Binocular vision loss
 persistent, 430
 transient, 429–30
Bioterrorism agents, 348–49
BiPAP (bilevel positive airway pressure), 212, 236, 313–14
Bitemporal (heteronymous) hemianopia, 22–27, 67, 430
Bladder
 flaccid, 460–61
 spastic, 460, 461, 462*t*
Bladder continence, 458
Bladder incontinence. *See* Urinary incontinence
Blepharospasm, 292–93
Blindness. *See* Vision loss
Blocadren (timolol), 420*t*
Blood flow: restoration of, 134–36
Blood pressure
 decreased or low (*see* Hypotension)
 increased or high (*see* Hypertension)
Blood pressure control, 138, 140*t*, 142–43, 148, 152–53
Blown pupil, 383–84
Body position, 410
 case histories, 486–87, 494
Body temperature. *See* Temperature
Bone density, 185
Borrelia burgdorferi, 342
Botulinum toxin (BOTOX)
 for back pain, 452
 for dystonia, 294, 501
 for headache, 420*t*
 for incontinence, 461
 for tremor, 276–77
 for trigeminal neuralgia, 421*t*
Botulism, 224, 225–26, 349
 infantile, 472

Bovine spongiform encephalopathy (BSE), 264
BPPV. *See* Benign paroxysmal positional vertigo
Brachial plexus, 206, 215
Brachial plexus tumors, 332
Brachioradialis reflex testing, 59
Bradykinesia
  in AD, 251–52
  case histories, 271–72, 302–3
  in CBD, 285
  definition of, 273
  in DLB, 257
  in PD, 278
Brain biopsy, 264–65, 330–31, 392
Brain death, 392–93
Brain edema, 331
Brain fog, 347–48
Brain imaging. *See also* Computed tomography; Imaging; Magnetic resonance imaging (MRI); Positron emission tomography
  in AD, 253
  in comatose patients, 385, 387
  in dizziness, 438
  in HIV infection, 338
  in IIH, 405–6
  indications for, 389–90
  in Wilson disease, 295–96
Brain lesions
  HIV-associated, 337–38
  structural, 377
Brain metastasis, 329–31
Brainstem gaze centers, 42, 80
Brainstem lesions, 42–43, 80
  extra-axial, 432–33
  intra-axial, 432
  signs suggesting, 445
Brain stimulation, responsive, 187
Brain tumors, 244, 329–31
Branch retinal artery occlusion, 428
Breakaway weakness, 100*t*
Breast cancer
  commonly associated antibodies, 364*t*
  metastatic, 329–30, 331–32
Breath-holding spells, 476–77
Breathing, 381–82
Breathing disorders, sleep-related, 311
Briumvi (ublituximab), 366*t*
Brivaracetam (Briviact), 192*t*, 194*t*
Broca aphasia, 30*f*, 30–33, 63
Bronchodilators, 384*t*
Brown-Séquard syndrome, 39

Bruxism, 322
BSE (bovine spongiform encephalopathy), 264
Bulbar lesions, 82
Bulk, 58
Bupropion, 299*t*
Butalbital/caffeine/acetaminophen (Fioricet, Esgic), 419*t*
Butalbital/caffeine/aspirin (Fiorinal), 419*t*
Butorphanol (Stadol), 420*t*
Butyrophenones, 279–80

C9ORF72 (*chromosome 9 open reading frame 72*), 211–12, 259–60
Caffeine, 276, 279, 310, 406–7
Caffeine/acetaminophen/aspirin (Excedrin, Excedrin Migraine), 419*t*
Caffeine/acetaminophen/butalbital (Fioricet, Esgic), 419*t*
Caffeine/aspirin/butalbital (Fiorinal), 419*t*
Calan (Verapamil), 420*t*
Calcitonin gene-related peptide (CGRP), 397–98
Calcitonin gene-related peptide (CGRP) antagonists (Gepants), 419*t*, 420*t*
Calcitonin gene-related peptide (CGRP) monoclonal antibodies, 420*t*
Calcium channel blockers, 269
  for headache, 407–8, 413–14, 420*t*
  for hypertension, 152–53
  side effects of, 279–80
Calcium channels, voltage-gated, 224, 364*t*
Calculation, 52
Caloric testing, 96–98
Canadian CT head rule, 389–90
Cancer. *See also* Lung cancer; Neoplastic disease(s); Paraneoplastic syndromes
  commonly associated antibodies, 364*t*
  dementia and, 245
  metastatic, 329–32, 333–34, 423, 449, 450, 454
  systemic, neurologic manifestations of, 329–33
Candesartan (Atacand), 420*t*
Cannabidiol (Epidiolex), 192*t*, 194*t*
Capillary telangiectasias, 126
Caplacizumab, 361–62
Capsaicin, 422*t*
Capsaicin cream, 230, 346
Captopril, 161–62

Carbamazepine (Tegretol, Carbatrol, Epitol)
  drug-drug interactions, 185
  for MS, 357
  for neuropathic pain, 230
  for seizures, 192t, 194t
  for shingles, 346
  side effects of, 185
  for trigeminal neuralgia, 415, 421t
  for vertigo, 443–44
Carbon monoxide exposure, 279–80
Carcinomatous meningitis, 331–32
Cardiac arrhythmias, 177, 226–27, 230
Cardioembolic disease, 144–45
Cardiomyopathy, hypertrophic, 287
Cardiovascular disease. See
  Atherosclerotic cardiovascular
  disease (ASCVD)
Cardizem (diltiazem), 271–72
Caregivers, 256
Carnitine palmitoyltransferase (CPT)
  deficiency, 227
Carotid angioplasty, 147, 156
Carotid endarterectomy, 140t, 146–47,
  155–56, 160t, 261–62
  case histories, 160–61
Carotid siphon, 148
Carotid stenosis
  cervical, 146–48, 155–56
  moderate, 147
  symptomatic, 146
Carotid ultrasound, 134, 140–41
Carpal tunnel syndrome, 358–59
Cataflam (diclofenac), 419t
Cataplexy, 178, 314, 315–16
Cataracts, 429, 494
  case histories, 436–37, 448, 486–87, 494
  early, 226–27
Catathrenia, 323–24
Catecholamine-depleting agents, 299t
Catechol O-methyltransferase (COMT)
  inhibitors, 281–82, 297t
Cavernomas, 126
Cavernous angiomas, 126
Cavernous hemangiomas, 126
CBD (corticobasal degeneration), 258–
  60, 285, 298t
CBIT (Cognitive Behavioral Intervention
  for Tics), 296–97
Cefepime, 399
Cefotaxime, 334, 342, 399
Ceftriaxone, 116–17, 334, 342, 399
Cell-based therapy, 282
Cenobamate (Xcopri), 192t, 194t

Central hypotonia, 472
Central lesions, 41, 82
  vs. peripheral lesions, 11, 22, 82, 105
Central nervous system (CNS)
  abscesses, 333–34
  focal diseases with multifocal
    propagation, 329–32
  incontinence and, 460–61
  infections, 333–49
  lesions, 8–11
  metastases, 329–32
  multifocal disorders, 327–73
  primary angiitis of, 360
Central retinal artery occlusion, 428
Central sleep apnea, 312, 313–14
Central vertigo
  differential diagnosis of, 439
  lesion localization, 437–38
  typical abnormalities in, 437–38
Cephalosporins, 334
Cerebellar degeneration, 332–33
Cerebellar lesions, 42, 445
Cerebellar testing, 70
Cerebral amyloid angiopathy, 126
Cerebral edema, 171, 423
Cerebral embolism, 334–35
Cerebral hemisphere dysfunction, 42–43
Cerebral hemorrhage, 151–52
Cerebral infarction, 125
Cerebral palsy, 473–74
Cerebral salt wasting, 137
Cerebral vasoconstriction, reversible,
  402, 407–8
Cerebral venous infarction, 136
Cerebral venous thrombosis, 125–26, 407
Cerebrospinal fluid (CSF). See also
    Lumbar puncture
  in AD, 253–54
  in CJD, 264–65
  in HIV infection, 338–39
  in HSE, 345
  in leptomeningeal metastasis, 331–32
  IgG index, 352–53
  in Lyme disease, 342
  in meningitis, 343–44, 399–400,
    401t, 403–4
  in MS, 352–53
  in neurosarcoidosis, 360–61
  in neurosyphilis, 340–41
  in paraneoplastic syndromes, 332–33
  in SAH, 399–402
Cerebrospinal fluid (CSF) leaks, 388–
  89, 406–7

Ceruloplasmin, 295–96
Cervical carotid stenosis, 146–48, 155–56
Cervical collars, 390
Cervical disc herniation, 453
Cervical dystonia, 292–93, 294
  case histories, 496–97, 500–1
Cervical manipulation, 148–49
Cervical myelopathy, 492–93, 494
Cervical spinal cord, 38*f*
Cervical spinal cord lesions, 34
  case histories, 436, 447–48
CGRP (calcitonin gene-related peptide), 397–98
CGRP antagonists (Gepants), 419*t*, 420*t*
CGRP monoclonal antibodies, 420*t*
CHA₂DS₂-VASc scale, 154–55
Charcot-Marie-Tooth (CMT) disease, 221
Checkpoint inhibitors, 222, 228, 330, 332
Chemotherapy, 330, 331–32
Chest pain, 109, 119–20
Chickenpox (varicella). *See* Herpes varicella-zoster
Children, 467–84
  ataxia, 468
  benign paroxysmal vertigo of childhood, 477
  breath-holding spells, 432–433, 476–77
  case histories, 306, 325, 467–69, 479–84
  childhood absence epilepsy, 180
  confusional arousals, 320–21
  developmental considerations, 469–70
  developmental delay, 472–75
  developmental regression, 472–75
  enuresis (bedwetting), 321
  epilepsy in, 180
  functional disorders, 479
  gait disturbances, 477–79
  hypotonic infants, 470–72, 471*f*
  night terrors, 306, 320, 325
  paroxysmal symptoms, 467, 468, 475–77, 479–81, 483
  school problems, 468–69, 483–84
  seizures, 476
  sleep disorders, 306
  sleep-related rhythmic movement disorder, 322
  sleepwalking, 320
  SMA, 214
  spells, 467, 483
  toe walking, 468, 482
Chiropractic manipulation, 148–49, 452
  case histories, 498, 503

Chlorambucil, 361
Chloramphenicol, 334, 349
Chlorpromazine (Thorazine), 419*t*
Cholinergics, 384*t*
Cholinesterase inhibitors
  for AD, 256, 269–70
  for DLB, 258
  for MSA, 286–87
  for PD, 281–83
  for PSP, 285
  and pupil size, 384*t*
  for vascular dementia, 262
Chorea, 57–58
  definition of, 273
  in Huntington disease, 290, 291
  medications for, 299*t*
  treatment of, 291
Choreoathetosis, 288, 294
Chromosome 9 open reading frame 72 (C9ORF72), 211–12, 259–60
Chronic alcohol use, 491
Chronic cluster headache, 416–17
Chronic degenerative diseases, 112
Chronic developmental disorders, 114
Chronic excessive daytime somnolence, 314
Chronic infections, 113, 243–44
Chronic inflammatory demyelinating polyradiculoneuropathy (CIDP), 220–22
  case histories, 235–36
  in HIV-positive patients, 336–37
Chronic inflammatory diseases, 113
Chronic lesions, 116, 117, 118, 119–20
Chronic Lyme disease, 342
Chronic neoplastic diseases, 112–13, 115*t*
Chronic nightmares, 323
Chronic obstructive pulmonary disease, 395–96
Chronic obstructive sleep apnea, 313
Chronic pain, 492
Chronic sinusitis, 408–9
Chronic symptoms, 112, 115*t*
Chronic toxic and metabolic diseases, 113–14
Chronic vision loss, 428–29
CIDP. *See* Chronic inflammatory demyelinating polyradiculoneuropathy
Cigarette smoking, 279
Cilostazol, 148
Ciprofloxacin, 348
Circadian rhythm generator, 310

Circadian rhythm sleep-wake disorders, 311
Circulation
ABCs (airway, breathing, circulation), 381–82
anterior, 125
posterior, 125
Cirrhosis, 280
CJD (Creutzfeldt-Jakob disease), 262–65, 267t
CK (creatine kinase), 209
Cladribine (Mavenclad), 356–57, 366t
Clasp-knife phenomenon, 69–70
case histories, 202
Clobazam (Onfi), 192t, 194t
Clonazepam (Klonopin)
for night terrors, 320
for REM sleep behavior disorder, 323, 501
for seizures, 192t, 194t
for sleepwalking and sleep talking, 320
Clonic activity, 168
Clonic movements, 168–69, 170
case histories, 166
Clonidine, 286–87, 299t
Clonus, 46, 59
case histories, 485–86
Clopidogrel, 136, 140t, 142, 148
Closed-loop (responsive) stimulation, 187
Clot evacuation, 136–37
Clot retrieval, 133–34
Clozapine (Clozaril), 258, 282, 292
Clumsiness, 349–50
Clumsy hand-dysarthria, 132
Cluster headaches, 416–17, 418
during sleep, 319, 323–24
treatment of, 422t
CMT (Charcot-Marie-Tooth) disease, 221
CMV (cytomegalovirus) infection, 214, 336–37
CNS. See Central nervous system
Coagulation disorders, 361–62
Coagulopathies, 149
Cocaine, 179, 384t, 387, 407–8
Codeine, 413–14
Codeine/acetaminophen, 419t
Coenzyme Q10, 413–14, 420t
Cogentin (benztropine), 297t
Cognition
mental status examination, 73–75
physiology of, 380

Cognitive Behavioral Intervention for Tics (CBIT), 296–97
Cognitive behavioral therapy, 299t, 317–18, 323, 363, 452
Cognitive delay, 227, 473–75
Cognitive impairment. See also Dementia
abnormal, 240–42
in AD, 251–52, 255
in ALS, 211
case histories, 237–39, 268–69
in CBD, 285
in CJD, 262–63
in COVID-19, 347–48
evaluation of, 240
generalized, 75
in Huntington disease, 290
mental status examination in, 75
mild (MCI), 253, 255, 278, 489
in MS, 349–50
in PSP, 284–85
reversible components, 242–45
vascular, 260–62, 269, 493
in Wilson disease, 294
Cogwheeling, 273
Cogwheel rigidity
case histories, 271, 497, 501
motor examination, 69–70
Cold (ice water) caloric procedure, 96–98, 392–93
Collagen vascular disorders, 218
Collapsing weakness, 100t
Colon cancer, 364t
Color Doppler ultrasound, 405
Coma, 380
case histories, 377, 394
definition of, 378
examination of, 98
Glasgow Coma Scale, 389–90, 389t
in HSE, 344–45
initial management of, 381–88
myxedema, 388
in tuberculous meningitis, 343
Common peroneal nerve, 89
Community resources, 256
Compazine (prochlorperazine), 419t
Complex partial seizures, 168
Comprehension, 50–51
Compression neuropathy
case histories, 497–98, 502
mononeuropathies, 215–18
Computed tomogram perfusion (CTP), 133–34, 135

Computed tomography (CT), xxiii. *See also* Brain imaging
Canadian CT head rule, 389–90
in comatose patients, 385, 389–90
in headache, 399–400, 402–3
indications for, 389–90
in metastatic cancer, 330–31, 333
New Orleans criteria for, 389–90
in progressive dementia, 244, 245
in SAH, 399–402
in seizures, 181
in stroke, 133–34, 150–51
Computed tomography angiography (CTA)
in endocarditis, 335
in SAH, 400–2
in stroke, 133–34, 140–41, 150–51
Computed tomography venography (CTV), 134
Comtan (entacapone), 297t
COMT (catechol O-methyltransferase) inhibitors, 281–82, 297t
Concussion, 114, 390
case histories, 378
post-concussion syndrome, 391, 409
Conduction aphasia, 30f, 30–33, 63
Confusion, 343, 492
Confusional arousals, 320–21
Congenital diseases
case histories, 118
characteristic spatial-temporal profiles, 115t
etiology, 114–15
Congenital myopathies, 234–35
Consciousness
altered level of (*see* Altered level of consciousness)
definition of, 378
level of (*see* Level of consciousness)
minimally conscious state, 379
physiology of, 43, 380–81
temporary loss of, 177–78
Constipation, 278, 472
Constraint-induced movement therapy, 138–39
Continuous positive airway pressure (CPAP), 313–14
Contusion, 114
Conversion disorder, 362–63
Convulsive status epilepticus, 166, 190, 200
Convulsive syncope, 177
Coordination testing, 57, 70

Copaxone (glatiramer acetate), 366t
Copolymer 1, xxiv–xxv
Copper deposition, 295–96
Coprolalia, 296
Corgard (nadolol), 420t
Corneal reflexes, 54–55, 68, 98
Coronary artery disease, 161–62
Corpus callosum section, 186
Corpus striatum, 273
Cortex, 34
Cortical gaze centers, 42, 80
Cortical infarcts, 149–50
Cortical lesions, 40, 42, 82, 116
Cortical spreading depression, 397–98
Corticobasal degeneration (CBD), 258–60, 285, 298t
Corticobasal ganglionic degeneration, 285
Corticobasal syndrome, 285
Corticospinal tract, 15
Corticosteroids
for CNS lymphoma, 338–39
for headache, 420t, 422t
for inflammatory myopathies, 228–29
for IRIS, 339
for neurosarcoidosis, 361
for nystagmus, 444–45
side effects of, 319
for spontaneous intracranial hypotension, 406–7
for tuberculous meningitis, 344
Counseling, 236, 291
COVID-19, 92, 126, 347–48, 407
CPT (carnitine palmitoyltransferase) deficiency, 227
Cramps, 227, 292–93
Cranial nerve III. *See* Oculomotor nerve
Cranial nerve IV, 430–32, 433
Cranial nerve V. *See* Trigeminal nerve
Cranial nerve VI. *See* Abducens nerve
Cranial nerve VII (facial nerve), 41, 98
Cranial nerve VIII (vestibular nerve), 96–98, 384
Cranial nerve IX (glossopharyngeal nerve), 82, 98
Cranial nerve X. *See* Vagus nerve
Cranial nerve XI (accessory nerve), 83
Cranial nerve XII (hypoglossal nerve), 83
Cranial nerve abnormalities, 343, 344–45, 346
Cranial nerve examination, 53–56
age-related changes in, 489
in altered level of consciousness, 96–98, 97f

case histories, 201–3
interpretation of, 75–83
screening examination, 91
technique for, 67–68
video examination, 92–94
Cranial nerve lesions
eye movements and, 67–68, 430–32
fourth nerve lesions, 430–32, 433
sixth nerve lesions, 430–32, 433
third nerve lesions, 430–32, 433
Cranial nerve palsies, 215–16, 341–42.
See also Facial nerve palsy
sixth nerve palsy, 405 6
third nerve palsy, 41–42, 130t
Cranial nerve pathways, 19
C-reactive protein, 405
Creatine kinase (CK), 209, 228
Cremasteric reflexes, 60
Creutzfeldt-Jakob disease (CJD), 262–65, 267t
Crus cerebri, 8–10
Crying, inappropriate, 209–10
Cryptococcal meningitis, 337–39, 403–4
CSF. See Cerebrospinal fluid
CT. See Computed tomography
Cubital tunnel syndrome, 497–98, 502
Cultural factors, 66
Cushing syndrome, 227, 388
Cyanosis, 166
Cyclical vomiting, 475–76
Cyclophosphamide, 361
Cyclosporine, 225, 276, 361
Cymbalta (duloxetine), 420t
Cyproheptadine (Periactin), 413 14, 420t
Cysticercosis, 227
Cystometrography, 461
Cytomegalovirus (CMV) infection, 214, 336–37
Cytosolic 5'-nucleotidase 1A (cN1A) antibodies, 229

Dabigatran, 140t, 144
Dalfampridine, 357
Dalmane (flurazepam), 237–38
DANG THERAPIST mnemonic, 219
Daridorexant (Quviviq), 317–18
Darifenacin (Enablex), 462t
DAT (dopamine transmitter) scans, 257–58, 280
Daydreaming, 468, 483
Daytime somnolence, 239, 270
excessive, 177–78, 283, 311–16 (See also Hypersomnia)

Dayvigo (lembrorexant), 317–18
Deamino-8-d-arginine vasopressin (DDAVP, Desmopressin), 321
Decadron (dexamethasone), 392, 420t, 450, 454
Decerebrate posturing, 95–96, 385
Decompressive surgery, 136–37, 421t, 454, 463, 502
Decorticate posturing, 95–96, 385
Decrement, 273, 277
Deep brain stimulation
for dystonia, 294
for epilepsy, 186
for PD, 282
for tardive dyskinesias, 292
for Tourette syndrome, 296–97
for tremor, 276–77
Deep tendon reflexes, 22, 84
age-related changes in, 490
examination of, 59, 98, 385
grading of, 71
hyperactive, 202
nerve roots, 85–88, 87f
Deep venous thrombosis, 138
Default mode network, 248–49
Defecation syncope, 177
Degenerative disease(s)
of brain, 246
case histories, 118, 486, 493
characteristic protein accumulations, 298t
characteristic spatial-temporal profiles, 115t
etiology, 112
joint disease, 486, 493
of spinal column, 457–58
Dehiscence of the superior semicircular canal, 443
Déjà vu, 168–69
Delayed sleep-wake phase disorder, 318
Delirium, 380
in anthrax meningoencephalitis, 348
case histories, 237–38, 239, 268–69, 270
definition of, 63, 243, 378–79
initial management of, 381
subacute, 239, 270
toxic, 237–38, 268–69
Delirium tremens, 383
Delta sleep, 308f, 308–9
Delta waves, 308
Delusions
case histories, 238, 269–70
in DLB, 257, 258
treatment of, 283

Dementia. *See also* Dementing illnesses
in AD, 238, 248, 252, 255, 269–70
in ALS, 211
case histories, 238, 269–70, 485–86,
492–93, 497, 501
in CJD, 262–63
definition of, 63, 242–43
vs. depression, 243
diagnosis of, 246, 265
frontotemporal (*see* Frontotemporal
dementia)
HIV-associated, 337
in Huntington disease, 291
incontinence and, 491–92
with Lewy bodies (*see* Dementia with
Lewy bodies (DLB))
memory-predominant, 262
mental status examination in, 75
neurologic diseases that produce, 265
in NPH, 244–45
in older people, 485–86, 492–93
in PD, 251–52, 265, 278, 283, 501
progressive, 244, 246, 270
vascular, 261–62
Dementia with Lewy bodies (DLB), 251–
52, 257–58, 284
case histories, 501
characteristic protein
accumulations, 298*t*
characteristic protein aggregates,
mutations when familial, and
clinical presentations, 267*t*
features characteristic of, 257
REM sleep behavior disorder and, 323
Dementing illnesses, 237–70
approach to, 240–48
case histories, 237–39, 268–70
characteristic protein accumulations
in, 298*t*
characteristic protein aggregates,
mutations causing familial forms,
and clinical presentations, 267*t*
degenerative, 298*t*
primary illnesses, 245–65
Demyelinating neuropathies, 220–21
Demyelination, 351, 352*f*
Dental appliances, 313–14
Depacon (valproic acid), 420*t*
Depakene. *See* Valproic acid
Depakote (valproate), 420*t*, 421*t*
Deprenyl (selegiline), 297*t*
Depression
in AD, 252

case histories, 271, 302
cortical spreading, 397–98
vs. dementia, 243
in DLB, 257
and early morning awakening, 318
in Huntington disease, 290
in older people, 491
and pain, 491
in PD, 278, 282, 302
pseudodementia of, 243
and sleep disorders, 324–25
in stroke, 137–38
in Tourette syndrome, 296–97
treatment of, 282, 296–97
Dermatomes, 88, 89*f*
Dermatomyositis, 227–28, 332–33
antibodies associated with, 233*t*
case histories, 201–2, 234–35
Desmopressin (DDAVP), 321
Detrol (tolterodine), 462*t*
Detrusor-external sphincter
dyssynergia, 460–61
Detrusor muscle, 458
Deutetrabenazine, 299*t*
Developmental delay, 472–75
case histories, 468, 482, 496, 499
Developmental diseases
case histories, 118
characteristic spatial-temporal
profiles, 115*t*
etiology, 114–15
Developmental plasticity, 469–70
Developmental regression, 472–75
Developmental venous anomalies, 126
Dexamethasone (Decadron), 116–17
for bacterial meningitis, 399
for brain metastasis, 331, 423
for headache, 420*t*, 422*t*, 423
for increased ICP, 392, 482
for spinal metastatic lesions, 450, 454
Dextroamphetamine (Dexedrine),
315–16
Dextroamphetamine-amphetamine,
468–69, 483
Dextromethorphan hydrobromide, 212
Dextrose solution, 382
DHE-45 (dihydroergotamine), 419*t*
Dhivy (levodopa/carbidopa), 297*t*
Diabetes insipidus, 460
Diabetes mellitus
case histories, 271–72, 302–3, 377
and compression
mononeuropathies, 218

and dementia, 243–44
  incontinence in, 460
  and lumbosacral plexus, 215
  movement disorders in, 271–72
  small-fiber neuropathies in, 209
  and stroke, 153
Diabetic polyneuropathy, 219–20, 221–22, 478
  case histories, 271–72, 302–3
Diagnostic categories, 115, 115t
Diagnostic reasoning, 107–20
3,4-Diaminopyridine, 225–26
Diamox (acetazolamide), 313–14, 405–6
Diazepam, 197t
Diclofenac (Cataflam), 419t
Didanosine (ddI), 336–37
Diencephalic lesions, 355–56
Diet, ketogenic, 187
Dietary factors, 156–57
Dietary modification, 152–53, 409, 500
Diffuse degenerative disease, 112
Diffuse developmental disorders, 114
Diffuse disease of peripheral nervous
  system, 84
Diffuse lesions, 109–10, 111, 115t
  case histories, 116–17, 118
  in inflammatory diseases, 113
  in toxic and metabolic
    diseases, 113–14
  in traumatic diseases, 114
  in vascular diseases, 113
Diffuse neuromuscular disorders, 206–8, 207f
Digital subtraction angiography, 400–2
Digit span, 51
Dihydroergotamine (DHE-45, Migranal,
  Trudhesa), 419t, 420t, 422t
Dilantin (phenytoin), 192t, 421t
Diltiazem (Cardizem), 161–62, 271–72
Dimethyl fumarate (Tecfidera), 366t
Diphenhydramine (Benadryl), 420t
Diplegia, 69
Diplopia, 430–33
  binocular, 42, 430–31
  in botulism, 349
  case histories, 234–35
  definition of, 426
  differential diagnosis of, 432–33
  lesion localization, 42, 430–32
  management of, 432–33
  in MS, 349–50
  in spontaneous intracranial
    hypotension, 406–7

Dipyridamole/aspirin, 140t, 142
Direct oral anticoagulants (DOACs), 144,
  151, 154–55
Diroximel fumarate (Vumerity), 366t
Discectomy, 453–54
Disc herniation, 450, 452–54, 463
Disease-modifying therapy, 356–57, 366t
Disequilibrium, 439, 445–46
  case histories, 436–37, 447–48, 486–87, 494
  in older people, 490–91, 494
Distal transcutaneous electrical
  stimulation (distal TENS), 413–14
Distal weakness, 84
Disuse atrophy, 494
Ditropan (oxybutynin), 462t
Diuretics, 460
Dix-Hallpike test, 440f, 440, 442,
  445, 446–47
Dizziness, 435–48
  approach to, 437
  case histories, 109, 435–37, 446–48
  differential diagnosis of, 438–45
  lesion localization, 437–38
  in older people, 490–91
  in spontaneous intracranial
    hypotension, 406–7
DLB. See Dementia with Lewy bodies
DOACs (direct oral anticoagulants), 144,
  151, 154–55
Documentation of subtle
  asymmetry, 71
Doll's eyes (oculocephalic) maneuver
  in brain death, 392–93
  in comatose patients, 96, 97f, 383–85
Dominant cerebral hemisphere
  lesions, 42, 74
Donanemab, 255
Donepezil (Aricept), 254, 299t, 313–14,
  323, 501
Dopamine agonists
  for DLB, 258
  for dystonia, 299t
  for PD, 281–83, 297t
  for PSP, 285
  for REM sleep behavior disorder, 323
  for restless legs syndrome, 321–22
  side effects of, 283, 286
Dopaminergic agents, 319. See also
  Dopamine agonists; Levodopa/
  carbidopa
Dopamine transmitter (DAT) scans,
  257–58, 280

Dopa-responsive dystonia
  DYT/PARK-*GCHI* dystonia (DYT5
    dystonia), 293–94, 299*t*
  DYT/PARK-*TH* dystonia, 293–94, 299*t*
Double simultaneous stimulation, 62, 91
  case histories, 395–96
Double vision. *See also* Diplopia
  case histories, 201–2, 234–35, 497, 501
Downgaze palsy, 284–85
Doxycycline, 342, 348–49
Dressing apraxia, 129–32
Driving assessment, 270
Driving restrictions
  drunk-driving test, 56–57
  in epilepsy, 189
Dronabinol, 313–14
Drop attacks, 170, 442–43
Droperidol (Inapsine), 419*t*
Droxidopa (Northera), 283, 286–87
Drug-induced parkinsonism, 271–72,
    279–80, 302–3
Drug overdose, 382, 389–90
Drugs. *See also specific drugs*
  medication overuse headache,
    412–13
  polypharmacy, 237–38, 268–69, 491
  and seizures, 171, 179
  side effects of, 491
Drug toxicity, 182, 336–37
Drug withdrawal, 383, 386–87
Drunk-driving test, 56–57
Dual antiplatelet therapy, 148
Duchenne muscular dystrophy, 226
  case histories, 468, 482
Duloxetine (Cymbalta), 420*t*
Duopa (levodopa/carbidopa), 297*t*
Duplex carotid ultrasound, 150–51
Durable power of attorney, 230, 256–57
Dysarthria, 42, 66, 82, 275
  in AD, 252
  in botulism, 349
  case histories, 495–96, 499
  in CBD, 285
  clumsy hand-dysarthria, 132
  cranial nerve examination, 56
  in Huntington disease, 290
  management of, 230
  in MS, 349–50
  in PD, 277
  in stroke, 130*t*, 132
  in Wilson disease, 294
Dysdiadochokinesis, 275
Dysesthesias, 204–5, 230, 349–50

Dysexecutive syndrome, 247, 251, 285
Dyskinesia, tardive, 292, 299*t*
Dyslexia, 468–69
Dyslipidemia, 153–54
Dysmetria, 275
Dysnomia, 63
  case histories, 496, 499–500
Dysphagia, 82
  in AD, 252
  in botulism, 349
  in CBD, 285
  in Huntington disease, 290, 291
  in IBM, 229
  management of, 230
  in MS, 349–50
  in MSA, 286–87
  in PSP, 284–85
  in stroke, 130*t*, 132
  in Wilson disease, 294
Dysphasia, 42, 63
Dysrhythmokinesis, 275
Dyssomnia, 307
Dystonia, 57–58, 275, 292–94
  cervical, 292–93, 294, 496–97, 500–1
  classification of, 275
  definition of, 273
  dopa-responsive, 293–94
  faciobrachial dystonic seizures, 332–33
  focal, 275, 294
  hemidystonia, 275, 292–93
  manifestations of, 276
  medications for, 299*t*
  in MS, 349–50, 357
  multifocal, 275
  in PSP, 284–85
  segmental, 275
  in Wilson disease, 294
Dystrophin, 226
DYT/PARK-*GCHI* dystonia (dopa-
    responsive dystonia, DYT5
    dystonia), 293–94, 299*t*
DYT/PARK-*TH* dystonia (dopa-
    responsive dystonia, DYT5
    dystonia), 293–94, 299*t*
DYT-*TORIA* dystonia (dystonia
    musculorum deformans, DYT1
    dystonia), 293–94

Early morning awakening, 316, 318–19
ECG. *See* Electrocardiography
Echocardiography
  transesophageal (TEE), 140–41, 150–51
  transthoracic (TTE), 140–41, 150–51

"Ecstasy" (methylenedioxy-
methamphetamine, MDMA), 179
Eculizumab, 225, 357
Edaravone, 212
Edema
around mass lesions, 331, 383–84
brain, 331, 383–84
cerebral, 171, 423
optic disc, 425, 429–30
papilledema, 343, 405–6, 410
Edoxaban, 140t, 144
Edrophonium (Tensilon) test, 224
Educational factors, 66
EEG. *See* Electroencephalography
Efavirenz, 337
Effexor (venlafaxine), 420t
Efgartigimod, 225
EKG. *See* Electrocardiography
Elbow extension
nerve roots and peripheral nerves
corresponding to, 85, 86f
testing, 58
Elbow flexion
nerve roots and peripheral nerves
corresponding to, 85, 86f
testing, 58
Eldepryl (selegiline), 297t
Elderly. *See* Older people
Electrical neuromodulation, remote, 413–14
Electrical stimulation. *See also* Deep brain
stimulation
distal transcutaneous (distal TENS),
413–14
for incontinence, 461
Electrocardiography (ECG or EKG), 140–
41, 310–11
Electrodiagnostic studies, 208–9
Electroencephalography (EEG), 172–74
in absence seizures, 173, 483
in acute mental status changes, 387
evoked potentials, 353–54
in HSE, 345
ictal, 172–73
interictal, 173, 181
in MS, 353–54
in polysomnography, 310–11
in SeLECTS, 480
during sleep, 307–9
in status epilepticus, 190
Electrolytes, 181, 243–44, 386
Electromyography (EMG)
in disc herniation, 452–53
in myopathy, 228

needle, 208–9, 236
in neuromuscular disorders, 208–9
in polysomnography, 310–11
single-fiber, 208–9
Eletriptan (Relpax), 419t
ELISA (enzyme-linked immunosorbent
assay), 342
Embolism, cerebral, 334–35
Emergencies
diagnostic evaluation in ED, 187–88
headache, 398–402, 420t
neuromuscular disease, 203, 229–30
EMG. *See* Electromyography
Emgality (alcanezumab), 420t
Emotional incontinence, 209–10, 212
Enablex (darifenacin), 462t
En bloc turning, 277
Encephalitis, 333
acute mental status changes and, 387–88
autoimmune, 332–33, 345
case histories, 116–17
cognitive impairment and, 245
herpes simplex (HSE), 116–17, 344–
45, 403
LGI1-associated, 332–33
viral, 402–3
Encephalomalacia, 114
Encephalomyelitis, 348, 355
Encephalopathy
autoimmune, 265
in COVID-19, 347
definition of, 379
limbic-predominant age-related TDP-
43 (LATE), 262, 267t
paraneoplastic, 265
posterior reversible syndrome (PRES),
387, 407–8
spongiform, 262–63, 264
Endarterectomy, carotid, 140t, 146–47,
155–56, 160t, 261–62
Endocarditis, 115
bacterial, 144–45
infective, 334–36
Endocrine disorders, 227, 319
Endolymphatic hydrops, 442–43
Endovascular therapy, 147, 407
Entacapone (Comtan), 297t
Enteroviruses, 213, 403
Entrainment, 100t
Entrapment mononeuropathies, 215.
See also Carpal tunnel syndrome;
Nerve compression
Enuresis, 321

Environmental factors, 279
Enzyme-linked immunosorbent assay (ELISA), 342
Eosinophilic granulomatosis with polyangiitis, 359
EPAP (expiratory positive airway pressure), 313–14
Epidemiology, 110, 112
Epidiolex (cannabidiol), 192t
Epidural abscess, 450
Epidural blood patch, 406–7
Epidural hematoma, 378, 388–89, 394
Epilepsia partialis continua, 190
Epilepsy, 180–81
    benign, with centrotemporal spikes (BECTS), 180
    benign rolandic, 180
    case histories, 198–200
    childhood absence, 180
    classification of, 172
    definition of, 167
    dementia and, 265
    driving restrictions, 189
    frontal lobe, nocturnal, 322
    imaging in, 181
    juvenile myoclonic, 179, 194t, 476
    management of, 182–87, 194t
    pathophysiology of, 174–75
    patient education, 187–88
    resolved, 167
    restrictions, 189
    vs. seizure, 171–72
    self-limited, with centrotemporal spikes (SeLECTS), 180, 322, 467, 476, 479–80
    sudden unexplained death in (SUDEP), 189
Epileptic cry, 170
Epileptiform abnormalities, 173
Episodic ataxias, 289
Epitol (carbamazepine), 192t
Epley maneuver, 441f, 441–42
Epstein-Barr virus, 338, 351
Eptinezumab (Vyepti), 420t
Erections, penile, 323–24
Erenumab (Aimovig), 420t
Ergots, 419t, 420t
Erythrocyte sedimentation rate (ESR), 245, 405
Esgic (acetaminophen/butalbital/caffeine), 419t
Eslicarbazepine (Aptiom), 192t, 194t, 421t
ESR (erythrocyte sedimentation rate), 245
Essential tremor, 276–77, 280

Estrogen, 411–12
Eszopiclone (Lunesta), 317–18
Etanercept, 361
Ethambutol, 344
Ethical issues, 392
Ethionamide, 344
Ethosuximide (Zarontin), 179, 192t, 194t, 198, 483
Etiology, 112–15
Evoked potentials, 353–54
Excedrin, Excedrin Migraine (aspirin/acetaminophen/caffeine), 419t
Excessive daytime somnolence, 177–78, 283, 311–16. See also Hypersomnia
Exelon (rivastigmine), 254
Exercise, 221–22, 500
Exercise intolerance, 227
Expiratory groaning, 323–24
Expiratory positive airway pressure (EPAP), 313–14
Expressive aphasia, 64
Extavia (interferon beta-1b), 366t
Extensor plantar responses, 59. See also Babinski sign
External sphincter, 458, 460–61
External trigeminal nerve stimulation (eTNS), 414
External ventricular drain, 391
Extracranial arteries, 134
Extracranial-intracranial bypass, 148
Eye movement(s)
    in altered level of consciousness, 96–98, 97f
    conjugate, 80
    cranial nerve examination, 67–68, 78–81
    examination of, 54, 67–68
    rapid (see Rapid eye movement (REM) sleep)
    screening examination, 91
Eye movement abnormalities, 78–81
    case histories, 234–35
    in cranial nerve lesions, 430–32
    in Huntington disease, 290
Ezetimibe, 140t

Facial nerve (cranial nerve VII), 41, 98
Facial nerve palsy, 341–42, 360. See also Bell palsy
    case histories, 495, 498
    idiopathic, 217–18
Facial numbness, 117

Facial pain
  atypical, 418
  persistent idiopathic, 418
Facial sensation
  pathway for, 19, 20f
  reduced, 19, 20f, 41, 435–36
Facial strength, 55, 91
Facial weakness
  in Bell palsy, 217–18, 495, 498
  case histories, 108, 116, 117, 123–24,
    328
  example problem, 45, 105
  ipsilateral to body weakness, 41, 116
  lesion localization, 41, 81–82, 108
  pathway for, 19, 24f
  in Ramsay Hunt syndrome, 346
  in stroke, 123–24, 129–32, 130t
Faciobrachial dystonic seizures, 332–33
Factor V Leiden, 361–62
Factor Xa inhibitors, 142, 144
Famciclovir, 119, 346
Family support, 256, 270
Fasciculations, 84, 210
  case histories, 202, 235–36, 495–96, 499
  individual muscle testing, 58
Fatigability, 223, 234–35
Fatigue, 347–48, 349–50, 357
FDG-PET (fluorodeoxyglucose-positron
  emission tomography), 253, 260
Febrile seizures, 179–80, 181
Feeding tubes, 212
Feet
  joint position sense, 34, 35f, 36f, 37–39
  numbness in, 271–72, 302–3, 457–58
Femoral nerve, 85
Fenestration, optic nerve sheath, 405–6
Fesoterodine (Toviaz), 462t
Festination, 56–57
  case histories, 271–72
  definition of, 273
  in PD, 277
Fever
  in anthrax meningoencephalitis, 348
  with headache, 410
  in HSE, 344–45
  seizures and, 165–66, 171, 179–80
  in tuberculous meningitis, 343
  in viral meningitis or encephalitis, 403
Feverfew (Tanacetum parthenium), 420t
Fine touch discrimination, 46
Finger abduction
  nerve roots and peripheral nerves
    corresponding to, 85, 86f
  testing, 58

Finger chase, 57
Finger extension
  nerve roots and peripheral nerves
    corresponding to, 85, 86f
  testing, 58
Finger flexion
  nerve roots and peripheral nerves
    corresponding to, 85, 86f
  testing, 58
Finger tapping, 57, 91
Finger-to-nose testing
  age-related changes in, 490
  motor examination, 57
  screening examination, 91
Fingolimod (Gilenya, Tascenso), 366t
Fioricet (acetaminophen/butalbital/
  caffeine), 419t
Fiorinal (aspirin/butalbital/caffeine),
  419t
Fistula, perilymphatic, 443
Flaccid bladder, 460–61
FLAIR. See Fluid attenuated inversion
  recovery imaging
Flexor plantar response, 59
Floppy baby, 470, 471f
Florinef (fludrocortisone), 286–87
Flow cytometry, 331–32
Fluconazole, 338–39
Flucytosine, 338–39
Fludrocortisone (Florinef), 286–87
Fluency, 50, 63
Fluid attenuated inversion recovery
  (FLAIR) imaging, 286, 352f
Flumazenil, 382
Flunarizine, 420t
Fluorescent treponemal antibody (FTA),
  243–44, 340–41
Fluorodeoxyglucose-positron emission
  tomography (FDG- PET), 253, 260
Fluoroquinolones, 225, 349
Fluphenazine, 299t
Flurazepam (Dalmane), 237–38, 269
FMRP (fragile X messenger
  ribonucleoprotein), 473
Focal aware seizures, 167, 169
Focal disease, with multifocal
  propagation, 329–49
Focal dystonia
  cervical, 496–97, 500–1
  classification of, 275
  diagnosis of, 294
  treatment of, 294, 501
Focal impaired awareness seizures, 167,
  169, 197t

Focal lesions, 74, 109–10, 115*t*
  case histories, 116, 117–20, 162–63
  in congenital and developmental
    diseases, 114
  HIV-associated, 337–38
  in inflammatory diseases, 113
  localization of, 111
  in peripheral nervous system, 84
  in traumatic diseases, 114
  in vascular diseases, 113
Focal mental status changes, 379
Focal myelitis, 333
Focal neoplastic diseases, 112–13
Focal-onset seizures (focal seizures)
  in AD, 252
  case histories, 198–200, 467, 479–80
  clinical characteristics of, 168–69
  definition of, 167
  management of, 183, 189–90, 194*t*, 197*t*
Folate supplementation, 165–66, 199
Folic acid supplements, 191, 199–200
Foot
  joint position sense, 34, 35*f*, 36*f*, 37–39
  numbness in, 271–72, 302–3, 457–58
Foot drop, 327–28
Forced vital capacity (FVC), 229
Forehead numbness, 19, 20*f*
Fosphenytoin, 197*t*, 421*t*
Fourth nerve lesions, 430–32, 433
Fractures
  hip, 486–87, 494
  skull, 388–89
Fragile X-associated tremor/ataxia
    syndrome (FXTAS), 289–90, 473
Fragile X messenger ribonucleoprotein
    (FMRP), 473
Fragile X syndrome, 289–90, 473
  case histories, 496, 499
Frataxin, 287
Fremanezumab (Ajovy), 420*t*
Friedreich ataxia, 287, 299*t*, 479
Frontal lobe epilepsy, nocturnal, 322
Frontal release signs, 60
Frontoparietal cortex, 8–11, 12*f*
Frontotemporal dementia (FTD), 211,
    258–60
  case histories, 496, 499–500
  characteristic protein accumulations,
    298*t*
  characteristic protein aggregates,
    mutations when familial, and
    clinical presentations, 267*t*
  neurologic diseases that produce, 265

Frovatriptan (Frova), 419*t*
FTA (fluorescent treponemal antibody),
    243–44, 340–41
FTD. *See* Frontotemporal dementia
Functional disorders, xxi, 362–64
  in children, 479
  exam findings typical of, 99, 100*t*
Functional imaging, 380–81
Functional incontinence, 459–60
  case histories, 457, 462
  in older people, 491–92
Funduscopic examination, 53, 481
Fungal infections, 339
Fungal meningitis, 401*t*, 403–4
Fused in sarcoma (FUS) protein, 259–60
Fused in sarcoma/translated in
    liposarcoma gene (*FUS/TLS*),
    259–60
FXTAS (fragile X-associated tremor/
    ataxia syndrome), 289–90, 473
Fycompa (perampanel), 192*t*

Gabapentin (Neurontin), xxiv–xxv
  for back pain, 452
  for headache, 420*t*
  for MS, 357
  for neuropathic pain and dysesthesia,
    230
  for numbness or paresthesias, 231
  for restless legs syndrome, 321–22, 325
  for seizures, 192*t*, 194*t*
  for shingles, 346
  for tardive dyskinesia, 299*t*
  for tremor, 276–77
  for trigeminal neuralgia, 421*t*
Gabitril (tiagabine), 192*t*
Gag reflex, 68, 98
Gait
  motor examination, 49, 56–57
  screening examination, 91
Gait disturbances
  age-related changes, 488, 489–90
  case histories, 203, 237–38, 271–72,
    436, 448, 485–87, 492–94
  in children, 477–79
  in HIV-associated neurocognitive
    disorder, 337
  in Huntington disease, 290, 291
  in MSA, 286–87
  in NPH, 244–45
  in older people, 486–87, 488, 489–90,
    491, 494
  in PSP, 284–85

psychological factors, 486–87, 494
treatment of, 291, 446
unstable gait, 275
in Wilson disease, 294
Galantamine (Razadyne), 254
Galcanezumab (Emgality), 421t, 422t
γ-hydroxybutyrate, 315–16
γ-secretase, 249–50, 250f
Ganglionopathy, 205
Gastroesophageal reflux, 305, 324–25
Gastrointestinal tumors, 329–30
Gaze centers, 80, 430–31
Gaze-evoked nystagmus, 438, 442
Gaze impairment
case histories, 497, 501
in older people, 489
in stroke, 130t
Gaze palsy, 42, 80, 284–85, 430–31
Gaze preference, 80, 123–24, 162–63
GCH1 (guanosine triphosphate
cyclohydrolase-1), 293–94
Gegenhalten, 69–70
Gemtesa (vibegron), 462t
Generalized cognitive impairment, 75
Generalized-onset seizures (generalized
seizures)
ASMs for, 194t
clinical characteristics of, 169–71
definition of, 167
Generalized tonic-clonic seizures
ASMs for, 183, 194t
case histories, 165–66
clinical characteristics of, 170
Gene therapy, 482
Genetic disorders
conditions associated with large-
fiber sensory neuropathy or
neuronopathy, 231t
conditions associated with small-fiber
sensory neuropathy, 231t
mutations causing familial dementing
illnesses, 267t
Genetic testing, 181, 209, 291
Genetic therapy, xxi, 226
Genitourinary tract tumors, 329–30
Gentamicin, 442–43
Gepants (CGRP antagonists), 419t, 420t
Geriatric neurology, 485–94. See also
Aging; Older people
case histories, 485–87, 492–94
Gerstmann syndrome, 64
GFAP (glial fibrillary acidic protein),
355–56

Giant cell (temporal) arteritis, 404–5,
428, 492
case histories, 425, 434
dementia and, 245
vision loss in, 425, 434
Gilenya (fingolimod), 366t
Give-way weakness, 100t
Glasgow Coma Scale, 389–90, 389t
Glatiramer acetate (Copaxone, Glatopa),
366t
Glaucoma, 428, 429, 494
Glial fibrillary acidic protein (GFAP),
355–56
Glioma, 116
Global aphasia, 30f, 30–33
Global developmental delay, 473
Glossopharyngeal nerve (cranial nerve
IX), 82, 98
Glossopharyngeal neuralgia, 415–16
Glucocorticoids, 346, 356–57, 361–62, 392
Glucose, 243–44, 382–83. See also
Hyperglycemia; Hypoglycemia
Glucose control, 221–22
Glucose tolerance, impaired, 226–27,
496, 500
Glucose tolerance test, 500
Glutamate, 251, 309
Glyburide, 123
Glycerol injection, 421t
Glycogen, 227
Gocovri (amantadine), 297t
Gowers sign, 468, 482
Granulomas, 360
Granulomatosis with polyangiitis, 359
Graphesthesia, 62
Grasp reflex, 60, 490
Groaning, expiratory, 323–24
Guanfacine, 299t
Guanosine triphosphate cyclohydrolase-1
(GCH1), 293–94
Guillain-Barré syndrome, 220–21, 232t,
347

H2-blockers, 269
Haemophilus influenzae, 399
Hallucinations, 168–69
in AD, 252
in DLB, 257
hypnagogic (hypnopompic), 315
in PD, 283
in seizures, 168–69
treatment of, 258, 283
Haloperidol, 299t

Hand
  innervation of, 88–89, 90*f*
  joint position sense, 34, 35*f*, 36*f*, 37–39
  mechanic's hands, 227–28
  pinprick sensation, 8–15, 9*f*, 10*f*, 12*f*,
    14*f*, 18*f*, 19–33, 21*f*, 34, 37–39
HANDs (HIV-associated neurocognitive
    disorders), 337
Hand weakness, 123, 160–61, 497–98, 502
Handwriting
  sloppy, 435–36
  small, 277
Headache, 395–423. *See also* Migraine
  abortive agents for, 412–14, 419*t*, 420*t*,
    423
  after seizure, 178
  in anthrax meningoencephalitis, 348
  approach to, 396
  case histories, 108, 109, 377, 394, 395–
    96, 423, 468, 497, 502
  in children, 468
  cluster, 319, 323–24, 416–17, 418,
    422*t*
  in COVID-19, 347–48
  emergencies, 398–402
  in HSE, 344–45
  ice-pick, 418
  medication overuse, 412–13
  primary, 396, 410–18
  prophylactic agents for, 412–14, 420*t*
  rebound, 412–13
  secondary, 396, 398, 402–9
  short-lasting unilateral neuralgiform,
    with conjunctival injection and
    tearing (SUNCT), 417–18
  short-lasting unilateral neuralgiform
    attacks (SUNHAs), 417–18
  short-lasting unilateral neuralgiform
    attacks with cranial autonomic
    symptoms (SUNAs), 417–18
  stabbing, 418
  tension, 410–14, 419*t*, 423
  thunderclap, 402, 407–8
  in tuberculous meningitis, 343
Head impulse test, 55
Head rotation, 56
Head thrust maneuver, 55
Head trauma, 388–91
  case histories, 377–78, 394
  and seizures, 181
Health care reform, xxiii
Hearing loss, 19, 82, 494
  age-related changes, 489

anomalous or inconsistent exam
    findings, 100*t*
  case histories, 108, 117, 328, 435–36,
    447, 486–87, 494
  cranial nerve examination, 55, 68
  and dementia, 244
  in Ramsay Hunt syndrome, 346
Heat therapy, 452
Heavy metals, 479
Heel-knee-shin testing, 489–90
Heel-to-shin testing, 57, 91
Hemangiomas, cavernous, 126
Hematologic disorders, 149, 243–44
Hematoma, 450
  epidural, 378, 388–89, 394
  subdural (SDH), 117, 244, 491
Hemianopia
  case histories, 107, 116, 123, 161–62
  heteronymous (bitemporal), 22–27,
    67, 430
  homonymous, 107, 123, 161–62
Hemicrania, paroxysmal, 417, 418
Hemicrania continua, 417, 418
Hemicraniectomy, 136–37
Hemidystonia, 275, 292–93
Hemiparesis, 69
  anomalous or inconsistent exam
    findings, 100*t*
  case histories, 107, 116, 162–63, 327,
    370–71, 395–96
  delayed contralateral, 346
  in herpes simplex encephalitis, 344–45
  in stroke, 132, 143
  in tuberculous meningitis, 343
Hemiplegia, 69
Hemispherectomy, 186
Hemodilution, 149
Hemorrhage, 113, 114
  cerebral, 151–52
  intraparenchymal, 137, 152
  lobar, 126
  in stroke, 133, 136–37
  subarachnoid (*see* Subarachnoid
    hemorrhage (SAH))
Hemorrhagic conversion, 126
Hemorrhagic stroke
  classification by etiology, 125–26
  definition of, 125
  differential diagnosis of, 133
  pathophysiology of, 127–28
Hemorrhagic transformation, 126
Hemotympanum, 388–89
Heparin, 136, 407

Hepatic abnormalities, 243–44, 294, 386
Hepatic failure, 171, 179
Herbal supplements, 420t
Hereditary ataxias, 287–90
Hereditary neuropathies, 221–22
    in children, 478
    with liability to pressure palsies, 218
Herniated discs. See Disc herniation
Heroin, 179, 327
Herpes simplex, 338
Herpes simplex encephalitis (HSE), 116–
    17, 344–45, 403
Herpes simplex virus type 1 (HSV1),
    344–45
Herpes simplex virus type 2 (HSV2),
    344–45
Herpes varicella-zoster virus (VZV),
    345–46
    and ataxia, 478–79, 481
    case histories, 468, 481
    and radiculopathy, 214
    reactivation, 336–37
Herpesviruses, 344–46
Herpes zoster reactivation, 119
Heteronymous (bitemporal) hemianopia,
    22–27, 67, 430
Hiccups, 355–56
Hip extension
    nerve roots and peripheral nerves
        corresponding to, 85, 87f
    testing, 58
Hip flexion
    in altered level of consciousness, 98
    nerve roots and peripheral nerves
        corresponding to, 85, 87f, 105
    testing, 58
    weakness, 45
Hip fracture, 486–87, 494
HIV. See Human immunodeficiency virus
HIV-associated neurocognitive disorders
    (HANDs), 337
HMG-CoA reductase inhibitors, 139–40
Hoarseness, 328
Hodgkin lymphoma, 109
Home sleep apnea tests, 310–11
Homocysteine, 156–57
Homonymous hemianopia, 107
    case histories, 123, 161–62
Hoover sign, 100t
Hormonal contraceptives, 411–12
Hormonal therapy, 191–92
Horner syndrome, 41–42, 76
    ipsilateral, 130t, 132

HSE (herpes simplex encephalitis), 116–
    17, 344–45, 403
HSV1 (Herpes simplex virus type 1),
    344–45
HSV2 (Herpes simplex virus type 2),
    344–45
Human immunodeficiency virus (HIV)
    CNS infection, 336–39
    HIV-associated neurocognitive
        disorders (HANDs), 337
    testing for, 245
Huntingtin, 291
Huntington disease, 290–91, 299t
Hydrocephalus
    normal pressure (NPH), 244–45, 491,
        493
    obstructive, 244
    in tuberculous meningitis, 344
Hydrochlorothiazide, 123–24
Hydrocortisone, 420t
Hydroxymethylglutaryl coenzyme A (HMG-
    CoA) reductase inhibitors, 139–40
Hyperactive reflexes, 22, 33–34, 84, 108
    hyperactive, 202
Hyperactivity. See Attention-deficit
    hyperactivity disorder (ADHD)
Hyperalgesia, 204–5
Hypercoagulability, 361–62
Hyperesthesia, 204–5
Hyperglycemia
    seizures and, 171, 179
    stroke and, 138
Hyperkinetic movement disorders, 274–75
Hypernatremia, 386
Hyperosmolar agents, 391
Hyperparathyroidism, 227
Hyperreflexia, 46–49
    case histories, 108, 116–17, 327–28,
        371–73, 395–96, 436, 495–96, 499
    example neurologic deficits, 33–34
    at knee, 33–34
    in myelopathy, 460
Hypersomnia, 311–16
    case histories, 108, 109, 239, 305, 324
    definition of, 307
Hypersomnolence. See Hypersomnia
Hypertension, 152–53
    case histories, 237–38, 268–69, 305,
        395–96
    idiopathic intracranial (IIH), 405–6,
        429–30, 497, 502
    permissive, 142–43
    in SAH, 400–2

Hypertension-related intraparenchymal hemorrhage, 152
Hyperthermia, 138
Hyperthyroidism
    acute mental status changes and, 388
    case histories, 118–19
    and myopathy, 227
    and tremor, 276
Hypertrophic cardiomyopathy, 287
Hyperventilation
    for increased ICP, 136–37, 391–92, 482
    provocation of absence seizures by, 165, 198, 483
Hypesthesia, 204–5
Hypnagogic hallucinations, 315
Hypnic jerks, 322
Hypnogenic neurons, 309
Hypnopompic hallucinations, 315
Hypoactive reflexes, 22
Hypocalcemia, 171, 179, 386
Hypocretin (orexin), 309–10
Hypocretin (orexin) receptor antagonists, 317–18
Hypoglossal nerve (cranial nerve XII), 83
Hypoglossal nerve stimulators, 313–14
Hypoglycemia
    acute mental status changes and, 382–83
    seizures and, 171, 179
    stroke and, 138
Hypokinesia, 273
Hypokinetic movement disorders, 274–75
Hypomagnesemia, 171, 179, 386
Hyponatremia, 137, 171, 179, 386–87
Hypoperfusion, transient, 115
Hyporeflexia, 271–72, 302–3
Hypotension
    acute mental status changes and, 383
    drug-induced, 490–91
    emergency measures for, 230
    orthostatic (see Orthostatic hypotension)
    spontaneous intracranial, 405–6
    stroke and, 138
Hypothermia, 386–87
Hypothyroidism, 219, 227, 316, 380, 388, 472
Hypotonia
    central, 472
    in infants, 470–72, 471f
    peripheral, 472
Hypoxia
    acute mental status changes and, 382–83
    seizures and, 171, 179

    stroke and, 138
Hysteria, 362–63

IBM (Inclusion body myositis), 229, 234–35, 478
Ibrutinib, 338–39
Ibuprofen (Advil, Motrin, Nuprin), 419t
ICA. See Internal carotid artery
Ice-pick headache, 418
Ice water (cold) caloric procedure, 96–98, 392–93
ICP. See Intracranial pressure
Idiopathic intracranial hypertension (IIH), 405–6, 429–30
    case histories, 497, 502
IgG index, 352–53
ILAE. See International League Against Epilepsy
Imaging. See also specific modalities
    amyloid-related abnormalities (ARIA), 255
    functional techniques for, 380–81
    vascular, 150–51
Imipramine (Tofranil), 321
Imitrex (sumatriptan), 419t, 423
Immobility, 291
Immune checkpoint inhibitors, 222, 228, 330, 332
Immune-mediated necrotizing myopathy, 227–29, 233t, 234–35
Immune reconstitution inflammatory syndrome (IRIS), 339
Immunoglobulin
    for autoimmune neuropathies, 221–22
    for CIDP, 236
    intravenous (IVIG), 221–22, 225–26, 236, 333
    for LEMS, 225–26
    for myasthenia gravis, 225
    for paraneoplastic syndrome, 333
Immunoglobulin G (IgG) index, 352–53
Immunomodulation, 225
Immunosuppressants, 265
    for autoimmune neuropathies, 221–22
    for myasthenia gravis, 225
    for myopathies, 228–29
    for paraneoplastic antibodies, 333
    side effects of, 279–80
Impersistence, 75
Impotence, 224
Improving symptoms, 111
    in traumatic diseases, 114
    in vascular diseases, 113

Inapsine (droperidol), 419*t*
Inbrija (levodopa), 297*t*
Inclusion body myositis (IBM), 229,
    234–35, 478
Incontinence
    emotional, 212
    urinary (*see* Urinary incontinence)
Inderal (propranolol), 413–14, 420*t*, 423
Indomethacin (Indocin)
    for headache, 419*t*, 420*t*
    for MSA, 286–87
    for paroxysmal hemicrania, 417
Inebilizumab, 357
Infantile spasms, 170–71, 194*t*, 476
Infants
    breath-holding spells in, 476–77
    hypotonic, 470–72, 471*f*
    physical examination of, 470, 471*f*
Infarcts, infarctions, 161–62
    acute myocardial, 144–45
    cerebral, 125, 136
    cortical, 149–50
    lacunar, 125, 132 (*See also* Penetrating
        artery disease)
    venous, 133, 134, 136
Infection(s)
    associated with small-fiber sensory
        neuropathy, 231*t*
    central nervous system, 333–49
    chronic, 113, 243–44
    diffuse lesions in, 113
    focal lesions in, 113
    fungal, 339
    parasitic, 347
    postinfectious ataxia, 478–79, 480–81
    progressive, 113
    spirochetal, 339–42
    subacute, 113
    systemic, 243–44
    urinary tract, 138, 269, 387–88, 460,
        491–92
    viral, 214
Infective endocarditis, 334–36
Inflammation, neurogenic, 397–98
Inflammatory demyelinating
    polyradiculoneuropathy, 220–21,
    336–37
Inflammatory demyelination, 214
Inflammatory diseases
    case histories, 116–18, 119
    characteristic spatial-temporal profiles,
        115*t*
    dementia and, 265

etiology, 113
immune reconstitution syndrome
    (IRIS), 339
Inflammatory myopathy, 227–29
    antibodies associated with, 233*t*
    case histories, 234–35
Infliximab, 361
Infraclavicular pulse generator, 186
INO (internuclear ophthalmoplegia),
    81, 431
Insomnia
    case histories, 237–38, 305, 324–25
    classification of, 311
    definition of, 307
    main patterns of, 316
    paradoxical, 319
    psychophysiologic, 305, 316–18,
        324–25
Insufficient sleep, 312
Insulin, 271–72
Intellectual regression, 475
    case histories, 468–69, 483–84
Intention tremor, 273
Interferon beta-1a (Avonex, Rebif,
    Plegridy), 366*t*
Interferon beta-1b (Betaseron, Extavia),
    366*t*
Internal carotid artery (ICA), 128, 134
Internal carotid artery (ICA) occlusion,
    132
Internal carotid artery (ICA) stenosis,
    139–40, 140*t*, 155–56, 160*t*
    case histories, 160–61
Internal clock, 310
Internal sphincter, 458
International Classification of Sleep
    Disorders, 311
International League Against Epilepsy
    (ILAE)
    definition of epilepsy, 167
    definition of status epilepticus, 168
    system of epilepsy classification, 172
Internuclear ophthalmoplegia (INO),
    81, 431
Intra-arterial angiography, 134, 150–51
Intracranial arteries
    evaluation of, 134
    large, occlusive disease of, 148
Intracranial hypertension, idiopathic
    (IIH), 405–6, 429–30
    case histories, 497, 502
Intracranial hypotension, spontaneous,
    405–6

Intracranial lesions, 137
Intracranial pressure (ICP), decreased,
    405–6
Intracranial pressure (ICP), increased,
    391–92, 481, 502
    in children, 481–82
    in comatose patients, 385
    in stroke, 136–37
    in tuberculosis, 344
    visual symptoms of, 429–30
Intracranial tumors, 329–31
Intraocular pressure, increased. *See*
    Glaucoma
Intraparenchymal hemorrhage, 137, 152
Intravenous (IV) drug abuse, 327, 371
Intravenous immunoglobulin (IVIG)
    for autoimmune neuropathies, 221–22
    for CIDP, 236
    for LEMS, 225–26
    for myasthenia gravis, 225
    for paraneoplastic syndrome, 333
Involuntary movements, 57–58
    case histories, 496–97, 500–1
IRIS (immune reconstitution
    inflammatory syndrome), 339
Iritis, acute, 428
Iron deficiency, 321–22, 325
Iron-deficiency anemia, 476–77
Iron replacement, 321–22, 325
Iron supplements, 476–77
Ischemia, 113
Ischemic cascade, 127
Ischemic penumbra, 127, 138
Ischemic stroke
    case histories, 118–19, 162–63
    classification by etiology, 125–26
    clinical features of, 128*f*, 128, 129*f*, 130*t*
    definition of, 125
    dietary factors, 156–57
    in endocarditis, 335–36
    hemorrhagic conversion of, 126
    hemorrhagic transformation of, 126
    imaging, 133
    pathophysiology of, 127–28
    restoration of blood flow in, 134–36
    secondary prevention of, 139–51
Isoniazid, 344
Istradefylline (Nourianz), 297*t*
IV (intravenous) drug use, 327, 371
IVIG. *See* Intravenous immunoglobulin

Jacksonian march, 169
Jamais vu, 168–69

Jargon, 64
Jaw claudication, 404–5, 425, 434
Jaw weakness, 223
JC virus, 337–39
Jendrassik maneuver, 59, 436–37
Joint disease, degenerative, 486, 493
Joint position sense
    anomalous or inconsistent exam
        findings, 100*t*
    example neurologic deficits, 33–34,
        35*f*, 36*f*, 37–39, 38*f*
    foot, 34, 35*f*, 36*f*, 37–39
    hand, 34, 35*f*, 36*f*, 37–39
    lesion localization, 34
    sensory examination, 61
Juvenile myoclonic epilepsy, 180, 194*t*, 476

Kaposi sarcoma, 339
Kayser-Fleischer rings, 295–96
Keppra (levetiracetam), 192*t*, 420*t*, 421*t*
Kesimpta (ofatumumab), 366*t*
Ketamine, 197*t*
Ketogenic diet, 187
Ketorolac (Toradol), 419*t*, 420*t*
"Kinetic red target" method, 67
Kinetic tremor, 275, 276
    in CBD, 285
    definition of, 274
    in older people, 490
    in PD, 278
Klonopin (clonazepam), 192*t*
Knee extension
    nerve roots and peripheral nerves
        corresponding to, 85, 87*f*
    testing, 58
Knee flexion
    nerve roots and peripheral nerves
        corresponding to, 85, 87*f*, 105
    testing, 58
Knee flexion weakness, 45
Knee hyperreflexia, 33–34
Knee reflex testing, 59
Korsakoff syndrome, 245–46
Kuru, 263–64
Kynmobi (apomorphine), 297*t*

Labyrinthectomy, 442–43
Labyrinthitis, acute, 444
Lacerations, scalp, 388–89
    case histories, 378, 394
Lacosamide (Vimpat), 192*t*, 194*t*, 197*t*
Lacunar infarcts, 125, 132. *See also*
    Penetrating artery disease

Lacunar syndromes, 132
Lacune, 125
Lambert-Eaton myasthenic syndrome (LEMS), 208, 222–23, 224–26, 332–33, 364*t*
Lamotrigine (Lamictal), xxiv–xxv
    for seizures, 183, 191, 192*t*, 194*t*
    for TACs, 417–18
    for trigeminal neuralgia, 421*t*
Language, 50–51, 74. *See also* Speech
Language delay, 474
Language disturbances. *See also* Aphasia
    case histories, 108–9, 118
Language pathways, 30*f*, 30–33
Language processing, 30*f*, 30–33
Large-fiber sensory neuropathy, 231*t*
Large intracranial arteries: occlusive disease of, 148
Laryngeal weakness, 82
Lasmiditan (Reyvow), 419*t*
LATE (limbic-predominant age-related TDP-43 encephalopathy), 262, 267*t*
Lateral medullary stroke, 130*t*, 149–50
Lateral medullary syndrome, 132
Laughing, inappropriate, 209–10
LDL-C (low-density lipoprotein cholesterol), 141–42
L-dopa. *See* Levodopa
Lead-pipe rigidity, 69–70
Lecanemab, 255
Left afferent pupillary defect, 76–78, 79*f*
Left cerebral cortex, 160
Left gaze preference, 80
Left hemisphere strokes, 137–38
Left ventricular assist devices (LVADs), 144–45
Leg stiffness, 436
Leg weakness
    case histories, 108, 109, 117, 119–20, 123–24
    lesion localization, 45
    in stroke, 123–24, 129–32, 130*t*
Lembrorexant (Dayvigo), 317–18
LEMS (Lambert-Eaton myasthenic syndrome), 208, 222–23, 224–26, 332–33, 364*t*
Lemtrada (alemtuzumab), 366*t*
Lennox-Gastaut syndrome, 180, 194*t*
Lenticular nucleus, 273
Lentiform nucleus, 273
Leprosy, 218–19
Leptomeningeal lymphoma, 372–73
Leptomeningeal metastasis, 331–32

Lesion(s). *See also specific sites*
    case histories, 107–9, 116–20
    central, 22, 41, 82
    diffuse (*see* Diffuse lesions)
    example neurologic deficits with, 8–39, 9*f*, 10*f*, 12*f*, 13*f*, 14*f*, 17*f*, 18*f*, 38*f*
    focal (*see* Focal lesions)
    level of consciousness and, 42–43
    linguistics and, 30*f*, 30–33
    locating (*see* Lesion localization)
    mass (*see* Mass lesions)
    multifocal, 111, 113, 338–39
    nerve root, 119
    nondominant hemisphere, 74–75
    non-mass lesions, 114
    peripheral, 41, 82
    spinal cord, 119–20
Lesion localization, 3–43, 111
    abbreviated version, 15–39
    based on cranial nerve examination, 75–83
    based on mental status examination, 73–75
    based on motor examination, 84–88
    beyond localization, 109–12
    in diplopia, 430–32
    in dizziness, 437–38
    example problems, 3–4, 8–39, 9*f*, 10*f*, 12*f*, 13*f*, 17*f*, 18*f*, 25*f*, 45, 105
    principles of, 40–43
    rules for, 7–8, 39–43
    with visual field defects, 75
Leucine-rich glioma-inactivated protein 1 (LGI1), 332–33, 364*t*
Leukemia, metastatic, 331–32
Leukodystrophy, 478
Leukoencephalopathy
    progressive multifocal (PML), 337–39
    reversible posterior syndrome (RPLS), 387
Leukomalacia, periventricular, 473–74, 478, 482
Level of alertness. *See also* Level of consciousness
    mental status examination, 50
Level of consciousness
    acute changes in, 109, 377–94
    altered (*see* Altered level of consciousness)
    in DLB, 257
    lesions and, 42–43
    mental status examination, 73–75

temporary loss of consciousness, 177–78
Levetiracetam (Keppra)
for headache, 420*t*
for seizures, 183, 191, 192*t*, 194*t*, 200
for status epilepticus, 197*t*
for tardive dyskinesia, 299*t*
for trigeminal neuralgia, 421*t*
Levodopa (L-dopa, Inbrija)
for CBD, 285
for DLB, 258
for dystonia, 299*t*
for MSA, 286–87
for PD, 281, 297*t*
for PSP, 285
for REM sleep behavior disorder, 323
for restless legs syndrome, 321–22
side effects of, 286–87, 323
Levodopa, carbidopa, entacapone (Stalevo), 297*t*
Levodopa/carbidopa (Sinemet, Rytary, Parcopa, Dhivy, Duopa), 281, 297*t*
Levofloxacin, 344
Levothyroxine, 457
Lewy bodies, 258, 278–79
dementia with (*see* Dementia with Lewy bodies (DLB))
LGI1 (leucine-rich glioma-inactivated protein 1), 332–33, 364*t*
Lhermitte phenomenon, 349–50, 357
Lidocaine
for headache, 419*t*, 420*t*, 422*t*
side effects of, 179
topical, 230
for trigeminal neuralgia, 421*t*
Lidocaine patch, 346
Lifestyle changes, 143, 152–53
Lifestyle factors, 156–57
Light-headedness, 177
Lightning-like pains, 340
Light therapy, 256, 318
Light touch sensation, 60, 91
age-related changes in, 490
anomalous or inconsistent exam findings, 100*t*
Limb-girdle muscular dystrophy, 457
Limbic-predominant age-related TDP-43 encephalopathy (LATE), 262, 267*t*
Limb position, 70–71
Limbs. *See also* Lower extremities
increased reflexes in, 41
periodic movements of sleep, 321–22
principal movements in, 85

reduced pain/temperature sensation in, 40
reduced position/vibration sensation in, 40
reduced strength and pain/ temperature sensation in, 40
Limb weakness
case histories, 201–2, 234–35
in MS, 349–50
Linezolid, 348
Lioresal (baclofen), 420*t*, 421*t*
Lipid management, 141–42, 149
Lipids, 227
Lipohyalinosis, 125
Lipoprotein(a), 156–57
Lisinopril (Prinivil, Zestril)
case histories, 123, 237–38, 436–37, 448
for headache, 420*t*
Listeria monocytogenes, 399
Literal or phonemic paraphasia, 64
Lithium, 276, 422*t*
Liver abnormalities, 243–44, 294, 386
Liver biopsy, 295–96
Liver disease, 243–44
Living wills, 230, 256–57
LMNs. *See* Lower motor neurons
Lobar hemorrhage, 126
Localization. *See* Lesion localization
Logopenic progressive aphasia, 246–47, 251, 266*t*
Lone bilateral blindness, 429
Long-COVID, 347–48
Long-haul COVID, 347–48
Long-term memory, 52
Lopressor (metoprolol), 413–14, 420*t*
Lorazepam, 197*t*
Loss of consciousness
in DLB, 257
temporary, 177–78
Lovastatin, 123–24, 162–63
Low back pain. *See* Back pain
Low-density lipoprotein cholesterol (LDL-C), 141–42
Low-density lipoprotein-related protein 4 (LRP4), 222
Lower extremities. *See also* Limbs
ankle dorsiflexion, 33–34
muscle strength testing, 58
nerve roots, 85
sensory innervation, 88–89, 89*f*, 90*f*
vibration sense, 19, 23*f*
weakness, 45, 436, 457–58, 462–63

Lower extremity pain, 496, 500
Lower motor neuron (LMN) lesions, 84, 460–61
in ALS, 209, 211
case histories, 235–36, 457–58, 462–63
pattern of weakness, 84–88
Lower motor neurons (LMNs), 22, 81–82
Low-molecular-weight heparin, 136, 407
LRP4 (low-density lipoprotein-related protein 4), 222
LSD, 387
Lucid intervals, 388–89
case histories, 378, 394
Lumbar disc herniation, 453
Lumbar puncture (spinal tap), 116–17
in bacterial meningitis, 399–400
in headache, 399–402
in HIV infection, 338
in IIH, 405–6
in leptomeningeal metastasis, 331–32
in syphilis, 341
Lumbar spinal stenosis, 451
case histories, 496, 500
Lumbar spine disease, degenerative, 457–58
Lumboperitoneal shunting, 405–6
Lumbosacral disc herniation. See Disc herniation
Lumbosacral plexus, 206, 215
Lumbosacral plexus tumors, 332
Luminal (phenobarbital), 192t
Lunesta (eszopiclone), 317–18
Lung cancer
commonly associated antibodies, 364t
metastatic, 329–30, 331–32
non-small cell, 330, 423
small-cell, 225, 270, 364t
Lupus. See Systemic lupus erythematosus
Lupus anticoagulant, 361–62
LVADs (left ventricular assist devices), 144–45
Lyme disease, 214, 341–42
Lymphocytic meningitis, 339–40
Lymphocytic pleocytosis, 345
Lymphoma
CNS, 337–39
leptomeningeal, 372–73
metastatic, 331–32
Lyrica (pregabalin), 192t

Macular degeneration, 429
Mad cow disease, 264
Magnesium, 225
for headache, 413–14, 420t

hypomagnesemia, 171, 179, 386
Magnetic resonance angiography (MRA)
in endocarditis, 335
in stroke, 134, 140–41
Magnetic resonance-guided ultrasound, 276–77, 282
Magnetic resonance imaging (MRI), xxiii, 15–19. See also Brain imaging
in acute vestibular syndrome, 445
in back pain, 450, 451
in cerebral venous thrombosis, 407
in CJD, 264–65
of CNS abscesses, 333–34
in diplopia, 433
functional, 380–81
in headaches, 404
in HSE, 345
in hydrocephalus, 481–82
in ischemic stroke, 128f, 129f, 133
in metastatic cancer, 330, 331–32
in MS, 319–320, 320f–321f, 333, 385–386, 351–52, 352f
in MSA, 286
in neck pain, 450
in NMOSD, 355–56
in optic neuritis, 433–34
in PRES, 387
in progressive dementia, 244
in seizures, 181
of spinal cord, 448
in spontaneous intracranial hypotension, 406–7
in stroke, 133, 150–51
in toxoplasmosis, 338–39
in trigeminal neuralgia, 415
Magnetic resonance perfusion (MRP), 133–34
Magnetic resonance venography (MRV), 134, 407
Magnetic stimulation, transcranial, 414
Maintenance of wakefulness test, 310–11
Malaise, 343
Malignancy. See also Cancer
systemic, 228
Manganese poisoning, 279–80
Mannitol, 391, 482
MAO-B (monoamine oxidase type B) inhibitors, 281–83, 297t
Marcus-Gunn pupil, 76–78
Marijuana, 407–8
Masked face, 277
Mass lesions, 114, 481–82

Mass lesions (*cont.*)
case histories, 116, 117–18, 119–20
dementia and, 244
edema, 331, 383–84
headache due to, 404
in HIV, 337–38
Mastication muscles, 55
Mavenclad (cladribine), 366*t*
Maxalt, Maxalt-MLT (rizatriptan), 419*t*
Mayzent (siponimod), 366*t*
MCA (middle cerebral artery) occlusion, 128*f*, 129–32, 130*t*, 148
McArdle disease (myophosphorylase deficiency), 227
MCA (middle cerebral artery) stroke, 352*f*
MCI. *See* Mild cognitive impairment
MDMA. *See* Methylenedioxymethamphetamine
Mechanical heart valves, 145, 154
Mechanical thrombectomy, 134–36
Mechanic's hands, 227–28
Medial longitudinal fasciculus (MLF), 80, 81, 430–31
Medial medullary stroke, 130*t*
Median nerve, 88–89, 90*f*
Medical Research Council (MRC) scale, 68–69
Medication overuse headache, 412–13
Medications. *See* Drugs; *specific medications*
Mediterranean diet, 156–57
Medulla, 40, 118–19
Melanoma, metastatic, 329–30, 331–32
Melatonin
for cluster headache, 422*t*
for sleep disorders, 310, 318, 323
Melatonin agonists, 317–18
Memantine (Namenda)
for AD, 254, 256
for DLB, 258
for headache, 420*t*
Memory. *See also* Cognition; Mental status
assessment of, 51–52
immediate, 51
long-term, 52
recent, 52
remote, 52
short-term, 52
Memory loss
in AD, 238, 269–70, 485–86
case histories, 108–9, 118, 237–38, 239, 269–70, 485–86
in Korsakoff syndrome, 245–46

memory-predominant syndromes, 246, 262
in older people, 489
Ménière disease, 442–43
Meningeal carcinomatosis, 331–32
Meningioma, 119–20, 439
Meningitis, 333, 334–35
acute mental status changes and, 387–88
aseptic, 340–41, 358, 359
bacterial, 398–402, 401*t*
basilar, 343
carcinomatous, 331–32
case histories, 116–17
chronic, 245, 341–42
cryptococcal, 337–39, 403–4
fungal, 401*t*, 403–4
in Lyme disease, 341–42
lymphocytic, 339–40
plague, 349
TB, 342–44, 401*t*, 403–4
tularemia, 349
typical CSF patterns, 401*t*
viral, 401*t*, 402–3
Meningoencephalitis, anthrax, 348
Meningovascular syphilis, 340
Mental status changes, 73–75
acute, 109, 377–94, 410
age-related, 488
focal, 379
Mental status examination, 49–52, 108–9
age-related changes in, 95–96
cultural and educational factors, 66
interpretation of, 73–75
in normal aging, 489
patient cooperation, 64–65
reporting findings, 66
screening examination, 91
standardized screening tests, 66
tailoring to the patient, 65
terminology for, 62–64, 65–66
in urinary incontinence, 460
video examination, 92–94
Mercury, 479
Meropenem, 348, 399
Mesial temporal sclerosis, 174
Mestinon (pyridostigmine), 225
Metabolic abnormalities, 214, 316
Metabolic disease, 479
characteristic spatial-temporal profiles, 115*t*
conditions associated with large-fiber sensory neuropathy or neuronopathy, 231*t*

conditions associated with small-fiber sensory neuropathy, 231t
etiology, 113–14
Metals, heavy, 479
Metastatic cancer, 115, 329–32, 333–34, 423, 450
case histories, 449, 454
Methergine (methylergonovine), 420t
Methotrexate, 338–39, 361, 373
N-Methyl-D-aspartate (NMDA) receptor antagonists, 254, 281–82, 299t, 420t
N-Methyl-D-aspartate receptor (NMDAR) antibodies, 345, 364t
Methylenedioxymethamphetamine (MDMA, "ecstasy"), 179
Methylergonovine (Methergine), 420t
Methylphenidate (Ritalin), 299t, 315–16, 357
Methylprednisolone (Solumedrol)
for giant cell arteritis, 405
for headache, 420t
for MS, 356–57, 433–34
for optic neuritis, 427–28, 433–34
Methylxanthines, 179
Metoclopramide (Reglan)
for headache, 413–14, 419t
side effects of, 271–72, 279–80, 302–3
Metoprolol (Lopressor, Toprol XL), 237–38, 413–14, 420t
Metronidazole, 334
MHA-TP (microhemagglutination-Treponema pallidum), 243–44, 340–41
Microdiscectomy, 453–54
Micrographia, 277
Microhemagglutination-Treponema pallidum (MHA-TP), 243–44, 340–41
Microscopic polyangiitis, 359
Microsurgery, 447
Microvascular decompression, 421t
Micturition reflex, 458
Micturition syncope, 177
Midazolam, 197t
Middle cerebral artery (MCA): occlusion of, 128f, 129–32, 130t, 148
Middle cerebral artery (MCA) stroke, 352f
Mid-medulla pathways, 15–19, 18f
Midodrine, 286–87
Midurethral sling, 459–60
Migraine, 410–14, 418
abortive agents for, 419t
with aura, 411–12

case histories, 395, 423
in children, 475–76
differential diagnosis of, 178
pathophysiology of, 396–98
triggers for, 411–12
vestibular, 439
visual symptoms of, 429
Migraine equivalents, 178
Migranal (dihydroergotamine), 419t
Mild cognitive impairment (MCI)
brain imaging in, 253
due to AD, 255
in older people, 489
in PD, 278
Miller Fisher syndrome, 232t
Minimally conscious state, 379
Mini-Mental State Examination (MMSE), 66
Mirabegron (Myrbetriq), 462t
Mirapex (pramipexole), 297t
Mirtazapine (Remeron), 313–14
Mitoxantrone (Novantrone), 356–57, 366t
Mixed connective tissue disease, 359
Mixed transcortical aphasia, 30f, 30–33, 74
MLF (medial longitudinal fasciculus), 80, 81, 430–31
MMSE (Mini-Mental State Examination), 66
MoCA (Montreal Cognitive Assessment), 66
Modafinil (Provigil), 313–14, 315–16, 357
MOG (myelin oligodendrocyte glycoprotein), 355–56
MOG antibody disease (MOGAD), 355–56
Monoamine oxidase type B (MAO-B) inhibitors, 281–83, 297t
Monocular vision loss, 427–29
case histories, 425, 433–34
in older people, 428–29
transient, 429–30
in young people, 427–28
Monomethyl fumarate (Bafiertam), 366t
Mononeuropathies, 215–18
Mononeuropathy multiplex, 215, 216f, 218–19
flowchart for identifying, 207f
in HIV-positive patients, 336–37
in polyarteritis nodosa, 359
in rheumatoid arthritis, 358
in sarcoidosis, 360
in Sjögren syndrome, 358–59
in SLE, 358
Monoparesis, 69
Monoplegia, 69

Montreal Cognitive Assessment (MoCA), 66
Mood-stabilizing agents, 299t
Motivation deficits, 130t
Motor asymmetry, 383–85
Motor deficits, bilateral, 40–41
Motor development delay, 473–74
  case histories, 468, 482
Motor examination, 56–59
  age-related changes in, 489–90
  in altered level of consciousness, 98
  grading muscle strength, 68–69
  interpretation of, 84–88
  limb position for, 70–71
  modifications of strength testing, 70–71
  screening examination, 91
  selection of muscles to test, 70
  technique for, 68–71
  terminology for, 69–70
  video examination, 92–94
Motor nerves, 204
Motor neuron diseases, 205, 209–14
  case histories, 235–36
  dementia and, 258–59, 265
  flowchart for identifying, 207f
  principle clues, 205
  symptomatic treatment of, 230
Motor pathways, 22, 40
Motor regression, 475
  case histories, 468, 482
Motrin (ibuprofen), 419t
Movement disorders, 271–303
  anatomic definitions, 272–73
  approach to, 272
  ataxic, 274–75
  case histories, 271–72, 302–3
  characteristic protein accumulations in, 298t
  classification of, 274–75
  clinical definitions, 273–74
  hyperkinetic, 274–75
  hypokinetic, 274–75
  management of, 272
  medications for, 299t
  sleep-related, 311, 322
  specific disorders, 276–97
MRA. See Magnetic resonance angiography
MRC (Medical Research Council) scale, 68–69
MRI. See Magnetic resonance imaging
MRP (magnetic resonance perfusion), 133–34
MRV (magnetic resonance venography), 134, 407
MS. See Multiple sclerosis

MSA (multiple system atrophy), 286–87, 298t, 323
MSA-C (multiple system atrophy-cerebellar predominant), 286
MSA-P (multiple system atrophy-parkinsonism predominant), 286–87
MSLT (Multiple Sleep Latency Test), 310–11, 315
Muller's muscle, 76
Multifocal central nervous system disorders, 327–73
  approach to, 329
  case histories, 327–28, 370–73
  focal diseases with multifocal propagation, 329–49
  inherently multifocal diseases, 349–64
Multifocal dystonia, 275
Multifocal lesions
  in HIV, 338–39
  in inflammatory diseases, 113
  localization, 111
Multiple sclerosis (MS), xxiv–xxv, 115, 349–57
  case histories, 10P8, 371–72, 425, 433–34
  dementia with, 265
  diagnostic criteria for, 354, 365t, 366t
  disease-modifying therapy for, 356–57, 366t
  optic neuritis in, 354, 355–56, 427–28, 433–34
  primary-progressive, 350, 354–55, 357, 366t
  progressive-relapsing, 350, 366t
  relapsing-remitting, 350–51, 356, 365t
  secondary-progressive, 350, 356
Multiple Sleep Latency Test (MSLT), 310–11, 315
Multiple subpial transections, 186
Multiple system atrophy (MSA), 286–87
  characteristic protein accumulations, 298t
  REM sleep behavior disorder and, 323
Multiple system atrophy-cerebellar predominant (MSA-C), 286
Multiple system atrophy-parkinsonism predominant (MSA-P), 286–87
Muscle(s). See also specific muscles
  bulk, 58, 490
  of facial expression, 55
  of mastication, 55
  motor examination, 58–59
  selection to test, 70
Muscle atrophy
  case histories, 202, 235–36

individual muscle testing, 58
  progressive (PMA), 207*f*, 213
  spinal (SMA), 207*f*, 213–14
Muscle biopsy, 209, 228, 234–35
Muscle disorders (myopathies), 226–29
  case histories, 234–35
  dementia and, 265
  diagnosis of, 208–9
  flowchart for identifying, 207*f*
Muscle pain, 228
Muscle-specific kinase (MuSK)
  antibodies, 222, 223, 224, 225
Muscle strength, 40
  facial, 55, 91
  testing (*see* Strength testing)
Muscle stretch reflexes, 59
Muscle tone
  hypotonic infants, 470–72, 471*f*
  individual muscle testing, 58–59
  terminology for, 69–70
Muscle wasting, 228
Muscle weakness. *See* Weakness
Muscular dystrophy, 226–27, 234–35
  case histories, 457, 462, 468, 482
  in children, 468, 478, 482
  dementia and, 265
  limb-girdle, 457
Musculoskeletal pain, 451–55
MuSK (muscle-specific kinase)
  antibodies, 222, 223, 224, 225
Myasthenia gravis, 222–25
  case histories, 234–35, 497, 501
  diagnosis of, 208, 224
  Tensilon test for, 224
  treatment of, 225
Mycobacterial infections, atypical,
  339
Mycobacterium tuberculosis, 342–43
Mycophenolate, 225, 361
Mycotic aneurysms, 335
Myelin oligodendrocyte glycoprotein
  (MOG), 355–56
Myelitis
  acute, 355–56
  case histories, 117–18
  focal, 333
  in MS, 354
  transverse, 450–51
  VZV, 346
Myelography, 451
Myelopathy, 450–51, 460
  cervical, 492–93, 494
  HIV-associated, 337
  nonstructural causes of, 493

Myoclonic jerks
  after syncope, 177
  in CBD, 285
  juvenile myoclonic epilepsy, 179
Myoclonic seizures, 171, 194*t*
Myoclonus, 57–58
  in AD, 252
  in anthrax meningoencephalitis, 348
  definition of, 274
  in Huntington disease, 290
  paraneoplastic, 479
Myopathies. *See* Muscle disorders
Myophosphorylase deficiency (McArdle
  disease), 227
Myositis. *See also* Dermatomyositis
  inclusion body (IBM), 229, 234–35,
  478
  overlap, 227–28
  polymyositis, 227–28
Myotonia, 226–27
Myotonic dystrophy type 1, 226–27
Myotonic dystrophy type 2, 226–27
Myrbetriq (mirabegron), 462*t*
Mysoline (primidone), 192*t*
Myxedema coma, 388

Nadolol (Corgard), 420*t*
Naloxone (Narcan), 382, 394
Namenda (memantine), 254, 420*t*
Naming, 51
Naproxen (Aleve, Anaprox, Naprosyn),
  419*t*, 420*t*, 423
Naratriptan (Amerge), 419*t*
Narcan (naloxone), 382
Narcolepsy, 314–16, 355–56
Narcotics, 179
Natalizumab (Tysabri), 356–57
National Institutes of Health Stroke Scale
  (NIHSS), 135–36, 158*t*
Nausea
  case histories, 108, 109, 395, 435
  in migraine, 411
  in NMOSD, 355–56
  in presyncope, 177
  in tuberculous meningitis, 343
Neck pain, 449–55
  approach to, 450–51
  case histories, 109, 449, 454–55,
  498, 503
  emergencies, 450–51
  musculoskeletal, 451–52
  non-urgent indications for surgery, 451
  specific conditions causing, 451–54
Neck rigidity, 284–85

Neck stiffness, 343, 403, 410
Neck trauma, 148–49
Neck weakness, 83
Necrotizing myopathy, immune-mediated, 227–29, 233t, 234–35
Needle electromyography (EMG), 208–9, 236
Negative inspiratory force, 229
Negative phenomena, 168–69
Neglect, 74–75
    in stroke, 123–24, 129–32, 130t, 162–63
Neonatal seizures, 476
Neonatal white matter injury, 473–74, 482
Neoplastic disease(s), 115
    case histories, 116, 117, 118, 119–20, 447, 497–98, 502
    characteristic spatial-temporal profiles, 115t
    etiology, 112
    metastatic cancer, 329–32
Neostriatum, 273
Nerve biopsy, 209
Nerve compression, 215–18
    case histories, 497–98, 502
Nerve conduction studies, 208
Nerve root disorders (radiculopathies), 205–6, 214
Nerve root lesions, 205–6
    case histories, 119
Nerve roots
    C6 nerve root, 88
    C7 nerve root, 88
    C8 nerve root, 88
    for dermatomes, 88, 89f
    for lower extremities, 85, 87f, 89f
    T4 nerve root, 119–20
    for upper extremities, 85, 86f, 89f
Nervous system. See also Central nervous system (CNS); Peripheral nervous system
    subway map of, 5–7, 6f
Neupro (rotigotine), 297t
Neuralgia
    postherpetic, 345–46
    trigeminal (see Trigeminal neuralgia)
Neuralgiform headache, 417–18
Neuraxis
    lesion localization and, 20–28
    pupillary light reflex pathway and, 27–28, 28f
Neuroblastoma, 479
Neurocognitive disorders, HIV-associated (HANDs), 337

Neurofibrillary tangles
    in AD, 249
    in PSP, 284–85
Neurogenic claudication, 454
Neurogenic incontinence, 461
Neurogenic inflammation, 397–98
Neurologic examination, 45–105
    age-related changes in, 487–90
    in altered level of consciousness, 94–98
    components of, 46, 47t
    inconsistent or anomalous findings, 99, 100t
    screening examination, 90–91
    sequence of, 47t, 49
Neuromuscular disorders, 201–36
    approach to, 203–4
    case histories, 201–3, 234–36
    dementia with, 265
    diffuse, flowchart for identifying, 206–8, 207f
    emergency measures for, 229–30
    motor symptoms, 230
    sensory symptoms, 230–31
    specific diseases, 209–29
    symptomatic treatment of, 229–31
Neuromuscular junction disorders, 206, 222–26
    case histories, 234–35
    flowchart for identifying, 207f
    hereditary, 472
Neuromuscular junction transmission tests, 208
Neuromyelitis optica spectrum disorders (NMOSD), 355–56, 357
Neuron-specific enolase, 264–65
Neurontin (gabapentin), 192t, 420t, 422t
Neuropathic pain, 204–5, 230
Neuropathies, 215–22
    small-fiber, 209, 231t
    syndromes associated with HIV infection, 336–37
Neurosarcoidosis, 360–61
Neurosyphilis, 340–41, 493
Neurotoxins, 420t
New Orleans criteria, 389–90
Nightmares, 323
Night terrors, 320, 321
    case histories, 306, 325
NIHSS (National Institutes of Health Stroke Scale), 135–36, 158t
Nimodipine, 400–2
NMDAR (N-Methyl-D-aspartate receptor) antibodies, 345, 364t

NMDA (*N*-Methyl-D-aspartate) receptor antagonists, 254, 281–82, 299*t*, 420*t*
NMOSD (neuromyelitis optica spectrum disorders), 355–56, 357
Nocardiosis, 339
Nociceptive pain, 204–5
Nociceptors, 204–5
Nocturia, 461
Nocturnal frontal lobe epilepsy, 322
Nocturnal seizures, 322–23
Nondominant hemisphere lesions, 74–75
Nonfluency, 64
Nonfluent/agrammatic progressive aphasia, 246–47, 260, 266*t*, 284–85
case histories, 496, 499–500
Noninvasive vagus nerve stimulation (nVNS), 413–14, 422*t*
Non-mass lesions, 114
Nonorganic symptoms, 362–63
Nonrapid eye movement (NREM) sleep, 319
parasomnias, 320–22
physiology of, 307–10, 308*f*
Non-small cell lung cancer, 330, 423
Nonsteroidal anti-inflammatory drugs (NSAIDs), 269
for back pain, 452
for headache, 413–14, 419*t*, 420*t*
for musculoskeletal pain, 452, 454–55
side effects of, 413–14
Normal pressure hydrocephalus (NPH), 244–45, 491, 493
Northera (droxidopa), 283
Nortriptyline, 420*t*, 421*t*
Nourianz (istradefylline), 297*t*
Novantrone (mitoxantrone), 366*t*
Noxious stimulation, 98, 392–93
NPH (normal pressure hydrocephalus), 244–45, 491, 493
NREM sleep. *See* Nonrapid eye movement sleep
NSAIDs. *See* Nonsteroidal anti-inflammatory drugs
Nuclear gaze palsy, 80
Nucleus ambiguus, 82
Numbness
case histories, 108, 117, 203, 271–72, 302–3
facial, 19, 20*f*, 117
foot, 271–72, 302–3, 457–58
forehead, 19, 20*f*
in MS, 349–50
treatment of, 231

Nuplazid (pimavanserin), 258
Nurtec (rimegepant), 419*t*, 420*t*
Nusinersin, 214
Nutritional deficiencies, 221–22, 231*t*, 336–37
Nutritional supplements, 420*t*
Nuvigil (armodafinil), 315–16
Nystagmus
case histories, 435–36, 447
in childhood ataxia, 478–79
cranial nerve examination, 54
gaze-evoked, 438, 442
positionally induced, 442
in stroke, 130*t*, 132
in vertigo, 438, 444

Obesity
case histories, 305, 497, 502
and compression mononeuropathies, 218
and sleep disorders, 305
and stroke, 156–57
Obsessive-compulsive disorder, 296–97, 299*t*
Obstructive hydrocephalus, 244
Obstructive sleep apnea, 312–14
case histories, 305, 324
and stroke, 143, 156–57
Obtundation, 379, 380
Occipital nerve stimulation, 422*t*
Occlusive disease: of large intracranial arteries, 148
Occupational therapy, 230
Ocrelizumab (Ocrevus), 357, 366*t*
Octreotide, 422*t*
Ocular motor system, 426
Oculocephalic maneuver. *See* Doll's eyes maneuver
Oculomotor apraxia, 288
Oculomotor nerve (cranial nerve III), 27–28, 28*f*
assessment of, in altered level of consciousness, 96–98
compression of, 215–16
lesions of, 430–32, 433
third nerve palsy, 41–42, 130*t*
Ofatumumab (Kesimpta), 366*t*
Olanzapine (Zyprexa), 258, 299*t*
Older people, 347, 485–94. *See also* Aging
case histories, 485–87, 492–94
common neurologic symptoms, 490–92
monocular vision loss, 428–29
neurologic assessment of, 487

Olfaction, 53, 67
Olfactory dysfunction, 278, 347–48
Olfactory hallucinations, 257
Omaveloxolone, 287, 299*t*
Onasemnogene abeparvovec-xioi, 214
Oligoclonal bands, 353–356, 365*t*, 366*t*
Ondansetron, 292
Onfi (clobazam), 192*t*
Ongentsys (opicapone), 297*t*
Ophthalmic artery occlusion, 128
Opicapone (Ongentsys), 297*t*
Opioids/opiates
  for discomfort, 399
  for headache, 413–14, 420*t*
  overdose, 377, 382, 386–87, 394
  and pupil size, 384*t*
  for restless legs syndrome, 321–22
  for shingles, 346
Opsoclonus, 479
Optical coherence tomography, 353–54
Optic chiasm, 22–28
Optic chiasm lesions, 430, 433
Optic disc edema
  bilateral, 429–30
  case histories, 425
Optic nerve(s), 22–27
Optic nerve lesions, 76–78, 349–50, 427
Optic nerve sheath fenestration, 405–6
Optic neuritis, xxiv–xxv, 354, 355–56,
    427–28, 433–34
Oral appliances, 313–14
Oral contraceptives, 191–92, 407–8,
    411–12
Orexin (hypocretin), 309–10
Orexin (hypocretin) receptor antagonists,
    317–18
Organ donation, 393
Orthostatic hypotension, 177
  in MSA, 286–87
  in PD, 283
  treatment of, 283, 286–87
Osmolex (amantadine), 297*t*
Osmotic agents, 391
Osmotic therapy, 136–37
Ovarian cancer, 364*t*
Overflow incontinence, 460–61
Overlap myositis, 227–28
Oxcarbazepine (Trileptal)
  for seizures, 191, 192*t*, 194*t*
  for trigeminal neuralgia, 421*t*
  for vertigo, 443–44
Oxidative stress, 251, 254–55
Oxybutynin (Ditropan), 313–14, 462*t*

Oxygen therapy
  for acute mental status changes, 382–83
  for headache, 420*t*, 422*t*
Ozanimod (Zeposia), 366*t*

Pain control, 215
Pain management, 492
Pain sensation, 204–5
  age-related changes in, 490
  in altered level of consciousness, 98
  back pain, 109, 205–6, 449–55
  in Bell palsy, 217–18
  chest pain, 109, 119–20
  chronic pain, 492
  in comatose patients, 385
  facial, 19, 20*f*, 41, 418
  headache, 395–423
  jaw claudication, 404–5, 425, 434
  lesion localization and, 17*f*, 19, 40
  lightning-like, 340
  lower extremity, 496, 500
  muscle pain, 228
  musculoskeletal pain, 451–55
  neck pain, 109, 449–55, 498, 503
  neuropathic pain, 204–5, 230
  nociceptive, 204–5
  in older people, 492
  pathway for, 40
  in PD, 278
  persistent idiopathic facial, 418
  reduced, 40, 41, 109
  sciatica, 452
  sensory examination, 60–61, 100*t*, 385
Palatal movement, 56, 328
Palatal weakness, 82, 118–19
Pallidotomy, 282, 292
Palmomental reflex, 60, 490
PAN (polyarteritis nodosa), 359
PAP. *See* Positive airway pressure
Papilledema
  in headache, 410
  in IIH, 405–6
  in increased ICP, 481
  in mass lesions, 404
  in tuberculous meningitis, 343
Paradoxical insomnia, 319
Paradoxical IRIS, 339
Paralytic agents, 392
Paraneoplastic antibody panels, 332–33
Paraneoplastic syndromes, 265, 332–33, 479
  case histories, 239, 270
  commonly associated antibodies, 364*t*
Paraparesis, 69, 343

Paraphasia, 64
  case histories, 238
  literal or phonemic, 64
  semantic or verbal, 64
Paraplegia, 69
Parasitic infections, 347
Parasomnias
  classification of, 311
  definition of, 307
  NREM sleep, 320–22
  REM sleep, 319
Parasympathetic nervous system
  innervation of pupils, 27–28, 28f
  lesions of, 75–76, 77f
Paratonia, 69–70, 490
Parcopa (levodopa/carbidopa), 297t
Paresis, general, 340
Paresthesias, 204–5, 231, 349–50
Parietal lesions, 74–75
Parkinson disease (PD), 112, 277–83
  case histories, 271, 302
  characteristic protein accumulations,
    298t
  clinical features of, 277–78
  with dementia, 251–52, 265, 278, 501
  differential diagnosis of, 257–58, 278,
    279–80
  early, 271, 302
  etiology of, 278–79
  incidence of, 278
  medications for, 297t
  pathology of, 278–79
  REM sleep behavior disorder and, 323
  treatment of motor manifestations of,
    281–82
  treatment of nonmotor manifestations
    of, 283
Parkinsonian features, 251–52, 257
Parkinsonian syndromes, 283–87
Parkinsonism, 275, 488
  in AD, 251–52
  case histories, 271–72, 302–3, 501
  definition of, 274
  drug-induced, 271–72, 279–80, 302–3
  in Huntington disease, 290
  in Wilson disease, 294
Paroxysmal hemicrania, 417, 418
Paroxysmal positional vertigo. See Benign
    paroxysmal positional vertigo
    (BPPV)
Paroxysmal symptoms, in children,
    475–77
  case histories, 467, 468, 479–81, 483

Paroxysmal vertigo, benign, of childhood,
    477
Partial seizures, 168
PASC (postacute sequelae of COVID-19),
    347–48
Passive manipulation: resistance to, 69–
    70, 98, 385
  in infants, 470
Patellar reflex testing, 59, 91
Patent foramen ovale (PFO), 145
Patient cooperation, 64–65
Patient education, 187–88, 270, 291, 372,
    409
Patient history, 46–49
PCA-1 (Purkinje cell antibody), 364t
PCA (posterior cerebral artery) occlusion,
    129f, 130t, 132
PCR. See Polymerase chain reaction
PCSK9 inhibitor (proprotein convertase
    subtilisein/kexin type 9 inhibitor),
    140t, 141–42
PD. See Parkinson disease
Pediatric neurology, 467–84
  case histories, 467–69, 479–84
  developmental considerations, 469–70
  paroxysmal symptoms, 475–77
PEG (percutaneous endoscopic
    gastrostomy) tubes, 212
Pelvic parasympathetic plexus, 458
Penetrating artery disease, 148, 149–50
Penicillamine, 296, 299t
Penicillin, 179, 341
Penicillin G, 342
Penile erections, 323–24
Pentobarbital, 197t, 392
Pentoxifylline, 361
Perampanel (Fycompa), 192t, 194t
Percutaneous discectomy, 453–54
Percutaneous endoscopic gastrostomy
    (PEG) tubes, 212
Periactin (cyproheptadine), 420t
Periarteritis nodosa, 359
Perilymphatic fistula, 443
Periodic limb movements of sleep,
    321–22
Peripheral hypotonia, 472
Peripheral nerve disorders
    (neuropathies), 215–22
Peripheral nerve lesions, 39, 205–6
  vs. central lesions, 11, 22, 41, 82, 105
  diffuse, 84
  focal, 84
  reflexes and, 41

Peripheral nervous system, 12*f*, 15–19,
  18*f*
  diffuse disease, 84
  electrodiagnostic studies, 208–9
  functional divisions of, 204–5
  HIV syndromes, 336–37
  incontinence and, 460–61
  lesions in, 203–4
  for lower extremity movements, 85, 87*f*
  metastatic cancer in, 332
  primary angiitis of, 360
  proximal-to-distal organization of,
    205–8
  sensory innervation for, 88–89, 89*f*, 90*f*
  for upper extremity movements, 85,
    86*f*
Peripheral polyneuropathy, 39
  case histories, 235–36, 271–72, 302–3,
    436–37, 448
  in HIV, 336–37
  in Lyme disease, 341–42
Peripheral reflex arc, 22, 26*f*
Peripheral vertigo
  differential diagnosis of, 439–45
  lesion localization, 437–38
  recurrent episodes, 439–45
Peripheral vestibular system, 437–38
Peripheral vestibulopathy, acute, 444–45
Periventricular leukomalacia, 473–74,
  478, 482
Peroneal nerve, 90*f*
Perseveration, 75, 284–85
Persistent binocular vision loss, 430
Persistent idiopathic facial pain, 418
Persistent symptoms, 111
Personality changes
  case histories, 108–9, 118
  in Huntington disease, 290
  in primary dementing illness, 247
  in PSP, 284–85
  in tuberculous meningitis, 343
Pessaries, 459
PET. *See* Positron emission tomography
PFO (patent foramen ovale), 145
Pharyngeal weakness, 82
Phencyclidine, 179, 387
Phenobarbital (Luminal)
  drug-drug interactions, 185
  for seizures, 191, 192*t*, 194*t*
  side effects of, 185
  for status epilepticus, 197*t*
  teratogenic effects of, 191
Phenothiazines, 269, 279–80, 299*t*

Phenytoin (Dilantin, Phenytek)
  drug-drug interactions, 185, 192*t*
  for MS, 357
  for neuropathic pain and dysesthesia, 230
  for seizures, 165–66, 192*t*, 194*t*
  side effects of, 185
  for status epilepticus, 197*t*
  for trigeminal neuralgia, 421*t*
Phlebotomy, 149
Phonemic paraphasia, 64
Phonophobia, 411
Photophobia, 395, 411
Phrenic nerve stimulators, 313–14
Physical examination
  in comatose patients, 385
  of infants, 470, 471*f*
  neurologic examination, 45–105
Physical therapy
  for back pain, 452, 454
  for developmental delay, 482
  for disequilibrium, 494
  for Duchenne muscular dystrophy, 482
  for gait disturbances, 448
  for MS, 357
  for musculoskeletal pain, 452, 454–55
  for neuromuscular diseases, 230, 236
  for plexopathies, 215
  for stroke, 138–39
Pick disease, 259
Pill-rolling, 278
Pimavanserin (Nuplazid), 258, 282
Pimozide, 299*t*
Pinprick sensation
  example neurologic deficits, 8–15, 9*f*,
    10*f*, 12*f*, 13*f*, 14*f*, 17*f*, 18*f*, 33, 34, 35*f*,
    37–39, 38*f*
  left forehead: pathway for, 11–15, 13*f*,
    14*f*, 19–33, 20*f*, 21*f*
  reduced, 33, 34, 37–39, 109, 118–19
  right hand, 8–15, 9*f*, 10*f*, 12*f*, 14*f*, 18*f*,
    19–33, 21*f*, 34
  right upper extremity: pathway for,
    15–19, 17*f*
Pins and needles, 204–5
Pitolisant (Wakix), 315–16
Plague, 349
Plantar responses, 59, 91
Plasma exchange
  for autoimmune neuropathies, 221–22
  for LEMS, 225–26
  for myasthenia gravis, 225
  for paraneoplastic antibodies, 333
  for TTP, 361–62

Plasticity, developmental, 469–70
Plegridy (interferon beta-1a), 366*t*
Pleocytosis, 343–44, 345
Plexus disorders (plexopathies), 206,
  215, 360
PMA (progressive muscular atrophy),
  207*f*, 213
PML (progressive multifocal
  leukoencephalopathy), 337–39
PNEEs (psychogenic nonepileptic
  events), 178–79
PNESs (psychogenic nonepileptic spells),
  178–79, 363
Pneumonia, 138, 236, 387–88
Poliovirus, 213
Polyangiitis, 359
Polyarteritis nodosa (PAN), 359
Polycythemia vera, 149
Polymerase chain reaction (PCR) testing,
  340–41, 342
  for HSV, 345
  for JC virus, 338–39
  for meningitis, 343–44, 400, 402–3
Polymyalgia rheumatica, 404–5, 492
Polymyositis, 227–28
Polyneuropathy, 39, 206, 215, 217*f*, 218–19
  case histories, 235–36, 271–72, 302–3,
    436–37, 448, 486–87, 494
  causes of, 219
  DANG THERAPIST mnemonic for,
    219
  diabetic, 219–20, 221–22, 271–72,
    302–3, 478
  flowchart for identifying, 207*f*
  in older people, 486–87, 494
  paraneoplastic, 332–33
  patterns, 220–21
  peripheral (*see* Peripheral
    polyneuropathy)
  in Sjögren syndrome, 358–59
  in SLE, 358
Polypharmacy, 237–38, 268–69, 491
Polyradiculoneuropathy, 207*f*
Polyradiculopathy, 214
  case histories, 235–36
  flowchart for identifying, 207*f*
  progressive, 336–37
Polysomnography, 310–11, 313, 323
Ponesimod (Ponvory), 366*t*
Pons, 15
Positional therapy, 313–14
Positional vertigo, benign paroxysmal
  (BPPV), 435, 440–42, 446–47

Position sense
  age-related changes in, 490
  case histories, 486–87, 494
  example neurologic deficits, 33–34,
    35*f*, 36*f*
  neurologic examination, 46, 61
  pathway for, 19, 23*f*, 35*f*, 36*f*, 40
  reduced, 486–87, 494
Positive airway pressure (PAP)
  autoadjusting (APAP), 313–14
  bilevel (BiPAP), 212, 236, 313–14, 499
  continuous (CPAP), 313–14
  expiratory (EPAP), 313–14
Positive phenomena, 168–69
Positron emission tomography (PET),
  xxiii, 380–81
  in AD, 253
  in FTD, 260
  in progressive dementia, 245
  whole-body, 245
Postacute sequelae of COVID-19 (PASC),
  347–48
Postcentral gyrus of cortex, 38–39
Postcentral gyrus of cortex lesions, 34
Post-concussion syndrome, 391, 409
Post-COVID-19 syndrome, 347
Posterior cerebral artery (PCA) occlusion,
  129*f*, 130*t*, 132
Posterior circulation, 125
Posterior cortical atrophy, 247, 251, 267*t*
Posterior fossa surgery, 421*t*
Posterior fossa tumors, 479, 481
Posterior reversible encephalopathy
  syndrome (PRES), 387, 407–8
Postherpetic neuralgia, 345–46
Postinfectious ataxia, 478–79
  case histories, 468, 481
Post-traumatic stress disorder, 323
Post-traumatic syndrome, 391, 409
Posttreatment Lyme disease syndrome,
  342
Postural instability
  age-related changes in, 489–90
  case histories, 271–72
  in PSP, 284–85
Postural tremor, 275, 276
  in CBD, 285
  definition of, 274
  in older people, 490
  in PD, 278
PPA. *See* Primary progressive aphasia
Practice cases, 495–503
Pramipexole (Mirapex), 297*t*

Prediabetes, 219–20, 221–22
Prednisolone, 217–18, 498
Prednisone
  for CIDP, 221–22
  for cluster headache, 422t
  for Duchenne muscular dystrophy, 482
  for giant cell arteritis, 405, 434
  for MS, 356–57
  for myasthenia gravis, 225, 235
  for myopathy, 228–29
Predominantly distal weakness, 84
Prefrontal cortex lesions, 75
Pregabalin (Lyrica)
  for neuropathic pain and dysesthesia,
    230
  for restless legs syndrome, 321–22, 325
  for seizures, 192t, 194t
  for shingles, 346
Pregnancy
  headache in, 407–8, 410, 413–14
  seizures in, 165–66, 190–92, 199–200
PRES (posterior reversible
    encephalopathy syndrome), 387
Presbycusis, 489
Presbyopia, 489
Prescription drugs. *See also specific drugs*
  medication overuse headache, 412–13
  polypharmacy, 237–38, 268–69, 491
  and seizures, 171, 179
Presenilin-1, 250
Presenilin-2, 250
Presyncope, 177
Primary lateral sclerosis, 213
Primary progressive aphasia (PPA), 246–
    47, 258–59
  case histories, 496, 499–500
  logopenic variant, 246–47, 251, 266t
  nonfluent/agrammatic, 246–47, 260,
    266t, 284–85, 496, 499–500
  semantic variant, 246–47, 260, 266t
Primidone (Mysoline)
  drug-drug interactions, 185, 192t
  for seizures, 192t, 194t
  side effects of, 185
  for tremor, 276–77
Primitive reflexes, 60, 490
Prinivil (lisinopril), 420t
Prion protein, 263
Prochlorperazine (Compazine), 279–80,
    419t
Programmed cell death, 127, 136
Progressive apraxia of speech, 247
Progressive degenerative diseases, 112

Progressive developmental disorders, 114
Progressive multifocal
    leukoencephalopathy (PML), 337–39
Progressive muscular atrophy (PMA),
    207f, 213
Progressive neoplastic diseases, 112–13
Progressive polyradiculopathy, 336–37
Progressive supranuclear palsy (PSP),
    258–59, 284–85, 298t
Progressive symptoms, 111
  case histories, 116, 117–18, 119–20
  in inflammatory diseases, 113
  in toxic and metabolic diseases,
    113–14
  in traumatic diseases, 114
  in vascular diseases, 113
Progressive systemic sclerosis
    (scleroderma), 359
Promethazine (Phenergan), 279–80
Pronator drift, 58
Propofol, 197t
Propranolol (Inderal, Inderal LA)
  case histories, 123
  for headache, 413–14, 420t, 423
  for tardive dyskinesias, 299t
  for tremor, 276–77
Proprioception. *See* Position sense
Proprioceptive sense. *See* Position sense
Proprotein convertase subtilisein/kexin
    type 9 inhibitor (PCSK9 inhibitor),
    140t, 141–42
Prosody, 64
Prosopagnosia, 64
Prostate cancer, 364t
Prostatic hypertrophy, 491–92
Protriptyline (Vivactil), 313–14
Provigil (Modafinil), 315–16
Pseudoataxia, 205, 358–59
Pseudoathetosis, 205
Pseudobulbar affect, 212
Pseudobulbar palsy, 82
Pseudodementia, 243
Pseudotumor cerebri, 405–6, 429–30
PSP (progressive supranuclear palsy),
    258–59, 284, 298t
Psychogenic nonepileptic events
    (PNEEs), 178–79
Psychogenic nonepileptic spells (PNESs),
    178–79
Psychogenic symptoms, 362–63
Psychological factors, 486–87, 494
Psychophysiologic insomnia, 316–18
  case histories, 305, 324–25

Psychosis, 262–63
Ptosis
    anisocoria and, 75–76
    in botulism, 349
    case histories, 201–2, 497, 501
    cranial nerve examination, 54
    in Horner syndrome, 41–42, 76
    lesion localization, 41–42, 105
    in myasthenia gravis, 224
    in older people, 489
    with third nerve palsy, 41–42
Pulvinar sign, 264–65
Pupillary abnormalities, 75–78
    asymmetry, 41–42, 75–76, 77f, 105, 378
    lesion localization, 45, 105
    in syphilis, 340
Pupillary light reflex
    in comatose patients, 383–85
    cranial nerve examination, 53–54
    pathway for, 27–28, 28f
    screening examination, 91, 94
Pupillary size, 45
    determination of, 29f, 29–30, 75–76
    drugs that affect, 384–85, 384t
Pupils
    blown, 383–84
    in comatose patients, 383–85
    innervation of, 29f, 29–30
Purkinje cell antibody (PCA-1), 364t
Pyramidal weakness, 84
Pyrazinamide, 344
Pyridostigmine (Mestinon)
    for MSA, 286–87
    for myasthenia gravis, 225, 235, 501
Pyridoxine (vitamin B6), 344
Pyrimethamine, 338–39

Quadriparesis, 69
Quadriplegia, 69
Quetiapine (Seroquel)
    for DLB, 258
    for PD, 282
    for tardive dyskinesia, 292
    for tics, 299t
Quinidine sulfate, 212
Qulipta (atogepant), 420t
Quviviq (daridorexant), 317–18

Radial nerve, 88–89, 90f
Radiation therapy
    for metastatic cancer, 330, 331–32
    for vertebral metastasis, 450, 454
    whole-brain, 330

Radiculopathy, 205–6, 214
Radiofrequency thermocoagulation, 421t
Radiosurgery, 330, 421t, 423, 447
Ramelteon (Rozerem), 317–18
Ramsay Hunt syndrome, 346
Ranitidine (Zantac), 237–38
Rapid alternating movements, 57
Rapid eye movement (REM) sleep, 319
    parasomnias, 319, 323–24
    physiology of, 307–10, 308f
Rapid eye movement (REM) sleep
        behavior disorder, 323
    case histories, 497, 501
    in DLB, 257
    in MSA, 286
    in PD, 278
Rapid plasma reagin (RPR), 243–44,
        340–41
Rasagiline (Azilect), 297t
Ravulizumab, 225
Razadyne (galantamine), 254
RCVS (reversible cerebral
        vasoconstriction syndrome), 402,
        407–8
Reading assessment, 51
Real-time quaking-induced conversion
        (RT-QuIC), 264–65, 280
Rebif (interferon beta-1a), 366t
Rebound headache, 412–13
Recent memory, 52
Receptive aphasia, 64
Recombinant tissue plasminogen
        activator (rtPA), 134–36, 157t,
        162–63
Recreational drugs, 171, 179
Reflex(es). See also Deep tendon reflexes;
        Tendon reflexes
    age-related changes in, 490
    central lesion and, 41
    corneal, 54–55, 68, 98
    gag, 68, 98
    grading, 71
    hyperactive, 22, 33–34, 84,
        108, 202
    hypoactive, 22
    increased, 41
    peripheral lesion and, 41
    primitive, 60, 490
    pupillary, 53–54
    reduced, 41
    subtle asymmetry, 71–72
    superficial, 60
Reflex arc, 22, 26f, 41

Reflex examination, 59–60
  detection and documentation of subtle
    asymmetry, 71–72
  grading reflexes, 71
  interpretation of, 88
  relaxing the patient, 72
  screening examination, 91
  technique, 71–72
Refractory seizures, 186–87, 192
Reglan (metoclopramide), 271–72, 419t
Rehabilitation
  stroke, 138–39
  vestibular, 444–45
Relaxing the patient, 72
Relpax (eletriptan), 419t
Remeron (mirtazapine), 313–14
REM-on cells, 309, 323
Remote electrical neuromodulation,
  413–14
Remote memory, 52
REM sleep. See Rapid eye movement sleep
Renal abnormalities, 243–44, 386
Reperfusion therapy, 136
Repetition, 51
Repetitive movements, 467
Reporting findings, 66
Requip (ropinirole), 297t
Reserpine, 279–80, 299t
Respiratory failure, 203
Responsive brain stimulation, 187
Restless legs syndrome, 321–22
  case histories, 305, 324–25
Rest tremor
  case histories, 271–72, 302–3
  definition of, 274
  in PD, 278
Retina, 22–27
Retinal artery occlusion, 428
Retinal detachment, 428
Retinal lesions, 76
Reversible cerebral vasoconstriction
  syndrome (RCVS), 402, 407–8
Reversible posterior leukoencephalopathy
  syndrome (RPLS), 387
Reyvow (lasmiditan), 419t
Rheumatoid arthritis, 227–28, 358
Rheumatologic diseases, 357–60
Rhythmic movement disorder, sleep-
  related, 322
Riboflavin, 413–14, 420t
Rifampin, 344
Rigidity
  in AD, 251–52

case histories, 271
  in CBD, 285
  cogwheel, 69–70, 271
  definition of, 274
  in DLB, 257
  lead-pipe, 69–70
  motor examination, 69–70
  in PD, 278
  in PSP, 284–85
Riluzole, 212, 236, 299t, 499
Rimegepant (Nurtec), 419t, 420t
Rinne test, 68
Risdiplam, 214
Risperidone, 299t
Ritalin (methylphenidate), 315–16
Rituximab, 225, 338–39, 357, 361–62
Rivaroxaban, 140t, 144
Rivastigmine (Exelon), 254
Rizatriptan (Maxalt, Maxalt-MLT), 419t
Romberg test, 61, 445
Root reflex, 60, 490
Ropinirole (Requip), 297t
Rosuvastatin, 140t
Rotigotine (Neupro), 297t
Rozanolixizumab-noli, 225
Rozerem (ramelteon), 317–18
RPLS (reversible posterior
  leukoencephalopathy syndrome),
  387
RPR (rapid plasma reagin), 340–41
rtPA. See Recombinant tissue
  plasminogen activator
RT-QuIC (real-time quaking-induced
  conversion), 264–65, 280
Rufinamide (Banzel), 192t, 194t
Rytary (levodopa/carbidopa), 297t

Sabril (vigabatrin), 192t
Saccades, voluntary, 54
Safety issues, 256, 270
Safety restraints, 320
Safinamide (Xadago), 297t
Sagging brain, 405–6
SAH. See Subarachnoid hemorrhage
Saline infusion, 406–7
Sanctura (trospium), 462t
Saphenous nerve, 90f
Sarcoidosis, 227, 360–61
SARS-CoV-2, 347
Satralizumab, 357
Scalp lacerations, 388–89
  case histories, 378, 394
SCAs (spinocerebellar ataxias), 288–89

School problems: case histories, 468–69, 483–84
Schwannoma, 439
  case histories, 117, 447
Sciatica, 452
Sciatic nerve, 85
Scleroderma (progressive systemic sclerosis), 359
SCM (sternocleidomastoid) muscle, 56, 83
SCN (suprachiasmatic nuclei), 310
Scopolamine, 387
Screening examination, 46
  neurologic examination, 90–91
  standardized tests, 66
  video examination, 92–94
SDH. *See* Subdural hematoma
α-Secretase, 249–50, 250*f*
β-Secretase, 249–50, 250*f*
γ-Secretase, 249–50, 250*f*
Sedative-hypnotic medications
  for increased ICP, 392
  for insomnia, 317–18
  side effects of, 316, 320–21, 393–94
Sedimentation rate. *See* Erythrocyte sedimentation rate
Seizure disorder, 168. *See also* Epilepsy
Seizures, 165–200
  absence (*see* Absence seizures)
  acute mental status changes after, 387
  in AD, 252
  in anthrax meningoencephalitis, 348
  approach to, 166
  ASMs effective for, 194*t*
  atonic, 170, 194*t*
  brain disorders that can predispose to, 181
  in brain metastasis, 331
  case histories, 108, 116–17, 165–66, 198–200, 239, 270, 468, 483
  cause of, 179–82
  in children, 468, 476, 483
  clinical characteristics of, 168–71
  complex partial, 168
  definition of, 167
  diagnosis of, 175–79
  diagnostic evaluation of, 181–82
  differential diagnosis of, 178
  driving restrictions, 189
  EEG patterns, 173
  in encephalitis, 403
  vs. epilepsy, 171–72
  faciobrachial dystonic, 332–33
  febrile, 179–80, 181

focal (*see* Focal-onset seizures)
focal aware, 167
focal impaired awareness, 167
generalized, 116–17
generalized-onset, 167, 169–71, 194*t*
generalized tonic-clonic, 165–66, 170, 194*t*
in HSE, 344–45
in Huntington disease, 290
key conditions, 174
management of, 182–89
in meningitis, 343, 403
in MS, 349–50
myoclonic, 171, 194*t*
neonatal, 476
nocturnal, 322–23
in paraneoplastic syndromes, 332–33
partial, 168
pathophysiology of, 174–75
patient education for, 187–88
in pregnancy, 165–66, 190–92
provoked, 179–80
recurrent, 171–72
refractory, 186–87, 192
restrictions, 189
simple partial, 168
in SLE, 358
during sleep, 180, 322
in stroke, 137
surgery for, 185–86
tonic, 349–50
tonic-clonic, 189–90, 197*t*, 200
of unknown onset, 171
urgent, 181
withdrawal, 179
Selective serotonin reuptake inhibitors (SSRIs)
  for agitation, 256
  for cataplexy, 315–16
  for MS, 357
  for neuropathic pain and dysesthesia, 230
  for nightmares, 323
  for night terrors, 320
  side effects of, 276, 407–8
  for tics, 299*t*
Selegiline (Deprenyl, Eldepryl, Zelapar), 297*t*
Self-limited epilepsy with centrotemporal spikes (SeLECTS), 180, 322, 476
  case histories, 467, 479–80
Semantic or verbal paraphasia, 64
Semantic variant primary progressive aphasia, 246–47, 260, 266*t*

Semont-plus maneuver, 441–42
Sensorimotor polyneuropathy, 207*f*
Sensory deficits
  anomalous or inconsistent exam
    findings, 99, 100*t*
  bilateral, 40–41
  case histories, 327
  in distal limbs, 39
  in stroke, 123–24, 130*t*, 132
Sensory nerves, 204
Sensory neuronopathy, 205, 358–59
  flowchart for identifying, 207*f*
  large-fiber, 231*t*
Sensory neuropathy, 221
  large-fiber, 231*t*
  painful, 219–20
  paraneoplastic, 332–33
  in sarcoidosis, 360
  in Sjögren's syndrome, 358–59
Sensory pathway, 40
Sensory pathway lesions, 204–5
Sensory polyneuropathy, 207*f*
Sensory system examination, 49,
    60–62
  in altered level of consciousness, 98
  interpretation of, 88–89
  screening examination, 91, 94
  technique for, 72–73
Sepsis, 387–88
Septic emboli, 334–35
Serial sevens, 73–74
Seroquel (quetiapine), 258
Serotonin, 397
Serotonin-$_{1B/D}$ agonists (triptans)
  for headache, 419*t*, 420*t*
  side effects of, 407–8, 413–14
Serotonin-norepinephrine-reuptake
    inhibitors (SNRIs)
  for back pain, 452
  for cataplexy, 315–16
  for headache, 420*t*
  for neuropathic pain and dysesthesia,
    230
  side effects of, 407–8
  for tics, 299*t*
Shingles. *See* Herpes varicella-zoster
Short-lasting unilateral neuralgiform
    headache attacks (SUNHAs),
    417–18
Short-lasting unilateral neuralgiform
    headache attacks with cranial
    autonomic symptoms (SUNAs),
    417–18

Short-lasting unilateral neuralgiform
    headache with conjunctival
    injection and tearing (SUNCT),
    417–18
Short-term memory, 52
Shoulder abduction
  nerve roots and peripheral nerves
    corresponding to, 85, 86*f*
  testing, 58
Shoulder elevation, 56
Shunting, 245
  lumboperitoneal, 405–6
  ventriculoperitoneal, 405–6
Shy-Drager syndrome, 286
SIADH (syndrome of inappropriate
    secretion of antidiuretic hormone),
    137
Sickle cell disease, 149, 156
Simple partial seizures, 168
Simultaneous stimulation, double, 62
Sinemet (levodopa/carbidopa), 281, 297*t*
Single nerve root lesions, 119
Single-photon emission computed
    tomography (SPECT), xxiii, 253,
    280
Single-pulse transcranial magnetic
    stimulation (sTMS), 413–14
Sinus disease, 408–9
Sinusitis, 408–9
Siponimod (Mayzent), 366*t*
Sixth nerve lesions, 430–32, 433
Sixth nerve palsy, 405–6
Sjögren syndrome, 227–28, 358–59
Skeletal deformities, 287
Skeletal muscle relaxants, 452
Skin biopsy, 209
Skin care, 138
Skin color changes, 177
Skin rash, 345–46
Skull fracture, 388–89
SLE (systemic lupus erythematosus),
    227–28, 358
Sleep
  abnormal behaviors during, 178, 319–24
  abnormal movements during, 178
  definition of, 307
  delta, 308*f*, 308–9
  insufficient, 312
  NREM (*see* Nonrapid eye movement
    sleep)
  physiology of, 307–10
  REM (*see* Rapid eye movement sleep)
  seizures during, 180

slow-wave, 308*f*, 308–9
stages of, 308*f*, 308
Sleep apnea, 312–14
central, 312, 313–14
home tests, 310–11
obstructive (*see* Obstructive sleep apnea)
Sleep attacks, 177–78, 311–12
Sleep deprivation, 312
Sleep disorders, 305–25
in AD, 252, 256
approach to, 306–7
case histories, 305–6, 324–25
classification of, 311
in COVID-19, 347–48
definitions, 307
diagnostic tests, 310–11
differential diagnosis of, 178
in DLB, 258
in PD, 278, 283
trouble sleeping, 316–19
trouble staying awake, 311–16
Sleep fragmentation, 316, 319
Sleep hygiene, 315–16
Sleep-onset delay, 316–18
Sleep paralysis, 315
Sleep-related breathing disorders, 311
Sleep-related movement disorders, 311
Sleep-related rhythmic movement disorder, 322
Sleep state misperception, 319
Sleep studies, 310–11
Sleep talking, 320, 321
Sleep terrors, 320
Sleep-wake cycle, 310
Sleep-wake schedule disturbances
advanced sleep-wake phase disorder, 319
delayed sleep-wake phase disorder, 318
Sleepwalking, 320, 321
Slit-lamp examination, 295–96
Slow-wave sleep, 308*f*, 308–9
Slurred speech, 495–96, 499
SMA (spinal muscular atrophy), 207*f*, 213–14, 472
Small-cell lung cancer, 270, 364*t*
Small-fiber neuropathy, 209, 231*t*
Smallpox, 348
Smell discrimination, 489
SMN1 (survival motor neuron 1 gene), 213–14
SMN2 (survival motor neuron 2 gene), 213–14

Smoking, 153
Smoking cessation, 143
Smooth pursuit movements, 54
Snout reflex, 60, 490
SNRIs. *See* Serotonin-norepinephrine-reuptake inhibitors
Social developmental delay, 475
SOD (superoxide dismutase), 211–12
Sodium oxybate, 315–16, 323
Soft neurologic signs, 483
Soft tissue injections, 452
Solifenacin (Vesicare), 462*t*
Solriamfetol (Sunosi), 315–16
Solumedrol (methylprednisolone), 420*t*
Somatic nervous system, 204
Somatization, 362–63
Somatoform disorder, 362–63
Somnambulism, 320
Somnolence, daytime, 239, 270
excessive, 177–78, 283, 311–16 (*See also* Hypersomnia)
Sonata (zaleplon), 317–18
Spasmodic torticollis, 496–97, 500–1
Spasms, infantile, 170–71, 194*t*, 476
Spastic bladder, 460, 461, 462*t*
Spasticity, 69–70, 473–74, 478
in AD, 252, 485–86
case histories, 202, 436, 485–86
interventions for, 482
motor examination, 69–70, 84
SPECT (single-photon emission computed tomography), xxiii, 253, 280
Speech
Broca's area and, 30*f*, 30–33
progressive apraxia of, 247
slurred, 495–96, 499
Speech deterioration, 223
Speech discrimination, 489
Speech pathologists, 230
Spells
breath-holding, 476–77
case histories, 467, 483
daydreaming, 468, 483
nonepileptic, 173–74, 176–79
Sphenoid sinusitis, 408
Spinal cord
cervical, 38*f*
compression of, 448, 450, 463
degenerative disease of, 214, 457–58
joint position sense and, 34, 35*f*
lesion localization, 15–19
pathways, 19, 21*f*, 40

Spinal cord lesions, 15–19, 40–41, 119–20
  case histories, 436, 447–48
  cervical, 34, 436, 447–48
  HIV-associated, 337–38
  incontinence and, 457–58
Spinal fluid analysis, 245, 345, 355–56.
  See also Cerebrospinal fluid (CSF)
Spinal metastasis, 329–30, 449, 454
Spinal muscular atrophy (SMA), 207f,
  213–14, 472
Spinal nerve root lesions, 205–6
Spinal stenosis, 454
  case histories, 496, 500
  lumbar, 451, 496, 500
Spinal tap. See Lumbar puncture
Spinocerebellar ataxias (SCAs), 288–89
Spirochetal infections, 344–46
Splitting the midline, 100t
Spongiform encephalopathy, 262–63
  bovine (BSE), 264
Spontaneous intracranial hypotension,
  405–6
SSRIs. See Selective serotonin reuptake
  inhibitors
Stabbing headache, primary, 418
Stadol (butorphanol), 420t
Stalevo (levodopa, carbidopa,
  entacapone), 297t
Standardized screening tests, 66
Staphylocccus aureus endocarditis, 335
Static (stationary) symptoms, 111
  in congenital and developmental
    diseases, 114
  in toxic and metabolic diseases,
    113–14
  in traumatic diseases, 114
  in vascular diseases, 113
Statin therapy
  and myopathy, 227–28
  for stroke prevention, 139–40, 140t,
    148, 153
Stationary symptoms. See Static
  symptoms
Status epilepticus, 137, 189–90
  case histories, 166, 200
  convulsive, 166, 190, 200
  definition of, 168
  in Lennox-Gastaut syndrome, 180–81
  management of, 182, 189–90, 197t
  nonconvulsive, 190
Stavudine (d4T), 336–37
Stenting, 140t, 147, 156, 261–62
Stereognosis, 62

Stereotactic radiosurgery, 330–31, 421t,
  423
Sternocleidomastoid (SCM) muscle, 56, 83
Steroids, xxiv–xxv. See also
  Corticosteroids; specific steroids
  for compression mononeuropathies, 215
  for dermatomyositis, 234–35
  for musculoskeletal pain, 452
  and myopathy, 227
  for paraneoplastic antibodies, 333
  side effects of, 228–29
Stiffness, 349–50, 403, 404–5, 410
  case histories, 436
Stimulants, 316
Stocking-glove distribution, 206, 217f,
  218–19
  case histories, 235–36
Straight leg raising sign, 449, 452–53
Strength testing. See also Motor
  examination
  in altered level of consciousness, 98
  grading muscle strength, 68–69
  individual muscles, 58
  in infants, 470
  limb position for, 70–71
  modifications of, 70–71
  screening examination, 91
Streptococcus pneumoniae, 399
Streptomycin, 344
Stress incontinence, 457, 459, 462
Striatum, 273, 274–75
Stroke, 123–63
  acute, 134–39
  in AIDS, 339
  anticoagulation therapy for, 136, 144,
    145, 148–49, 154–55, 161
  antiplatelet therapy for, 136, 140t, 142,
    144, 148–49, 154
  antithrombotic therapy for, 154–55
  approach to, 124
  case histories, 118–19, 123–24, 160–63,
    498, 503
  classification by etiology, 125–26
  clinical features of, 128f, 128–33, 129f
  definition of, 125
  diagnosis of, 128–34
  dietary factors, 156–57
  in endocarditis, 335–36
  gait changes and, 491
  hemorrhagic, 125, 127–28
  imaging in, 133–34
  ischemic (see Ischemic stroke)
  lateral medullary, 130t, 149–50

left hemisphere, 137–38
lifestyle factors, 156–57
limitation of deficits in, 136–38
mechanisms of, 149–51
medial medullary, 130*t*
multiple, 280
pathophysiology of, 127–28
PD and, 280
primary prevention of, 124, 139–40,
    152–57, 160*t*
risk factors for, 445
secondary prevention of, 124, 139–51,
    140*t*, 160*t*
seizures and, 181
statin therapy for, 139–40, 140*t*, 148,
    153
systemic factors, 138
in young people, 498, 503
Stroke rehabilitation, 138–39
Stupor, 108, 380
after seizure, 387
definition of, 379
in HSE, 344–45
initial management of, 381
in tuberculous meningitis, 343
Subacute delirium, 239, 270
Subacute infections, 113
Subacute inflammatory diseases, 113
Subacute monocular vision loss
in older people, 428–29
in young people, 427–28
Subacute neoplastic diseases, 112–13
Subacute symptoms, 112, 115*t*
case histories, 116–18, 119
Subacute toxic and metabolic diseases,
    113–14
Subarachnoid hemorrhage (SAH), 133,
    387–88, 398–402
case histories, 118
diagnosis of, 398–400
secondary prevention of, 151–52
Subdural hematoma (SDH)
case history, 117
dementia and, 244
gait changes and, 491
Subpial transections, 186
Subway map of nervous system, 5–7, 6*f*
Suck reflex, 490
Sudden unexplained death in epilepsy
    (SUDEP), 189
Sulfadiazine, 338–39
Sumatriptan (Imitrex), xxiv–xxv, 419*t*,
    420*t*, 421*t*, 422*t*, 423

SUNAs (short-lasting unilateral
    neuralgiform headache attacks
    with cranial autonomic symptoms),
    417–18
SUNCT (short-lasting unilateral
    neuralgiform headache with
    conjunctival injection and tearing),
    417–18
Sundowning, 256
SUNHAs (short-lasting unilateral
    neuralgiform headache attacks),
    417–18
Sunosi (solriamfetol), 315–16
Superficial reflexes, 60
Superior semicircular canal dehiscence,
    443
Superoxide dismutase (SOD), 211–12
Suprachiasmatic nuclei (SCN), 310
Supranuclear gaze palsy, 80
Supranuclear palsy, progressive (PSP),
    258–59, 284, 298*t*
Surgery
ablative, 185–86, 282
for back pain, 453–54
decompressive, 136–37, 421*t*, 454,
    463, 502
for disc herniation, 453–54
extracranial-intracranial bypass, 148
for metastatic cancer, 330
microsurgery, 447
non-urgent indications for, 451
for PD, 282
radiosurgery, 447
for seizures, 185–86
for sleep apnea, 313–14
spine stabilization, 450
stereotactic radiosurgery, 330–31,
    421*t*, 423
for temporomandibular
    disorders, 409
for tremor, 276–77
for trigeminal neuralgia, 421*t*
for tuberculoma, 344
for urinary incontinence, 459–60
valve replacement, 336
Survival motor neuron 1 gene (SMN1),
    213–14
Survival motor neuron 2 gene (SMN2),
    213–14
Suvorexant (Belsomra), 317–18
Swallowing problems, 138, 291
Swinging flashlight test, 76, 427
Symmetrel (amantadine), 297*t*

Sympathetic nervous system
    innervation of pupils, 29f, 29–30
    lesions of, 75–76, 77f
Sympathomimetics, 384t, 407–8
Syncope, 177, 411, 416, 475
    convulsive, 177
    defecation, 177
    micturition, 177
    vasodepressor, 177
    vasovagal, 177
Syndrome of inappropriate secretion of
    antidiuretic hormone (SIADH), 137
α-Synuclein, 278–79, 280, 283, 298t, 323
Syphilis, 243–44, 338–41
    meningovascular, 340
    neurosyphilis, 340–41, 493
    primary, 339–40
    secondary, 339–40
Systemic conditions, 408
Systemic lupus erythematosus (SLE),
    227–28, 245, 358
Systemic sclerosis, 227–28, 359

Tabes dorsalis, 340
Tacrine, xxiv–xxv
Tacrolimus, 276
TACs (trigeminal autonomic
    cephalalgias), 417–18
Tactile hallucinations, 257
Tamoxifen, 276
Tardive dyskinesia, 292, 299t
TAR (transactivation response region)-
    DNA binding protein 43 (TDP-43),
    211–12, 229, 259–60, 262
Tascenso (fingolimod), 366t
Task-specific tremor, 274
Tasmar (tolcapone), 297t
Taste discrimination, 489
Taste sensation, 217–18, 347–48
Tau protein
    accumulations in AD, 253–54, 298t
    accumulations in CJD, 264–65
    accumulations in degenerative
        dementing illnesses and movement
        disorders, 298t
    accumulations in FTD, 259–60, 298t
    accumulations in parkinsonian
        syndromes, 283–85
    hyperphosphorylated, 229
TCAR (transcarotid artery
    revascularization), 147
TCD (transcranial Doppler) ultrasound,
    150–51, 156

TDP-43 (TAR-DNA binding protein of 43
    kDa), 211–12, 229, 259–60, 262
Tecfidera (dimethyl fumarate), 366t
TEE (transesophageal echocardiography),
    140–41, 150–51
Tegretol (carbamazepine), 192t, 422t
Telangiectasias, 288
Temperature abnormalities, 386
Temperature sensation
    facial, 19, 20f, 41
    lesion localization, 40
    neurologic examination, 46
    pathways for, 19, 20f, 40
    reduced, 41
    sensory examination, 60–61
Temporal (giant cell) arteritis, 404–5,
    428, 492
    case histories, 425, 434
    dementia and, 245
    vision loss in, 425, 434
Temporal artery biopsy, 405, 434
Temporal profile, 110, 111–12
Temporomandibular disorders, 409
Tendon reflexes, 22
    absent, 203
    examination of, 59, 94
    grading of, 71
    hyperactive, 202
Tenecteplase (TNK), 134
Tenormin (atenolol), 420t
TENS (transcutaneous electrical nerve
    stimulation), distal, 413–14
Tensilon test, 224
Tension headache, 410–14, 419t, 423
Teriflunomide (Aubagio), 366t
Terminal tremor, 274
Terminology
    acute mental status changes, 378–79
    anatomic definitions, 272–73
    aphasia, 65–66
    mental status examination, 62–64,
        65–66
    motor examination, 69–70
    movement disorders, 273–74
    muscle tone, 69–70
    patterns of weakness, 69
    seizures, 167–68
    sleep disorders, 307
    visual symptoms, 426
Testicular atrophy, 226–27
Testicular cancer, 364t
Testicular germ cell tumors, metastatic,
    330

Tetrabenazine, 279–80, 299t
Thalamotomy, 282
Thalamus: lesions in, 42–43
Thalidomide, 361
Theophylline, 406–7
Thermocoagulation, radiofrequency, 421t
Thiamine, 219–20, 231t, 245, 382
Thiazide diuretics, 140t, 152–53
Thiopental, 197t
Third nerve lesions, 430–32, 433
Third nerve palsy, 41–42, 130t
Thorazine (chlorpromazine), 419t
Thrombectomy, 134–36
Thrombin inhibitors, 142
Thrombolytic therapy, 136
Thrombosis, cerebral venous, 407
Thrombotic thrombocytopenic purpura
    (TTP), 361–62
Thunderclap headache, 402, 407–8
Thymectomy, 225, 235
Thymoma, 222, 225
Thymus gland, 222
Thyroglobulin antibodies, 332–33, 364t
Thyroid disease, 218, 243–44, 269, 493,
    494
Thyroid hormone replacement, 271–72
Thyroid peroxidase, 332–33
Thyroxine, 276
TIA. See Transient ischemic attack
Tiagabine (Gabitril), 192t, 194t
Tibial nerve, 89, 90f
Ticagrelor, 136, 140t, 142, 148
Tic douloureux. See Trigeminal neuralgia
Ticlopidine, xxiv–xxv
Tics, 57–58, 479–81
    in children, 467, 480–81
    classification of, 275
    definition of, 274
    therapy for, 296–97, 299t
    in Tourette syndrome, 296
Timed voiding, 461
Timolol (Blocadren), 420t
Tinel sign, 497–98
Tingling
    case histories, 108, 203, 496, 497–98,
        500, 502
    in MS, 349–50
Tinnitus
    case histories, 108, 117, 435–36, 447
    in presyncope, 177
    in Ramsay Hunt syndrome, 346
Tissue plasminogen activator (tPA),
    recombinant, 134–36, 157t, 162–63

TMS (transcranial magnetic stimulation),
    single-pulse (sTMS), 413–14
TNK (tenecteplase), 134
TNS (trigeminal nerve stimulation),
    external (eTNS), 414
Tocilizumab, 405
Toddlers. See Children
Toe walking, 482
    case histories, 468, 482
Tofersen, 212
Tolcapone (Tasmar), 297t
Tolterodine (Detrol), 462t
Tone. See Muscle tone
Tongue movement, 56
Tongue weakness, 83, 130t
Tonic activity, 167, 168–69
Tonic-clonic seizures. See also
    Generalized tonic-clonic seizures
    case histories, 165–66, 200
    management of, 189–90, 197t
Tonic seizures, 349–50
Tooth grinding, 322
Topiramate (Topamax, Trokendi)
    for headache, 420t
    for IIH, 405–6
    for neuropathic pain and dysesthesia,
        230
    for seizures, 183, 192t, 194t
    teratogenic effects of, 191
    for tics, 299t
    for tremor, 276–77
    for trigeminal neuralgia, 421t
Toprol XL (metoprolol), 237–38, 420t
Toradol (ketorolac), 419t
Torticollis, 292–93
    spasmodic, 496–97, 500–1
Tourette syndrome, 296–97, 299t, See
    also Tics
Toviaz (fesoterodine), 462t
Toxic delirium, 237–38, 268–69
Toxic exposures, 479
    drug or alcohol, 182, 389–90
Toxic-metabolic disorders
    case histories, 116–17, 118
    characteristic spatial-temporal profiles,
        115t
    conditions associated with large-
        fiber sensory neuropathy or
        neuronopathy, 231t
    etiology, 113–14
Toxoplasmosis, 337–39
tPA. See Tissue plasminogen activator
Tramadol (Ultram), 419t

Transactivation response DNA binding protein of 43 kDa (TAR DNA binding protein of 43 kDa, TDP-43), 211–12, 229, 259–60, 262
Transcarotid artery revascularization (TCAR), 147
Transcortical aphasia, 64, 74
Transcortical motor aphasia, 30*f*, 30–33, 74
Transcortical sensory aphasia, 30*f*, 30–33, 74
Transcranial Doppler (TCD) ultrasound, 150–51, 156
Transcranial magnetic stimulation, single-pulse (sTMS), 414
Transcutaneous electrical stimulation, distal (distal TENS), 413–14
Transcutaneous supraorbital nerve stimulation, 414
Transesophageal echocardiography (TEE), 140–41, 150–51
Transient global amnesia, 379
Transient hypoperfusion, 115
Transient ischemic attack (TIA)
    case histories, 160–61, 425, 434
    definition of, 125
    differential diagnosis of, 132–33, 178
    secondary stroke prevention after, 139–41, 140*t*, 151
    visual symptoms of, 429
Transient symptoms, 111, 115
Transient vision loss, 429–30
Transition tremor, 274
Transtentorial herniation, 215–16, 383–84
Transthoracic echocardiography (TTE), 140–41, 150–51
Transverse myelitis, 450–51
Trapezius muscle, 83
Trauma. *See also* Post-traumatic stress disorder
    head, 181, 388–91
    neck, 148–49
    post-traumatic syndrome, 391, 409
Traumatic diseases
    case histories, 118–19
    characteristic spatial-temporal profiles, 115*t*
    etiology, 114
Tremor(s), 57–58, 275
    action, 273, 276
    anomalous or inconsistent exam findings, 100*t*
    bilateral, 271–72, 302–3
    case histories, 271–72, 302–3

definition of, 274
essential, 276–77, 280
fragile X-associated tremor/ataxia syndrome (FXTAS), 289–90
initial, 274
intention, 273
kinetic (*see* Kinetic tremor)
in MS, 349–50, 357
in older people, 490
in PD, 278, 280
postural (*see* Postural tremor)
in PSP, 284–85
rest, 271–72, 274, 278, 302–3
task-specific, 274
terminal, 274
transition, 274
treatment of, 282
in Wilson disease, 294
Triceps reflex, 59, 91
Trichinosis, 227
Tricyclic antidepressants
    for ADHD, 299*t*
    for cataplexy, 315–16
    for enuresis, 321
    for headache, 413–14, 420*t*
    for musculoskeletal pain, 452, 454–55
    for neuropathic pain, 230
    for nightmares, 323
    for night terrors, 320
    for numbness or paresthesias, 231
    for PSP, 285
    for shingles, 346
    side effects of, 269, 276, 387, 413–14
    for sleepwalking and sleep talking, 320
Trientine, 296, 299*t*
Trigeminal autonomic cephalalgias (TACs), 417–18
Trigeminal nerve (cranial nerve V), 11–13, 98
Trigeminal nerve stimulation, external (eTNS), 414
Trigeminal neuralgia, 414–15
    in MS, 349–50, 357
    treatment of, 421*t*
Trigeminal sensory neuropathy, 358–59
Trigeminocervical complex, 396–98
Trihexyphenidyl (Artane), 297*t*
Trileptal (oxcarbazepine), 192*t*, 422*t*
Trimethoprim/sulfamethoxazole, 269
Triple flexion, 98
Triptans (serotonin-$_{1B/D}$ agonists)
    for headache, 419*t*, 420*t*
    side effects of, 407–8, 413–14
Trokendi (topiramate), 192*t*

Trospium (Sanctura), 462*t*
Trudhesa (dihydroergotamine), 419*t*
TTE (transthoracic echocardiography),
140–41, 150–51
TTP (thrombotic thrombocytopenic
purpura), 361–62
Tuberculin skin test, 343–44
Tuberculoma, 342–43, 344
Tuberculosis, 338, 342–44
Tuberculous meningitis, 342–44, 403–4
Tuberculous (TB) meningitis, 401*t*
Tularemia, 349
Tullio phenomenon, 443
Tumors
commonly associated antibodies, 364*t*
dementia and, 243–44
increased ICP and, 392
intracranial, 329–31
Turn en bloc, 277
Tylenol (acetaminophen), 419*t*
Tyrosine hydroxylase, 293–94
Tyrosine kinase inhibitors, 330, 331–32,
338–39
Tysabri (natalizumab), 366*t*

Ubiquitin, 259, 278–79
Ubiquitin-proteasome system, 278–79
Ublituximab (Briumvi), 366*t*
Ubrogepant (Ubrelvy), 419*t*
Ulnar nerve, 11, 12*f*, 88–89, 90*f*
Ulnar nerve compression, 497–98, 502
Ultram (tramadol), 419*t*
Ultrasound
carotid, 134, 150–51
color Doppler, 405
magnetic resonance-guided, 276–77,
282
for musculoskeletal pain, 452
transcranial Doppler (TCD), 150–51,
156
UMNs. *See* Upper motor neurons
Uncal herniation, 383–84, 433
Unilateral peripheral vestibulopathy,
acute idiopathic, 444–45
Unilateral prefrontal cortex disease, 75
Unmasking IRIS, 339
Upgaze palsy, 284–85
Upper extremities
muscle strength testing, 58
muscle weakness in, 15–19, 16*f*
nerve roots, 85, 86*f*, 89*f*
reflex arcs, 22, 26*f*
sensory innervation, 88–89, 89*f*, 90*f*
Upper extremity tremor, 271–72

Upper motor neuron (UMN) lesions, 84
in ALS, 209–10, 211
case histories, 235–36
pattern of weakness, 84, 105
Upper motor neurons (UMNs), 22,
81–82
Upward gaze impairment, 489
case histories, 497, 501
Uremia, 171, 179, 325, 386
Urge incontinence, 460
Urgencies
seizures, 181
visual symptoms, 425, 434
Urinary incontinence, 457–63
in AD, 252, 256
approach to, 458–61
case histories, 166, 237–38, 436, 457–
58, 462–63, 485–86, 492–93
causes of, 459–61
in dementia, 491–92
functional, 457, 459–60, 462, 491–92
in HIV-associated neurocognitive
disorder, 337
neurogenic, 461
in NPH, 244–45
in older people, 485–86, 491–93
overflow incontinence, 460–61
stress incontinence, 457, 459, 462
in syphilis, 340
urge incontinence, 460
Urinary tract infections, 138, 269, 387–
88, 460, 491–92
Urodynamic studies, 461
Uvulopalatopharyngoplasty, 313–14

Vagus nerve (cranial nerve X)
assessment of, in altered level of
consciousness, 98
pathway, 82
Vagus nerve stimulation (VNS), 186
noninvasive (nVNS), 413–14, 422*t*
Valacyclovir, 217–18
Valacyclovir, 346
Valbenazine, 299*t*
Valproic acid (Depakote, Depacon,
Depakene)
drug-drug interactions, 185
for headache, 413–14, 420*t*
for seizures, 183, 191, 192*t*, 194*t*
side effects of, 185, 191, 276, 279–80
for status epilepticus, 197*t*
for tardive dyskinesia, 299*t*
for trigeminal neuralgia, 421*t*
Valve replacement surgery, 336

Vancomycin, 116–17, 334, 371, 399
Varicella (chickenpox). *See* Herpes
 varicella-zoster
Varicella-zoster virus (VZV). *See* Herpes
 varicella-zoster virus
Vascular claudication, 454
Vascular cognitive impairment, 260–62,
 269, 493
Vascular dementia, 261–62
Vascular diseases
 case histories, 116, 118–19
 characteristic spatial-temporal profiles,
  115*t*
 etiology, 113
Vascular imaging, 150–51
Vasculitis, 115, 214, 218
Vasoconstriction, cerebral, 402, 407–8
Vasodepressor syncope, 177
Vasovagal syncope, 177
VDRL (Venereal Disease Research
 Laboratory) test, 243–44, 340–41
Vegetative state, 379
Venereal Disease Research Laboratory
 (VDRL) test, 243–44, 340–41
Venlafaxine (Effexor), 420*t*
Venous angiomas, 126
Venous infarcts, 133, 134
Ventriculoperitoneal shunting, 405–6
Verapamil (Calan, Verelan), 420*t*, 422*t*
Verbal paraphasia, 64
Verelan (Verapamil), 420*t*
Vertebral artery dissection, 445, 503
Vertebral artery stenosis, 148
Vertebrobasilar artery occlusion, 130*t*
Vertigo, 437
 benign paroxysmal, of childhood, 477
 benign paroxysmal positional (BPPV),
  435, 440–42, 446–47
 central, 437–38, 439
 definition of, 437
 differential diagnosis of, 438
 drug-induced, 490–91
 lesion localization, 82, 437–38
 in Ménière disease, 442–43
 in MS, 349–50
 peripheral, 437–38, 439–45
 in Ramsay Hunt syndrome, 346
 recurrent episodes, 439–45
 single episode, 444–45
 in stroke, 130*t*, 132
Vesicare (solifenacin), 462*t*
Vestibular function, 55
Vestibular migraine, 439

Vestibular nerve (cranial nerve VIII),
 96–98, 384
Vestibular nerve schwannoma, 439, 447
Vestibular paroxysmia, 443–44
Vestibular pathway, 19
Vestibular rehabilitation, 444–45
Vestibulo-ocular reflex, 55, 80, 96, 383–
 85, 489
Vibegron (Gemtesa), 462*t*
Vibration sense
 age-related changes in, 490
 pathway for, 19, 23*f*, 40
 reduced, 23*f*, 40, 203, 271–72, 302–3,
  486–87, 493
 screening examination, 91
 sensory examination, 61–62
Video examination, 92–94
Vigabatrin (Sabril), 192*t*, 194*t*
Vimpat (lacosamide), 192*t*
Viral encephalitis, 402–3
Viral infections, 214
Viral meningitis, 401*t*, 402–3
Vision loss
 age-related changes, 489
 case histories, 123, 161–62, 327–28,
  425, 486–87, 494
 in giant cell arteritis, 404–5, 425, 434
 in homonymous hemianopia, 161–62
 in ICA occlusion, 128
 lone bilateral blindness, 429
 monocular, 427–29
 persistent, 430
 transient, 429–30
Vision testing, 53
Visual acuity
 cranial nerve examination, 53
 reduced, 37
Visual field deficits
 in altered level of consciousness, 96
 cranial nerve examination, 53, 67, 75
 in HSE, 344–45
 screening examination, 91, 94
 in spontaneous intracranial
  hypotension, 406–7
 in stroke, 123–24, 128–32, 130*t*,
  162–63
Visual hallucinations, 257
Visual illusions, 168–69
Visual pathways, 22–27, 27*f*
Visual symptoms, 425–34
 approach to, 426–27
 case histories, 425, 433–34, 497, 501–2
 definitions, 426

restricted to one eye, 42
urgencies, 425, 434
Visual system, 426
Visuospatial deficits
case histories, 238, 269–70
in stroke, 130t
Visuospatial function, 52
Vitamin B2, 420t
Vitamin B6 (pyridoxine), 344
Vitamin B12 deficiency, 243–44, 269,
349–50, 450–51, 493, 494
Vitamin E, 254–56, 299t
Vitamin supplements, prenatal, 165–66
Vivactil (Protriptyline), 313–14
VNS (vagus nerve stimulation), 186,
413–14, 422t
Voltage-gated calcium channels, 224, 364t
Voluntary saccades, 54
Vomiting. See also Nausea
in anthrax meningoencephalitis, 348
case histories, 108, 109
cyclic, 475–76
in migraine, 411
in NMOSD, 355–56
in tuberculous meningitis, 343
Vumerity (diroximel fumarate), 366t
Vyepti (eptinezumab), 420t

Wakix (pitolisant), 315–16
Wallenberg syndrome, 132
Wandering behavior, 252
Warfarin, 140t, 142, 144–45, 151, 154–55
Weakness, 46–49
ankle dorsiflexion, 33–34, 45, 327–28,
457–58, 462–63
ankle plantar flexion, 449
anomalous or inconsistent exam
findings, 100t
with areflexia, 235–36
arm, 45, 107–8, 117, 123–24, 129–32,
130t, 327
breakaway, 100t
case histories, 108, 109, 116, 117, 118–
20, 123–24, 160–61, 201–3, 234–36,
271–72, 302–3, 327–28, 370–73,
436–37, 449, 457–58, 462–63, 495,
497–98, 502
in children, 478
collapsing, 100t
corticospinal tract and, 15
example neurologic deficits, 8–11, 9f,
10f, 12f, 15–19, 16f, 17f, 18f, 33–34,
105

facial, 19, 24f, 41, 45, 81–82, 105, 108,
116, 117, 123–24, 129–32, 130t,
217–18, 328, 346, 495, 498
give-way, 100t
hand, 123, 160–61, 497–98, 502
hip flexion, 45
jaw, 223
knee flexion, 45
laryngeal, 82
leg, 45, 108, 109, 117, 119–20, 123–24,
129–32, 130t
lesion localization, 45, 105
LMN patterns, 84–88
lower extremity, 436, 457–58,
462–63
in MS, 349–50
in muscle disorders, 227, 229
in myasthenia gravis, 223–24
neck, 83
palatal, 82, 118–19
patterns of, 69
pharyngeal, 82
predominantly distal, 84
pyramidal, 84
in Ramsay Hunt syndrome, 346
in stroke, 123–24, 129–32, 130t
tongue, 83, 130t
UMN pattern, 84
upper extremity muscles, 15–19, 16f
in VZV, 346
Weber syndrome, 132
Weber test, 68
Weight loss
case histories, 239, 270, 271–72, 454–
55, 502
for sleep apnea, 313–14
Wernicke aphasia, 30f, 30–33, 64, 74
Wernicke's area, 30f, 30–33
Western blot assay, 342
West Nile virus, 213, 403
White blood cells, 401t
White matter lesions, 427–28,
433–34
Whole-brain radiation therapy, 330
Wilson disease, 294–96, 299t
Withdrawal seizures, 179
Word-finding problems
case histories, 123, 160–61, 485–86
in older people, 489
Wrist extension
nerve roots and peripheral nerves
corresponding to, 81, 86f
testing, 58

Wrist flexion
   nerve roots and peripheral nerves
      corresponding to, 81, 86f
   testing, 58
Writer's cramp, 292–93
Writing assessment, 51

Xadago (safinamide), 297t
Xcopri (cenobamate), 192t

Yawning, 209–10
Yoga, 452
Young people. See also Children
   monocular vision loss, 427–28
   stroke, 498, 503

Zalcitabine (ddC), 336–37
Zaleplon (Sonata), 317–18

Zantac (ranitidine), 237–38
Zarontin (ethosuximide), 192t
Zavegepant (Zavzpret), 419t
Zelapar (selegiline), 297t
Zeposia (ozanimod), 366t
Zestril (lisinopril), 237–38, 420t
Zilucoplan, 225
Zinc therapy, 296, 299t
Zolmitriptan (Zomig), 419t, 422t
Zolpidem (Ambien), 317–18
Zomig (zolmitriptan), 419t
Zonisamide (Zonegran), 192t, 194t, 420t
Zoster. See Herpes varicella-zoster
Zoster auricularis, 346
Zoster cephalicus, 346
Zoster ophthalmicus, 345–46
Zoster oticus, 346
Zyprexa (olanzapine), 258